Sleep Disorders in Children

Soňa Nevšímalová • Oliviero Bruni

Editors

Sleep Disorders in Children

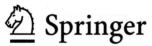 Springer

Editors
Soňa Nevšímalová
Department of Neurology
Charles University and General Teaching
Hospital
Prague
Czech Republic

Oliviero Bruni
Sapienza University
S. Andrea Hospital, Department of
Developmental and Social Psychology
Rome
Roma
Italy

ISBN 978-3-319-28638-9   ISBN 978-3-319-28640-2   (eBook)
DOI 10.1007/978-3-319-28640-2

Library of Congress Control Number: 2016954802

Printed on acid-free paper

This Springer imprint is published by Springer Nature
The registered company is Springer International Publishing AG Switzerland

To my mother, who infinitely loved me even if I was a "sleepless infant" She soothed me every night of my infancy and childhood with loving kindness that only a mother could give (Oliviero Bruni).

This book is dedicated to my best teacher of sleep medicine prof. Bedřich Roth, and to my family, particularly to my sons Radan and Petr (Soňa Nevšímalová).

Preface

Sleep has often been an interesting subject for novelists, poets, painters, and other artists. From the antiquities to the Middle Ages up to the last centuries, several of them acknowledged the importance and the impact of sleep on behavior, emotions, performance, and overall health. Sleep was depicted as a mysterious part of life, bringing suggestions and premonitions, and always beneficial for the humans by Aristotle, Cicero, Dante, and Shakespeare, among many others.

After the Middle Ages, some interest on the functions of sleep emerged and some specific pathologies linked to sleep were described, but little understanding of the physiology of sleep occurred until the twentieth century.

The beginning of sleep medicine as a scientific field is linked to the discovery of the EEG by Hans Berger in 1929, which allowed the identification of sleep stages by Loomis et al. in 1937, followed by the discovery of REM sleep in 1953 by Aserinsky and Kleitman, and has impressively progressed over the past 60 years, highlighting the importance of sleep for several physiological functions and stressing the negative effects of sleep deprivation or disruption.

In the nineteenth century, doctors and pediatricians began to characterize sleep disorders in infants and children, but children's sleep has been neglected until the end of the last century with the main textbooks of pediatrics reporting no chapters but only few paragraphs devoted to pediatric sleep.

Pediatric sleep medicine arose as an autonomous entity about 30 years ago, due to the huge increase of studies and publications in different fields of sleep disorders: obstructive sleep apnea and other sleep-related breathing disorders, sudden infant death syndrome (SIDS), insomnia, narcolepsy, parasomnias, etc. However, it was the gradual identification of the importance of sleep for daytime dysfunction, such as neurobehavioral problems, learning difficulties, and growth failure, which started to raise awareness on the importance of sleep in infancy and childhood development.

The link between sleep-disordered breathing or sleep-related movement disorders and attention deficit hyperactivity disorder (ADHD) or between sleep and depression or substance abuse in adolescence or between sleep deprivation and cognitive dysfunctions and poor school performance has been widely recognized.

Furthermore, the vicious circle and interplay involving sleep apnea, inflammation, and childhood obesity has been emphasized. Finally, recent research has identified the specific features of hypersomnia and narcolepsy in children.

Sleep during the first months of life occupies more than 50% of the time of infants, and the brain and body maturation and changes are mainly driven by the sleep hours (i.e., synaptic reorganization or growth hormone secretion), highlighting the fundamental role of sleep for optimal development.

Thus the proper diagnosis and treatment of sleep disorders in infancy and childhood is a priority for pediatricians or physicians in order to maintain an adequate growth of the brain and body.

Although the importance of sleep for development is now widely recognized, in the pediatric clinical practice, the evaluation and assessment of sleep problems continues to be neglected by most pediatricians, linked probably also to insufficient education programs in medical school and training courses.

The goal for this book is to review the clinical disorders of sleep for child neurologists, psychiatrists, pulmonologists, pediatricians, and clinical practitioners of any specialty with an interest in sleep medicine.

Prague, Czech Republic   Soňa Nevšímalová
Rome, Italy   Oliviero Bruni

Contents

Contributors

Marco Angriman, MD Department of Pediatrics—Child Neurology and Neurorehabilitation Unit, Regional Hospital of Bolzano, Bolzano, South Tyrol, Italy

Irene Aricò, MD, PhD Department of Neurosciences, AOU G. Martino, Messina, Messina, Italy

Kate Bartel, BPsych (Hons) School of Psychology, Flinders University, Adelaide, SA, Australia

Oliviero Bruni, MD Department of Developmental and Social Psychology, Sapienza University, Rome, Italy

Raffaele Ferri, MD Department of Neurology IC, Oasi Research Institute (IRCCS), Troina, Enna, Italy

David Gozal, MD, MBA Neuroscience and Neurobiology, Department of Pediatrics, The University of Chicago, Chicago, IL, USA

Michael Gradisar, PhD, MPsych (Clin), BSc (Hons) School of Psychology, Flinders University, Adelaide, SA, Australia

Madeleine Marie Grigg-Damberger, MD Department of Neurology, University of New Mexico Medical Center, Albuquerque, NM, USA

Pamela E. Hamilton-Stubbs, BSN, MD Dr. Hamilton-Stubbs' Sleep and Total Wellness Institute, LLC, Richmond, VA, USA

Rosemary S.C. Horne, PhD The Ritchie Centre and Department of Paediatrics, The Ritchie Centre, Hudson Institute of Medical Research and Monash University, Clayton Melbourne, VIC, Australia

Sejal V. Jain, MD Department of Neurology, Cincinnati, OH, USA

Leila Kheirandish-Gozal, MD, MSc Department of Pediatrics, The University of Chicago, Chicago, IL, USA

Suresh Kotagal, MB, BS Department of Neurology, Department of Neurology and Pediatrics, May Clinic, Rochester, MN, USA

Sanjeev V. Kothare, MD Department of Neurology, New York University School of Medicine, New York, NY, USA

Silvia Miano, MD, PhD Neurocenter of Italian Switzerland, Sleep and Epilepsy Center, Civic Hospital of Lugano, Lugano, Ticino, Switzerland

Soňa Nevšímalová, MD, DSc Department of Neurology, Charles University and General Teaching Hospital, Prague, Czech Republic

Lino Nobili, MD, PhD Department of Neuroscience, Niguarda Hospital, Milan, Italy

Luana Novelli, PsyD Department of Psychology, Sapienza University of Rome, Rome, Rome, Italy

Teresa Paiva, MD, PhD CENC, Sleep Medicine Center, Lisbon, Portugal

Paola Proserpio, MD Department of Neuroscience, Niguarda Hospital, Milan, Italy

Stephen H. Sheldon, DO, FAAP Ann & Robert H. Lurie Children's Hospital of Chicago, Chicago, IL, USA

Rosalia Silvestri, MD Department of Neurosciences, AOU G. Martino, Messina, Messina, Italy

Hui-Leng Tan, MBBChir, MD (res) Department of Paediatric Respiratory Medicine, Royal Brompton Hospital, London, UK

Arthur S. Walters, MD Sleep Division, Department of Neurology, Vanderbilt University Medical Center, Nashville, TN, USA

Part I
Introduction

Chapter 1
Ontogeny of Sleep and Its Functions in Infancy, Childhood, and Adolescence

Madeleine Marie Grigg-Damberger

Abstract We have long understood sleep as an active, not passive, process that serves many functions, some of which vary in importance across the human lifespan. Ontogeny is the study of how a living organism develops from conception to birth and across its lifespan. This chapter reviews the ontogeny of sleep and its functions from infancy through adolescence. Sleep in humans serves many functions including: (1) fostering optimal brain growth and development; (2) enhancing learning, attention, memory, synaptic efficiency, and plasticity; (3) regulation of emotion, appetite, feeding, body weight, risk-taking, and pleasure-seeking behaviors; (4) strengthening immune function; and (5) providing optimal time for clearing the brain of cellular debris and neurotoxins. The chapter provides summaries of growing evidence for each of these. Sleep/wake states are scored in polysomnography using electroencephalography (EEG), electromyography (EMG), and electrooculography (EOG), and the ontogeny of these is also reviewed here.

Keywords NREM disorder of arousal (DoA) • Parasomnias • Polysomnography • Polysomnogram (PSG) • REM sleep behavior disorder (RBD) • REM sleep without atonia (RSWA) • Sleepwalking

Introduction

We have long understood sleep is an active, not passive, process that serves many functions. The importance of one function or another varies with age and development. Ontogeny (also called morphogenesis or ontogenesis) is the study of how a living organism develops from conception to birth and across its lifespan. This

M.M. Grigg-Damberger, MD
Department of Neurology, University of New Mexico School of Medicine,
MSC10 5620, One University of NM, Albuquerque, NM 87131-0001, USA
e-mail: mgriggd@salud.unm.edu

© Springer International Publishing Switzerland 2017
S. Nevšímalová, O. Bruni (eds.), *Sleep Disorders in Children*,
DOI 10.1007/978-3-319-28640-2_1

chapter provides a review of the ontogeny of sleep and its functions in infancy, childhood, and adolescence.

The word "ontogeny" comes from the Greek word *ontos* (ὄντος, a present participle genitive singular neuter of εἶναι, "to be") and the suffix *-geny*, which means a "mode of production". The concept that "ontogeny recapitulates phylogeny" is a hypothesis that humans particularly during early embryonic development exhibit physical features or behaviors which resemble those seen during the stages of development of other animal species.

Ontogeny of the Functions of Sleep

Sleep in humans serves many functions including: (1) fostering optimal brain growth and development [1–5]; (2) enhancing learning, attention, memory, synaptic efficiency, and plasticity [6–17]; (3) regulating emotion, appetite, feeding, body weight, risk-taking, and pleasure-seeking behaviors [6, 18–26]; (4) strengthening immune function [27–30]; and (5) providing optimal time for clearing the brain of cellular debris and neurotoxins [31–33].

Sleep Fosters Optimal Brain Growth and Development

Perhaps the most important function of sleep from an ontogenetic perspective is the role sleep plays in early brain development. Piaget thought play was the major "work" of children [34–36], but it is sleep for neonates and young infants. Term infants sleep 16–18 h per day, 50 % of it in REM sleep [37, 38]. Premature infants spend even more time sleep, 80 % of it in REM sleep. By age 2 years, the average child has spent 10,000 h asleep compared to 7,500 h awake [24].

The greater time spent sleeping in infants and early childhood reflects the crucial role sleep (especially REM sleep) plays in optimal brain development. The time course of REM sleep development (and decline) in humans corresponds well with critical periods of brain maturation [39]. From a historical perspective, Roffwarg et al. [38] were the first to hypothesize that brain stem mechanisms that produce REM sleep provide direct ascending stimulation to the forebrain which promote brain development at ages when wake-related stimulation is low [2]. The time course of REM sleep development (and decline in the percentage of time spent in it) in humans corresponds well with critical periods of brain maturation [39].

Recent animal and human studies confirm that sleep in early life promotes optimal neural and cognitive brain development, cortical maturation, and brain connectivity [40–57]. Premature infants are seemingly whirling dervishes in REM sleep, constantly moving and twitching, far more than when they are nearer to term, and much more than adults do when sleeping. These myoclonic twitches of skeletal muscles (often tens of thousands per day) are neither random nor purposeless [4, 58, 59]. Evidence from studies in human infants and infant animal models show that proprioceptive feedback from a twitching limb triggers bursts of oscillatory electrical activity in the appropriate regions of the developing somatosensory cortex [1–4]. Blumberg et al. [60] argue that myoclonic twitches during REM sleep in infants represent a form of motor exploration which help human infants and other mammals explore limb biomechanics, build motor synergies, and lay a foundation for complex, automatic, and goal-directed movements when awake [4].

Furthermore, studies show proprioceptive feedback from a twitching limb trigger bursts of oscillatory electrical activity in the appropriate regions of the developing somatosensory cortex [1–4]. These bursts of EEG activity are none other than the quintessential EEG signature of premature infants, delta brushes. Scalp EEG recorded delta brushes reflect bursts of 8–25 Hz electrical activity within the cortex which is most prominent and prevalent during the third trimester of gestation. Simultaneously recording scalp EEG and limb electromyographic (EMG) activity, Milh et al. showed that sporadic hand and foot movements in premature infants 29–31 weeks CA herald the appearance of delta brushes in the corresponding areas of the lateral and medial contralateral central cortex, respectively [5]. Moreover, direct hand and foot stimulation reliably provoked the delta brushes in the same regions.

Still other studies have shown similar mapping of auditory [61], touch, pain, and smell in early development correlating delta brush activity with different sensory stimuli in premature infants [4, 44, 58–61]. For example, a longitudinal study evaluated delta brush activity in 46 healthy premature infants between 31 and 38 weeks CA in response to low level auditory clicks and human voices during both quiet/NREM and active/REM sleep [61]. Before 34 weeks, low volume auditory clicks or human voices evoked similar scalp-recorded EEG responses: delta brushes which localized particularly to the temporal scalp regions. Whereas, after 34 weeks CA, voices evoked delta brushes localized to the temporal region while auditory clicks elicited diffuse delta brushes.

Reduced time spent in REM sleep during early infancy has been shown to have lasting effects on later cognitive functioning [41, 54, 62]. Less REM sleep time in premature infants (32–36 weeks CA) was associated with poorer developmental outcomes on the Bayley II at 6 months in a prospective study of 81 infants born premature [41]. Whereas, better cognitive outcomes appeared in infants who had longer periods of sustained sleep, more time spent in REM sleep, and more periods of REM sleep with rapid eye movements. Another prospective study of 65 infants born premature found that those who slept poorly as neonates exhibited poorer attention and greater distractibility at 4 and 18 months than those who slept well [62]. Another study found sleep/wake transitions from NREM to wake were associated with greater neonatal neuromaturation, less negative emotionality, and better verbal, symbolic, and executive competences at age 5 in 143 infants born premature (mean age 32 weeks CA) [54]. REM sleep and cry, short episodes of REM, and NREM sleep were associated with poorer outcomes.

Such findings have prompted interventions to improve premature sleep in neonatal intensive care units including environmental noise reduction, ear muffs when sleeping, lights on only from 7 am to 7 pm, and non-pharmacological treatments for pain less likely to disrupt REM sleep [63–68].

Sleep Crucial for Learning, Memory, and Attention

In order to learn a memory, task or skill, we must first be trained, then encode and consolidate it if is to be retained. A wealth of research and medical literature has recently been published on the importance of sleep on learning using a variety of different tasks or particular types of memory. These and other studies have shown that consolidation of declarative/episodic, motor, emotional, sensory, and olfactory memories occur preferentially during sleep [6–13]. Sleep within a few hours after learning a new task, skill, or information enhances retention. New learning and memories acquired during wakefulness is initially stored (encoded) in the hippocampus. Some of these newly encoded memories are selected, reactivated, replayed, and redistributed during sleep toward other neuronal networks (neocortex) where they are processed. Processing of memories during sleep includes: (1) selecting some memories for retention, discarding others, (2) integrating new memories into preexisting networks of associated memories, (3) abstracting gist and rules from new memories, and (4) modifying memories to facilitate discovery of creative insights and future utilities [69, 70].

Studies in adults have shown the sufficient quantities and temporal sequences of NREM 2, 3 and REM sleep are needed to learn novel tasks and new memories [69] and reorganize memories [70]. For example, learning a visual texture discrimination task improved significantly after a night's sleep which contained sufficient NREM 3 in the first half and REM sleep in the second [71]. Another study found NREM 2 sleep spindles especially late in the night correlated with learning a particular motor task [72]. Even more intriguing are a handful of recent studies which correlate sleep spindles (or EEG power in the sigma band of sleep spindles) with cognitive and intellectual abilities in adolescents and adults [73–75]. Spindles and sigma power in children and adolescents have been linked to speed [76], full-scale and fluid intelligence [73, 77], and overnight enhancement of motor task accuracy [74].

Studies demonstrating sleep-related memory consolidation in infants and toddlers are few but the results interesting [78, 79]. Fifteen-month-olds were better at recognizing previously presented auditory strings of an artificial language if they napped after these were first presented [80]. Infants who napped after learning recognized the artificial language 25 h later, whereas the infants who did not nap did not [81]. Another study confirmed 9- to 16-months old infants were able to better learn word pairs if they napped after training [82]. Three- to 5-year-olds who habitually nap (≥5 days per week) were compared with those who usually napped less [79]. Nonhabitual nappers remembered less accurately in more challenging encoding conditions suggesting they may still need naps to consolidate more fragile forms of learning.

Studies of memory consolidation in older children and adolescents have shown the beneficial effects of sleep on consolidating declarative memories including vocabulary [83–86]. However, experimental studies evaluating where procedural memory is enhanced by sleep (as has been demonstrated in adults) have shown negative results in children. Learning of a visual-motor sequence in children improved less after post-training sleep than in wakefulness [87], or worse yet deteriorated with sleep in another study [88]. More studies may unravel these discrepancies and inconsistencies between sleep and learning, particularly the impact of age upon them [89].

Sleep deprivation preferentially affects creative, divergent, and innovative thinking and cognitive systems that rely upon emotional data learning [90]. Neuroimaging studies have shown the prefrontal cortex is particularly susceptible to the effects of sleep loss. Shortened sleep duration in children and adolescents predisposes them to inattention, hyperactivity, easy irritability, risk-taking, reward-seeking, distracted driving, accidental injuries, negative attitudes, poor appetite control, and frontal lobe executive dysfunction. Insufficient sleep particularly impairs alertness and attention, thereby impeding learning [90].

Experimental studies in other mammalian species have confirmed post-learning reactivation of learning-elicited neuronal network activity occurs during subsequent sleep. Processing of memories during sleep has also been demonstrated in nonmammalian species (e.g., filial imprinting in chicks and song learning in birds) suggesting memory consolidation during sleep may be an evolutionary conserved function of sleep [91].

Sleep Enhances Synaptic Strength, Efficiency, and Plasticity

Enhancing synaptic strength, efficiency and plasticity is another increasingly recognized function of sleep. As we learn new things awake, we add synaptic connections. If all synapses acquired awake were saved, over time synaptic efficiency would be reduced. Sleep is the optimal time to maintain synaptic efficiency by integrating new neuronal firing patterns while pruning unneeded synapses [14–17]. Neuronal activity during learning triggers cortical plasticity that allows for reorganization of the neuronal network and integration of new information [92].

Sleep appears to play an important role in synaptic plasticity particularly in children and adolescents [50, 89, 93–97]. At birth, an infant's brain contains 100 billion neurons and the number of synapses per neuron is 2,500. As the infant learns, new synapses are added so by age 2 or 3 years, the number of synapses to neurons has grown to 15,000 per neuron. Such synaptic density places the brain at risk for synaptic overload and reduced synaptic efficiency. During adolescence, a massive pruning of synapses occurs, and again preferentially during sleep. Insufficient sleep during adolescence may lead to improper refinement of neural circuits. If chronic, it may result in aberrant wiring (e.g., schizophrenia, autistic spectrum disorders) or inadequate consolidation of memory and learning [98–101]. Chronic sleep disruption in rats during critical periods of development impair synaptic pruning preventing proper refinement of mature neural circuits [14, 15].

The quantity and amplitude of SWA (0.5–4 Hz) of NREM 3 sleep across a night of sleep decreases throughout adolescence and has been thought to reflect synaptic pruning which occurs then [50]. Synaptic pruning first begins at 8 months in the visual cortex and 24 months in the frontal cerebral cortex during which unnecessary excitatory and inhibitory synaptic connections are removed to enhance synaptic efficiency. Pruning is usually complete by age 11 with 40% of synapses in the brain eliminated. NREM SWA is believed to reflect the number of cortical neurons that participate, as well as the number and strength of the synaptic connections between them [102–105].

Absolute values of SWA (EEG power between 0.5 and 4 Hz during NREM sleep) follow an inverted U curve in human development with a progressive increase between ages 6 and 8 years, a peak around 8 years of age, and a decline by more than 60% with the highest decline between ages 12 and 16.5 years [106–108]. The massive decline in SWA reflects extensive elimination of unnecessary cortical synapses which occurs during adolescence, the final step in brain neurodevelopment. Parallel declines in synaptic density, delta wave amplitude, and cortical metabolic rate during adolescence would suggest this. More evidence is needed to confirm this.

Sleep and Emotional Brain Regulation

Another more recently recognized function of sleep is regulation of emotion. The amygdala and prefrontal cortex regulate and process emotional feelings, behaviors, reactions, and memories, and this appears to occur preferentially in sleep, especially REM sleep [6, 18–22]. REM sleep appears to play an important role in strengthening emotional memories but weakens their emotional overtones and recalibrates perceptions of complex social signals such as social threat [6, 20, 109–111].

One study found young adults kept awake for approximately 35 h showed heightened responses when shown pictures of threatening faces which correlated with a 60% increase in amygdala responses in functional magnetic resonance imaging (fMRI) [111]. Sleep deprivation particularly affects frontal lobe executive functions, impairing inhibition (ability to act on choice rather than impulse, resisting inappropriate behaviors and responding appropriately) and cognitive flexibility (adapting behavior to changing conditions) [19]. Insufficient sleep, especially of REM sleep, weakens these processes.

Self-control is an important developmental skill acquired in early childhood. A recent study explored the effect of afternoon nap restriction on ability of 12 healthy toddlers to control their attention, behavior, and emotions when challenged by an unsolvable puzzle [112]. Depriving the children of an approximately 90 min nap resulted in moderate to large effects with the children resorting to less mature self-regulation strategies. Analysis of data from a large longitudinal multi-city cohort study of adolescents who were followed from birth through age 15 recently found sleep deprivation was positively related to low self-control; low self-control is positively related to delinquency even when accounting for common confounders [113].

Another recent longitudinal study found bidirectional associations between better sleep quality and more effective emotion regulation in college students [18].

Poor sleep affects emotional well-being and certain emotions or negative moods may compromise sleep [19]. Better sleep quality led to more positive social relationships and more positive relationships to more effective emotion regulation and less sleep problems. It seems we sleep not only to remember but also to forget.

Sleep Regulates Appetite, Feeding, Body Weight, Risk-Taking, and Pleasure-Seeking Behaviors

Sleep regulates appetite and feeding. Animals faced with starvation or need to store food sleep less. Animals who suffer prolonged sleep deprivation markedly increase their food intake. Humans when sleep deprived or sleep restricted have: (1) impairment in decision-making centers of brain, (2) increased stimulation of pleasure-seeking regions of brain, (3) glucose dysregulation, and (4) increased cravings and consumption of high-caloric foods, simple sugars, starch, and salty snacks [114–116]. Insufficient or poor sleep in adolescents appears to exaggerate the normal balance between affective and cognitive control systems, leading to greater risk taking, diminished attentional and behavioral control, and poor emotion regulation [23–25]. Using functional MRI imaging, Telzer et al. demonstrated that adolescents who reported poorer sleep exhibited greater risk taking [26]. Moreover, this was associated with diminished recruitment of the dorsolateral prefrontal cortex during cognitive control, greater insular activation during reward processing, and reduced functional coupling between prefrontal cortex and affective regions in the insula and ventral striatum during reward processing.

Sleep Can Strengthen Immune Function

Less known even among sleep specialists is the close bidirectional reciprocal relationships between sleep and immune function [27–30]. Sleep (especially NREM 3) has an important role in the formation of immunologic memory. NREM 3 sleep and SWA are enhanced during infection, and REM sleep inhibited. Insufficient sleep can weaken immunity and increase susceptibility to bacterial, viral, and parasitic infections [29]. Cytokines (particularly interleukin-1 (IL-1) appear to regulate this.

Different immune cell types (macrophages, natural killer cells, and lymphocytes) exhibit circadian rhythms [30]. Insufficient and disrupted sleep in children secondary to obstructive sleep apnea, eczema, and asthma create pro-inflammatory states [117–119]. Problematic internet use sufficient to be called an addiction is an increasingly common problem among adolescents and is associated with sleep problems and reduced self-reported immune function [120, 121]. Chronic misalignment with one's internal circadian clock predisposes to a higher incidence of cancer and exacerbation of autoimmune illnesses [122].

Preferential Cleaning of Brain Toxins During Sleep

The most recent proposed (and least confirmed) sleep function is cleaning of neuro-toxins and cellular debris by convective flow from the brain to the circulation occurs preferentially during sleep [33, 123]. This attribute resides in the newly discovered glymphatic system which clears endogenous neurotoxic waste products from the brain [32]. Regulated by astroglia, the glymphatic system appears to operate prefer-entially during sleep [31–33]. This may be of more importance to middle-aged and older adults [33, 124–129]. For example, chronic complaints of inadequate and/or insufficient sleep increase the risk and severity of Alzheimer's disease, limiting the time the brain has to clear amyloid-beta and tau from the brain [33, 130, 131].

Parasomnias and Local Sleep: Humans Sleep with Only Parts of Their Brain

Ontogeny may contribute to the appearance and/or disappearance of both normal and abnormal parasomnias in humans. Parasomnias are unusual or undesirable motor, behavioral, and/or experiential events which occur during (or in the transi-tions from and to) sleep. Parasomnias are more common in young children and decrease with increasing age.

Parasomnias in humans may reflect the protective role of sleeping with only parts of our brains at one time. So-called unihemispheric sleep in NREM is a phyloge-netic adaptation observed in some marine mammals and birds. Sleeping with only one half of their brain at a time permits bottle-nosed dolphins, seals, beluga whales, and killer whales to surface to breathe. Moreover, their eye contralateral to the awake hemisphere is kept open and out of the water monitoring the environment while they continue to swim; the eye contralateral to the sleeping hemisphere remaining closed. Mallard ducks will sleep standing in a line with a duck on each end sleeping with the eye to outside open to guard the flock from invaders. The sentinel ducks have more unihemispheric sleep than those who sleep in the middle of the flock, and they can react to threatening stimuli seen by the one open eye.

Many parasomnias in humans may represent release or expression of neocortical inhibition of brain stem and spinal cord central pattern generators (CPGs) during sleep [132]. After infancy, CPGs are usually suppressed by the cerebral neocortex awake. Release or lack of inhibition of CPGs during sleep (combined with youth, a familial/genetic predisposition, made worse by sleep restriction, noise or light) per-mit sleepwalking and sleep terrors. CPGs may underlie other sleep-related phenom-ena such as periodic limb movements during sleep, sleep bruxism, sleep-related expiratory groaning, sleep-related eating, nocturnal tongue biting, faciomandibular myoclonus, and nocturnal hypermotor seizures [133, 134].

Recent studies confirm only parts of our brain sleep at a time (this termed local sleep) [135–138]. Which part sleeps depends upon which area got the most work or which cognitive tasks were performed in prior wakefulness [135, 139]. Which part of the brain is activated during sleep in the process of memory consolidation has been shown to correlate with which cognitive tasks were performed in the period before sleep [139]. Using magnetoencephalography (MEG), the intensity of parietal-occipital SWA during NREM 3 sleep was recently shown in adult subjects to correlate with their post-sleep performance of learning a novel visual-motor task [92].

Functional MRI studies in human subjects showed particular and similar localized patterns of brain activity when they learned a motor task and later during subsequent periods of REM sleep [140]. Moreover, the intensity of reactivation correlated with how well they performed the newly learned task following sleep [141]. Using high-density EEG recording techniques, another study showed a marked increase in SWA during NREM 3 sleep localized to the left frontoparietal region in 14 healthy 10- to 16-year-olds' sleep following 3 weeks of intensive working memory training [135]. The percentage increase in SWA correlated positively with increased working memory performance assessed immediately and 2–5 months after the training. The investigators suggested mapping of sleep SWA using high-density EEG recordings could be used to longitudinally monitor the effects of working memory training in children and adolescents with working memory deficiencies [135].

Ontogeny of Polysomnographic Measures of Sleep/Wake States

Developmental sleep researchers continue to argue whether sleep at first is an undifferentiated behavioral state (pre-sleep). Leaving this unresolved debate aside, sufficient evidence has demonstrated that active sleep in human infants at 32 weeks GA is an immature form of REM sleep seen in older children and adults [142–144]. Elegant experimental studies have demonstrated that all the REM sleep generator mechanisms and connections are present in neonatal rats equivalent in developmental age to human infants 32 weeks CA and are similar to those seen in adult cats [145]. Whether quiet sleep is an immature form of NREM sleep remains undetermined [146, 147]. For the sake of simplicity, I will usually use the term REM sleep for active sleep and NREM for quiet sleep. This section summarizes the development of the biomarkers of sleep/wake states which are used to score sleep/wake states in polysomnography. The first biomarkers to develop in utero are body, then limb, and finally eye movements; EEG correlates of sleep and wake appear last.

Ontogeny of Body and Limb Movements and Rest-Activity Cycles In Utero

The earliest signs of life in utero besides the beating heart are body and limb movements. Fetal ultrasound studies show a human embryo by 6 weeks gestational age (GA) can arch its back and neck after striated muscle fibers have developed. Reflex-driven limb movements are first seen by 7 weeks CA, independent limb movements by 9 weeks after the spinal cord motor neurons controlling them have developed. Stretches and yawning are first observed at 10 weeks, mouth opening and finger sucking by 11 weeks, and swallowing of amniotic fluid by 12 weeks. The first purposeful fetal movements are observed by 18–20 weeks GA after the thalamus has completely formed.

Cycles of "rest-activity" are present as early as 20–21 weeks GA. These typically last 40–60 min at 24 weeks CA. Of note, the majority of kicking or jabbing movements after 32–34 weeks CA occur when the fetus is sleeping. Premature infants spend more time moving than when nearer to term; median percent time spent in fetal body movements at 24 weeks was 17 %, decreasing to 7 % near term. Somewhat surprising is that the rest/activity periods of the fetus in utero do *not* correspond with those of the mother; fetuses in utero tend to be most active from 9 a.m. to 2 p.m. and again from 7 p.m. to 4 a.m.

As mentioned earlier, premature infants move much more than when they are nearer to term, still move a lot when sleeping as infants, and far more than adults do when sleeping [148, 149]. A longitudinal study examining the ontogeny of gross, localized, and phasic (twitches lasting <0.5 s) movements in healthy normal subjects between age 30 weeks CA and 18 months term found: (1) all types of body movements decrease with increasing age; (2) phasic muscle activity was the first to decrease, localized body movements next, but the frequency of gross body motor movements during sleep remained unchanged until a basal level of 9–13 months term; and (3) the number of epochs without body movements increased steadily until about 8 months term [150].

Ontogeny of Sleep-Related Eye Movements

Studies using fetal ultrasound have demonstrated that eye repositioning is observed as early as 16 weeks GA, rapid eye movements (REMs) as early as 18–20 weeks [151]. Eye movements occur almost continuously but at slow frequencies (1–4 per minute) between 28 and 30 weeks CA and unrelated to body movements, breathing, or heart rate patterns [152, 153]. By 32 weeks CA, REMs are much more frequent and occur in clusters with interburst intervals <1/s. These have been called REM storms or the burst pattern of REMs. They are first seen after 28 weeks, maximal 33–36 weeks, and decrease across the first year of life [152–155].

Ontogeny of Chin Axial Muscle Tone Present During NREM Sleep

Loss of chin EMG activity is one of the most important PSG measures which identifies REM sleep in a PSG (so-called REM sleep without atonia). Increased or preserved chin EMG tone during quiet/NREM sleep is first seen in PSG of infants at 34 weeks CA, but then becomes less reliably present between 37 and 40 weeks, and then usually present after 40 weeks CA [152, 156]. Other studies have shown that 15–20 % of 30-s epochs of PSG in infants at age 6 months of age have inappropriate absence of chin EMG during NREM sleep (when by scoring criteria it should be present) [152, 156–159] and comparable to values of 20 % of NREM sleep in adults [160]. These studies suggest chin EMG will be absent when it should be present during 15–20 % of NREM sleep time from term to adulthood.

Ontogeny of Sleep/Wake EEG in Infants from 25 to 48 Weeks Conceptional Age

EEG background activity between 24 and 25 weeks GA are very discontinuous with bursts of higher amplitude (>50 μV) EEG activity lasting <60 s alternating with periods of relatively lower amplitude (15–50 μV) lasting 20–25 s. This EEG pattern is called trace discontinue. Cycles of rest and activity are seen, last 40–60 min, and are unrelated to those of the mother. EEG background does not change (unreactive) in relation to rest/activity cycles, tactile, or painful stimuli.

The EEG between 26 and 27 weeks CA cannot be used to distinguish active/REM from quiet/NREM sleep [161]. Behavioral correlates better identify these: frequent eye movements and muscle twitches are present during active periods, no eye movements or muscle twitches during rest periods. The bursts of trace discontinue at this CA last longer than earlier (80 s) as do the periods of inactivity (up to 29–46 s).

By 28–29 weeks CA, three behavioral states are identifiable (wakefulness, REM and NREM sleep) but not by EEG criteria [161, 162]. The EEG is more continuous with runs of EEG activity lasting up 160 s alternating with periods of inactivity (interburst intervals [IBIs] which now only last ≤30 s). Most time is spent in active/REM sleep, very little awake. Finally, by 30–31 weeks CA, the EEG can help distinguish wakefulness from active/REM and quiet/NREM sleep. The EEG during active/REM sleep is continuous, while in NREM sleep it remains discontinuous with bursts of activity lasting ≥3 s alternating with IBIs lasting ≤20 s. EEG now correlates with behavioral correlates of wakefulness, active/REM and quiet NREM sleep. Wakefulness is best recognized by muscle artifacts. Reactivity of EEG noted to stimuli.

By 32 and 35 weeks CA, the EEG is continuous both during wakefulness and REM sleep so these two states can only be distinguished by behavioral correlates. The EEG in NREM sleep remains discontinuous with lower values of normal for interburst intervals during NREM sleep at 32 weeks are ≤15 s and ≤10 s at 34 weeks GA. By 36 weeks CA, two different EEG patterns of REM sleep are seen; both are continuous but the EEG before a period of NREM sleep contains generous amounts of intermixed delta activity, REM sleep after a period of NREM sleep characterized by a predominance of theta activity.

By 37 and 38 weeks GA (beginning maturational age for term infants), the EEG in wake and REM sleep is characterized by a continuous mixture of different frequencies (*activité moyene*). Because the EEG activity in wakefulness and REM sleep are so similar in appearance, behavioral correlates are needed to differentiate them. Two EEG patterns of NREM sleep are seen by 38 weeks CA: *trace alternant* characterized by synchronous symmetrical bursts of 1–3 Hz delta on a continuous background of lower amplitude activity and high-voltage slow characterized by 50–150 µV 1–3 Hz activity often with an occipital predominance. At this maturational age, trace alternant is the dominant pattern of NREM sleep.

By 42–44 weeks CA, the bursts of trace alternant shorten to 1–2 s and the amplitude difference between bursts and interburst intervals shortens. Trace alternant usually disappears by 44 to as late as 46 weeks CA, replaced by high-voltage slow activity. By 46 weeks CA, high-voltage slow in NREM sleep is characterized by continuous synchronous 100–150 µV 1–2 Hz delta activity, no (or rare vertical) eye movements, regular respiration and heart rates, and periodic chin EMG activation related to sucking. REM sleep is best identified by reduced chin EMG, rapid eye movements, irregular respiration and heart rate, and continuous mixed frequencies especially near 3 Hz.

Many epochs of sleep in premature and term infants until 3 months post-term are best scored as indeterminate or transitional sleep. Transitional sleep represents "discordant" sleep where mixtures of two or more sleep/wake states are seen within a given PSG epoch. The percentage of transitional sleep rapidly falls beginning after 36 weeks CA. Regular heart rate and respiration, no eye movements and elevated chin EMG tone are observed in epochs of well-differentiated NREM sleep in infants at 40 weeks CA [152, 156, 163]. Parmalee et al. (1967) reported that 67 % of total sleep time was best scored as indeterminate in an infant 30 weeks CA, 38 % at 40 weeks CA, and falls to 29 % 3 months term [164].

In 2010, Andre et al. published their definitive current review of developmental features of EEG in premature and full-term infants [165]. It provides the most current comprehensive descriptions of the EEG features and neonatal behavioral states at different gestational ages for both normal and pathological EEGs based upon evidence and consensus. I recommend using this as a reference when reading and interpreting neonatal EEG and PSG.

Ontogeny of the Sleep/Wake EEG from Infancy to Young Adulthood

The first major EEG feature of mature sleep to appear after birth are sleep spindles [166]. Sleep spindles are an EEG signature of NREM 2 sleep. They are sometimes seen as early as 43–44 weeks CA, often present by 46–48 weeks, and should be present by 3 months term [147, 167–170]. Spindles first appear at a frequency of

12–14 Hz over the midline central derivations. Infants born premature show earlier development of spindles relative to their CA. Delayed appearance or abnormal appearing sleep spindles are an early biomarker of metabolic and/or brain abnormalities.

Fifty percent of sleep spindles are synchronous at 6 and 9 months, 70% at 12 months. Sleep spindles are usually symmetric by 2 years. Sleep spindles have a sharp surface negativity in central regions between ages 6 and 24 months. Sleep spindles in children can occur independently at two different EEG frequencies and maximal over two different scalp locations: 11–12.75 Hz maximal over the frontal and 12–14.75 Hz over the centroparietal regions. Frontal spindles decreased dramatically in power around age 13; they can be seen on occasion in young adults.

Development of the Dominant Posterior Rhythm

The next EEG marker to develop is a dominant posterior rhythm (DPR) of relaxed wakefulness. The frequency of the DPR increases from birth until young adulthood. The amplitude of the DPR increases after birth, reaches a maximum during adolescence, and decreases thereafter [171]. The DPR is first seen in 75% of normally developing infants by 3–4 months term and then characterized by an irregular greater than 50–100 μv 3.5–4.5 Hz activity over occipital areas which is reactive (i.e., blocks with eye opening, appears with passive eye closure) [167]. Most infants by age 5–6 months have a DPR of 5–6 Hz. Seventy percent of typically developing children have 6 Hz by 12 months of age. By age 3 years, 82% of normal term infants show a mean occipital frequency of 8 Hz (range 7.5–9.5 Hz). After age 3, the mean alpha frequency increases only 2 Hz over the next 6 years reaching 9 Hz by 9–10 year. The mean alpha rhythm is 9 Hz in 65% of 9-year-olds and 10 Hz in 65% of normal 15-year-old controls. Reactivity of the DPR to eye opening (so-called reactivity of the EEG) is not observed until 2–6 months of age.

Age-Related Appearance of Other EEG Patterns of NREM and REM Sleep

Other EEG signatures of NREM sleep which develop with increasing age are: vertex sharp waves, K-complexes, hypnagogic hypersynchrony, slow-wave activity (SWA), bioccipital delta slow activity, and fast activity of light sleep. The ages these appear (and sometimes disappear) and their EEG features are summarized in Table 1.1.

Table 1.1 Age-related appearance of other EEG patterns of NREM and REM sleep

EEG feature	Developmental and EEG features
Vertex sharp waves	Seen in late NREM 1 and 2 sleep, maximal over the central EEG derivations, and predominantly surface electronegative. Infrequent broad immature vertex waves over the central derivations have been reported to be observed as early as 6 months term. However, vertex waves resembling those seen in older children and adults first appear later at 16 months term [172]. Beginning around 30 months of age, vertex waves in young children often occur in repetitive runs. Around 36 months of age, vertex waves are more often high amplitude (>250 μV) and sharply peaked, occasionally misidentified as epileptiform. Vertex waves at this age have an initial negative phase (which only lasts 1/8th of a second followed by an aftercoming positive wave approximately 1/6th of a second, occasionally ending with slow negative afterswing. Between ages 3–13 years, vertex waves evolve to sharply peaked primarily surface waveforms similar to those seen in adults [173–175]
K-complexes	K-complexes are (1) typically first appear about 5 months term; (2) are usually present by 5–6 months and then characterized by a surface-negative 50–100 μV wave lasting 200 ms followed by a surface-positive 30–50 μV 300–500 ms wave maximal over the prefrontal and frontal EEG derivations; (4) well-established by age 18 months; (5) the surface-negative component is of highest amplitude and most sharply contoured between ages 3–5 years; (5) occur in runs of 3–8 K-complexes in 1–3 s between ages 3 to years and later in the run the may consist primarily of an initial surface-negative component; (6) by adolescence, typically repeat at rates of one every 1–3 s permitting full expression of the biphasic or triphasic waveform [173–180]
Slow-wave activity of NREM 3 sleep	NREM 3 sleep is scored when ≥20% of a 30-s PSG epoch contains SWA in infants and children which is usually >150 μV [39]. SWA is often ≥300 μV in amplitude in young children [39, 181]. SWA can often be scored in a PSG as early as 3 months, more often 4–4.5 months, and usually is present by 5–6 months of age [146, 147, 168, 182–186]. NREM 1, 2, and 3 sleep can usually be distinguished between 3 and 6 months term [183, 187–190]. A study recording 24-h PSG in 31 normal infants ≤6 months of age found that sleep spindles first appeared approximately 8–12 weeks term and "true slow wave with delta waves" of slow-wave sleep between 3 and 6 months term [183]
Hypnagogic hypersynchrony	Paroxysmal bursts or runs of diffuse rhythmic high amplitude 75–350 μV 3–5 Hz waves which typically begin abruptly and can occur intermittently or continuously for several minutes [174, 191–194]. Their appearance signals drowsiness and NREM 1 sleep. Widely distributed but often maximal over central, frontal, or frontocentral regions, HH typically disappears with deeper stages of NREM sleep, can be seen in NREM 2 sleep, but when seen in NREM 2 sleep, some call it hypersynchronous theta [195]. Hypnagogic hypersynchrony first appears about age 3 months term (seen in about 30% of infants at this age), tends to be most prominent between ages 3 and 11 months, present in 95% of all normal infants and children between ages 6–8 months and 2–4 years, gradually disappearing (seen in only 10% of 11-year-olds and rare after age 12 or 13 years of age) [174, 192, 193]

Table 1.1 (continued)

EEG feature	Developmental and EEG features
Post-arousal hypersynchrony	Paroxysmal runs or bursts of diffuse bisynchronous 75–350 μV 3–5 Hz waves which signal arousal from sleep in young children [174, 191, 192, 196, 197]. Often maximal over the central, frontal, or frontocentral derivations, it is most often seen between ages 3–4 months and 3–4 years with a peak incidence 1–2 years. Similar runs of hypnagogic hypersynchrony are seen when attempting to arouse infants and young children from sleep and have been called in the past hypnopompic hypersynchrony, more recently termed post-arousal hypersynchrony
Bioccipital delta slowing in NREM sleep	Runs of high voltage 1–2 Hz delta slowing over the occipital regions bilaterally. It is most often seen between ages 6 months and 4 years; may be seen as early as 2–3 months and uncommon after age 6 [198]
Fast activity of early NREM sleep	The abrupt onset of prominent 20–25 Hz beta activity typically maximal over the central and postcentral EEG derivations which appears with drowsiness and often persists into NREM 1 and 2 sleep is sometimes called fast activity of early sleep [173]. It first appears 5–6 months term as 5 μV 20–25 Hz activity, reaches maximal expression between ages 12 and 18 months when it averages 30–50 μV, declines after 30–60 months, and is rarely seen after age 7 years [174, 175]
Rhythmic anterior theta activity	Rhythmic runs of sinusoidal 6–7 Hz theta activity maximal over the frontal or frontocentral regions and first seen around 5 years. It is common across the first decade of life, maximal between 9 and 12 years of age, and still seen in 15 % of 16-year-olds
EEG of REM sleep	EEG in REM sleep in infants resembles that of adults but the dominant EEG frequency is slower and higher voltage than that seen in adults. The dominant frequency of REM sleep increases with age: 3 Hz at 7–8 weeks post-term, 4–5 Hz with bursts of saw tooth waves by about by 5 months of age, 4–6 Hz by 9 months, and prolonged runs of notched 5–7 Hz activity at 1–5 years of age [199]. After age 5–10 years, the EEG background of REM sleep resembles that seen in adults (although often of higher amplitude) and is characterized by mixed frequency activity with bursts of often notched 4–6 per second saw tooth waves usually maximal over the midline central region (Cz)

Developmental Changes in Sleep Architecture

In normal healthy infants, sleep cycles typically last a mean of 50–60 min (range 30–70 min). Wakefulness represents only 8–10 % of a 24-h day in infants up to 8 weeks post-term [200]. Until approximately 44 weeks CA, sleep cycles repeat in a polyphasic pattern across the 24-h day interrupted approximately every 3–4 h by an awakening for care and feeding [200]. Within a given sleep cycle, REM sleep lasts 10–45 (mean 25) minutes, NREM near to 20 min, and transitional about 10 min [200, 201]. The distribution of NREM and REM sleep are typically evenly distributed during the night [187].

The most conspicuous changes in sleep architecture during infancy and early childhood are: (1) decrease in total sleep time; (2) gradual consolidation of periods of sleep at night, wakefulness in the day; (3) decrease in the intensity of (EEG power) of NREM 3 slow-wave activity (SWA); and (4) a steady decline in the percentage of sleep time spent in REM sleep [202].

Changes in Total Sleep Time, Sleep Cycle Length, Sleep Efficiency, and Sleep Stage Distribution

The distribution of NREM and REM sleep are typically evenly distributed during the night in infants younger than 3 months of age [187] and sleep polyphasic. Until approximately 44 weeks CA, sleep cycles repeat in a polyphasic pattern across the 24-h day interrupted approximately every 3–4 h by an awakening for care and feeding [200]. Sleep cycles typically last a mean of 50–60 min (range 30–70 min). Wakefulness represents only 8–10% of a 24-h day in infants up to 8 weeks postterm [200]. Within a given sleep cycle, REM sleep lasts 10–45 (mean 25) minutes, NREM near to 20 min, and transitional about 10 min [200, 201]. The distribution of NREM and REM sleep are typically evenly distributed during the night [187]. By age 6 months, NREM 3 sleep is preferentially present toward the beginning of the night and REM sleep in the latter.

The timing of different sleep stages changes from infancy to adolescence. Between 4 and 12 weeks term, most sleep onsets are REM sleep. However, NREM sleep onsets begin to occur more often beginning 10–12 weeks post-term [203]. After 3 months post-term, NREM sleep onsets are more frequent, and infrequent after age 6 months. Two-thirds of sleep onsets were REM sleep in infants 3 weeks term but only 18% at age 6 months [204, 205]. REM latencies of 20–40 min are typical in infants 3–12 months and sleep cycles average 50 min (compared to 100 min in adults) [203]. REM latencies increased from 15 ± 20 min at 3 months to 70 ± 29 min at 24 months although sleep latencies did not change. REM latencies averaged 116 min in children ages 1–10 and 136 min ages 11–18 years.

Total sleep time also decreases across infancy, early childhood, and adolescence. The number and duration of naps decrease such that 82% of children 18 months or older do not take naps on some or all days. Sleep cycle length increases from an average of 69 min in infants at term, 85–115 min between ages 8–12, and 90 min in adults. This results in fewer sleep cycles across a sleep period. Sleep efficiency (percentage of time in bed spent sleeping) remains constant across infancy to adolescence.

Sleep stage distribution changes with age across the pediatric years. Premature infants spend 80% of their sleep time in REM sleep, 50% at term. The percentage of sleep time spent in REM sleep falls to 30% at 1 year and reaches adult percentages of 20–25% by age 5. The proportion of sleep spent in NREM sleep increases while REM sleep decreases such that NREM 3 sleep occupies a greater proportion of sleep time than REM sleep at age 12 months. From ages 5 to 19 years, the percentage of REM sleep remains relatively stable while the percentage of NREM 2 sleep increases with a concomitant decrease in NREM 3 sleep.

Scholle et al. [206] published normative values for one-night PSG in children ages 1–18 years using AASM sleep scoring criteria [206]. They found sleep macroarchitecture showed significant changes with increasing age. REM latency, awakening index, sleep efficiency, mean sleep cycle duration, and number of sleep stage shifts increased with age. Total sleep time, wake after sleep onset, movement time, number of sleep cycles, NREM 3, and REM sleep decreased. Sleep parameters which showed a dependency on Tanner staging as well as corresponding age were: total sleep time, awakening index, REM latency, NREM 2, NREM 3, number of sleep cycles, and mean sleep cycle duration. No gender dependencies were found. The delta power of NREM 3 sleep activity decreases by more than 60 % between ages 10 and 20 years [207]. SWA also declines across recurring periods of NREM sleep within a night. Longitudinal studies have shown delta power of the sleep EEG begins to decrease around age 11.5, reduced by 60 % by age 16 years. The fall in delta power begins earlier in girls than boys (consistent with observed age-related changes in gray matter volume) but then slows so that the overall rate decline is similar between girls and boys at age 16.

Ontogeny of Circadian Rhythm

In the last 10 weeks of gestation, the circadian rhythm of the fetus is synchronized with the mother's maternal rest-activity cycle, heart rate, cortisol, melatonin, and body temperature rhythms [39]. Newborn infants exhibit no rest-activity circadian rhythm independent of their mother before 1 month of age. By 5–6 weeks following birth, sleep is more concentrated during the night and wakefulness more prevalent during the day [208]. By 12–14 weeks, a diurnal pattern is established with a long nocturnal sleep period, shorter daytime naps and 1–3 h of wakefulness preceding the nocturnal sleep period . By 6 months of age, infants display a circadian pattern with period, amplitude, and phase activity similar to an adult. Providing cycles of dark and light in neonatal intensive care units may foster development of the rest-activity circadian rhythm [209, 210].

Ontogeny of Dreaming

Despite evidence that REM sleep appears early in utero and infancy we have no evidence or knowledge about whether infants dream. A recent review analyzing findings of different studies of the ontogeny of dreaming found different methods for collecting dreams in children often result in highly variable and sometimes contradictory assessments and outcomes [211]. Fairly consistent observations are that: (1) dream narratives in younger children are often shorter and simpler than those reported by older children and adults; (2) preschoolers when reporting their dreams often verbalize only one relevant aspect of the dream and may have difficulty distinguishing between internal and external events; (3) the highest prevalence of nightmares is between ages 6 and 10 years [212]. Schoolchildren in whom nightmares are reported to occur often are more likely to have emotional problems or anxiety.

In Closing

We have long understood sleep as an active, not passive, process that serves many functions, some of which vary in relative importance at different ages across the human lifespan. Sleep in humans serves many functions including: (1) fostering optimal brain growth and development; (2) enhancing learning, attention, memory, synaptic efficiency and plasticity; (3) regulating of emotion, appetite, feeding, body weight, risk-taking, and pleasure-seeking behaviors; (5) strengthening immune function; and (4) providing optimal time for clearing the brain of cellular debris and neurotoxins. Myoclonic twitches of skeletal muscles and delta brushes in premature infants appear to: (1) construct sensory and motor maps for auditory, motor, touch, and noxious topographic regions of brain; (2) sculpt nascent neuronal circuits in cerebral cortex and connecting neural circuits linking muscle, spinal cord, and brain; and (3) guide the formation, rearrangement, and elimination of synapses. Ontogeny often underlies the relative importance of a sleep function at particular age. Changes in sleep across infancy, childhood, and adolescence reflect ongoing development of brain networks. The time course of REM sleep development (and decline) in humans corresponds well with critical periods of brain maturation [39].

References

1. Sorribes A, Thornorsteinsson H, Arnardottir H, Johannesdottir I, Sigurgeirsson B, de Polavieja GG, et al. The ontogeny of sleep-wake cycles in zebrafish: a comparison to humans. Front Neural Circ. 2013;7:178.
2. Blumberg MS. Ontogeny of sleep. In: Kushida CA, editor. Encyclopedia of sleep, Elsevier, Boston, MA. 1st ed. 2013. p. 32–7.
3. Corner M, van der Togt C. No phylogeny without ontogeny: a comparative and developmental search for the sources of sleep-like neural and behavioral rhythms. Neurosci Bull. 2012;28(1):25–38.
4. Blumberg MS, Marques HG, Iida F. Twitching in sensorimotor development from sleeping rats to robots. Curr Biol CB. 2013;23(12):R532–7.
5. Milh M, Kaminska A, Huon C, Lapillonne A, Ben-Ari Y, Khazipov R. Rapid cortical oscillations and early motor activity in premature human neonate. Cereb Cortex. 2007;17(7):1582–94.
6. Kaida K, Niki K, Born J. Role of sleep for encoding of emotional memory. Neurobiol Learn Mem. 2015;121:72–9.
7. Genzel L, Spoormaker VI, Konrad BN, Dresler M. The role of rapid eye movement sleep for amygdala-related memory processing. Neurobiol Learn Mem. 2015;122:110–21.

8. Barnes DC, Wilson DA. Sleep and olfactory cortical plasticity. Front Behav Neurosci. 2014;8:134.
9. Weber FD, Wang JY, Born J, Inostroza M. Sleep benefits in parallel implicit and explicit measures of episodic memory. Learn Mem. 2014;21(4):190–8.
10. Inostroza M, Born J. Sleep for preserving and transforming episodic memory. Annu Rev Neurosci. 2013;36:79–102.
11. van der Helm E, Gujar N, Nishida M, Walker MP. Sleep-dependent facilitation of episodic memory details. PLoS ONE. 2011;6(11), e27421.
12. Walker MP, Stickgold R, Alsop D, Gaab N, Schlaug G. Sleep-dependent motor memory plasticity in the human brain. Neuroscience. 2005;133(4):911–7.
13. Fischer S, Nitschke MF, Melchert UH, Erdmann C, Born J. Motor memory consolidation in sleep shapes more effective neuronal representations. J Neurosci Off J Soc Neurosci. 2005;25(49):11248–55.
14. Tononi G, Cirelli C. Sleep and the price of plasticity: from synaptic and cellular homeostasis to memory consolidation and integration. Neuron. 2014;81(1):12–34.
15. Tononi G, Cirelli C. Perchance to prune. During sleep, the brain weakens the connections among nerve cells, apparently conserving energy, and paradoxically, aiding memory. Sci Am. 2013;309(2):34–9.
16. Frank E, Sidor MM, Gamble KL, Cirelli C, Sharkey KM, Hoyle N, et al. Circadian clocks, brain function, and development. Ann N Y Acad Sci. 2013;1306:43–67.
17. Frank MG. Sleep and synaptic plasticity in the developing and adult brain. Curr Top Behav Neurosci. 2015;25:123–49.
18. Tavernier R, Willoughby T. A longitudinal examination of the bidirectional association between sleep problems and social ties at university: the mediating role of emotion regulation. J Youth Adolesc. 2015;44(2):317–30.
19. Gruber R, Cassoff J. The interplay between sleep and emotion regulation: conceptual framework empirical evidence and future directions. Curr Psychiatry Rep. 2014;16(11):500.
20. Deliens G, Gilson M, Peigneux P. Sleep and the processing of emotions. Exp Brain Res. 2014;232(5):1403–14.
21. Desseilles M, Duclos C. Dream and emotion regulation: insight from the ancient art of memory. Behav Brain Sci. 2013;36(6):614; discussion 34–59.
22. van der Helm E, Walker MP. Sleep and emotional memory processing. Sleep Med Clin. 2011;6(1):31–43.
23. Holm SM, Forbes EE, Ryan ND, Phillips ML, Tarr JA, Dahl RE. Reward-related brain function and sleep in pre/early pubertal and mid/late pubertal adolescents. J Adolesc Health. 2009;45(4):326–34.
24. Dahl RE. The impact of inadequate sleep on children's daytime cognitive function. Semin Pediatr Neurol. 1996;3(1):44–50.
25. Harrison Y, Horne JA. The impact of sleep deprivation on decision making: a review. J Exp Psychol Appl. 2000;6(3):236–49.
26. Telzer EH, Fuligni AJ, Lieberman MD, Galvan A. The effects of poor quality sleep on brain function and risk taking in adolescence. NeuroImage. 2013;71:275–83.
27. Kurien PA, Chong SY, Ptacek LJ, Fu YH. Sick and tired: how molecular regulators of human sleep schedules and duration impact immune function. Curr Opin Neurobiol. 2013;23(5):873–9.
28. Ingiosi AM, Opp MR, Krueger JM. Sleep and immune function: glial contributions and consequences of aging. Curr Opin Neurobiol. 2013;23(5):806–11.
29. Ibarra-Coronado EG, Pantaleon-Martinez AM, Velazquez-Moctezuma J, Prospero-Garcia O, Mendez-Diaz M, Perez-Tapia M, et al. The bidirectional relationship between sleep and immunity against infections. J Immunol Res. 2015;2015:678164.
30. Hurtado-Alvarado G, Pavon L, Castillo-Garcia SA, Hernandez ME, Dominguez-Salazar E, Velazquez-Moctezuma J, et al. Sleep loss as a factor to induce cellular and molecular inflammatory variations. Clin Dev Immunol. 2013;2013:801341.

31. Xie L, Kang H, Xu Q, Chen MJ, Liao Y, Thiyagarajan M, et al. Sleep drives metabolite clearance from the adult brain. Science. 2013;342(6156):373–7.
32. Jessen NA, Munk AS, Lundgaard I, Nedergaard M. The glymphatic system: a beginner's guide. Neurochem Res. 2015;40:2583–99.
33. Mendelsohn AR, Larrick JW. Sleep facilitates clearance of metabolites from the brain: glymphatic function in aging and neurodegenerative diseases. Rejuvenation Res. 2013;16(6):518–23.
34. Piaget J. Play, dreams, and imitation in childhood, vol. ix. New York: Norton; 1951. 296 p. p.
35. Piers MW, Piaget J, Erikson Institute., Loyola University Chicago. School of Education., Loyola University Chicago. Department of Psychology. Play and development; a symposium. 1st ed. New York: Norton; 1972. 176 p. p.
36. Montessori M. The Montessori method; scientific pedagogy as applied to child education in the Children's Houses, with additions and revisions by the author, vol. xli. Cambridge, MA: R. Bentley; 1964. 377 p. p.
37. Parmelee Jr AH, Wenner WH, Schulz HR. Infant sleep patterns: from birth to 16 weeks of age. J Pediatr. 1964;65:576–82.
38. Roffwarg H, Muzio J, Dement W. Ontogenetic development of the human sleep-dream cycle. Science. 1966;152:604–19.
39. Mirmiran M, Maas YG, Ariagno RL. Development of fetal and neonatal sleep and circadian rhythms. Sleep Med Rev. 2003;7(4):321–34.
40. Mirmiran M. The function of fetal/neonatal rapid eye movement sleep. Behav Brain Res. 1995;69(1–2):13–22.
41. Arditi-Babchuk H, Feldman R, Eidelman AI. Rapid eye movement (REM) in premature neonates and developmental outcome at 6 months. Infant Behav Dev. 2009;32(1):27–32.
42. Aton SJ, Seibt J, Dumoulin M, Jha SK, Steinmetz N, Coleman T, et al. Mechanisms of sleep-dependent consolidation of cortical plasticity. Neuron. 2009;61(3):454–66.
43. Tikotzky L, DE Marcas G, Har-Toov J, Dollberg S, Bar-Haim Y, Sadeh A. Sleep and physical growth in infants during the first 6 months. J Sleep Res. 2010;19(1 Pt 1):103–10.
44. Graven S. Sleep and brain development. Clin Perinatol. 2006;33(3):693–706, vii.
45. Dionne G, Touchette E, Forget-Dubois N, Petit D, Tremblay RE, Montplaisir JY, et al. Associations between sleep-wake consolidation and language development in early childhood: a longitudinal twin study. Sleep. 2011;34(8):987–95.
46. Frank MG, Issa NP, Stryker MP. Sleep enhances plasticity in the developing visual cortex. Neuron. 2001;30(1):275–87.
47. Aton SJ, Suresh A, Broussard C, Frank MG. Sleep promotes cortical response potentiation following visual experience. Sleep. 2014;37(7):1163–70.
48. Jha SK, Jones BE, Coleman T, Steinmetz N, Law CT, Griffin G, et al. Sleep-dependent plasticity requires cortical activity. J Neurosci Off J Soc Neurosci. 2005;25(40):9266–74.
49. Scher MS, Johnson MW, Holditch-Davis D. Cyclicity of neonatal sleep behaviors at 25 to 30 weeks' postconceptional age. Pediatr Res. 2005;57(6):879–82.
50. Ringli M, Huber R. Developmental aspects of sleep slow waves: linking sleep, brain maturation and behavior. Prog Brain Res. 2011;193:63–82.
51. Scher A. Infant sleep at 10 months of age as a window to cognitive development. Early Hum Dev. 2005;81(3):289–92.
52. Scher A, Tse L, Hayes VE, Tardif M. Sleep difficulties in infants at risk for developmental delays: a longitudinal study. J Pediatr Psychol. 2008;33(4):396–405.
53. Scher MS, Loparo KA. Neonatal EEG/sleep state analyses: a complex phenotype of developmental neural plasticity. Dev Neurosci. 2009;31(4):259–75.
54. Weisman O, Magori-Cohen R, Louzoun Y, Eidelman AI, Feldman R. Sleep-wake transitions in premature neonates predict early development. Pediatrics. 2011;128(4):706–14.
55. Shellhaas RA, Burns JW, Barks JD, Chervin RD. Quantitative sleep stage analyses as a window to neonatal neurologic function. Neurology. 2014;82(5):390–5.

56. Thomas AJ, Erokwu BO, Yamamoto BK, Ernsberger P, Bishara O, Strohl KP. Alterations in respiratory behavior, brain neurochemistry and receptor density induced by pharmacologic suppression of sleep in the neonatal period. Brain Res Dev Brain Res. 2000;120(2):181–9.
57. Touchette E, Petit D, Seguin JR, Boivin M, Tremblay RE, Montplaisir JY. Associations between sleep duration patterns and behavioral/cognitive functioning at school entry. Sleep. 2007;30(9):1213–9.
58. Blumberg MS, Coleman CM, Gerth AI, McMurray B. Spatiotemporal structure of REM sleep twitching reveals developmental origins of motor synergies. Curr Biol CB. 2013;23(21):2100–9.
59. Blumberg MS. Beyond dreams: do sleep-related movements contribute to brain development? Front Neurol. 2010;1:140.
60. Blumberg MS, Gall AJ, Todd WD. The development of sleep-wake rhythms and the search for elemental circuits in the infant brain. Behav Neurosci. 2014;128(3):250–63.
61. Chipaux M, Colonnese MT, Mauguen A, Fellous L, Mokhtari M, Lezcano O, et al. Auditory stimuli mimicking ambient sounds drive temporal "delta-brushes" in premature infants. PLoS ONE. 2013;8(11), e79028.
62. Geva R, Yaron H, Kuint J. Neonatal sleep predicts attention orienting and distractibility. J Atten Disord. 2016;20(2):138–50.
63. Almadhoob A, Ohlsson A. Sound reduction management in the neonatal intensive care unit for preterm or very low birth weight infants. Cochrane Database Syst Rev. 2015;1:Cd010333.
64. Voos KC, Terreros A, Larimore P, Leick-Rude MK, Park N. Implementing safe sleep practices in a neonatal intensive care unit. J Matern Fetal Neonatal Med. 2015;28(14):1637–40.
65. Guedj R, Danan C, Daoud P, Zupan V, Renolleau S, Zana E, et al. Does neonatal pain management in intensive care units differ between night and day? An observational study. BMJ Open. 2014;4(2), e004086.
66. Hwang SS, O'Sullivan A, Fitzgerald E, Melvin P, Gorman T, Fiascone JM. Implementation of safe sleep practices in the neonatal intensive care unit. J Perinatol Off J Calif Perinat Assoc. 2015;35(10):862–6.
67. Szymczak SE, Shellhaas RA. Impact of NICU design on environmental noise. J Neonatal Nurs JNN. 2014;20(2):77–81.
68. Mason B, Ahlers-Schmidt CR, Schunn C. Improving safe sleep environments for well newborns in the hospital setting. Clin Pediatr. 2013;52(10):969–75.
69. Rasch B, Born J. About sleep's role in memory. Physiol Rev. 2013;93(2):681–766.
70. Landmann N, Kuhn M, Piosczyk H, Feige B, Baglioni C, Spiegelhalder K, et al. The reorganisation of memory during sleep. Sleep Med Rev. 2014;18(6):531–41.
71. Stickgold R, James L, Hobson JA. Visual discrimination learning requires sleep after training. Nat Neurosci. 2000;3(12):1237–8.
72. Walker MP, Brakefield T, Morgan A, Hobson JA, Stickgold R. Practice with sleep makes perfect: sleep-dependent motor skill learning. Neuron. 2002;35(1):205–11.
73. Geiger A, Huber R, Kurth S, Ringli M, Jenni OG, Achermann P. The sleep EEG as a marker of intellectual ability in school age children. Sleep. 2011;34(2):181–9.
74. Astill RG, Piantoni G, Raymann RJ, Vis JC, Coppens JE, Walker MP, et al. Sleep spindle and slow wave frequency reflect motor skill performance in primary school-age children. Front Hum Neurosci. 2014;8:910.
75. Lustenberger C, Maric A, Durr R, Achermann P, Huber R. Triangular relationship between sleep spindle activity, general cognitive ability and the efficiency of declarative learning. PLoS ONE. 2012;7(11), e49561.
76. Nader RS, Smith CT. Correlations between adolescent processing speed and specific spindle frequencies. Front Hum Neurosci. 2015;9:30.
77. Geiger A, Huber R, Kurth S, Ringli M, Achermann P, Jenni OG. Sleep electroencephalography topography and children's intellectual ability. Neuroreport. 2012;23(2):93–7.
78. Maski KP. Sleep-dependent memory consolidation in children. Semin Pediatr Neurol. 2015;22(2):130–4.

79. Gomez RL, Edgin JO. Sleep as a window into early neural development: shifts in sleep-dependent learning effects across early childhood. Child Dev Perspect. 2015;9(3):183–9.
80. Gomez RL, Bootzin RR, Nadel L. Naps promote abstraction in language-learning infants. Psychol Sci. 2006;17(8):670–4.
81. Hupbach A, Gomez RL, Bootzin RR, Nadel L. Nap-dependent learning in infants. Dev Sci. 2009;12(6):1007–12.
82. Friedrich M, Wilhelm I, Born J, Friederici AD. Generalization of word meanings during infant sleep. Nat Commun. 2015;6:6004.
83. Backhaus J, Hoeckesfeld R, Born J, Hohagen F, Junghanns K. Immediate as well as delayed post learning sleep but not wakefulness enhances declarative memory consolidation in children. Neurobiol Learn Mem. 2008;89(1):76–80.
84. Prehn-Kristensen A, Goder R, Chirobeja S, Bressmann I, Ferstl R, Baving L. Sleep in children enhances preferentially emotional declarative but not procedural memories. J Exp Child Psychol. 2009;104(1):132–9.
85. Henderson LM, Weighall AR, Brown H, Gareth GM. Consolidation of vocabulary is associated with sleep in children. Dev Sci. 2012;15(5):674–87.
86. Wilhelm I, Metzkow-Meszaros M, Knapp S, Born J. Sleep-dependent consolidation of procedural motor memories in children and adults: the pre-sleep level of performance matters. Dev Sci. 2012;15(4):506–15.
87. Wilhelm I, Diekelmann S, Born J. Sleep in children improves memory performance on declarative but not procedural tasks. Learn Mem. 2008;15(5):373–7.
88. Fischer S, Wilhelm I, Born J. Developmental differences in sleep's role for implicit off-line learning: comparing children with adults. J Cogn Neurosci. 2007;19(2):214–27.
89. Urbain C, Galer S, Van Bogaert P, Peigneux P. Pathophysiology of sleep-dependent memory consolidation processes in children. Int J Psychophysiol Off J Int Organ Psychophysiol. 2013;89(2):273–83.
90. Killgore WD. Effects of sleep deprivation on cognition. Prog Brain Res. 2010;185:105–29.
91. Vorster AP, Born J. Sleep and memory in mammals, birds and invertebrates. Neurosci Biobehav Rev. 2015;50:103–19.
92. Piantoni G, Van Der Werf YD, Jensen O, Van Someren EJ. Memory traces of long-range coordinated oscillations in the sleeping human brain. Hum Brain Mapp. 2015;36(1):67–84.
93. Tesler N, Gerstenberg M, Huber R. Developmental changes in sleep and their relationships to psychiatric illnesses. Curr Opin Psychiatry. 2013;26(6):572–9.
94. Damaraju E, Caprihan A, Lowe JR, Allen EA, Calhoun VD, Phillips JP. Functional connectivity in the developing brain: a longitudinal study from 4 to 9 months of age. NeuroImage. 2014;84:169–80.
95. Kurth S, Ringli M, Lebourgeois MK, Geiger A, Buchmann A, Jenni OG, et al. Mapping the electrophysiological marker of sleep depth reveals skill maturation in children and adolescents. NeuroImage. 2012;63(2):959–65.
96. Arain M, Haque M, Johal L, Mathur P, Nel W, Rais A, et al. Maturation of the adolescent brain. Neuropsychiatr Dis Treat. 2013;9:449–61.
97. Wang G, Grone B, Colas D, Appelbaum L, Mourrain P. Synaptic plasticity in sleep: learning, homeostasis and disease. Trends Neurosci. 2011;34(9):452–63.
98. Tang G, Gudsnuk K, Kuo SH, Cotrina ML, Rosoklija G, Sosunov A, et al. Loss of mTOR-dependent macroautophagy causes autistic-like synaptic pruning deficits. Neuron. 2014;83(5):1131–43.
99. Boksa P. Abnormal synaptic pruning in schizophrenia: urban myth or reality? J Psychiatry Neurosci. 2012;37(2):75–7.
100. Saugstad LF. Infantile autism: a chronic psychosis since infancy due to synaptic pruning of the supplementary motor area. Nutr Health. 2011;20(3–4):171–82.
101. Paolicelli RC, Bolasco G, Pagani F, Maggi L, Scianni M, Panzanelli P, et al. Synaptic pruning by microglia is necessary for normal brain development. Science. 2011;333(6048):1456–8.
102. Vyazovskiy VV, Olcese U, Lazimy YM, Faraguna U, Esser SK, Williams JC, et al. Cortical firing and sleep homeostasis. Neuron. 2009;63(6):865–78.

103. Esser SK, Hill SL, Tononi G. Sleep homeostasis and cortical synchronization: I. Modeling the effects of synaptic strength on sleep slow waves. Sleep. 2007;30(12):1617–30.
104. Riedner BA, Vyazovskiy VV, Huber R, Massimini M, Esser S, Murphy M, et al. Sleep homeostasis and cortical synchronization: III. A high-density EEG study of sleep slow waves in humans. Sleep. 2007;30(12):1643–57.
105. Vyazovskiy VV, Riedner BA, Cirelli C, Tononi G. Sleep homeostasis and cortical synchronization: II. A local field potential study of sleep slow waves in the rat. Sleep. 2007;30(12): 1631–42.
106. Feinberg I, Campbell IG. Longitudinal sleep EEG trajectories indicate complex patterns of adolescent brain maturation. Am J Physiol Regul Integr Comp Physiol. 2013;304(4): R296–303.
107. de Vivo L, Faraguna U, Nelson AB, Pfister-Genskow M, Klapperich ME, Tononi G, et al. Developmental patterns of sleep slow wave activity and synaptic density in adolescent mice. Sleep. 2014;37(4):689–700, A-B.
108. Feinberg I, Campbell IG. Sleep EEG changes during adolescence: an index of a fundamental brain reorganization. Brain Cogn. 2010;72(1):56–65.
109. Walker MP, van der Helm E. Overnight therapy? The role of sleep in emotional brain processing. Psychol Bull. 2009;135(5):731–48.
110. Goldstein-Piekarski AN, Greer SM, Saletin JM, Walker MP. Sleep deprivation impairs the human central and peripheral nervous system discrimination of social threat. J Neurosci Off J Soc Neurosci. 2015;35(28):10135–45.
111. Goldstein AN, Walker MP. The role of sleep in emotional brain function. Annu Rev Clin Psychol. 2014;10:679–708.
112. Miller AL, Seifer R, Crossin R, Lebourgeois MK. Toddler's self-regulation strategies in a challenge context are nap-dependent. J Sleep Res. 2015;24(3):279–87.
113. Meldrum RC, Barnes JC, Hay C. Sleep deprivation, low self-control, and delinquency: a test of the strength model of self-control. J Youth Adolesc. 2015;44(2):465–77.
114. Hart CN, Carskadon MA, Demos KE, Van Reen E, Sharkey KM, Raynor HA, et al. Acute changes in sleep duration on eating behaviors and appetite-regulating hormones in overweight/obese adults. Behav Sleep Med. 2015;13(5):424–36.
115. St-Onge MP, O'Keeffe M, Roberts AL, RoyChoudhury A, Laferrere B. Short sleep duration, glucose dysregulation and hormonal regulation of appetite in men and women. Sleep. 2012;35(11):1503–10.
116. Morselli L, Leproult R, Balbo M, Spiegel K. Role of sleep duration in the regulation of glucose metabolism and appetite. Best Pract Res Clin Endocrinol Metab. 2010;24(5):687–702.
117. Kim J, Hakim F, Kheirandish-Gozal L, Gozal D. Inflammatory pathways in children with insufficient or disordered sleep. Respir Physiol Neurobiol. 2011;178(3):465–74.
118. Jernelov S, Lekander M, Almqvist C, Axelsson J, Larsson H. Development of atopic disease and disturbed sleep in childhood and adolescence – a longitudinal population-based study. Clin Exp Allergy J Br Soc Allergy Clin Immunol. 2013;43(5):552–9.
119. Hon KL, Ching GK, Ng PC, Leung TF. Exploring CCL18, eczema severity and atopy. Pediatr Allergy Immunol Off Publ Eur Soc Pediatr Allergy Immunol. 2011;22(7):704–7.
120. Reed P, Vile R, Osborne LA, Romano M, Truzoli R. Problematic internet usage and immune function. PLoS ONE. 2015;10(8), e0134538.
121. An J, Sun Y, Wan Y, Chen J, Wang X, Tao F. Associations between problematic internet use and adolescents' physical and psychological symptoms: possible role of sleep quality. J Addict Med. 2014;8(4):282–7.
122. Cermakian N, Lange T, Golombek D, Sarkar D, Nakao A, Shibata S, et al. Crosstalk between the circadian clock circuitry and the immune system. Chronobiol Int. 2013;30(7):870–88.
123. Hui FK. Clearing your mind: a glymphatic system? World Neurosurg. 2015;83(5):715–7.
124. Iliff JJ, Lee H, Yu M, Feng T, Logan J, Nedergaard M, et al. Brain-wide pathway for waste clearance captured by contrast-enhanced MRI. J Clin Invest. 2013;123(3):1299–309.
125. Pahnke J, Langer O, Krohn M. Alzheimer's and ABC transporters – new opportunities for diagnostics and treatment. Neurobiol Dis. 2014;72(Pt A):54–60.

126. Porter VR, Buxton WG, Avidan AY. Sleep, cognition and dementia. Curr Psychiatry Rep. 2015;17(12):97.
127. Tsapanou A, Gu Y, Manly J, Schupf N, Tang MX, Zimmerman M, et al. Daytime sleepiness and sleep inadequacy as risk factors for dementia. Dement Geriatr Cogn Dis Extra. 2015;5(2):286–95.
128. Guarnieri B, Sorbi S. Sleep and cognitive decline: a strong bidirectional relationship. It is time for specific recommendations on routine assessment and the management of sleep disorders in patients with mild cognitive impairment and dementia. Eur Neurol. 2015;74(1–2): 43–8.
129. Cross N, Terpening Z, Rogers NL, Duffy SL, Hickie IB, Lewis SJ, et al. Napping in older people 'at risk' of dementia: relationships with depression, cognition, medical burden and sleep quality. J Sleep Res. 2015;24(5):494–502.
130. Tarasoff-Conway JM, Carare RO, Osorio RS, Glodzik L, Butler T, Fieremans E, et al. Clearance systems in the brain-implications for Alzheimer disease. Nat Rev Neurol. 2015;11(8):457–70.
131. Kress BT, Iliff JJ, Xia M, Wang M, Wei HS, Zeppenfeld D, et al. Impairment of paravascular clearance pathways in the aging brain. Ann Neurol. 2014;76(6):845–61.
132. Kotagal S. Seminars in pediatric neurology. Sleep-wake disorders of childhood. Introduction. Semin Pediatr Neurol. 2008;15(2):41.
133. Tassinari CA, Cantalupo G, Hogl B, Cortelli P, Tassi L, Francione S, et al. Neuroethological approach to frontolimbic epileptic seizures and parasomnias: the same central pattern generators for the same behaviours. Rev Neurol. 2009;165(10):762–8.
134. Tassinari CA, Rubboli G, Gardella E, Cantalupo G, Calandra-Buonaura G, Vedovello M, et al. Central pattern generators for a common semiology in fronto-limbic seizures and in parasomnias. A neuroethologic approach. Neurol Sci. 2005;26 Suppl 3:s225–32.
135. Pugin F, Metz AJ, Wolf M, Achermann P, Jenni OG, Huber R. Local increase of sleep slow wave activity after three weeks of working memory training in children and adolescents. Sleep. 2015;38(4):607–14.
136. Fisher SP, Vyazovskiy VV. Local sleep taking care of high-maintenance cortical circuits under sleep restriction. Sleep. 2014;37(11):1727–30.
137. Mascetti L, Muto V, Matarazzo L, Foret A, Ziegler E, Albouy G, et al. The impact of visual perceptual learning on sleep and local slow-wave initiation. J Neurosci Off J Soc Neurosci. 2013;33(8):3323–31.
138. Nobili L, De Gennaro L, Proserpio P, Moroni F, Sarasso S, Pigorini A, et al. Local aspects of sleep: observations from intracerebral recordings in humans. Prog Brain Res. 2012;199:219–32.
139. Drummond SP, Brown GG, Stricker JL, Buxton RB, Wong EC, Gillin JC. Sleep deprivation-induced reduction in cortical functional response to serial subtraction. Neuroreport. 1999;10(18):3745–8.
140. Maquet P, Laureys S, Peigneux P, Fuchs S, Petiau C, Phillips C, et al. Experience-dependent changes in cerebral activation during human REM sleep. Nat Neurosci. 2000;3(8):831–6.
141. Maquet P, Peigneux P, Laureys S, Boly M, Dang-Vu T, Desseilles M, et al. Memory processing during human sleep as assessed by functional neuroimaging. Rev Neurol. 2003;159(11 Suppl):6S27–9.
142. Corner MA. Sleep and the beginnings of behavior in the animal kingdom – studies of ultradian motility cycles in early life. Prog Neurobiol. 1977;8(4):279–95.
143. Corner M. Ontogeny of brain sleep mechanisms. In: McGinty D, editor. Brain mechanisms of sleep. New York: Raven; 1985. p. 175–97.
144. Morrison AR. Paradoxical sleep without atonia. Arch Ital Biol. 1988;126(4):275–89.
145. Karlson K, Gall A, Mohns E, Seelke A, Blumberg M. The neural substrates of infant sleep in rats. PLoS Biol. 2005;3(5), e143.
146. Bes F, Schulz H, Navelet Y, Salzarulo P. The distribution of slow-wave sleep across the night: a comparison for infants, children, and adults. Sleep. 1991;14(1):5–12.

147. Jenni OG, Borbely AA, Achermann P. Development of the nocturnal sleep electroencephalogram in human infants. Am J Physiol Regul Integr Comp Physiol. 2004;286(3):R528–38.
148. Roffwarg H, Dement W, Fisher C. Preliminary observations of the sleep-wake pattern in neonates, infants, children, and adults. In: Harms E, editor. Problems of sleep and dreams in children. 2. New York: Macmillan; 1964. p. 60–72.
149. Passouant P, Cadilhac J, Delange M. The sleep of the newborn. Considerations on the period of ocular movements. Arch Fr Pediatr. 1965;22(9):1087–92.
150. Fukumoto M, Mochizuki N, Takeishi M, Nomura Y, Segawa M. Studies of body movements during night sleep in infancy. Brain Dev. 1981;3(1):37–43.
151. Prechtl HF, Nijhuis JG. Eye movements in the human fetus and newborn. Behav Brain Res. 1983;10(1):119–24.
152. Parmelee AH, Stern E, Harris MA. Maturation of respiration in prematures and young infants. Neuropadiatrie. 1972;3(3):294–304.
153. Parmalee Jr A, Akiyama Y, Stern E, Harris M. A periodic cerebral rhythm in newborn infants. Exp Neurol. 1969;35:575.
154. Scholle S, Schafer T. Atlas of states of sleep and wakefulness in infants and children. Somnologie. 1999;3:163–241.
155. Becker PT, Thoman EB. Rapid eye movement storms in infants: rate of occurrence at 6 months predicts mental development at 1 year. Science. 1981;212(4501):1415–6.
156. Dreyfus-Brisac C. Ontogenesis of sleep in human prematures after 32 weeks of conceptional age. Dev Psychobiol. 1970;3(2):91–121.
157. Eliet-Flescher J, Dreyfus-Brisac C. The sleep of the full-term newborn and premature infant. II. Electroencephalogram and chin muscle activity during maturation. Biol Neonatorum Neonatal Stud. 1966;10(5):316–39.
158. Schloon H, O'Brien MJ, Scholten CA, Prechtl HF. Muscle activity and postural behaviour in newborn infants. A polymyographic study. Neuropadiatrie. 1976;7(4):384–415.
159. Curzi-Dascalova L, Peirano P, Morel-Kahn F. Development of sleep states in normal premature and full-term newborns. Dev Psychobiol. 1988;21(5):431–44.
160. Salzaulo P. L'atonie msculaire pendant le sommeil chez l'homme. Riv Psicol. 1968;62:201–20.
161. Okai T, Kozuma S, Shinozuka N, Kuwabara Y, Mizuno M. A study on the development of sleep-wakefulness cycle in the human fetus. Early Hum Dev. 1992;29(1–3):391–6.
162. Curzi-Dascalova L, Figueroa JM, Eiselt M, Christova E, Virassamy A, d'Allest AM, et al. Sleep state organization in premature infants of less than 35 weeks' gestational age. Pediatr Res. 1993;34(5):624–8.
163. Kahn A, Dan B, Groswasser J, Franco P, Sottiaux M. Normal sleep architecture in infants and children. J Clin Neurophysiol. 1996;13(3):184–97.
164. Parmelee Jr AH, Wenner WH, Akiyama Y, Schultz M, Stern E. Sleep states in premature infants. Dev Med Child Neurol. 1967;9(1):70–7.
165. Andre M, Lamblin MD, d'Allest AM, Curzi-Dascalova L, Moussalli-Salefranque F, S Nguyen The T, et al. Electroencephalography in premature and full-term infants. Developmental features and glossary. Neurophysiologie clinique=Clinical neurophysiology. 2010;40(2):59–124.
166. MacLean JE, Fitzgerald DA, Waters KA. Developmental changes in sleep and breathing across infancy and childhood. Paediatr Respir Rev. 2015;16:276–84.
167. Grigg-Damberger M, Gozal D, Marcus CL, Quan SF, Rosen CL, Chervin RD, et al. The visual scoring of sleep and arousal in infants and children. J Clin Sleep Med JCSM Off Publ Am Acad Sleep Med. 2007;3(2):201–40.
168. Louis J, Zhang J, Revol M, et al. Ontogenesis of nocturnal organization of sleep spindles: a longitudinal study during the first six months of life. Electroencephalogr Clin Neurophysiol. 1992;83:289–96.
169. Iglowstein I, Jenni OG, Molinari L, Largo RH. Sleep duration from infancy to adolescence: reference values and generational trends. Pediatrics. 2003;111(2):302–7.

170. Lutter WJ, Maier M, Wakai RT. Development of MEG sleep patterns and magnetic auditory evoked responses during early infancy. Clin Neurophysiol Off J Int Fed Clin Neurophysiol. 2006;117(3):522–30.

171. Danker-Hopfe H. Growth and development of children with a special focus on sleep. Prog Biophys Mol Biol. 2011;107(3):333–8.

172. Hughes JR. The development of the vertex sharp transient. Clin Electroencephalogr. 1998;29(4):183–7.

173. Werner SS, Stockard JE, Bickford RG. The ontogenesis of the electroencephalogram of prematures. Atlas of neonatal electroencephalography. 1st ed. New York City: Raven; 1977. p. 47–91.

174. Kellaway P, Fox BJ. Electroencephalographic diagnosis of cerebral pathology in infants during sleep. I. Rationale, technique, and the characteristics of normal sleep in infants. J Pediatr. 1952;41(3):262–87.

175. Kellaway P. Ontogenetic evolution of the electrical activity of the brain in man and animal. Acta Med Belg. 1957:141–54.

176. Anders T, Emde R, Parmelee A. A manual of standardized terminology, techniques and criteria for scoring states of sleep and wakefulness in newborn infants. Los Angeles: UCLA Brain Information Service, NINDS Neurological information Network; 1971.

177. Metcalf DR, Mondale J, Butler FK. Ontogenesis of spontaneous K-complexes. Psychophysiology. 1971;8(3):340–7.

178. Fisch BJ. Fisch and Spehlmann's EEG Primer. 3rd printing revised and enlarged ed. New York: Elsevier; 2002. 621 p.

179. Halasz P. K-complex, a reactive EEG graphoelement of NREM sleep: an old chap in a new garment. Sleep Med Rev. 2005;9(5):391–412.

180. Niedermeyer E. In: Niedermeyer E, Lopes da Silva F, editors. Electroencephalography: basic principles, clinical applications and related fields. 4th ed. Philadelpha: Lippincott, Williams and Wilkins; 1999. p. 189–214.

181. Ferber R. In: Ferber R, Kryger M, editors. Introduction to pediatric sleep disorders medicine. Philadelphia: W.B. Saunders; 1995. Pg. 1 p.

182. Schechtman VL, Harper RM. The maturation of correlations between cardiac and respiratory measures across sleep states in normal infants. Sleep. 1992;15(1):41–7.

183. Coons S, Guilleminault C. Development of sleep-wake patterns and non-rapid eye movement sleep stages during the first six months of life in normal infants. Pediatrics. 1982;69(6):793–8.

184. Salzarulo P, Fagioli I, Salomon F, Ricour C, Raimbault G, Ambrosi S, et al. Sleep patterns in infants under continuous feeding from birth. Electroencephalogr Clin Neurophysiol. 1980;49(3–4):330–6.

185. Liefting B, Bes F, Fagioli I, Salzarulo P. Electromyographic activity and sleep states in infants. Sleep. 1994;17(8):718–22.

186. Ficca G, Fagioli I, Salzarulo P. Sleep organization in the first year of life: developmental trends in the quiet sleep-paradoxical sleep cycle. J Sleep Res. 2000;9(1):1–4.

187. Hoppenbrouwers T, Hodgman JE, Harper RM, Sterman MB. Temporal distribution of sleep states, somatic activity, and autonomic activity during the first half year of life. Sleep. 1982;5(2):131–44.

188. Samson-Dolfuss D, Nogues B, Verdure-Poussin A, Mallevile F. Electroencephalogramme du sommeil de l'enfant normal entre 5 mois et 3 ans. Rev EEG Neurophysiol. 1977;7:335–45.

189. Lenard H. The development of sleep behavior in babies and small children. Electrocephalogr Clin Neurophysiol. 1972;32:710.

190. Tanguay PE, Ornitz EM, Kaplan A, Bozzo ES. Evolution of sleep spindles in childhood. Electroencephalogr Clin Neurophysiol. 1975;38(2):175–81.

191. Brandt S, Brandt H. The electroencephalographic patterns in young healthy children from 0 to five years of age; their practical use in daily clinical electroencephalography. Acta Psychiatr Neurol Scand. 1955;30(1–2):77–89.

192. Gibbs EL, Lorimer FM, Gibbs FA. Clinical correlates of exceedingly fast activity in the electroencephalogram. Dis Nerv Syst. 1950;11(11):323–6.

193. Dale PW, Busse EW. An elaboration of a distinctive EEG pattern found during drowsy states in children. Dis Nerv Syst. 1951;12(4):122–5.
194. Westmoreland B, Stockard J. The EEG in infants and children: normal patterns. Am J EEG Technol. 1977;17(4):187–207.
195. Sheldon S. Evaluating sleep in infants and children. Evaluating sleep in infants and children. Philadelphia: Lippincott-Raven; 1996. p. 228.
196. Nekhorocheff I. Electroencephalogram of sleep in children. Rev Neurol (Paris). 1950;82(6):487–95.
197. Hess R. The electroencephalogram in sleep. Electroencephalogr Clin Neurophysiol. 1964;16:44–55.
198. Niedermeyer E. Sleep and EEG. In: Niedermeyer E, Lopes da Silva F, editors. Electroencephalography: basic principles, clinical applications, and related fields. 5th ed. Philadelphia: Lippincott, Williams & Wilkins; 2005.
199. Sheldon SH. Development of sleep in infants and children. In: Sheldon SH, Ferber R, Kryger MH, Gozal D, editors. Principles and practice of pediatric sleep medicine. 2nd ed. London: Elsevier Saunders; 2014. p. 17–24.
200. Lamblin MD, Walls Esquivel E, Andre M. The electroencephalogram of the full-term newborn: review of normal features and hypoxic-ischemic encephalopathy patterns. Neurophysiol Clin Clin Neurophysiol. 2013;43(5–6):267–87.
201. Monod N, Pajot N. The sleep of the full-term newborn and premature infant. I. Analysis of the polygraphic study (rapid eye movements, respiration and E.E.G.) in the full-term newborn. Biologia neonatorum Neo-natal studies. 1965;8(5):281–307.
202. Galland BC, Taylor BJ, Elder DE, Herbison P. Normal sleep patterns in infants and children: a systematic review of observational studies. Sleep Med Rev. 2012;16(3):213–22.
203. Schulz H, Salzarulo P, Fagioli I, Massetani R. REM latency: development in the first year of life. Electroencephalogr Clin Neurophysiol. 1983;56(4):316–22.
204. Anders TF, Keener M. Developmental course of nighttime sleep-wake patterns in full-term and premature infants during the first year of life. I. Sleep. 1985;8(3):173–92.
205. Coons S. In: Guilleminault C, editor. Development of sleep and wakefulness during the first 6 months of life. New York: Raven Press; 1987. p. 7–27.
206. Scholle S, Beyer U, Bernhard M, Eichholz S, Erler T, Graness P, et al. Normative values of polysomnographic parameters in childhood and adolescence: quantitative sleep parameters. Sleep Med. 2011;12(6):542–9.
207. Campbell IG, Darchia N, Higgins LM, Dykan IV, Davis NM, de Bie E, et al. Adolescent changes in homeostatic regulation of EEG activity in the delta and theta frequency bands during NREM sleep. Sleep. 2011;34(1):83–91.
208. McMillen IC, Kok JS, Adamson TM, Deayton JM, Nowak R. Development of circadian sleep-wake rhythms in preterm and full-term infants. Pediatr Res. 1991;29(4 Pt 1):381–4.
209. Erren TC, Trautmann K, Salz MM, Reiter RJ. Newborn intensive care units and perinatal healthcare: on light's imprinting role on circadian system stability for research and prevention. J Perinatol Off J Calif Perinat Assoc. 2013;33(10):824–5.
210. Tsai SY, Thomas KA, Lentz MJ, Barnard KE. Light is beneficial for infant circadian entrainment: an actigraphic study. J Adv Nurs. 2012;68(8):1738–47.
211. Sandor P, Szakadat S, Bodizs R. Ontogeny of dreaming: a review of empirical studies. Sleep Med Rev. 2014;18(5):435–49.
212. Schredl M, Fricke-Oerkermann L, Mitschke A, Wiater A, Lehmkuhl G. Longitudinal study of nightmares in children: stability and effect of emotional symptoms. Child Psychiatry Hum Dev. 2009;40(3):439–49.

Chapter 2
The Discovery of Pediatric Sleep Medicine

Oliviero Bruni and Raffaele Ferri

Abstract The aim of this chapter is to depict the discovery of sleep physiology in infants and the emergence of the discipline of pediatric sleep as relatively autonomous entity.

The gradual awareness regarding sleep disorders in infants and children begins in the nineteenth century when the first doctors and pediatricians begin to classify infants and children sleep disorders. The process that leads to the increasing understanding and knowledge of pediatric sleep disorders was not easy. Children's sleep has been neglected until the end of the last century with the main textbook of pediatrics reporting no chapters or only few paragraphs devoted to pediatric sleep.

It is interesting to note that the first observation that leads to the discovery of rapid eye movement (REM) sleep was made on neonates and infants, and the first study on the negative behavioral consequences of sleep apnea has been reported in children.

The story of the infants' and children's sleep behavior during the antiquity is briefly delineated, and subsequently the first recommendations on the sleep time duration are reported with surprisingly data.

This chapter also briefly lists the fundamental contribution of researchers from different countries and their role in the development of pediatric sleep medicine.

Finally, the history and the establishment of the scientific associations related to the pediatric sleep medicine are delineated.

O. Bruni, MD (✉)
Center for Pediatric Sleep Disorders, Department of Social and Developmental Psychology, Sapienza University, Via dei Marsi 78, 00185 Rome, Italy

S. Andrea Hospital, Rome, Italy
e-mail: oliviero.bruni@uniroma1.it

R. Ferri
Sleep Research Centre, Department of Neurology, I.C., Oasi Institute for Research on Mental Retardation and Brain Aging (IRCCS), Troina, Italy

© Springer International Publishing Switzerland 2017
S. Nevšímalová, O. Bruni (eds.), *Sleep Disorders in Children*,
DOI 10.1007/978-3-319-28640-2_2

31

This historical overview has limitations, and some fundamental researchers that greatly contributed to the birth of pediatric sleep medicine as an independent field probably have been forgotten. However the last few years have acknowledged the growing interest on pediatric sleep, and different health providers (pediatric pulmonologists, otolaryngologists, neurologists, orthodontists, and psychologists) become interested in recognizing the negative consequence of sleep disorders for child health and development.

Keywords Sleep • Infant • Child • Adolescent • Development • Pediatric sleep associations

General Overview

Sleep medicine in adult as a scientific field begins in the 1950s and has greatly and speedily evolved over the past 60 years.

The appearance of pediatric and adolescent sleep medicine as an autonomous entity begins about 30 years ago related to several important researches in different clinical fields: obstructive sleep apnea and other sleep-related breathing disorders, sudden infant death syndrome (SIDS), insomnia, and narcolepsy. However, it was the gradual identification of the importance of sleep for several daytime dysfunctions like neurobehavioral problems, learning difficulties, growth failure, etc., which began to raise awareness on the importance of sleep in infancy and childhood development [1].

Beginning from the 1980s, there was a huge growth of pediatric and adolescent sleep medicine starting with two important publications. The first book for parents entitled *Solve Your Child's Sleep Problems* was written in 1985 by Richard Ferber [2] of the Boston Children's Hospital that for the first time described the behavioral treatment for pediatric insomnia and highlighted the developmental and behavioral aspects of pediatric sleep. Just 2 years later, Christian Guilleminault edited the book *Sleep and Its Disorders in Children* [3] that represented the reference for the pediatric sleep for clinicians and healthcare providers involved with infants and children. The contributions presented in that book provided the basis for the future development of a knowledge base for understanding normal and pathological sleep in infants and children.

The first comprehensive pediatric sleep textbook *Pediatric Sleep Medicine* was published by Sheldon, Spire, and Levy in 1992 [4], followed in 1995 by the reference book *Principles and Practice of Sleep Medicine in the Child* by Richard Ferber and Meir Kryger [5]; then the revised edition *Principles and Practice of Pediatric Sleep Medicine* by Sheldon, Ferber, and Kryger in 2005 [6]); and finally the second edition of this book published in 2014 [7].

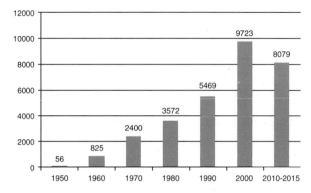

Fig. 2.1 Number of publications for each decade in PubMed with search word "sleep" limited to humans and all children (0–18 years)

Notwithstanding the awareness of the importance of sleep for development, pediatricians slowly begin to recognize the importance of sleep physiology and sleep structure to human development and behavior. Gradually, over the past decade, pediatric pulmonologists, otolaryngologists, neurologists, orthodontists, and psychologists have acknowledged the negative consequence of sleep disorders for child health and development and have integrated this into their clinical practice.

Although the growth of pediatric sleep medicine was tremendous, the classical pediatric textbooks almost ignored the topics of sleep disturbances with very few parts of the books dedicated to sleep disorders.

In 2002, the American Academy of Sleep Medicine (AASM) applied to the Accreditation Council on Graduate Medical Education (ACGME) for the establishment of sleep medicine training programs, and in 2003 sleep medicine was accepted as an independent medical specialty with a new multidisciplinary specialty examination in sleep medicine. In the first examination in 2007, considerations and disorders unique to childhood comprised 2 % of the first examination. Several efforts have been made to increase the presence of childhood sleep, and actually many schools of sleep medicine, hospitals, and academic clinics set up training programs, residencies, and fellowships in pediatric sleep medicine and recognized the peculiarity and uniqueness of sleep during human development [1].

This acknowledgment leads to a gradual and huge growth of scientific papers in pediatric sleep, with special emphasis on respiratory disturbances during sleep, as revealed by the amount of publications indexed on PubMed from the 1980s.

Figure 2.1 shows the number of publications that can be found in PubMed with the search word "sleep" limited to humans and all children (01–18 years). There was a steep increase in papers, especially in the last decade.

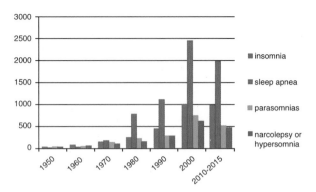

Fig. 2.2 Number of publications for each decade in PubMed search on the major sleep disorders of childhood limited to humans and all children (0–18 years)

In Fig. 2.2 the total number of publications on the major groups of sleep disturbances of childhood is reported based on PubMed search with the different words for each disorder limited to humans and all children (01–18 years).

As reported above, over the past 30 years, there has also been an increasing awareness of pediatric pulmonologists and pediatric otolaryngologists on the role of respiratory sleep disturbances in their clinical work, with an increasing understanding of the importance of a comprehensive knowledge of sleep medicine, since without a global view of the different physiological parameters during sleep it is extremely difficult to perform a correct diagnosis and a therapeutic decision.

Paralleling this consciousness, there was an increase of pediatric sleep centers in the USA and in Europe, and more and more countries are building up their own sleep centers. The need for specialized sleep laboratories is mandatory for the clear differences in sleep physiology and disturbances between adults and infants or children.

Besides the sleep medicine field, sleep research in childhood has been greatly developed by psychologists especially related to the neurobehavioral and psychosocial consequences of sleep disorders, with population studies on the effect of disturbed sleep on mental and physical health.

The changes in the society and especially the advent of the new technologies have had a great impact on sleep and could have been an addictive role in the progressive decrease of sleep duration in the modern societies.

In the following paragraphs, we will describe how pediatric sleep medicine evolved beginning from the description of the studies on infant and child sleep that helped the discovery of rapid eye movement (REM) sleep and of the efforts of the researchers for defining the different sleep structures in newborns, infants, and children. In the second part, we will review the clinical picture, analyzing studies on insomnia, parasomnias, respiratory disturbances, narcolepsy, disorders of movements during sleep, and sudden infant death syndrome (SIDS). The third part will illustrate the fascinating stories of sleep researchers that made this process possible and that built the history of pediatric sleep medicine. The final section will be devoted to the description of the birth of different pediatric sleep associations.

Infant's Eyes and the Discovery of REM Sleep

In 1926, during the Russian Academy of Sciences congress, the pediatricians Denisova and Figurin presented the results of their first formal pediatric sleep research showing that, several times during sleep, infants presented episodes, lasting for 10–15 min every half an hour, during which respiration and pulse became irregular and fast and small muscles presented numerous twitches. This periodic instability of physiological functions was present in healthy children, and the authors concluded that "normal sleep is not a state of rest" [8].

As reported by William Dement, this research inspired Kleitman and ultimately led to his decision to observe eye motility during sleep [9]:

> Kleitman had become very interested in what he termed the "basic rest-activity cycle". Being able to read Russian, he was aware of the report of Denisova and Figurin (1926) which described an impressively regular respiratory cycle in infants with a period of 50 minutes . He hypothesized that this short term periodicity ensured that a newborn infant would have frequent opportunities to respond to the stimulus of hunger pangs by waking up and crying, and would therefore get adequate nutrition…
>
> …All of this suggested to Kleitman that eye motility could be the most sensitive measure of the basic rest-activity cycle and also be more representative of changing brain activity, i.e. changing depth of sleep. He then assigned graduate student, Eugene Aserinsky, to observe eye and body motility in infants.

However, the first description that eye movements occur in sleep was reported by de Toni (1933) describing slow rolling eye movements at the onset of sleep which appeared to decrease as sleep continued and presumably deepened [10]. This observation precedes the landmark study that suggested that rapid eye movements represented a "lightening" of sleep and might indicate dreaming, due to the close association with irregular respiration and an increase in heart rate [11].

Before the discovery of REM sleep in 1953, between 1949 and 1952, Aserinsky observed that sleeping infants exhibited a recurring "motility cycle manifested by ocular and gross bodily activity" paralleling the observation of Denisova and Figurin in 1926.

Aserinsky described "periods of motility" (writhing or twitching of the eyelids) and "periods of no motility." The average duration of the periods of quiescence was about 23 min and of the entire motility cycle was approximately 50–60 min. This observation led Aserinsky and Kleitman to look for a similar phenomenon in adults and they discovered REM sleep.

After the description of REM sleep, the French school of Dreyfus-Brisac and Monod [12, 13] begins to study neonates and infants' sleep. Since infants can be easily studied during daytime, Dreyfus-Brisac and Monod attempted to define the specific sleep electroencephalographic (EEG) patterns of infants. N. Monod, invited to the USA by Parmelee, introduced neonatal polygraphic recording to the latter's laboratory and highlighted the need of a full polygraphic investigation including the recording of eye movements, respiration rate, and the electromyogram in addition to the ECG.

At the same time, sleep researchers in Prague described the development of sleep in infancy showing that "quiet" sleep (QS) (regular breathing with frequency of 30/min, closed eyes without movements, disappearance of body movements, spindles, and slow waves in EEG) alternated with "active" sleep (AS) (irregular respiration, eyes alternatively closed, half-open, or there were movements of bulbus oculi, increased frequency of body movements) in about 50–60 min intervals. These authors stated that the most striking changes took place in the first 12 weeks of life [14].

In the following years, Parmelee [15, 16] first showed two distinctive EEG patterns of sleep in infants called "active" sleep (AS) and "quiet" sleep (QS). QS is characterized by preserved chin EMG, few body movements, regular respiration and heart rate, and no eye movements; AS is characterized by rapid eye movements, frequent small face and limb movements, irregular respiration and heart rate, and the absence of or minimal chin EMG activity [17].

The same authors subsequently reported the changes of EEG in infants according to maturation related to conceptional age [18, 19] showing that QS in newborns at term is characterized by one of two EEG patterns: *tracé alternant* or high-voltage slow (HVS) activity:

> Tracé alternant is an EEG pattern in which 3–8 second bursts of moderate to high voltage 0.5–3.0 Hz slow waves intermixed with 2–4 Hz sharply contoured waveforms alternate with 4- to 8-second intervals of attenuated mixed frequency EEG activity; because this pattern alternates between activity and much less activity it is considered to be "discontinuous." In contrast, HVS consists of continuous moderately rhythmic 50–150 μV 0.5–4 Hz slow activity, without the bursting activity of the tracé alternant. HVS represents the more mature pattern of quiet sleep in infants.

Soon after the publication of the standards recommended by Rechtschaffen and Kales for the scoring of sleep stages in adults, it was clear that they were inappropriate for the scoring sleep stages in newborn infants. Therefore, a committee cochaired by Anders, Emde, and Parmelee worked on the definition of criteria for sleep scoring in infants that led to the publication of *A Manual for Standardized Techniques and Criteria for Scoring of States of Sleep and Wakefulness in Newborn Infants* in 1971 [20]. Afterward, Guilleminault and Souquet published a manual on the scoring of sleep and respiration during infancy [21].

In 1970, Dreyfus-Brisac [19] observed that active (REM) sleep could be identified in polygraphic tracings by 32 weeks of gestation because of the presence of frequent body movements, irregular respiration, and rapid eye movements while the eyes were closed.

In 1966 Roffwarg, Muzio, and Dement (1966) firstly described the ontogenesis of sleep states. They also tried to answer the question at what age do humans start having dreams. By observing infants, they confirmed the richness of their rapid eye movements; they therefore supposed that REM sleep was fundamental for the optimal development of the CNS. Roffwarg and colleagues found infants spent half of their total sleep time in REM sleep, leading to the theory that REM sleep must play an important role in the development and maturation of the immature brain [22].

Petre-Quadens in 1970 [23] described for the first time a decrease of REM sleep time and of rapid eye movements in mentally retarded subjects vs. normal children, supporting the hypothesis of the importance of REM sleep for CNS development and learning. This and other observations led the researchers to investigate the relationships between REM sleep and cognition and memory for the next two decades.

Later on, a better definition of the evolution of different physiological parameters during sleep in infants was achieved by Curzi-Dascalova leading to the publication of a manual of methods for recordings and analyzing sleep-wakefulness states in preterm and full-term infants [24].

The difficulties of the definition of scoring rules for infants, children, and adolescents are mainly related to rapid and dynamic changes that occur during the first two decades of life and to the extreme interindividual variability. The comparison of polysomnographic variables needs serial longitudinal assessments linked to the normal progression of maturation, rather than a single polygraphic study at a single point in time [1].

Besides these difficulties, standards for evaluating sleep in older infants, toddlers, children, and preadolescents have been published in the new American Academy of Sleep Medicine (AASM) manual in 2007 [25] in which a specific pediatric task force was appointed. Not clearly in the manual, but in the associated papers published in the Journal of Clinical Sleep Medicine, a critical review and collection of data defined better the features of the sleep structure during development [26]. Finally, a German group headed by Dr. Sabine Scholle published three papers attempting to define the normative polysomnographic data during development [27–29].

The Gradual Discovery of Sleep Disorders in Infants and Children

There are very few reports on the infant and child's sleep in the antiquity. Aristotle's treatises on sleep and dreaming reported only that "Children sleep more than other people" and that "Very young children do not dream at all" or "Children begin to dream from ages 4 or 5" [30].

In the Roman era, the children were not allowed to get much sleep since it was believed that too much sleep decreased intelligence and stunted growth [31].

According to medieval beliefs about beds and sleeping, between 7 and 9 h of sleep were recommended, but this depended upon individual body types; with all people categorized according to the Galenic four humors, too much or too little sleep could cause dangerous imbalances and lead to illness. Nor did children require more sleep: one late fifteenth-century manual suggested 7 h was sufficient. This would roughly equate to summertime daylight hours, with an extra hour in the winter. In the mid-sixteenth century, physician Andrew Boorde was recommending two periods of sleep at night, with people rising briefly between them. Sleepers should lie first on one side and then on the other, in dry rooms to which snails, spiders, rats, and mice had no access [32].

During the Renaissance, children went to bed early, often before sunset. In boarding school, they slept two in a bed until the age of 14 when they were adults and slept alone. Poor children slept at home in the same bed with their siblings or parents. Children's beds were more like a hay pillow in a frame called a crib or they slept on hay mattresses on the floor. After the age of 7, children only slept with siblings of the same sex, a dog or two on cold nights. Even the aristocrat's children shared their bedrooms with their siblings and their servants. Sleeping alone was considered odd, lonely, and sad. Until the industrial era, sharing the bed with infants and children was the norm: families in the lower ranks routinely slept two, three, or more to a mattress, with overnight visitors included to generate welcome warmth and even brought farm animals within sleeping quarters at night. Besides protecting cows, sheep, and other livestock from predators and thieves, boarding with beasts allowed greater warmth, notwithstanding the "nastiness of their excrement" [33].

In the nineteenth century, there was an increasing interest for pediatric medicine, but the first books published devoted no chapters or even paragraphs to sleep. Child-rearing manuals did not deal with sleep as a problem, despite or perhaps because of extensive health advice in other categories. Sleep was not considered as a problem at that time probably because most activities went on during the night and there were much more possibilities to recover sleep during daytime than actually in modern societies. Surely, individual parents faced children with unusual sleep difficulties, but a sense of a larger category of issues did not emerge.

The reasons why people and doctors did not pay much attention to children's sleep can be different: (a) naps were common; (b) sleep patterns were less rigid; (c) many parents undoubtedly used opiates or alcohol to help the child sleep; and (d) the absence of much artificial light reduced nighttime stimulation and facilitated getting children off to bed.

From the late nineteenth century onward, there have been specific changes in sleeping arrangements with babies increasingly placed in cribs at a fairly young age, rather than rocked in cradles as their parents worked or relaxed. The infants and children had to learn to sleep alone as soon as possible.

Recurrent advices in health columns in popular journals dealt primarily with health precautions during sleep, rather than with sleep itself. There was a discussion of how much covering to place on the child, with concern both about overheating and underprotection; it is interesting to read that cold feet were to be avoided: "neglect of this has often resulted in a dangerous attack of croup, diphtheria, or fatal sore throat."

The first generic recommendations and guidelines about infant sleep and expectations with regard to "normal sleep" can be found in the medical books of the nineteenth century (e.g., "newborns don't sleep for more than 2 hours at a time," "children won't sleep through regularly until about 17 months," "by about six months of age, babies could get used to sleeping at specific times of the day and that mothers should not rush to comfort the baby immediately but should instead see if it resettles on its own).

Contrary to what is expected, the recourse to drug treatment was frequent: for children troubled in sleep, the easy access to and wide use of opiates surely reduced the need for extensive expert comment on what to do to fight insomnia. At that time, however, there were recurrent warnings focused on the danger of opiates administered to children with fatal events [34].

Looking at the great debate on the adequate amount of sleep need for children, we could be really surprised in reading that in the nineteenth century, attitudes toward sleep involved surprisingly modest requirements of amount: (a) authorities urging early rising recommended going to bed by 10 pm, but then getting up as soon as the infant was compatible with not feeling sleepy or lethargic the next day; (b) infants, having slept uninterruptedly for 9 months in the womb, should sleep at least 12 h; (c) afternoon naps could be abandoned around 2 years of age; (d) by age 3, children should sleep no more than 12 h, and after this, sleep time should be shortened by 1 h per year; thus a 7-year-old should sleep 8 h and certainly no more than 9; (e) adolescents required less sleep still, and authorities explicitly discussing sleep sometimes advocated no more than 6–7 h for adults [35, 36].

With the advent of the industrial revolution, the artificial light, and the regulation of working and school hours, a disrupted night became a highly disturbing event. Social habits have dramatically changed, and obtaining a healthy night sleep was mandatory for optimal social and work functioning. At the same time, sleep has become more and more consolidated into one single bout per night, and also the possibility of ad hoc naps in children was limited by the new social and school rules.

At the end of nineteenth century, doctors noted the importance of sleep in building up "nerve force" in neurasthenic patients. Hypnotics were particularly recommended for sleepless patients, though drugs were often prescribed in the period as well, coming under more critical scrutiny by physicians only in the 1890s.

Problems of children's insomnia began to receive explicit attention, with recommendations of special feeding. The frequency and fervor of advice against using opiates for children increased; parents who assimilated this warning become more concerned about what other remedies to employ. The first tables with indications of sleep timing and duration begun to be published. The 1910 table, backed by the Bureau of Education, insisted on 13 h of sleep for children 5–6, 12 for those 6–8, 11 for those 10–12, 10 1/2 for those 12–14, 10 for those 14–16, and still 9 1/2 for those up to 18. These recommendations were strikingly different from the approach of the nineteenth century. A 1931 table called for 14–16 h for infants, 13–14 for toddlers, 12–13 still until 8 years of age, and on clown to 9 for 16-year-olds.

It was not until the 1920s that child-rearing manuals picked up the question of children's sleep and doctors dispensed sleep advice and recommend increasing amounts of sleep. Establishing a nighttime routine became important with rituals like daily bathing, story reading, toys, or night lights.

The importance of sleep and naps routine was greatly emphasized in the 1920s and 1930s. The American Medical Association highlighted the significance of a regular sleep schedule and even claimed that a "half-hour variation from this schedule … may induce masturbation, surreptitious reading in bed, restlessness, and inability to concentrate in school."

Children's sleep became a new kind of issue from around the 1920s. Nineteenth-century parents had undoubtedly worried about their charges' sleep, at least in particularly difficult cases.

After 1920, specific advice increased the amount of sleep held to be essential and the explicit scheduling required. Children had been sleeping for hundreds of thousands of years, with considerable apparent success. Why the new fuss, and new directives, early in this century?

An interesting paper tried to answer to these questions [34].

An important contributing factor was the increase of specialists in children that delivered the guidelines for the "correct behavior of infants and children" and were eager to export the findings of science to a parental audience. Further, the major improvements in infant health with the decrease of deaths in childbirth as well as the possibility of a novel arrangement for children's beds determined that infants were increasingly isolated from adults for sleep, placed in their own bedrooms, and early separated not only from parents but also from the nurse. This leads to a decrease of parental controls on infant's sleep behavior with the difficulty to interpret the nighttime behavior (crying, awakenings).

Due to the decrease of the use of opiates, parental concerns about children's sleep increased, and the opiates have been substituted by over-the-counter soporifics that had become the most widely prescribed of all drugs, as of today.

The First Scientific Publications on Sleep in Infants and Children

A specific search in PubMed looking at the first scientific publications on pediatric sleep found some interesting papers that could give us a picture of how sleep in infants and children was considered in the first decades of the last century. In one of these papers, *Sleep Requirements of Children* published in the California State Journal of Medicine in 1921, there were recommendations for the amount of sleep for each age and several statements of common sense that would have been demonstrated scientifically several years later by the literature [37]:

> The Service commends the following precepts just issued by the London County Council: School children aged four years need twelve hours' sleep a day; aged five to seven, eleven to twelve hours; eight to eleven, ten to eleven hours; and twelve to fourteen, nine to ten hours.
>
> Children grow mainly while sleeping or resting; do you want yours to grow up stunted?
>
> Tired children learn badly and often drift to the bottom of the class; do you want yours to grow up stupid?
>
> When children go to bed late their sleep is often disturbed by dreams and they do not get complete rest; do you want yours to sleep badly and become nervous?
>
> Sufficient sleep draws a child onward and upward in school and in home life; insufficient sleep drags it backward and downward. Which way do you want your child to go?
>
> Tiresome children are often only tired children; test the truth of this.

> That a neighbor's child is sent to bed late is not a good reason for sending your child to bed late; two wrongs do not make a right. Going to bed late is a bad habit which may be difficult to cure; persevere till you succeed in curing it.

In a meeting of the British and Canadian Medical Associations, in 1931, Dr. Cameron categorized sleep disturbances as follows: (1) sleeplessness and continuous crying in young infants, (2) sleeplessness in older children, (3) night terrors, and (4) enuresis. He identified three causative factors for sleeplessness in infants: (a) pain (mainly colic or dyspepsia or aerophagy treated with chloral hydrate 10 min before each feed) or discomfort (nasal obstruction treated with few drops of adrenaline solution in the nostrils before the child is put to the breast), (b) inherited or constitutional neuropathy (which resembles the description of neonatal hyperexcitability), and (c) faulty management (which resembles the description of behavioral insomnia of childhood) [38].

Dr. Cameron affirmed that most infants who are sleepless and who cry constantly without any specific pain or discomfort do so because the management is faulty. Dr. Cameron also suggested practices to help crying infants, such as the primitive habit in all countries of putting the crying infant in the swaddling clothes and enveloped in the steady pressure of a light and porous shawl or putting him up against the mother's back (as in the African culture), so that he takes no part in the expression of her emotions, and divulging her thoughts from the child would lead the restless infant to soundly fall asleep. He finally expounded on a theory by which hypoglycemia or the presence of ketone bodies in the blood leads to enuresis, sleepwalking, and night terrors.

In a paper published in 1936 [39], the causes of disturbances of sleep in children had been classified as:

1. *Constitutional neuropathy* that included restless children who did not fall asleep easily and who were easily aroused by even trivial environmental stimuli; this was attributed to a calcium deficiency and treated with calcium.
2. *Sleep disturbances accompanying disease*: in infants painful conditions like otitis media, pain of colic and intestinal disturbances, hunger, teething, and eczema and in older children, renal colic, rheumatic fever, cardiomyopathies, and respiratory difficulties. Preferred treatments were narcotics (codeine very effective) and the barbiturates were given freely, especially when there was considerable restlessness.
3. *Faulty physical and mental hygiene*: disturbed sleep or failure to fall asleep may be due to uncomfortable or too much clothing or emotional disturbances. The author suggested that in infancy, faulty sleeping habits are easily established and difficult to overcome. Overstimulation, as represented by a too ambitious school program, too many extracurricular activities (dancing, music lessons, etc.), premature and untimely participation in social affairs and pleasures of the adult, unsuitable movies, and radio programs, is not conducive to restful sleep.
4. *Temperatures on the child*: the high temperature would determine a tremendous increase of the child's motor activity.

5. *Heavy meals*: a heavy meal at night is prone to cause not only excessive motor
   activity but terrifying dreams, crying out in sleep, and a constant turning in bed.

The famous pediatrician Benjamin Spock, in the late 1940s, made recommendations that have been greatly influential throughout the next several decades. The
advices for getting the baby to sleep were "The cure is simple: Put the baby to bed
at a reasonable hour. Say goodnight affectionately but firmly, walk out of the room,
and don't go back…" [40].

In a following paper in pediatrics [41], Spock stated that chronic resistance to
sleep in infancy is a behavior problem which was formerly rare but was becoming
more frequent, and its frequency seems related to the trend toward self-regulation to
babies and to confusion in how to apply this philosophy. The treatment of sleep
problem in the baby less than 1 year of age with the crying out method showed that
most of these babies would cry indignantly from 10 to 20 min the first night and
perhaps 5–10 min the second night, but a great majority of them would be cured of
sleep disturbance within two nights. Spock emphasized that this policy of letting the
baby "cry it out" is recommended only for chronic resistance to sleep in the infant
up to the age of 1 or 1.5 years.

In 1949, an interesting paper analyzed for the first time sleep disturbances in 100
children (5–14 years old) with primary behavior and emotional disorders at Rockland
State Hospital, Children's Group. Sleep disorders were grouped into five categories:

- 1. Restlessness and minor disturbed states of sleep were found in 46 cases,
  divided into two subgroups: (a) restlessness such as rolling, rocking, tossing, and
  jerky movements and (b) talking, mumbling, crying, and swearing.
- 2. Nightmares were found in seven cases.
- 3. Night terrors in two cases.
- 4. Sleep walking in one case.
- 5. Enuresis in 26 cases.

The most frequent disorders were restlessness and minor disturbed states of
sleep and enuresis that apparently occurred frequently in rejected children, while
nightmares, night terrors, and sleep walking were relatively infrequent [42].

Kleitman in a paper entitled "Mental hygiene of sleep in children" [43] described
perfectly for the first time the features of behavioral insomnia of childhood stating
that "the child is born with certain capacities for learning, including the ability to
synchronize, with ease or difficulty, the primitive sleep-wakefulness cycle with
diurnal periodicity in his physical and social environment. To establish good sleep
habits in children it is necessary to cooperate with the natural tendency to develop a
persistent 24-hour rhythm, reinforcing the latter by the customary methods of conditioning." Moreover, he acknowledged the individual variability for the need of
sleep and warned about the recommendations on the amount of sleep needed for the
infants and children. He affirmed that "the total time spent in sleep, out of each
diurnal period, decreases with age, but not uniformly in all children nor in a particular child at different ages. Tables of hours of sleep provided as a guide to parents are
misleading in that the figures suggested for all ages are arbitrarily high. Even if

more realistic, such figures could stand only for averages, which, by and large, are meaningless when the individual child is considered."

During the period 1950–1970, the literature on sleep problems in children increased steadily. Ronald Illingworth published several papers attempting to categorize sleep disturbances in infants and children [44, 45].

Concluding one paper on sleep problems in the first 3 years of age, he indicated the difficulties in treating sleep problems reporting that it is not sufficient to instruct on sleep hygiene rules or to give a drug and finally acknowledged the complexities of the treatment of sleep problems.

In the 1966 paper [45], Illingworth summarized the causes of sleep problems in children as follows:

1. Problems Related to Parents.
2. Habit Formation
3. The Child's Ego and Negativism
4. Sleep Needs.
5. Developmental Patterns.
6. The Child's Love for His Parents.
7. Causes of awakenings
8. Errors Concerning Bedtime
9. Other Emotional Factors
10 Unknown Causes

The treatment of sleep problems at that time was based on common sense and on the beliefs of a single pediatrician. Illingworth suggested that it is wrong to pick a child up at the first whimper but also that it is essential to go immediately to his room when a child wakens with a sudden scream because at these times it would be not only cruel but possibly dangerous not to go to him. He stated that drugs have little place in sleep problems and phenobarbital is useless with these children and suggests chloral hydrate given 0.5 h before bedtime as the best drug for this problem. Finally, he reported that, in some cases, unfortunately, the parents should accept the early morning awakenings as one of the penalties of having children.

In the 1950–1960s, different studies attempted to define the normative parameters of sleep in children as well as the frequency of sleep disturbances. A paper analyzed the frequency of night awakenings in 1957, finding a prevalence of 17 % at 6 months and 10 % at 12 months [46]. In a longitudinal study, Klackenberg in 1968 defined the sleep behavior of children up to 3 years of age [47].

The New Era of Pediatric Sleep: Contribution by Researchers from Different Countries

There is no doubt that pediatric sleep medicine received a strong initial input from European researchers 50 years ago. In France, Belgium, Italy, and Germany, researchers begun to publish on the early development of the sleep cycle, sleep EEG, and sleep behavior in infants [48].

The French group (Dreyfus-Brisac, Monod, Curzi-Dascalova) worked on the definition of the features of the sleep EEG and respiratory and cardiovascular parameters in newborns and infants. The studies by the Italian group of Salzarulo and Fagioli shed light on sleep organization and sleep states during development. The French researchers also contributed to the characterization of sleep apnea, parasomnias, and narcolepsy (Marie Jo Challamel) together with Sona Nevsimalova, from Prague (Czech Republic). In Belgium, André Kahn and his group (Patricia Franco and José Groswasser) made important advancements in clarifying the mechanisms of the sudden infant death syndrome (SIDS) and infant sleep apnea.

Thanks to André Kahn, in the 1990's a medial campaign was launched about infant's sleeping position ("back is best"), and therefore, the SIDS risk was greatly diminished.

In Germany, Prechtl described sleep patterns before and after birth, emphasizing the concept of "state"; other German groups made a big effort to characterize the features of sleep EEG during development (Schölle), as well as the characterization of infant sleep apnea (Poets). In the UK, Stores investigated mainly sleep in children with mental retardation; other sleep researchers were also involved in the research in pediatric sleep (Wiggs, Gringras, Hill, Fleming, and others).

Halasz from Hungary published several papers on the neurophysiology of sleep and on the relationship between sleep and epilepsy in children.

Another group of Italian researchers (Bergonzi, Gigli, and Ferri) started to explore sleep neuro- and psychophysiology in children with mental retardation, in an international collaboration with Grubar in France and Petre-Quadens in Belgium.

The first specific sleep questionnaires have been published in the last 1990s: the Sleep Disturbance Scale for Children by Oliviero Bruni [49], the Child Sleep Habits Questionnaire by Judith Owens [50], the Pediatric Sleep Questionnaire by Ronald Chervin [51], and several others.

In Italy, Oliviero Bruni and his group, in strict collaboration with Raffaele Ferri, made a great effort to advance the definition of sleep microstructure in children, characterizing the alterations of the cyclic alternating pattern in normal children and in those with neurodevelopmental disabilities. Giannotti and Cortesi explored the sleep habits in adolescents and the sleep problems in children with neurodevelopmental disabilities such as autism and epilepsy. In Sicily, Silvestri has contributed to the definition of sleep disorders in children with ADHD. Contributions on sleep apnea in children and on the treatment with orthodontic apparels have been reported by the group of Maria Pia Villa. In Spain an enthusiastic group of researchers gave a big contribution in the different fields of pediatric sleep. Among them, Rosa Peraita-Adrados, co-founder of the Iberian Association of Sleep Pathology and research fellow at the Stanford University, made contributions on infants' sleep and neurological disorders and was editor of a Book "Trastornos de Sueño en la Infancia" (1992), with an important dissemination in the Spanish speaking community worldwide. Eduard Estivill was a pioneer for treatment of pediatric insomnia; Teresa Sagales made contributions on epidemiology and pediatric neurology; Gonzalo Pin Arboledas as well as many other Spanish researchers on consensus documents for common pediatric sleep disorders.

In Israel, following the input by Peretz Lavie, Avi Sadeh studied how to investigate sleep in infants objectively and less invading and developed the actigraph and characterized the algorithm for scoring actigraphic recordings in infants and children. Further, his studies on normative sleep data in children and on the relationships between sleep and academic achievement made a great advancement in the pediatric sleep field.

In the USA, Richard Ferber, from the Children's Hospital of Boston, was the first to publish a comprehensive book for treating behavioral insomnia in infants and children which had an enormous success, so that the acronym "ferberize the child" is currently used to indicate the application of the behavioral techniques to solve insomnia of infants and children.

At the University of California, Los Angeles, a child psychiatrist, Thomas Anders (coauthor of the manual for sleep scoring in infants together with Emde and Parmalee) focused his research on ontogenesis of sleep-wake states from infancy through early childhood and on sleep disorders in children with autism and other neurodevelopmental disorders. He classified infants as self-soothers or signalers, depending upon whether they cry following a nighttime awakening or whether they put themselves back to sleep without signaling to their parents.

Christian Guilleminault at Stanford University is the researcher who established the branch of sleep medicine in childhood; he can be considered as a pioneer of pediatric sleep medicine, and there is no branch of pediatric sleep medicine to which he has not contributed.

Mary Carskadon started her career at the Stanford University and, along with Dr. William Dement, she developed the Multiple Sleep Latency Test. Her research on adolescent sleep-wake behavior and consequences of insufficient sleep in adolescents raised public health issues and determined some changes in the public policy, such as a later school start time in secondary schools.

Another huge contributor to the field of pediatric sleep is David Gozal with fundamental researches in the last 20 years that have revolutionized the studies on sleep apnea in children. He studied, in particular, the relationships between respiratory sleep disorders and neurobehavioral, cardiovascular, and metabolic diseases and the mechanisms that mediate defense responses that lead to complications from low oxygen levels, disrupted sleep, and long-term health and developmental consequences of chronic sleep and breathing problems during childhood.

Carole Marcus' studies shed light on diagnosis and management of childhood OSAS and on the use of positive airway pressure therapy in children heading the publication of several clinical practice guidelines on OSAS.

In the field of insomnia in childhood, Judith Owens made significant contributions on the pharmacologic treatment of sleep disorders in children and on the interaction between sleep and ADHD, as well as on the impact of delaying school start time on adolescent sleep, mood, and behavior. Jodi Mindell, a clinical psychologist specializing in pediatric sleep medicine, has published many papers on the treatment of behavioral insomnia in childhood, on pharmacologic treatment of pediatric sleep disorders, on cultural issues impacting sleep, and on the cultural differences in sleep patterns and behaviors.

Ronald Chervin made several important contributions on neurological and behavioral effects of sleep disorders; his studies highlighted the importance of disrupted sleep and described an association between inattentive, hyperactive behavior and symptoms of two primary sleep disorders: OSAS and RLS.

In Canada, Brouillette, over the past 30 years, made major contributions to the understanding of childhood OSAS and other controls of breathing disorders; he also developed a specific scale to assess the clinical severity of OSAS and evaluated the utility of oximetry for the diagnosis of OSAS in children.

More recently, Gruber, from McGill University in Montreal, showed the importance of an adequate sleep duration for optimal functioning in children, demonstrating that even a small sleep deprivation has serious consequences for health and daytime functioning in normal and ADHD children.

Pediatric sleep researchers in Australia in the last years (Horne, Blunden, Matricciani, Olds, Lushington, Kennedy, Kohler, Gradisar, and others) have produced significant and important papers on the cardiovascular control during sleep in neonates and children, on the declining trend of sleep duration in children and adolescents, on cognitive functioning in normal children and in children and infants with sleep-disordered breathing, on the behavioral treatment of sleep disorders in children, and on the impact of technology in adolescents' sleep.

South America, Brazil, and Chile had several prolific researchers: in Chile, Peirano and Algarin conducted several studies on the effect of iron deficiency anemia on sleep in children; in Brazil, several researchers such as Tufik, Lahorgue-Nuñes, Lopes, and Alvés also made substantial contributions.

In Japan, Segawa, in collaboration with Nomura, after the discovery of dopamine-responsive dystonia, explored the body movements during sleep in infancy as indicators for the detection of normal or abnormal CNS development. At the same time, Okawa defined the disorders of the circadian rhythm in brain-damaged children, while other sleep researchers such as Kohyama, Komada, Kato, and many others continued to work in the pediatric sleep medicine field.

Many Asian countries are actually growing in the pediatric sleep medicine field, as acknowledged by the increasing number of publications especially from China, Hong Kong, Taiwan, Singapore, and Thailand, and probably new insights and new developments from other developing countries should be expected [48].

The Establishment of the Pediatric Sleep Associations

The rise of pediatric sleep medicine as a specific field was not an easy process. The marginal place in the sleep congresses in the 1970s was clear too strict for this emerging area, linked to the evidence that most of the adult sleep disorders begin in childhood or even in infancy with specific age-related clinical expressions. Therefore, it was immediately evident that a specific "pediatric sleep knowledge" would have been required in order to identify and treat correctly the different sleep disorders of infants and children. Starting with small symposia or satellite meetings during the congresses of the main sleep adult societies like the European Sleep Research Society (ESRS) and the Associated Professional Sleep Societies (APSS), the exponential and huge growth of contributions by pediatric sleep researchers rise the exigency to develop independent pediatric sleep associations.

The European Pediatric Sleep Club

Pediatric sleep medicine in Europe started within the ESRS and paralleled the development of this society. In the late 1980s, a group of pediatricians, child neurologists, psychiatrists, and psychologists interested in sleep during development began to join in informal meetings during the early ESRS congresses. They were represented by most eminent sleep researchers that made the history of pediatric sleep medicine: Dreyfus-Brisac, Monod, Curzi-Dascalova, Dittrichova, Mirmiran, Prechtl, Salzarulo, Fagioli, and Kahn worked together to start the European research of infant sleep. Other researchers joined this initial group like Navelet, Challamel, Guilleminault, Vecchierini, Gaultier, Stores, Peraita-Adrados, Nevsimalova, Katz Salomon, Poets, and many other scientists. After the preliminary informal meetings, this group of scientists subsequently constituted the European Pediatric Sleep Club (EPSC) as a part of the ESRS, aimed at consolidating the area of pediatric sleep medicine, with the goal to bring together clinicians and researchers from different disciplines. The EPSC had its own meeting every year since the first one in 1991 in Paris and joins the ESRS Congress every 2 years.

The EPSC meetings were held in Paris (1991), Helsinki (1992), Prague (1993), Firenze (1994), Messina (1995), Brussels (1996), Lyon (1997), Madrid (1998), Dresden (1999), Istanbul (2000), Bled (2001), Reykjavik (2002), Rome (2003), and Prague (2004). Following the efforts by André Kahn, the International Pediatric Sleep Association (IPSA) blossomed in 2005 from the EPSC.

The Pediatric Sleep Medicine Conference

The inaugural Pediatric Sleep Medicine Conference was held in Amelia Island, Florida, in February 2005. The meeting was cofounded by Jodi Mindell and Judith Owens, with the objective of bringing together pediatric sleep experts from around the world to share sleep science. The meeting also sought to define priorities for basic and clinical research, patient care, and public policy for the emerging field of pediatric sleep medicine. The conferences included pediatricians, pulmonologists, psychologists, psychiatrists, and neurologists, as well as social workers and nurses. The meeting was held yearly until 2009, at which time it became a biannual meeting offset by biannual meetings of the IPSA. The meeting continues to be held in Amelia Island, Florida, and now includes courses on best practices in pediatric sleep medicine and pediatric polysomnography.

The International Pediatric Sleep Association

The story of IPSA is strictly linked to the EPSC, as mentioned above. The creation of this international association was the dream of André Kahn and was initiated in 2003 by his efforts and by his dedication to the field of pediatric sleep medicine. The author of this chapter has been involved in this project by Dr. Kahn and was honored to work with him. Unfortunately, shortly before his 61st birthday, André Kahn abruptly died on September 1, 2004, in Brussels, at the end of his usual karate training session. Despite his absence, but following his inspiration, during the last EPSC meeting in 2004 in Prague, it was decided to build up a new international association. It was not an easy step, since there were long debates about the nature of this association which was initially intended as a "clinically oriented" organization. Also there were other uncertainties about the lack of the strength and the power to build this association and several uncertainties about scientific and financial support.

However, the following year, during the World Association of Sleep Medicine (WASM) meeting in Berlin, the IPSA was founded on October 13, 2005, with the crucial contribution of Christian Guilleminault. The bylaws were created stating the mission of IPSA: (a) to promote basic and applied research in all areas of sleep in infants, children, and adolescents, (b) to provide topical information to the public about pediatric sleep, (c) to increase the knowledge of pediatric sleep problems and their consequences, (d) to promote teaching programs on pediatric sleep, (e) to hold scientific meetings, and (f) to provide information to the public about perspectives and applications of pediatric sleep research.

The first board was elected and appointed in 2007, with the aim to represent nearly all the countries in the world in which pediatric sleep medicine was pursued, for a 4-year term, consisting of Oliviero Bruni as president, Christian Guilleminault as vice-president, and Patricia Franco as secretary. The Board of Directors comprised Ronald Chervin, David Gozal, Avi Sadeh, Patricio Peirano, Magda Lahorgue-Nuñes, Rosemary Horne, and Daniel Ng.

In 2007, IPSA has been affiliated with the Elsevier's journal *Sleep Medicine*, an affiliate of the World Association of Sleep Medicine (WASM), and in 2009, it joined the Pediatric Sleep Medicine Conference.

From 2007 to 2009, IPSA meetings were held as part of the WASM congresses, but in 2010 the first independent IPSA congress was organized by Oliviero Bruni in Rome. The congress was a huge success in terms of participants and high scientific quality, with 203 abstracts, 64 symposia, 1 pediatric sleep course, 1 keynote lecture, and 34 countries represented worldwide.

After this successful meeting, it was decided to continue to have an IPSA meeting every 2 years in different parts of the world. The second IPSA meeting was held in Manchester (UK) in December 2012, and the third IPSA meeting was held in Porto Alegre (Brazil) in 2014. The next meetings will be in Taiwan in 2016 and in Lille (France) in 2018.

The IPSA congresses aim to lead to a substantial advancement of pediatric sleep medicine, collecting the most renowned international speakers and giving to all participants the opportunity to share knowledge in sleep medicine and research.

In 2012, with the help of Allan O'Bryan (WASM), the IPSA Foundation (a non-profit organization) has been created to raise funds from different sources, such as industries and pharmaceutical companies, in order to allow fund-raising for scientific and charity purposes.

Conclusions

The historical overviews always have limitations, and also this representation of the birth of pediatric sleep medicine as an independent field probably has forgotten to cite some fundamental researchers. The aim was to delineate the emergence of pediatric sleep depicting the progressive awareness on sleep of infants, children, and adolescents.

A huge amount of studies in the last decades have demonstrated that almost all sleep disorders have a negative impact on the child health.

The field of pediatric sleep medicine is currently growing in the different countries with huge possibilities of expansion. Innovative researches will highlight the role of sleep in brain plasticity and in integrating neural networks required for early brain development. Further, new studies will lead to a better knowledge of the development of sleep and of the effects of sleep disruption on behavioral disorders, problems of attention, and learning disabilities.

References

1. Sheldon SH. History of pediatric sleep medicine. In: Sheldon SH, Kryger MH, Ferber R, Gozal D, editors. Principles and practice of pediatric sleep medicine. 2nd ed. London: Elsevier Saunders; 2014. p. 13–16.
2. Ferber R. Solve your child's sleep problems. New York: Simon & Schuster; 1985.
3. Guilleminault C. Sleep and its disorders in children. New York: Raven; 1987.
4. Sheldon SH, Spire JP, Levy HB. Pediatric sleep medicine. Philadelphia: WB Saunders; 1992. p. 185–240.
5. Ferber R, Kryger MH. Principles and practice of sleep medicine in the child. Philadelphia: Saunders; 1995.
6. Sheldon SH, Ferber R, Kryger MH. Principles and practice of pediatric sleep medicine. Amsterdam: Elsevier; 2005.
7. Sheldon SH, Ferber R, Kryger MH, Gozal D, editors. Principles and practice of pediatric sleep medicine. 2nd ed. London: Elsevier Saunders; 2014.
8. Denisova MP, Figurin NL. Periodic phenomena in the sleep of children. Nov Refl Fiziol Nerv Syst. 1926;2:338–45.
9. Dement WE. Remembering Nathaniel Kleitman. Arch Ital Biol. 2001;13(9):11–7.

10. De Toni G. I movimenti pendolari dei bulbi oculari dei bambini durante il sonno fisiologico, ed in alcuni stati morbosi. Pediatria. 1933;41:489–98.
11. Aserinsky E, Kleitman N. Regularly occurring periods of eye motility, and concomitant phenomena, during sleep. Science. 1953;118(3062):273–4.
12. Dreyfus-Brisac C, Fischgold H, Samson-Dollfus D, et al. Veille, sommeil et réactivité sensorielle chez le prématuré, le nouveauné et le nourisson. Clin Neurophysiol 1957;Suppl 6:417–40.
13. Monod N, Pajot N. The sleep of the full-term newborn and premature infant. I. Analysis of the polygraphic study (rapid eye movements, respiration and E.E.G.) in the full-term newborn. Biol Neonat. 1965;8:281–307.
14. Dittrichová J. Development of sleep in infancy. J Appl Physiol. 1966;21:1243–6.
15. Parmelee Jr AH, Schulte FJ, Akiyama Y, et al. Maturation of EEG activity during sleep in premature infants. Electroencephalogr Clin Neurophysiol. 1968;24:319–29.
16. Parmelee Jr A, Akiyama Y, Stern E, et al. A periodic cerebral rhythm in newborn infants. Exp Neurol. 1969;35:575.
17. André M, Lamblin MD, d'Allest AM, Curzi-Dascalova L, Moussalli-Salefranque F, Nguyen The Tich S, et al. Electroencephalography in premature and full-term infants. Developmental features and glossary. Neurophysiol Clin. 2010;40:59–124.
18. Parmelee AH, Stern E. Development of states in infants. In: Clemente CD, Purpura DP, Mayer FE, editors. Sleep and the maturing nervous system. New York: Academic; 1972. p. 199–215.
19. Dreyfus-Brisac C. Ontogenesis of sleep in human prematures after 32 weeks of conceptional age. Dev Psychobiol. 1970;3:91–121.
20. Anders TF, Emde R, Parmelee AH, eds. A manual of standardized terminology, techniques and criteria for scoring of states of sleep and wakefulness in newborn infants. UCLA Brain Information Service, NINDS Neurological Information Network, Los Angeles; 1971.
21. Guilleminault C, Souquet M. Sleep states and related pathology. In: Guilleminault C, Korobkin R, editors. Advances in neonatal neurology. 1st ed. New York: Spectrum Publications; 1979. p. 225–47.
22. Roffwarg HP, Muzio JN, Dement WC. Ontogenetic development of the human sleep-dream cycle. Science. 1966;152(3722):604–19.
23. Petre-Quadens O, De Lee C. Eye-movements during sleep: a common criterion of learning capacities and endocrine activity. Dev Med Child Neurol. 1970;12:730–40.
24. Curzi-Dascalova L, Mirmiran M. Manual of methods for recordings and analyzing sleep-wakefullness states in preterm and full-term infant. Les Editions INSERM; 1996.
25. Iber C, Ancoli-Israel S, Chesson AL, et al. The AASM manual for the scoring of sleep and associated events: rules, terminology, and technical specifications. 1st ed. Westchester: American Academy of Sleep Medicine; 2007.
26. Grigg-Damberger M, Gozal D, Marcus CL, et al. The visual scoring of sleep and arousal in infants and children. J Clin Sleep Med. 2007;3:201–40.
27. Scholle S, Beyer U, Bernhard M, Eichholz S, Erler T, Graness P, Goldmann-Schnalke B, Heisch K, Kirchhoff F, Klementz K, Koch G, Kramer A, Schmidtlein C, Schneider B, Walther B, Wiater A, Scholle HC. Normative values of polysomnographic parameters in childhood and adolescence: quantitative sleep parameters. Sleep Med. 2011;12(6):542–9.
28. Scholle S, Wiater A, Scholle HC. Normative values of polysomnographic parameters in childhood and adolescence: cardiorespiratory parameters. Sleep Med. 2011;12(10):988–96.
29. Scholle S, Wiater A, Scholle HC. Normative values of polysomnographic parameters in childhood and adolescence: arousal events. Sleep Med. 2012;13(3):243–51.
30. van der Eijk PJ. Medicine and philosophy in classical antiquity: Doctors and Philosophers on nature, soul, health and disease. Cambridge: Cambridge University Press; 2005.
31. Aldrete GS. Daily life in the Roman City: Rome. Pompeii: Greenwood Publishing Group; 2004.
32. License A. Sleep tight! Going to bed in Medieval and Tudor England. http://authorherstorian-parent.blogspot.it/2012/10/sleep-tight-going-to-bed-in-medieval.html.

33. Ekirch's R. Sleep we have lost: pre-industrial sleep in the British Isles. Am Hist Rev. 2001;106(2):343–86.
34. Stearns PN, Rowland P, Giarnella L. Children's sleep: sketching historical change. J Soc Hist. 1996;30:345–66.
35. Godey's Lady's Book. Hints about health: sleepless nights. (Dec 1865): 448.
36. Godey's Lady's Book. Health department: early rising. (Mar 1875): 285.
37. No Authors Listed. Sleep requirements of children. Cal State J Med. 1921;19:418.
38. Cameron HC. Sleep and its disorders in childhood. Can Med Assoc J. 1931;2(4):239–44.
39. No Authors Listed. Disorders of sleep in children. Cal West Med. 1936;45:65–8.
40. Spock B. The common sense book of baby and child care. New York: Duell, Sloan and Pearce; 1946.
41. Spock B. Chronic resistance to sleep in infancy. Pediatrics. 1949;4:89–93.
42. Clardy ER, Hill BC. Sleep disorders in institutionalized disturbed children and delinquent boys. Nerv Child. 1949;8:50–3.
43. Kleitman N. Mental hygiene of sleep in children. Nerv Child. 1949;8:63–6.
44. Illingworth RS. Sleep problems in the first three years. BMJ. 1951;1(4709):722–8.
45. Illingworth RS. Sleep problems of children. Clin Pediatr. 1966;5:45–8.
46. Moore T, Ucko LE. Night waking in early infancy. Arch Dis Child. 1957;32:333.
47. Klackenberg G. The development of children in a Swedish urban community. A prospective longitudinal study. VI. The sleep behaviour of children up to three years of age. Acta Paediatr Scand Suppl. 1968;187:105–21.
48. Bruni O, Ferri R. The emergence of pediatric sleep medicine. In: Chokroverty S, Billiard M, editors. Sleep medicine: a comprehensive guide to its development, clinical milestones and advances in treatment. New York: Springer; 2015. p. 473–86.
49. Bruni O, Ottaviano S, Guidetti V, et al. The Sleep Disturbance Scale for Children (SDSC). Construction and validation of an instrument to evaluate sleep disturbances in childhood and adolescence. J Sleep Res. 1996;5:251–61.
50. Owens JA, Spirito A, McGuinn M. The Children's Sleep Habits Questionnaire (CSHQ): psychometric properties of a survey instrument for school-aged children. Sleep. 2000;23(8):1043–51.
51. Chervin RD, Hedger K, Dillon JE, Pituch KJ. Pediatric sleep questionnaire (PSQ): validity and reliability of scales for sleep-disordered breathing, snoring, sleepiness, and behavioral problems. Sleep Med. 2000;1(1):21–32.

Chapter 3
Epidemiology of Sleep Disorders in Children and Adolescents

Teresa Paiva

Abstract Epidemiologic analysis of sleep disorders (SDs) in children and adolescents faces several difficulties. There is a marked interindividual variability during the first years of life, which is more relevant in the first 2 years, and consequently the definition of what is "normal" can become a difficult issue to which cultural and ethnic differences might add clear complexity. Furthermore many available survey lack objective data; this issue is particularly relevant whenever data are provided by the caregivers, since known discrepancies do exist between children and caregivers information, and the fact that data obtained from younger individual are subjected to important ethical regulations is likely to reduce the number of available studies. Other contributing issues are the position of pediatric sleep in the field of sleep medicine and the successive classifications of sleep disorders and the methodologic modifications, rendering difficult comparisons across decades.

In spite of all difficulties, robust data are essential both to understand disease mechanisms, comorbidities, and treatments and to plan strategic and healthcare plans.

Keyword Epidemiology • Sleep disorders • Children • Adolescents • Insomnia • Hypersomnia • Sleep-related breathing disorders • Sleep-related movement disorders • Parasomnias • Circadian disorders

Epidemiologic analysis of sleep disorders (SDs) in children and adolescents faces several difficulties. There is a marked interindividual variability during the first years of life, which is more relevant in the first 2 years, and consequently the definition of what is "normal" can become a difficult issue to which cultural and ethnic differences might add clear complexity. Furthermore many available studies are based in qualitative survey and lack objective data; this issue is particularly relevant whenever data are provided by the caregivers, since known discrepancies do exist between children and caregivers information, and the fact that data obtained from

T. Paiva, MD, PhD
CENC, Sleep Medicine Center, Rua Conde das Antas 5, Lisbon 1070-068, Portugal
e-mail: teresapaiva0@gmail.com

© Springer International Publishing Switzerland 2017
S. Nevšímalová, O. Bruni (eds.), *Sleep Disorders in Children*,
DOI 10.1007/978-3-319-28640-2_3

younger individual are subjected to important ethical regulations is likely to reduce the number of available studies. Other contributing issues are the position of pediatric sleep in the field of sleep medicine and the successive classifications of sleep disorders and the methodologic modifications, rendering difficult comparisons across decades.

In spite of all difficulties, robust data are essential both to understand diseases mechanisms, comorbidities, and treatments and to plan strategic and healthcare plans.

In what concerns pediatric sleep disorders (PSDs), three aspects must be taken into account: one is the dimension of the problem itself, and the other is the already available knowledge of long-term effects of infancy, childhood, and adolescence disturbances and finally the impact of family behavior upon children sleep.

This is illustrated in the following examples:

- The global percentage of sleep problems and sleep complaints in children and adolescents is very high, reaching 80 % in some world regions [1].
- Sleep problems of the newborn predict sleep problems in school age [2].
- Persistent sleep difficulties in childhood predict psychiatric problems in adult life [3].
- Caregivers' behaviors at sleep onset predict sleep patterns in babies and toddlers [4].
- Parents' sleep-wake patterns predict their children sleep-wake profile [5].
- Parents stress is associated with behavioral problems in insomniac children [6].
- Sleep deprivation and irregular sleep habits increase the risk of health complaints and health and mental disorders, together with the risk of falls and domestic accidents and poor academic performance [7].
- Most medical, neurologic, and psychiatric disorders in children are associated with an increased risk of SD [7].

The subsequent text presents the prevalence of the pediatric SD according to the ICSD2 [8]: insomnias, hypersomnias of central origin, sleep-related breathing disorders (SRBDs), parasomnias, sleep-related movement disorders (SRMDs), and circadian disorders. Furthermore, epidemiologic data concerning comorbidities and prevalence data of the different SDs in other pathologies will also be discussed.

Insomnia

In toddlers and preschoolers, insomnias express themselves either as "sleep-onset association or night wakings" or "insufficient limits and sleep resistance," and with age progression chronic insomnia develops.

- Sleep-onset association type or night wakings
  It is present in 25–50 % between 6 and 12 months, in 30 % with 1 year, and in 15–20 % between 1 and 3 years of age.
  The risk factors are co-bedding, breastfeeding, colic, medical disorders, bad temper, parent anxiety, and maternal depression.

Table 3.1 Insomnia in adolescents

Authors	N	Age	Country	Prevalence	PSG	Gender differences
Roberts et al. (2008) [9]	4175	11–17	USA	26.8% wave 2 W1 –26.48 5.08% W2 W1 –6.55	No	
Siomos et al. (2009) [10]	2195	13–18	Greece	11.43%	No	No
Zhang et al. (2009) [11]	5695	6–13	Hong Kong	4% preceding year	No	No
Pan et al. (2012) [12]	816	12–18	Guangdong	22.9	No	
	618		Macao	16.5	No	
Amaral et al. (2013) [13]	6919	12–18	Portugal	Symptoms of insomnia – 21.4 Insomnia – 8.3	No	Yes
Calhoun et al. (2014) [14]	700	5–12	USA	19.3%	Yes	Yes Girls from 11–12: 30.6%

- Limit-setting type or bed resistance.
  They occur in 10–30% of the children.
  The risk factors are parents' permissiveness, parental conflicts concerning child education, unrealistic parents' expectations, age, bad temper, daytime-opposing behaviors, unstable domestic or family environment, and errors in circadian organization.
- Insomnia in school children and adolescents occurs in 9–13% of the adolescents (see Table 3.1).
  The risk factors are sleep hygiene errors, sleep perception difficulties, errors concerning knowledge about sleep, personality characteristics, medical disorders, health perception and somatic complaints [9], psychiatric problems (insomnia occurs in 53.5% of depressive adolescents [15], psychologic problems [9, 10], female gender after puberty, familial history of insomnia, low socioeconomic status, tobacco and alcohol consumption, TV in the room, insufficient communication with the parents [11, 16, 17], and excessive Internet use [10].

Hypersomnias of Central Origin

Narcolepsy and Kleine-Levin syndrome start/occur during the first two decades. The Kleine-Levin syndrome is a rare disorder with unknown prevalence.

The prevalence of narcolepsy is also low but it is increasing in the last decades. Narcolepsy affects 3–16 in 10,000 children/adolescents, and the prevalence of narcolepsy with cataplexy is still lower 0.2–0.5 per 10,000; in Japan the prevalence is six times higher.

Narcolepsy is currently considered an autoimmune disorder; the prevalence of autoimmune disorders, exception made for celiac disease, is rare among children. However, the narcolepsy prevalence, for not clarified reasons, is increasing in the last decade. A clear risk factor was the vaccination against H1N1 flu virus with Pandemrix, due to the adjuvant used (AS03) [18], with described cases in China [19], Sweden, Finland, Norway [20], and Portugal. During the 6 months following the winter vaccination, there was a significant increase of the narcolepsy prevalence (13 times higher), mostly among children.

In China, even without vaccination, there was a significant increase of the narcolepsy prevalence during March, April, and May, suggesting a seasonal fluctuation and the winter viral infections as risk factors; these fluctuations are superimposed in a positive trend of increased prevalence across the years [19].

HLA-DQB1 *06:02 positivity is a risk factor for narcolepsy. Recently, in a multicenter study, an association between narcolepsy and allergic diseases has been observed but there are differences between patients with and without cataplexy since the frequency of allergic conditions, particularly asthma and allergic rhinitis, was markedly lower in narcolepsy with cataplexy (58/275) when compared with patients without cataplexy (94/193; $P < 0.0001$) [21].

Sleep-Related Breathing Disorders

The prevalence of primary snoring is 8 %; it varies with ethnicity and age, but it can be present since birth and it may occur in premature infants.

Snoring prevalence studies in children are usually based in parents/caregivers reports and lack objective confirmation.

The snoring prevalence has been evaluated in several studies in infants, toddlers, and schoolchildren [22–26]; the prevalence of "habitual snoring" varies enormously between 3.2 % and 34.6 % of the children, although for most studies the prevalence varies between 3 % and 10 % [22–26]; the prevalence is higher in Italy [27] and in the USA [28] (see Table 3.2).

Among Asian countries there are regional differences, with higher snoring prevalence in the first years of life in Australia, New Zealand, and the Philippines [26].

The prevalence of "habitual snoring" among schoolers and adolescents varies between 3.3 % and 15.1 % [23, 29–32] (see Table 3.3).

The OSAS prevalence is lower than snoring prevalence and varies between 0.69 % and 4.7 % [29, 32]; in most studies there are no gender differences (see Table 3.4). It is relevant since birth and it assumes special relevance in premature children [39]. The association with asthma has been proven in large epidemiologic studies and systematic reviews [40, 41].

The risk factors of SRBD are:

- Upper airway obstruction, namely, adenotonsillar hypertrophy; improper diagnosis of OSAS before adenotonsillectomy (the prevalence of OSAS raises to 38%) [32, 42]; allergies [41]; craniofacial abnormalities, namely, Pierre Robin

Table 3.2 Prevalence of snoring in infants, toddlers, and preschoolers

Authors	N	Age	Country	% snoring
Gislason et al. (1995) [22]	454	6 months–6 years	Iceland	3.2 – habitual
Brunetti et al. (2001) [23]	895	3–11 years	Italy	4.9 – habitual
Castronovo et al. (2003) [27]	604	3–6 years	Italy	34.6 – habitual 12.0 – pathological?
Montgomery Downs et al. (2003) [28]	1010	3–5.3 years	USA	22 – habitual
Montgomery Downs et al. (2006) [24]	944	2W–2 years	USA	5.3 – habitual
Liukkonen (2008) [25]	1471	1–6 years	Finland	6.3 – habitual
Li et al. (2013) [26]	23,481	From birth to 3 years	ASIA 14 countries	Caucasian – 6.2 No Caucasian – 5.1 Au, NZ, Fil > 10 %; Korea=2.4 %

Table 3.3 Prevalence of snoring in schoolers and adolescents

Authors	N	Age	Country	% snoring
Auntaseree et al. (2001) [29]	1142	6–13	Thailand	8.5 – habitual
Ersu et al. (2004) [33]	2147	5–13	Turkey	7.0 – habitual
Kaditis et al. (2004) [34]	3680	1–18	Greece	5.3 – habitual
Sogut et al. (2005) [30]	1215	3–11	Turkey	3.3 – habitual
Gozal et al. (2008) [35]	16,321	5–7	USA	11.3 – habitual
Ferreira et al. (2009) [36]	976	6–10	Portugal	8.6 – habitual
Tafur et al. (2009) [37]	890	6–12	Ecuador	15.1 – habitual
Sogut et al. (2009) [38]	1030	12–17	Turkey	4.0 – habitual
Kitamura et al. (2014) [31]	170	6–8	Japan	12.9 – habitual

Table 3.4 Prevalence of OSAS

Authors	N	Age	Country	Prevalence	Gender differences
Auntaseree et al. (2001) [29]	1142	6–13	Thailand	0.69 %	No
Brunetti et al. (2001) [23]	895	3–11	Italy	1 %	Yes/males
Rosen et al. (2003) [32]	850	8–11	USA	4.7 % 2.2 of the population	
Sogut et al. (2005) [30]	1215	3–11	Turkey	0.9 % among snorers	No
Kitamura et al. (2014) [31]	170	6–8	Japan	3.5	–

syndrome, etc.; gastroesophageal reflux; nasal deviation; chronic nasal obstruction and mouth breathing; obesity; cleft palate; and laryngomalacia since its prevalence in OSAS is 3.9 % [43].

- Floppy airway either due to neuromuscular disorders or due to hypothyroidism

- Reduced central ventilatory drive, as observed in Arnold-Chiari malformation, myelomeningocele, brain stem injuries, or tumors.
- Medical/developmental disorders such as Down syndrome (it affects 50–80% of the patients [44], Prader-Willi syndrome (central apnea is more prevalent in infants, with a good response to oxygen therapy, while obstructive apnea is more common in older children) [45], and sickle cell anemia since OSAS occurs in 10.6% of the patients and has significant negative correlations with the mean annual level of hemoglobin and with the total sleep time [46].

Data related to the long-term consequences of OSAS point to the increased prevalence of recurrent otitis in children from 5 to 7 years of age, with a prevalence of 44.8%, with a predominance of boys [35]. Furthermore, hypertension and obesity have been proved in a prospective study in 334 children: hypertension was present in 3.6% of the children at the initial observation and in 4.2% 5 years' later; the same pattern was observed for obesity 15.0% initially and 19.5% latter on [47].

Parasomnias

This item will focus in NREM parasomnias, enuresis, and nightmares

NREM Parasomnias

Epidemiologic studies in parasomnias must take into account the frequency of the complaint by family members and the accuracy of the report, since confusion with other disorders is likely to occur as it is the case for epilepsy [48, 49], together with the occurrence of several parasomnias in the same individual; about one-third of the children with sleep terrors in younger ages will develop sleepwalking some years later [50]. The misdiagnosis with epilepsy is common in confusional arousals, sleep terrors, and sleepwalking.

Using the Quebec Longitudinal Study of Child Development, the peak age of occurrence for sleep terrors was 1.5 (34.4% of the children) and 10 years (13.4%) for sleepwalking [50]. The prevalence of sleep terrors and sleepwalking in children with ages ranging from 3 to 10 years is 14.7% for sleep terrors and 9.2 for sleepwalking [51]. Both parasomnias tend to cluster in the first decade of life disappearing in the first years of the second decade. For sleepwalking their average age of onset is from 3 to 10 for 66.4% of the children 17.2% at 11 years of age, 12.9% at 12, and 3.5% at 13; these values for sleep terrors are 84.6%, 9.4%, 4.0%, and 2%, respectively. The opposite trend occurs for the age of disappearance, which for 23.8% of the children is between 3 and 10 years of age, 18.1% at 11, 34.5% at 12, and 24.1% at 13 years for sleepwalking, while for sleep terrors, the trend of disappearance is similar to the onset trend with 67.1 % of the children having no more sleep terrors between 3 and 10 years, 14.8 % at 11, 11.4 % at 12, and 6.7 % at 13 years [51].

Another important issue of NREM parasomnias is the familial aggregation pattern; in fact for sleepwalking, the prevalence increases with the degree of parental history: 22.5 % for children without a parental history, 47.4 % for children who had one parent with a history of sleepwalking, and 61.5 % for children whose both parents had a history of sleepwalking [50].

Sleep terrors are usually associated with anxiety [52], other sleep disorder, or psychiatric problems [50].

Enuresis

Enuresis prevalence values range from 4.6 % to 24.4 %, but in most studies, the prevalence value is close to 10 % (see Table 3.5). It is more common in boys [53, 56–59], and the prevalence increases when there is a familial history of enuresis (OR = 2.8) [53, 58], when there are confusional arousals (OR = 2.4), or whenever the child is confused during night awakenings (OR = 3.4) and also whenever there is also daytime incontinence (OR = 3.0) [53].

The prevalence of enuresis is significantly higher in children with attention deficit/hyperactivity disorder and oppositional defiant disorder in preschool children [56] and sickle cell anemia [60].

Table 3.5 Prevalence of enuresis

Author	Country	N	Age	Prevalence
Neveus et al. (1999) [53]	Sweden	1390	6.2–10.9 years	Boys – 10.8 Girls – 5.3
Laberge et al. (2000) [51]	Canada	1353	3–13 years	15.7 % 12.4 (persisting)
Su et al. (2011) [54]	Hong Kong	6147	6–11 years 117	4.6 % 1.9 (at 11)
Mota et al. (2014) [55]	Brazil	3602	7 years	Boys – 11.7 Girls – 9.3
Niemczyk et al. (2015) [56]	Germany	1676	Mean 5.7 years	9.1 %
Sarici et al. (2015) [57]	Turkey	4250	6–13 years	9.52 Boys – 12.4 Girls – 6.5
Esezebor et al. (2015) [58]	Nigeria	928	5–17	24.4
Doganer et al. (2015) [59]	Turkey	2314	6–14	9.9 Boys – 10.7 Girls – 9.2

Nightmares

Nightmares are quite common since 75 % of the children had at least one nightmare in their lifetime.

Chronic nightmare occurrence increases with age in the first decade: it affects 25 % of the children between 2 and 5 years of age and 41 % between 6 and 10 years. In younger ages there are no gender differences, but after age 12, nightmares are more common in girls; the peak prevalence is usually at age 10 [61].

The risk factors include the previous existence of nightmares and bad dreams, stress or traumatic events, anxiety and anxiety disorders, sleep deprivation, insomnia, and REM-enhancing medication [5].

Other risk factors to be considered are suicidal ideation, sleepwalking and sleep terrors, and behavioral dysfunction [62]. Furthermore, familial aggregation [63, 64], low family income, and the presence of comorbid insomnia affecting 20 % of the children with high nightmare frequency have been described [64].

Many studies point to higher prevalence in girls, but some authors found it was higher in boys [63].

Significant short-term nightmare consequences are poor academic performance, mood disturbances and temper outbursts, and hyperactivity [64]. In spite of that, emotional features in nightmares are stable in longitudinal studies [65].

There are many studies focused on nightmare prevalence in children; however methodologic issues are common especially in its exact definition, in the great variability of questionnaires used, and in the utilization of parents' reports [62]. Table 3.6 summarizes several nightmare epidemiologic studies in children and adolescents [63, 64, 66–78].

Sleep-Related Movement Disorders

The REST study provided strong epidemiologic data of restless legs syndrome in children and adolescents; it was carried out in 10,000 families from the USA and the UK. The prevalence of definitive RLS was 2 % between 8 and 11 years and 3 % between 12 and 17 years; moderate-to-severe symptoms affected one-fourth to one-half of the children with no gender differences at these ages; female preponderance was only found after 15 years [79].

In clinical samples the prevalence varies between 1.3 % and 5.9 % [80, 81].

The risk factors are familial history since 70–80 % of the children have at least one parent with RLS while 16 % have both parents, sleep deprivation, medical conditions with a special reference to renal insufficiency with prevalence ranging between 15.3 % and 35 % [82, 83], iron deficiency, association with periodic limb movement of sleep (PLMS) in 74 % of the patients from sleep clinics [84], and association with growing pains (23 % of the twins with growing pains fulfill the criteria for RLS diagnosis [85] and 54.5 % of the RLS patients fulfill the criteria for growing pains) [86].

Table 3.6 Prevalence of nightmares

Authors	N	Age	% nightmares	% high frequency	Gender diff
Simonds and Parraga (1982) [66]	309	5–18	17	1.7	No
Velabueno et al. (1985) [67]	487	6–12	22	–	No
Fischer & Wilson (1987) [68]	1695	5–18	55	16	No
Fischer et al. (1989) [69]	870	6–13	6.0–8.5 years – 65 8.5–11.5 – 72 >11.5 – 65	>12	Yes
Hawkins and Williams (1992) [70]	163	3–5	33	14	–
Schredl et al. (1996) [71]	624	10–16	62	11	–
Smejde et al. (1998) [72]	378	5–6	62	3	–
Smejde et al. (1999) [73]	1844	5–7	62	3	Yes (frequent)
Nielsen et al. (2000) [74]	610	13–16	13y – 79M/90F 16y – 73M/90F	13 – 25M/37F 16 – 40M/20F	Yes
Liu (2004) [75]	1362	12–18	49	7	Yes
Abdel-Khalek (2006) [76]	6767	10–18	10y – 46M/38F 13y – 53M/49F 18y – 51M/51F	10 – 9M/12F 13 – 18M/15F 18 – 6M/18F	Yes at 15
Shang et al. (2006) [77]	1319	4–9	Past month 8 Lifetime 49		No
Schredl et al. (2008) [78]	4531	8–11	44	2.3	Yes
Coolidge et al. (2010) [63]	1318	4–17	–	6.4	Yes, higher in boys
Li et al. (2011) [64]	6359	Mean 9.2	–	5.2	–

The determination of PLMS implies polysomnography recordings; therefore epidemiologic data are obtained mostly in clinical populations and reach values between 5 % and 27 % [87–89]; they are associated with RLS (in 28 % of the cases) [85] but the prevalence does not present gender differences; they are more prevalent in Caucasian and in attention deficit and hyperactivity disorder (ADHD).

The PLMS risk factors are medical disorders (uremia and leukemia); iron deficiency; neurologic and developmental disorders (ADHD, Williams syndrome, spinal cord lesions); migraine [90]; sleep disturbances (OSAS and narcolepsy); medication, namely, the selective of serotonin reuptake inhibitor (SSRI); and positive familial history of RLS [85].

Bruxism prevalence varies between 14 % and 25 % until 11 years of age, without gender differences [4, 51, 91]. The risk factors are anxiety, depression, stress, temporomandibular dysfunction, allergic conditions and nasal obstruction, cerebral palsy and mental retardation, toxics, stimulating medication and drugs, SSRIs, OSAS [91], positive familial history of bruxism, and ADHD [4, 51].

Circadian Disorders

Circadian preferences in Italian children and adolescents with ages ranging between 8 and 14 years showed that 10.3 % are clearly evening types and 10.9 % clearly morning types [92].

According to the ICSD2, the prevalence of sleep phase delay syndrome is 10 % (ICSD2) but the data vary in different studies: it affects 0. 4 % of the Europeans aged between 15 and 18 years [93], 0.13–3.1 % of the US population [94], and in the same country 7–16 % of the adolescents [4]; in Norway it affects 3.3 % of the youngsters between 16 and 18 years and has a higher prevalence in girls (3.7 %) and lower in boys (2.7 %) [95]. The syndrome often starts during adolescence.

Insomnia is commonly associated with circadian disorders (30 % of the subjects with sleep phase delay syndrome have at least one insomnia symptom) [93]; furthermore, insomnia is present in 53.8 % of the boys and in 57.1 % of the girls [95].

The short- and long-term consequences are quite relevant: missing classes (OR = 3.22 for boys and 1.87 for girls) [95], academic failure, loss of job, social and familiar difficulties, and depression.

References

1. Sadeh A, Mindell J, Rivera L. "My child has a sleep problem": a cross-cultural comparison of parental definitions. Sleep Med. 2011;12(5):478–82. doi:10.1016/j.sleep.2010.10.008. Epub 2011 Apr 7.
2. Tikotzky L, Shaashua L. Infant sleep and early parental sleep-related cognitions predict sleep in pre-school children. Sleep Med. 2012;13(2):185–92. doi:10.1016/j.sleep.2011.07.013. Epub 2011 Dec 3.
3. Gregory AM, Caspi A, Eley TC, Moffitt TE, Oconnor TG, Poulton R. Prospective longitudinal associations between persistent sleep problems in childhood and anxiety and depression disorders in adulthood. J Abnorm Child Psychol. 2005;33(2):157–63.
4. Mindell J, Owens J. A clinical guide to pediatric sleep: diagnosis and management of sleep problems. 2nd ed. Philadelphia: Lippincott WW; 2010.
5. Zhang J, Li AM, Fok TF, Wing YK. Roles of parental sleep/wake patterns, socioeconomic status, and daytime activities in the sleep/wake patterns of children. J Pediatr. 2010;156(4):606–12.e5.
6. Byars KC, Yeomans-Maldonado G, Noll JG. Parental functioning and pediatric sleep disturbance: an examination of factors associated with parenting stress in children clinically referred for evaluation of insomnia. Sleep Med. 2011;12(9):898–905.

7. Ferreira R, Paiva T. Clínica do Sono da Criança e do Adolescente. In: Paiva T, Andersen M, Tufik S, editors. O Sono e a Medicina do Sono. São Paulo: Editora Manole; 2014.
8. AASM. The international classification of sleep disorders. Diagnostic and coding manual. 2nd ed. Westchester, IL, American Academy of Sleep Medicine. 2005.
9. Roberts RE, Roberts CR, Duong HT. Chronic insomnia and its negative consequences for health and functioning of adolescents: a 12-month prospective study. J Adolesc Health. 2008;42(3):294–302.
10. Siomos KE, Braimiotis D, Floros GD, Dafoulis V, Angelopoulos NV. Insomnia symptoms among Greek adolescent students with excessive computer use. Hippokratia. 2010;14(3):203–7.
11. Zhang J, Li AM, Kong AP, Lai KY, Tang NL, Wing YK. A community-based study of insomnia in Hong Kong Chinese children: prevalence, risk factors and familial aggregation. Sleep Med. 2009;10(9):1040–6.
12. Pan JY, Chou MF, Zhang J, Liu YP. Sleep patterns, insomnia and daytime sleepiness between Guangdong and Macau Chinese adolescents: a cross-cultural comparison study. Biol Rhythm Res. 2012;43(5):527–39.
13. Amaral MO, de Figueiredo Pereira CM, Silva Martins DI, de Serpa CR, Sakellarides CT. Prevalence and risk factors for insomnia among Portuguese adolescents. Eur J Pediatr. 2013;172(10):1305–11.
14. Calhoun SL, Fernandez-Mendoza J, Vgontzas AN, Liao D, Bixler EO. Prevalence of insomnia symptoms in a general population sample of young children and preadolescents: gender effects. Sleep Med. 2014;15(1):91–5.
15. Chong SA, Vaingankar J, Abdin E, Subramaniam M. The prevalence and impact of major depressive disorder among Chinese, Malays and Indians in an Asian multi-racial population. J Affect Disord. 2012;138(1–2):128–36.
16. dos Reis DC, de Almeida TA, Miranda MM, Alves RH, Madeira AM. Health vulnerabilities in adolescence: socioeconomic conditions, social networks, drugs and violence. Rev Lat Am Enfermagem. 2013;21(2):586–94.
17. Malta DC, Mascarenhas MD, Porto DL, Barreto SM, Morais Neto OL. Exposure to alcohol among adolescent students and associated factors. Rev Saude Publica. 2014;48(1):52–62. Portuguese.
18. Poli F, Overeem S, Lammers GJ, Plazzi G, Lecendreux M, Bassetti CL, Dauvilliers Y, Keene D, Khatami R, Li Y, Mayer G, Nohynek H, Pahud B, Paiva T, Partinen M, Scammell TE, Shimabukuro T, Sturkenboom M, van Dinther K, Wiznitzer M, Bonhoeffer J. Narcolepsy as an adverse event following immunization: case definition and guidelines for data collection, analysis and presentation. Vaccine. 2013;31(6):994–1007.
19. Han F, Lin L, Warby SC, Faraco J, Li J, Dong SX, An P, Zhao L, Wang LH, Li QY, Yan H, Gao ZC, Yuan Y, Strohl KP, Mignot E. Narcolepsy onset is seasonal and increased following the 2009 H1N1 pandemic in China. Ann Neurol. 2011;70(3):410–7.
20. Heier MS, Gautvik KM, Wannag E, Bronder KH, Midtlyng E, Kamaleri Y, Storsaeter J. Incidence of narcolepsy in Norwegian children and adolescents after vaccination against H1N1 influenza A. Sleep Med. 2013;14(9):867–71.
21. Aydinoz S, Huang YS, Gozal D, Inocente CO, Franco P, Kheirandish-Gozal L. Allergies and disease severity in childhood narcolepsy: preliminary findings. Sleep. 2015;38(12):1981–4.
22. Gislason T, Janson C, Tómasson K. Epidemiological aspects of snoring and hypertension. J Sleep Res. 1995;4(S1):145–9.
23. Brunetti L, Rana S, Lospalluti ML, Pietrafesa A, Francavilla R, Fanelli M, Armenio L. Prevalence of obstructive sleep apnea syndrome in a cohort of 1,207 children of southern Italy. Chest. 2001;120(6):1930–5.
24. Montgomery-Downs HE, Gozal D. Sleep habits and risk factors for sleep-disordered breathing in infants and young toddlers in Louisville, Kentucky. Sleep Med. 2006;7(3):211–9.
25. Liukkonen K, Virkkula P, Aronen ET, Kirjavainen T, Pitkäranta A. All snoring is not adenoids in young children. Int J Pediatr Otorhinolaryngol. 2008;72(6):879–84.

26. Li AM, Sadeh A, Au CT, Goh DY, Mindell JA. Prevalence of habitual snoring and its correlates in young children across the Asia Pacific. J Paediatr Child Health. 2013;49(2):E153–9.
27. Castronovo V, Zucconi M, Nosetti L, Marazzini C, Hensley M, Veglia F, Nespoli L, Ferini-Strambi L. Prevalence of habitual snoring and sleep-disordered breathing in preschool-aged children in an Italian community. J Pediatr. 2003;142(4):377–82.
28. Montgomery-Downs HE, Jones VF, Molfese VJ, Gozal D. Snoring in preschoolers: associations with sleepiness, ethnicity, and learning. Clin Pediatr (Phila). 2003;42(8):719–26.
29. Anuntaseree W, Rookkapan K, Kuasirikul S, Thongsuksai P. Snoring and obstructive sleep apnea in Thai school-age children: prevalence and predisposing factors. Pediatr Pulmonol. 2001;32(3):222–7.
30. Sogut A, Altin R, Uzun L, Ugur MB, Tomac N, Acun C, Kart L, Can G. Prevalence of obstructive sleep apnea syndrome and associated symptoms in 3–11-year-old Turkish children. Pediatr Pulmonol. 2005;39(3):251–6.
31. Kitamura T, Miyazaki S, Kadotani H, Suzuki H, Kanemura T, Komada I, Nishikawa M, Kobayashi R, Okawa M. Prevalence of obstructive sleep apnea syndrome in Japanese elementary school children aged 6–8 years. Sleep Breath. 2014;18(2):359–66.
32. Rosen G. Identification and evaluation of obstructive sleep apnea prior to adenotonsillectomy in children: is there a problem? Sleep Med. 2003;4(4):273–4.
33. Ersu R, Arman AR, Save D, Karadag B, Karakoc F, Berkem M, Dagli E. Prevalence of snoring and symptoms of sleep-disordered breathing in primary school children in istanbul. Chest. 2004;126(1):19–24.
34. Kaditis AG, Finder J, Alexopoulos EI, Starantzis K, Tanou K, Gampeta S, Agorogiannis E, Christodoulou S, Pantazidou A, Gourgoulianis K, Molyvdas PA. Sleep-disordered breathing in 3,680 Greek children. Pediatr Pulmonol. 2004;37(6):499–509.
35. Gozal D, Kheirandish-Gozal L, Capdevila OS, Dayyat E, Kheirandish E. Prevalence of recurrent otitis media in habitually snoring school-aged children. Sleep Med. 2008;9(5):549–54. Epub 2007 Oct 24.
36. Ferreira AM, Clemente V, Gozal D, Gomes A, Pissarra C, César H, Coelho I, Silva CF, Azevedo MH. Snoring in Portuguese primary school children. Pediatrics. 2000;106(5), E64.
37. Tafur A, Chérrez-Ojeda I, Patiño C, Gozal D, Rand C, Ronnie M, Thomas G, Jaime S, Jacquelin C. Rhinitis symptoms and habitual snoring in Ecuadorian children. Sleep Med. 2009;10(9):1035–9.
38. Sogut A, Yilmaz O, Dinc G, Yuksel H. Prevalence of habitual snoring and symptoms of sleep-disordered breathing in adolescents. Int J Pediatr Otorhinolaryngol. 2009;73(12):1769–73.
39. Huang YS, Paiva T, Hsu JF, Kuo MC, Guilleminault C. Sleep and breathing in premature infants at 6 months post-natal age. BMC Pediatr. 2014;14(1):303.
40. Li L, Xu Z, Jin X, Yan C, Jiang F, Tong S, Shen X, Li S. Sleep-disordered breathing and asthma: evidence from a large multicentric epidemiological study in China. Respir Res. 2015;16:56.
41. Brockmann PE, Bertrand P, Castro-Rodriguez JA. Influence of asthma on sleep disordered breathing in children: a systematic review. Sleep Med Rev. 2014;18(5):393–7.
42. Jiang N, Muhammad C, Ho Y, Del Signore AG, Sikora AG, Malkin BD. Prevalence of severe obstructive sleep apnea in pediatric adenotonsillectomy patients. Laryngoscope. 2014;124(8):1975–8.
43. Thevasagayam M, Rodger K, Cave D, Witmans M, El-Hakim H. Prevalence of laryngomalacia in children presenting with sleep-disordered breathing. Laryngoscope. 2010;120(8):1662–6.
44. Dyken ME, Lin-Dyken DC, Poulton S, Zimmerman MB, Sedars E. Prospective polysomnographic analysis of obstructive sleep apnea in down syndrome. Arch Pediatr Adolesc Med. 2003;157(7):655–60.
45. Cohen M, Hamilton J, Narang I. Clinically important age-related differences in sleep related disordered breathing in infants and children with Prader-Willi syndrome. PLoS One. 2014;9(6), e101012.
46. Salles C, Ramos RT, Daltro C, Barral A, Marinho JM, Matos MA. Prevalence of obstructive sleep apnea in children and adolescents with sickle cell anemia. J Bras Pneumol. 2009;35(11):1075–83.

47. Archbold KH, Vasquez MM, Goodwin JL, Quan SF. Effects of sleep patterns and obesity on increases in blood pressure in a 5-year period: report from the Tucson Children's Assessment of Sleep Apnea Study. J Pediatr. 2012;161(1):26–30.
48. Derry CP. Sleeping in fits and starts: a practical guide to distinguishing nocturnal epilepsy from sleep disorders. Pract Neurol. 2014;14(6):391–8.
49. Manni R, Terzaghi M. Comorbidity between epilepsy and sleep disorders. Epilepsy Res. 2010;90(3):171–7.
50. Petit D, Pennestri MH, Paquet J, Desautels A, Zadra A, Vitaro F, Tremblay RE, Boivin M, Montplaisir J. Childhood sleepwalking and sleep terrors: a longitudinal study of prevalence and familial aggregation. JAMA Pediatr. 2015;169(7):653–8.
51. Laberge L, Tremblay RE, Vitaro F, Montplaisir J. Development of parasomnias from childhood to early adolescence. Pediatrics. 2000;106(1 Pt 1):67–74.
52. Gau SF, Soong WT. Psychiatric comorbidity of adolescents with sleep terrors or sleepwalking: a case-control study. Aust N Z J Psychiatry. 1999;33(5):734–9.
53. Nevéus T, Hetta J, Cnattingius S, Tuvemo T, Läckgren G, Olsson U, Stenberg A. Depth of sleep and sleep habits among enuretic and incontinent children. Acta Paediatr. 1999;88(7):748–52.
54. Su MS, Li AM, So HK, Au CT, Ho C, Wing YK. Nocturnal enuresis in children: prevalence, correlates, and relationship with obstructive sleep apnea. J Pediatr. 2011;159(2):238–42.e1.
55. Mota DM, Barros AJ, Matijasevich A, Santos IS. Prevalence of enuresis and urinary symptoms at age 7 years in the 2004 birth cohort from Pelotas, Brazil. J Pediatr (Rio J). 2015;91(1):52–8.
56. Niemczyk J, Equit M, Braun-Bither K, Klein AM, von Gontard A. Prevalence of incontinence, attention deficit/hyperactivity disorder and oppositional defiant disorder in preschool children. Eur Child Adolesc Psychiatry. 2015;24(7):837–43.
57. Sarici H, Telli O, Ozgur BC, Demirbas A, Ozgur S, Karagoz MA. Prevalence of nocturnal enuresis and its influence on quality of life in school-aged children. J Pediatr Urol. 2015 Dec 24; pii: S1477-5131(15)00450–7.
58. Esezobor CI, Balogun MR, Ladapo TA. Prevalence and predictors of childhood enuresis in southwest Nigeria: findings from a cross-sectional population study. J Pediatr Urol. 2015;11(6):338.e1–6.
59. Doganer YC, Aydogan U, Ongel K, Sari O, Koc B, Saglam K. The prevalence and sociodemographic risk factors of enuresis nocturna among elementary school-age children. J Family Med Prim Care. 2015;4(1):39–44.
60. Eneh CI, Okafor HU, Ikefuna AN, Uwaezuoke SN. Nocturnal enuresis: prevalence and risk factors among school-aged children with sickle-cell anaemia in a South-East Nigerian city. Ital J Pediatr. 2015;41:66.
61. Mindell JA, Barrett KM. Nightmares and anxiety in elementary-aged children: is there a relationship. Child Care Health Dev. 2002;28(4):317–22.
62. Gauchat A, Séguin JR, Zadra A. Prevalence and correlates of disturbed dreaming in children. Pathol Biol (Paris). 2014;62(5):311–8.
63. Coolidge FL, Segal DL, Coolidge CM, Spinath FM, Gottschling J. Do nightmares and generalized anxiety disorder in childhood and adolescence have a common genetic origin? Behav Genet. 2010;40(3):349–56.
64. Li SX, Yu MW, Lam SP, Zhang J, Li AM, Lai KY, Wing YK. Frequent nightmares in children: familial aggregation and associations with parent-reported behavioral and mood problems. Sleep. 2011;34(4):487–93.
65. Schredl M, Fricke-Oerkermann L, Mitschke A, Wiater A, Lehmkuhl G. Longitudinal study of nightmares in children: stability and effect of emotional symptoms. Child Psychiatry Hum Dev. 2009;40(3):439–49.
66. Simonds JF, Parraga H. Prevalence of sleep disorders and sleep behaviors in children and adolescents. J Am Acad Child Adolesc Psychiatry. 1982;21(4):383–8.
67. Velabueno A, Bixler EO, Dobladezblanco B, Rubio ME, Mattison RE, Kales A. Prevalence of night terrors and nightmares in elementary-school children – a pilot study. Res Commun Psychiatr Psychol. 1985;10(3):177–88.

68. Fisher BE, Wilson AE. Selected sleep disturbances in schoolchildren reported by parents – prevalence, interrelationships, behavioral-correlates and parental attributions. Percept Mot Skills. 1987;64(3):1147–57.
69. Fisher BE, Pauley C, McGuire K. Children's sleep behavior scale – normative data on 870 children in grade 1 to grade 6. Percept Mot Skills. 1989;68(1):227–36.
70. Hawkins C, Williams TI. Nightmares, life events and behaviors problems in school-aged children. Child Care Health Dev. 1992;18(2):117–28.
71. Schredl M, Pallmer R, Montasser A. Anxiety dreams in school-aged children. Dreaming. 1996;6(4):265–70.
72. Smedje H, Broman JE, Hetta J. Sleep disturbances in Swedish pre-school children and their parents. Nordic J Psychiatry. 1998;52(1):59–67.
73. Smedje H, Broman JE, Hetta J. Parents' reports of disturbed sleep in 5–7-year old Swedish children. Acta Paediatr. 1999;88(8):858–65.
74. Nielsen TA, Laberge L, Paquet J, Tremblay RE, Vitaro F, Montplaisir J. Development of disturbing dreams during adolescence and their relation to anxiety symptoms. Sleep. 2000;23(6):727–36.
75. Liu X. Sleep and adolescent suicidal behavior. Sleep. 2004;27(7):1351–8.
76. Abdel-Khalek AM. Nightmares: prevalence, age and gender differences among Kuwaiti children and adolescents. Sleep Hypn. 2006;8(1):33–40.
77. Shang CY, Gau SSF, Soong WT. Association between childhood sleep problems and perinatal factors, parental mental distress and behavioral problems. J Sleep Res. 2006;15(1):63–73.
78. Schredl M, Anders A, Hellriegel S, Rehm A. TV viewing, computer game playing and nightmares in school children. Dreaming. 2008;18(2):69–76.
79. Picchietti D, Allen RP, Walters AS, Davidson JE, Myers A, Ferini-Strambi L. Restless legs syndrome: prevalence and impact in children and adolescents—the Peds REST study. Pediatrics. 2007;120(2):253–66.
80. Turkdogan D, Bekiroglu N, Zaimoglu S. A prevalence study of restless legs syndrome in Turkish children and adolescents. Sleep Med. 2011;12(4):315–21. doi:10.1016/j.sleep.2010.08.013. Epub 2011 Feb 19.
81. Kinkelbur J, Eckart R, Rothenberger A. Indications for sleep laboratory studies in psychiatrically symptomatic children and adolescents. Kinderkrankenschwester. 2003;22(4):166–9. German.
82. Kotagal S, Silber MH. Childhood-onset restless legs syndrome. Ann Neurol. 2004;56(6):803–7.
83. Riar SK, Leu RM, Turner-Green TC, Rye DB, Kendrick-Allwood SR, McCracken C, Bliwise DL, Greenbaum LA. Restless legs syndrome in children with chronic kidney disease. Pediatr Nephrol. 2013;28(5):773–95.
84. Applebee GA, Guillot AP, Schuman CC, Teddy S, Attarian HP. Restless legs syndrome in pediatric patients with chronic kidney disease. Pediatr Nephrol. 2009;24(3):545–8.
85. Picchietti DL, Rajendran RR, Wilson MP, Picchietti MA. Pediatric restless legs syndrome and periodic limb movement disorder: parent-child pairs. Sleep Med. 2009;10(8):925–31.
86. Champion D, Pathirana S, Flynn C, Taylor A, Hopper JL, Berkovic SF, Jaaniste T, Qiu W. Growing pains: twin family study evidence for genetic susceptibility and a genetic relationship with restless legs syndrome. Eur J Pain. 2012;16(9):1224–31.
87. Kirk VG, Bohn S. Periodic limb movements in children: prevalence in a referred population. Sleep. 2004;27(2):313–5.
88. Chervin RD, Archbold KH. Hyperactivity and polysomnographic findings in children evaluated for sleep-disordered breathing. Sleep. 2001;24(3):313–20.
89. Martinez S, Guilleminault C. Periodic leg movements in prepubertal children with sleep disturbance. Dev Med Child Neurol. 2004;46(11):765–70.
90. Esposito M, Parisi P, Miano S, Carotenuto M. Migraine and periodic limb movement disorders in sleep in children: a preliminary case-control study. J Headache Pain. 2013;14:57.
91. Ferreira NM, Dos Santos JF, Dos Santos MB, Marchini L. Sleep bruxism associated with obstructive sleep apnea syndrome in children. Cranio. 2015;29:1–5.

92. Russo PM, Bruni O, Lucidi F, Ferri R, Violani C. Sleep habits and circadian preference in Italian children and adolescents. J Sleep Res. 2007;16(2):163–9.
93. Ohayon MM, Roberts RE, Zulley J, Smirne S, Priest RG. Prevalence and patterns of problematic sleep among older adolescents. J Am Acad Child Adolesc Psychiatry. 2000;39(12):1549–56.
94. Wyatt JK. Delayed sleep phase syndrome: pathophysiology and treatment options. Sleep. 2004;27(6):1195–203. Review.
95. Sivertsen B, Harvey AG, Pallesen S, Hysing M. Mental health problems in adolescents with delayed sleep phase: results from a large population-based study in Norway. J Sleep Res. 2015;24(1):11–8.

Chapter 4
New Directions in the Link Between Technology Use and Sleep in Young People

Kate Bartel and Michael Gradisar

Abstract Young people have an affinity for technological devices. Several reviews of more than 70 studies over the past 15 years have shown consistent links between young people's use of technology and sleep. This has led the scientific and general communities to deduce that using technology before bed worsens sleep. However, the majority of studies performed have been correlational in nature, making causal inferences difficult. This chapter focuses on two important questions of "how" and "how much" technology use affects sleep. The former question details primarily experimental studies that have tested potential mechanisms, including technology use inducing physiological arousal, displacing bedtime, or screenlight disturbing sleep and circadian rhythms. While the latter question appears straightforward, new meta-analytic results suggest it is not. Furthermore, new studies are identifying important moderators for the link between technology use and sleep. Finally, we consider the reverse relationship – the possibility of technology use increasing in response to difficulty sleeping. Our chapter concludes with a research agenda that does not necessarily point the finger at technology use as the reason why so many young people are sleeping too late and too little.

Keywords Technology use • Sleep • Adolescents • Arousal • Screenlight • Displacement • Bedtimes

Introduction

Apple cofounder Steve Jobs once said "People did not know what they want, but we'll show them" [1]. Mr Jobs' vision for enhancing our lives was laudable – but do you think he considered the cost of his choices on young people? One could easily argue he, or Apple, did not. Just watch the scene in Apple's "Love" TV commercial where

K. Bartel, BPsych (Hons) • M. Gradisar, PhD, MPsych (Clin), BSc (Hons) (✉)
School of Psychology, Flinders University, GPO Box 2100, Adelaide 5001, SA, Australia
e-mail: kate.bartel@flinders.edu.au; michael.gradisar@flinders.edu.au

© Springer International Publishing Switzerland 2017
S. Nevšímalová, O. Bruni (eds.), *Sleep Disorders in Children*,
DOI 10.1007/978-3-319-28640-2_4

69

a young boy's room is brightly lit at night by the glow of his iPad 2. Sure he is loving his iPad, but when does he put it down to go to bed? How does he sleep afterward?

We should not be too unfair on Apple's iconic inventor, for in the early 2000s, parents were advised to position computer screens in areas visible by all [2]. This was when home Internet was hardwired – before domestic Wi-Fi made it possible for Apple to develop iDevices that can be placed in any corner of the household (including the bedroom, which can lead to its use after lights off [3–6]). But more than a decade beyond the invention of Wi-Fi, with the introduction of touch screen "gorilla glass" in iPads and iPods (and associated copycat devices), is there a cost of this accelerated technology on young people's sleep?

This chapter can only provide a snapshot in time of what we now know, but it does not pretend to assume that we know it all. Apple spent $1.68 billion in the 2014 September quarter on research and development [7], and Samsung invested $13.4 billion in 2013 [8], yet when one reviews the scientific literature of investigations into the harms to sleep health from technology use, the funding for such science pales in comparison. We will learn more over the next decade as the research attempts to catch up to the advances in technology. But what we aim to achieve in this chapter is to (1) convey what the data are currently telling us about the relationship between technology use and young people's sleep[1] (you may be surprised) and thus (2) provide direction to researchers for where future research should be focused.

In the hope of achieving these aims, we will concentrate on two key questions:

1. How much does technology use affect young people's sleep?
2. How does technology use affect young people's sleep?

However, before addressing the "how much" question, let us turn our attention to the possible mechanisms between technology use and sleep.

How Technology Affects Sleep?

In 2010, both van den Bulck [9] and Cain and Gradisar [10] performed reviews of the scientific literature reporting links between various technological devices and sleep in school-aged children and adolescents. These reviews were later updated by Gradisar and Short [11] and more recently with a systematic review by Hale and Guan [12]. At the end of this section, we present an update of the original model, which now incorporates new moderating factors for the relationship between technology use and sleep.

After reviewing 36 papers, Cain and Gradisar [10] concluded that the majority of studies that investigated various devices, including televisions, computers/the Internet, and phones, found significant relationships with primarily reduced total sleep time,

---

[1] By current data we mean that we wish to not provide an exhaustive review of studies in this area as this has already been performed; rather, we wish to focus on new studies that have provided new insights in this area.

but occasionally with a longer sleep latency and/or a later bedtime. The authors presented a model potentially explaining how technology use could affect sleep, which is not unlike the model presented at the end of this section. First was that technology use has been linked to a later bedtime. This was initially proposed by van den Bulck as the displacement hypothesis [13]. This hypothesis states that technology use displaces sleep by delaying bedtime. Second, some studies had provided evidence of increased physiological arousal (e.g., increased heart rate, body temperature, objective alertness via EEG trace) in the evening due to technology use (e.g., [14, 15]). This reduces the body's preparedness for sleep [16]. The third potential mechanism was that the bright light from screens could potentially decrease evening levels of melatonin and even delay its onset. Finally, and although not contained within the model, Cain and Gradisar alluded to some evidence that electromagnetic radiation from devices (e.g., phones) had shown effects with altered sleep architecture and suppressing endogenous melatonin [17, 18]. Cain and Gradisar [10] provided the first illustrative framework for future research to test these proposed mechanisms, yet explained:

> It would be useful for future studies to comprehensively test this model, using research designs that move beyond the correlational analyses which are prevalent in this area. (p.741)

Five years since this review, Hale and Guan [12] performed an updated systematic review of technology use and the sleep of children and adolescents. Their search results yielded a further 31 studies additional to those found in the Cain and Gradisar [10] review. This alone provided a clear indication of the popularity of researchers investigating this particular field. Unfortunately, the vast majority of new studies were correlational in nature. Yet there had been some advances that not only helped to test Cain and Gradisar's model but also began to find that there were important moderators that heightened, or dampened, the link between technology use and sleep.

Several experimental studies have attempted to test the mechanism of *physiological arousal* induced by technology use. For example, an increased heart rate was found in three studies [14, 19, 20], one testing Japanese young adults and two using older Swedish adolescents. However, the effects on sleep latency were anticlimactic, with an extension of objective sleep latency (via polysomnography [PSG]) of only 2.3 min and an extension of subjective sleep latency by up to 18 min. Two separate Australian studies could not detect differences in heart rate between their active and control conditions [15, 21], and both reported PSG sleep latency extensions of less than 5 min. It is worth noting that, for the exception of one study [14], studies asked participants to attempt sleep at their usual time. This avoids the confound of a buildup in sleep homeostatic pressure, which would decrease sleep latency the later young people attempted sleep. Thus, by holding bedtimes constant, researchers are able to more cleanly observe effects of physiological arousal on sleep due to technology use. However, as mentioned above, there has been little support for the physiological arousal-sleep mechanism.

The second mechanism to receive attention from experimental studies is the effect *screenlight* may have on the sleep of young people. Originally, Higuchi and colleagues [14] found little evidence for an effect on sleep from a dim vs bright screen, which was likely due to asking their young adult participants to attempt

sleep at 2 AM. In contrast, Cajochen et al. [22] found that compared to a dim lap-
top screen, using a bright screen for 5 h attenuated the natural rise in melatonin of
their young adults and increased both objective and subjective alertness in the pre-
bedtime period. This was possibly the first evidence to confirm bright screenlight's
effect on sleep. Unfortunately, sleep was not measured in this study. In 2012, Wood
et al. [23] measured possible melatonin suppression effects from the screenlight of
an iPad in their sample of young adults and adolescents. Although 1 h of screenlight showed no significant melatonin suppression, melatonin was significantly
suppressed after 2 h of bright screenlight. Again though, sleep was not measured.
In 2014, Heath and colleagues [24] compared the effects from 1-h use of a dim vs
bright iPad, as well as a filtered iPad screen (Fig. 4.1), on both pre-bedtime alertness and subsequent sleep and next-morning functioning. Compared to the dim
light condition, the bright screen induced greater cognitive alertness in the pre-
bedtime period, but no significant effects were found for sleep (e.g., sleep latency,
REM; or SWS sleep). However, the pre-bedtime alertness effects were of question-
able real-world significance, with only a 23-ms difference for speed processing
and 13 % difference in accuracy. Furthermore, pre-bedtime melatonin levels were
not measured. Recently though, van der Lely and colleagues [25] designed an
excellent study that measured the pre-bedtime alertness (subjective, objective,
melatonin) as well as sleep and next-morning functioning of older adolescents.

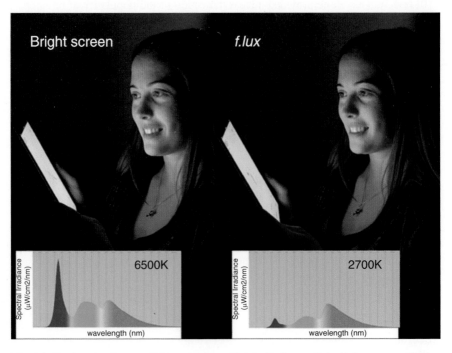

Fig. 4.1 Heath and colleagues [24] comparison of bright iPad screenlight (*left*) vs screen filtering
short-wavelength light using the *f.lux* app (*right*; stereopsis.com)

Their findings showed that 1.5 h (or more) of a bright screen attenuated the rise in evening melatonin and increased subjective alertness compared to wearing blue-blocking glasses (designed to filter alerting short-wavelength light). However, no effects were found on sleep. The abovementioned studies all tested young people in a controlled laboratory setting on single nights, which thus suffer from poor external validity, as many adolescents use technological devices frequently throughout the week [26]. A study by Chang and colleagues [27] overcame this limitation by securing young adults in the laboratory for 14 consecutive days (and nights) and exposed them to either a brightly lit e-book or a printed book in dim light for 5 h each night for 5 days (counterbalanced). Their findings not only confirmed a suppression of melatonin in the e-book condition but also a meaningful delay in circadian timing (by 1.5 h), providing the first support for a circadian delay mechanism. Interestingly, although significant effects were found for an increase in sleep latency from the e-book condition, this was only 10 min longer, which is not overly meaningful.

Taken together, the abovementioned studies suggest that at least 1 h of bright screenlight can induce increased alertness (whether perceived or objective); 1.5 h of screenlight can suppress the natural rise in melatonin, but does not affect the sleep of young people. Thus, there is limited support for this mechanism in the relationship between technology use and sleep. Chang et al. [27] have confirmed a delay in circadian timing, yet these findings require replication. Yet one question that remains is that if adolescents did use a bright screen and felt alert, would they continue to use their device beyond their usual bedtime?

There is a paucity of experimental research into the ability of technology use to *displace* young people's bedtimes. Indeed, to our knowledge only one study has done so. Reynolds and colleagues [28] allowed older adolescents to play a novel video game for as long as they wanted. More importantly, the researchers anticipated that the teenagers would differ in when they would "switch off" and thus explored what characteristics might determine a later vs earlier bedtime. They found those adolescents who reported more consequences of risk-taking were more likely to cease video gaming and retire for bed. This study reinforces others which have shown that the link between technology use and sleep may be moderated by other characteristics, including gamer experience/habituation [20] and more recently parental involvement and flow [29] (Fig. 4.2).

If we were asked to write this chapter a couple of years ago, this is where we would end, as we would not be considering the question: whether technology use affects the sleep of young people. However, our new work suggests otherwise.

How Much Technology Affects Sleep?

Much of the revised literature on technology use and sleep used binary significance testing (which reflects the nature of the science during this time). In other words, researchers were primarily testing whether there was a significant relationship

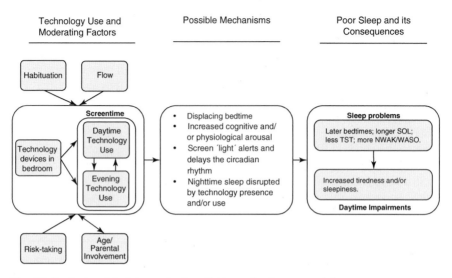

Fig. 4.2 Revised model of the mechanisms linking technology use and sleep

between technology use and sleep, and significance was usually defined as obtaining a significance level of $p < 0.05$. More recently, binary significance testing has been criticized [30]. For example, a relationship may occur between two variables, but it may be so small that it does not mean much in the real world.

The field of technology use and sleep seemingly neglected the size of the real-world effect between these two variables. However, a meta-analysis by Bartel et al. [31] was able to estimate the magnitude of the effects between various technological devices and teenagers' sleep, along with a multitude of other risk (and protective) factors. Surprisingly, the correlations between technological devices and sleep were negligible. The use of technology was not related to sleep latency, and only computer use was associated with a decrease in total sleep time. Technology did appear to correlate, to a small extent, with bedtime. Namely, as video gaming, phone use, computer use, and Internet use increased, bedtime became later [31]. Figure 4.3 provides an illustrative look of the relative protective and risk factors for adolescents' sleep, including "technology use." The segments of the pie chart demonstrate the percentage of variance from each factor. We have used the mean-weighted correlations between "technology use" and "sleep" (i.e., between Internet use and bedtime, which showed an $r = 0.212$) from the meta-analytical findings from Bartel and colleagues – thus, at best, technology use represents just a sliver of a contribution toward adolescents' sleep. At a glance, there appear other more important contributions, including family influences (i.e., parent-set bedtimes, family environment). The most obvious piece is represented by the question mark. Normally, this would mean we do not know what this extra contribution is and may elect to claim it is a measurement error, other methodological anomalies, or simply things we do not know. However, Bartel and colleagues were unable to

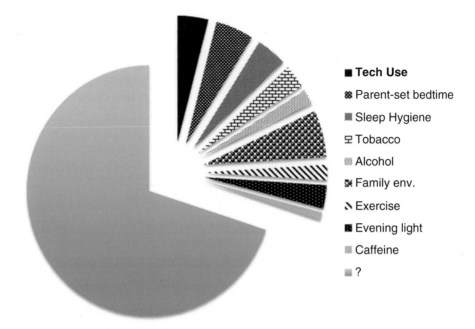

Fig. 4.3 Illustrative pie chart of the relative protective and risk factors for adolescents' sleep (Derived from meta-analytic data from Bartel et al. [31])

meta-analyze biological contributions to teenagers' sleep (i.e., circadian rhythm timing, sleep homeostasis, genetics), which are known to be major influences on teenagers' sleep.

Can Sleep Affect Technology Use?

At the outset of this chapter, we did state that we had two key questions, which we have addressed above. However, we knew, before the reader, that the current data are telling us that there is little effect between technology use and adolescents' sleep. It follows then that we should not close our minds to the possibility that the relationship may occur the other way round – that increased technology use occurs *after* sleep becomes more problematic. After all, the majority of the scientific literature to date are correlational, and the limited experimental studies available suggest when one manipulates technology use, the resultant effect on sleep is small to meaningless.

Our insight into whether the technology use of adolescents occurs after sleep becomes problematic comes from a cross-sectional study of 2,546 Belgian adolescents. The 2006 study, titled "Nodding off or switching off? The use of popular media as a sleep aid in secondary-school children," was likely ahead of its time. Eggermont and van den Bulck [32] asked seventh- (13.2 years) and tenth-grade

(16.4 years) adolescents how often they used either computer games, television, books,[2] or music to *help them fall asleep*. Respondents answered either *never*, *rarely*, *sometimes*, or *often*. One in five adolescents used television at least occasionally as a sleep aid, one in ten used computer games, and one in three used books, but it was music that was used the most, with almost one in every two adolescents using music to help them fall asleep. Despite that only books led to an earlier bedtime, more sleep, and less next-day tiredness (compared to other sleeping aids), this was the first study of teenagers exploring technology use as an aftereffect of trouble sleeping. We are likely overstating this claim, as technically adolescents were not asked to report if they had a sleep problem. We can only infer that by asking teenagers if sleep onset was assisted with an associated technological activity, that at least for some adolescents, difficulty initiating sleep may have occurred before the use of such technology.

Perhaps the best evidence to date attempting to answer the question about whether sleep can affect technology use comes from a prospective study of adults. Tavernier and Willoughby [33] followed 942 emerging adults (age at Time 1 = 19.0 years) for 3 years and measured their average weekly hours of TV watching and online social networking (e.g., Facebook, Myspace, Twitter, e-mail, Messenger), as well as their typical sleep duration, as well as an adapted version of the Insomnia Severity Index (items included difficulty initiating sleep, staying asleep, early morning awakening, and sleep satisfaction [34]), which provided a continuous variable known as "sleep problems." Cross-lagged analyses showed that sleep problems at Time 1 predicted Time 2 television watching and online social networking, but the reverse relationship (i.e., technology use predicting later sleep problems) was not supported. Interestingly, no prospective relationships existed between technology use and sleep duration, which supports the meta-analytical findings in adolescents [31]. Nevertheless, these prospective findings suggest young adults' perceptions of their sleep, including perceived sleep difficulties, are an important perspective for researchers to consider, as like bedtime data, difficulties in sleeping appear to show significant relationships with technology use (e.g., [35]).

Conclusions

When we began our first discussions on planning this chapter about technology and sleep, we knew we wanted to "spin readers' thinking" about this relationship. We do not mean to claim that using a technological device does not lead to sleep problems in young people. We have observed this, whether in our own children or

---

[2] Given the year of data collection, we presume the researchers referred to printed books as opposed to e-books.

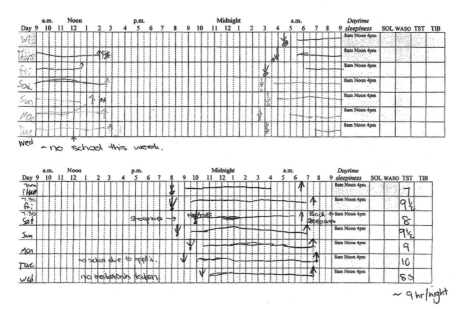

Fig. 4.4 (*Top*) Sleep diary of a 15-year-old male client who regularly plays online games in the evening. (*Bottom*) Sleep diary of the same client after treatment with motivational interviewing to reduce evening online gaming and a combination of evening melatonin and bright light therapy to phase advance his sleep timing

teenagers presenting with sleep problems to our Child and Adolescent Sleep Clinic at Flinders University (Fig. 4.4), albeit temporarily. Instead, we believe we need to work harder than usual to convince readers that, overall, the effect between technology use and sleep is small to negligible. If anything, we lack data to analyze whether technology use fills the void while young people wait for sleep onset to arrive [32]. Sleep problems may already exist in young people [36], and it is possibly better to avoid lying in the quiet darkness ruminating about past events and catastrophizing about future events [37, 38] by distracting oneself with a screen or the sound of music. The displacement hypothesis proposes that technology use may replace other activities, including sleeping [13]. So far, the data provide support for this hypothesis, as if anything, bedtime is related to technology use (more than sleep latency or sleep itself). However, there have been extremely few studies that have attempted to experimentally manipulate technology use and observe the effect on bedtimes [28]. If using technological devices accounts for at best 4 % of the variation in teenagers' sleep (or more accurately, bedtimes; Fig. 4.3), then doesn't this suggest we should turn our attention toward other culprits for why young people may sleep too little and too late [39]? We conclude this chapter by directing readers to Box 4.1, which lists areas for future research – including areas that do not involve technology use.

Box 4.1: Research Agenda
Future Research Directions

- Experimental studies to draw cause and effects between technology use and adolescent sleep
- Considering whether use of technology affects sleep beyond that of employing adequate sleep hygiene
- Designing experiments which focus on other factors which may contribute negatively to adolescent sleep (e.g., negative home environment, evening light)
- Designing experiments focusing on protective factors of sleep (e.g., sleep hygiene, parent-set bedtimes, exercise) and interventions (e.g., motivational interviewing)
- Research into contributions from biological factors (e.g., circadian delay, sleep homeostasis) to young people's sleep

References

1. Isaacson W. Steve jobs. London: Little Brown; 2011.
2. Slatalla M. Computing; parents' dilemma: a child's own PC? The New York Times, 1998. Retrieved from: http://www.nytimes.com/1998/02/26/technology/computing-parents-dilemma-a-child-s-own-pc.html on 23 Aug 2015.
3. Adams SK, Kisler TS. Sleep quality as a mediator between technology-related sleep quality, depression and anxiety. Cyberpsychol Behav Soc Netw. 2013;16:25–30.
4. Munezawa T, Kaneita Y, Osaki Y, Kanda H, Minowa M, Suzuki K, Higuchi S, Mori J, Yamamoto OT. The association between use of mobile phones after lights out and sleep disturbances among Japanese adolescents: a nationwide cross-sectional survey. Sleep. 2011;34:1013–20.
5. National Sleep Foundation. Sleep in America poll, communications technology in the bedroom: summary of findings. Washington, DC: National Sleep Foundation; 2011. p. 2011.
6. Van den Bulck J. Adolescent use of mobile phones for calling and for sending text messages after lights out: results from a prospective cohort study with a one-year follow-up. Sleep. 2007;30:1220–3.
7. Hughes N. Apple spent record $1.7B on research & development last quarter, $6B in fiscal 2014. Appleinsider, 2014.Retrieved from: appleinsider.com/articles/14/10/28/apple-spent-record-17b-on-research-development-last-quarter-6b-in-fiscal-2014 on 23 Aug 2015.
8. Casey M, Hackett R. The 10 biggest R&D spenders worldwide. Fortune, 2014. Retrieved from: http://fortune.com/2014/11/17/top-10-research-development/on 23 Aug 2015.
9. Van den Bulck J. The effects of media on sleep. Adolesc Med State Art Rev. 2010;21:418–29.
10. Cain N, Gradisar M. Electronic media use and sleep in school-aged children and adolescents: a review. Sleep Med. 2010;11:735–42.
11. Gradisar M, Short MA. Sleep hygiene and environment: the role of technology. In: Wolfson AR, Montgomery-Downs HE, editors. The Oxford handbook of infant, child, and adolescent sleep and behavior. Oxford: Oxford University Press; 2013. p. 113.
12. Hale L, Guan S. Screen time and sleep among school-aged children and adolescents: a systematic review of the literature. Sleep Med Rev. 2015;21:50–8. http://dx.doi.org/10.1016/j.smrv.2014.07.007.

13. Van den Bulck J. Television viewing, computer game playing, and internet use and self-reported time in bed and time out of bed in secondary-school children. Sleep. 2004;27: 101–4.
14. Higuchi S, Motohashi Y, Liu Y, Maeda A. Effects of playing a computer game using a bright display on presleep physiological variables, sleep latency, slow wave sleep and REM sleep. J Sleep Res. 2005;14:267–73.
15. Weaver E, Gradisar M, Dohnt H, Lovato N, Douglas P. The effect of presleep video-game playing on adolescent sleep. J Clin Sleep Med. 2010;6:184–9.
16. Freeman RR, Sattler HL. Physiological and psychological factors in sleep-onset insomnia. J Abnorm Psychol. 1982;91:380–9.
17. Loughran SP, Wood AW, Barton JM, Croft RJ, Thompson B, Stough C. The effect of electromagnetic fields emitted by mobile phones on human sleep. Neuroreport. 2005;16:1973–6.
18. Wood AW, Loughran SP, Stough C. Does evening exposure to mobile phone radiation affect subsequent melatonin production? Int J Radition Biol. 2006;82:69–76.
19. Ivarsson M, Anderson M, Akerstedt T, Lindblad F. Playing a violent television game affects heart rate variability. Acta Paediatr. 2009;98:166–72.
20. Ivarsson M, Anderson M, Akerstedt T, Lindblad F. The effect of violent and nonviolent video games on heart rate variability, sleep, and emotions in adolescents with different violent gaming habits. Psychosom Med. 2013;75:390–6.
21. King DL, Gradisar M, Drummond A, Lovato N, Wessel J, Micic G, Douglas P, Delfabbro P. The impact of prolonged violent video-gaming on adolescent sleep: an experimental study. J Sleep Res. 2013;22:137–43.
22. Cajochen C, Frey S, Anders D, Spati J, Bues M, Pross A, Mager R, Wirz-Justice A, Stefani O. Evening exposure to a light-emitting diodes (LED)-backlit computer screen affects circadian physiology and cognitive performance. J Appl Physiol. 2011;110:1432–8.
23. Wood B, Rea MS, Plitnick B, Figuerio MG. Light level and duration of exposure determine the impact of self-luminous tablets on melatonin suppression. Appl Ergon. 2013;44:237–40.
24. Heath M, Sutherland C, Bartel K, Gradisar M, Williamson P, Lovato N, Micic G. Does one hour of bright or short-wavelength filtered tablet screenlight have a meaningful effect on adolescents' pre-bedtime alertness, sleep and daytime functioning? Chronobiol Int. 2014;31: 496–505.
25. Van der Lely S, Frey S, Garbazza C, Wirz-Justice A, Jenni OG, Steiner R, Wolf S, Cajochen C, Bromundt V, Schmidt C. Blue blocker glasses as a countermeasure for alerting effects of evening light-emitting diode screen exposure in male teenagers. J Adolesc Health. 2015;56: 113–9.
26. Gamble AL, D'Rozario AL, Bartlett DJ, Williams S, Bin YS, Grunstein RR, Marshall NS. Adolescent sleep patterns and night-time technology use: results of the Australian Broadcasting Corporation's big sleep survey. PLoS ONE. 2014;9, e111700.
27. Chang A-M, Aeschbach D, Duffy JF, Czeisler CA. Evening use of light-emitting eReaders negatively affects sleep, circadian timing, and next-morning alertness. PNAS. 2015;112: 1232–7.
28. Reynolds CM, Gradisar M, Kar K, Perry A, Wolfe J, Short MA. Adolescents who perceive fewer consequences of risk-taking choose to switch off games later at night. Acta Paediatr. 2015;104:e222–7.
29. Smith LJ, Gradisar M, Short MA, King DJ. Intrinsic and extrinsic predictors between video gaming behavior and adolescent bedtimes. Sleep Med. In press.
30. Cumming G. Understanding the new statistics: effect sizes, confidence intervals, and meta-analysis. New York: Routledge; 2012.
31. Bartel KA, Gradisar M, Williamson P. Protective and risk factors for adolescent sleep: a meta-analytical review. Sleep Med Rev. 2015;21:72–85.
32. Eggermont S, van den Bulck J. Nodding off or switching off? The use of popular media as a sleep aid in secondary-school children. J Paediatr Child Health. 2006;42:428–33.
33. Tavernier R, Willoughby T. Sleep problems: predictor or outcome of media use among emerging adults. J Sleep Res. 2014. doi:10.1111/jsr.12132.

34. Morin CM. Insomnia: psychological assessment and management. New York: Guilford Press; 1993.
35. Gradisar M, Wolfson AR, Harvey AG, Hale L, Rosenberg R, Czeisler CA. The sleep and technology use of Americans: findings from the National Sleep Foundation's 2011 Sleep in America poll. J Clin Sleep Med. 2013;9:1291–9.
36. Short M, Gradisar M, Gill J, Camfferman D. Identifying adolescent sleep problems. PLoS ONE. 2013;8, e75301.
37. Danielsson NS, Harvey AG, MacDonald S, Jansson-Frojmark M, Linton SJ. Sleep disturbance and depressive symptoms in adolescence: the role of catastrophic worry. J Youth Adolesc. 2013;42:1223–33.
38. Hiller RM, Lovato N, Gradisar M, Oliver M, Slater A. Trying to fall asleep whilst catastrophising: what sleep-disordered adolescents think and feel. Sleep Med. 2014;15:96–103.
39. Stokes, K. Wired-up children need more sleep. The Advertiser, 2012. Retrieved from: http://www.adelaidenow.com.au/news/wired-up-children-need-more-sleep/story-fn3o6nna-1226343124338 on 23 Aug 2015.

Chapter 5
Sleep Laboratory Tests

Suresh Kotagal

Abstract The spectrum of childhood sleep–wake disorders extends from sleep-disordered breathing to parasomnia, hypersomnias, and circadian rhythm disorders. Clinical history and examination help select the most appropriate diagnostic test. Nocturnal polysomnography is the gold standard for obstructive and central sleep apnea, while the multiple sleep latency test combined with polysomnography is utilized for the investigation of hypersomnias. Nocturnal seizures may mimic parasomnias; hence, extended electroencephalographic monitoring may be required for investigating some nocturnal episodic phenomena. Practice parameters and evidence-based reviews on indications for polysomnography in children have been recently published. Actigraphy and sleep logs are helpful in investigating suspected circadian rhythm sleep disorders.

Keywords Nocturnal polysomnography • Multiple sleep latency test (MSLT) • Actigraphy • Sleep apnea • Hypersomnia • Parasomnias • Actigraphy

Introduction

Sleep disorders of infants and children are challenging to diagnose because of their diverse etio-pathology and changes in predilection of some disorders to specific age and developmental stage of the patient. Further, the clinical history varies in accuracy depending upon the perceptions, communication ability, and biases of the patient, or parent. Also, normal values for parameters of sleep–wake function tend to change with maturation of central nervous system (CNS) and respiratory control mechanisms. Clinical history and examination are often unable to enable accurate

S. Kotagal, MD
Division of Child Neurology, Department of Neurology, May Clinic,
200 First Street SW, Rochester, MN 55905, USA
e-mail: kotagal.suresh@mayo.edu

© Springer International Publishing Switzerland 2017
S. Nevšímalová, O. Bruni (eds.), *Sleep Disorders in Children*,
DOI 10.1007/978-3-319-28640-2_5

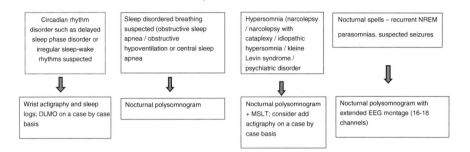

Circadian rhythm disorder such as delayed sleep phase disorder or irregular sleep-wake rhythms suspected	Sleep disordered breathing suspected (obstructive sleep apnea / obstructive hypoventilation or central sleep apnea	Hypersomnia (narcolepsy / narcolepsy with cataplexy / idiopathic hypersomnia / kleine Levin syndrome / psychiatric disorder	Nocturnal spells – recurrent NREM parasomnias, suspected seizures
⇩	⇩	⇩	⇩
Wrist actigraphy and sleep logs; DLMO on a case by case basis	Nocturnal polysomnogram	Nocturnal polysomnogram + MSLT; consider add actigraphy on a case by case basis	Nocturnal polysomnogram with extended EEG montage (16-18 channels)

Fig. 5.1 Matching sleep–wake disturbance to sleep laboratory tests

diagnosis. Consequently, the sleep specialist has to periodically resort to laboratory tests to confirm the diagnosis. The nature of the sleep laboratory test and specific, step-by-step instructions pertaining to the actual performance are heavily dependent upon the accuracy of the sleep history. Technological advances in sleep–wake monitoring systems hardware and software, combined with publication of adult and pediatric polysomnogram scoring guidelines [1], practice parameters on indications for polysomnography [2, 3], and older reviews of this topic [4] underscore the need for its reassessment. This chapter aims to provide an overview of tests commonly employed in the practice of pediatric sleep medicine. Figure 5.1 helps to match sleep–wake symptoms with the appropriate type of investigation.

Nocturnal Polysomnography

Technical Aspects

The test consists of the recording of multiple physiological parameters during sleep. Most often this includes two to three channels of electroencephalogram (EEG), eye movements, chin and leg electromyogram (EMG), oronasal airflow, nasal pressure, thoracic and abdominal respiratory effort, oxygen saturation, and end-tidal carbon dioxide. The scalp EEG montage generally consists of C4-M1, F4-M1, plus O2-M1. The International 10–20 system is utilized for appropriate placement of EEG electrodes over the scalp [5]. Backup electrodes are placed at similar locations over the opposite scalp sites. Electrodes are fixed using collodion or paste while ensuring that the electrode impedance is kept low, i.e., below 5 kΩ. This helps to minimize picking up of extraneous artifact by the electrodes. The centrally placed EEG electrodes help to sample vertex sharp transients and sleep spindles, while occipital leads help to distinguish the waxing and waning amplitude alpha rhythm of wakefulness from the alpha to theta transition that is typical of stage N1 sleep as well as the predominant delta rhythm of stage N3, which is usually <4 Hz and >75 uv amplitude. In case of suspected nocturnal seizures, placement of a minimum

16-channel EEG montage is recommend. The usual sensitivity for EEG recording is 7 uv/mm, though it may need to be decreased to 10–15 uv/mm if the amplitude of the activity is too high, as happens in preschool-age children. Eye movements are generally recorded using a left outer canthus–right outer canthus montage, with the electrodes being placed in a slightly oblique plane in order to capture both horizontal and vertical eye movements. The transition from wakefulness into N1 sleep is associated with the onset of slow rolling eye movements, while transition to REM sleep is associated with rapid eye movements. Monitoring of end-tidal CO_2 is essential in all patients to capture hypoventilation. If the $EtCO_2$ sensor (it yields breath by breath values) is not tolerated by infants and toddlers due to anxiety or increased perioral sensitivity, a transcutaneous CO_2 sensor can be utilized (this yields a trended value). For sampling the chin EMG, 2–3 electrodes need to be affixed under the chin. The absolute amplitude of the EMG is not relevant, but the relative changes in amplitude help distinguish wakefulness, NREM sleep, and REM sleep from each other.

Data are recorded and stored in a computerized polysomnogram system which is composed of preamplifiers for both alternative current (AC) and direct current (DC) input. The AC channels are useful for recording EEG, EMG, and eye movements, whereas the DC channels help record slow biopotentials like respiratory effort. Sleep is scored in 30 s epochs by the attending technologist, with subsequent verification of the scored record by a certified polysomnographer. Nap sleep studies are not recommended as the quantity and type of sleep sampled are variable. Only technician-attended, all night sleep studies are recommended. The technical guidelines for scoring sleep and sleep-related events have been published by the American Academy of Sleep Medicine.

For infants of age 2 months or less, sleep can be scored simply as active or quiet sleep, i.e., REM and NREM sleep. A low-voltage, irregular pattern is associated with active sleep while a high-voltage, slow pattern is characteristic of quiet sleep. After age 2 months, the standard criteria that are utilized in children and adults can be applied, with breakdown of NREM sleep into N1, N2, and N3 categories. For details about sleep scoring, the reader is again referred to the scoring manual of the American Academy of Sleep Medicine [1]. Parameters scored in polysomnography include start time, stop time, total time in bed, total sleep time, sleep efficiency, percentage of time spent in the various sleep stages, arousals per hour of sleep, percentage of arousals related to respiratory events, total number of apneas and hypopneas with attention to occurrence in REM or NREM sleep and relationship to body position, oxygen saturation nadir and mean, $EtCO_2$ nadir, high and mean, percent of time with $EtCO_2$ greater than 50 mm, frequency of periodic limb movements, and comments about any unusual events observed in the simultaneous video recording. A flattened contour on the nasal pressure tracing may be indicative of the upper airway resistance type of obstructive sleep apnea. The polysomnogram report should provide data in a tabular form, coupled with narrative about the overall impression and recommendations of the polysomnographer.

Indications

The definitions of levels of evidence utilized by the AASM and how emphatic the recommendation are for PSG in specific sleep disorders are shown in Table 5.1 [refs 2–4]. The investigation of sleep-disordered breathing is a major indication for PSG (Standard). This includes habitual snoring, suspected obstructive sleep apnea, obstructive hypoventilation, central sleep apnea, and congenital central hypoventilation syndrome. Monitoring of end-tidal carbon dioxide ($EtCO_2$) or, if this is not available, transcutaneous carbon dioxide is mandatory for assessing hypoventilation – this is a major component of sleep-disordered breathing in Down syndrome, Prader–Willi syndrome, obesity, neuromuscular disorders, and kyphoscoliosis. Reference values for respiratory parameters differ from those of adults. For instance, the duration of obstructive apneas in children is generally in the 5–10 s range (two-breath duration), whereas in adults, scored obstructive apnea events are invariably 10 s or longer in duration. The investigation of excessive daytime sleepiness, including suspected narcolepsy, requires a PSG followed the next day by the multiple sleep latency test (MSLT). This recommendation is also at Standard level (Table 5.1). A key tenet in narcolepsy is that there is excessive daytime sleepiness despite adequate sleep duration at night. PSG is also indicated in nonverbal children with suspected restless legs syndrome/periodic limb movement disorder in order to document

Table 5.1 AASM level of recommendation for polysomnography and sleep disorder

Level	Definition	Disorder
Standard	This is a generally accepted patient care strategy that reflects a high degree of clinical certainty and generally implies the use of level 1 evidence or overwhelming level 2 evidence	Periodic limb movement disorder Narcolepsy Diagnosis of obstructive sleep apnea, to evaluate for residual obstructive sleep apnea after adeno-tonsillectomy; follow-up of children on chronic PAP support, for PAP titration
Guideline	This is a patient care strategy that reflects a moderate degree of clinical certainty and implies the use of level 2 evidence or a consensus of level 3 evidence	NREM parasomnias, epilepsy, nocturnal enuresis, assessment of sleep-related hypoventilation, apparent life-threatening event
Option	This is a patient care strategy that reflects uncertain clinical use and implies either inconclusive or conflicting evidence or conflicting expert opinion	Restless legs syndrome, when supportive information is needed for diagnosis; hypersomnia from causes other than narcolepsy; follow-up of children needing oral appliance or rapid maxillary expansion; patients on mechanical ventilation for adjustment of their machine settings; tracheostomy patients being considered for decannulation, if there is suspicion of a sleep disorder in cystic fibrosis/asthma/kyphoscoliosis/pulmonary hypertension

presence of periodic limb movements in sleep. In this regard, preschool-age children are often candidates for PSG. Reference values for the periodic limb movement index in children have been extrapolated from adults at 5 or less. With regard to parasomnias, PSG is not indicated routinely as clinical history may be sufficient to make a diagnosis. If there are recurrent parasomnia-like events or if one is unable to exclude the diagnosis of nocturnal seizures, however, PSG is indicated. The investigation of nocturnal seizures requires the utilization of a 16–18 channel EEG montage. REM sleep behavior disorder may accompany daytime sleepiness in children with narcolepsy–cataplexy; hence, when PSG is being conducted for diagnosing narcolepsy, it is important to carefully examine segments of REM sleep for the presence of the electrophysiological marker of RBD, i.e., persistence of muscle tone during REM sleep, which is also called REM sleep without atonia.

Limitations

PSG is the gold standard procedure for the investigation of many childhood sleep disorders. It is however an expensive and labor-intensive tool. Patient and parent anxiety about the procedure may affect variables such as sleep latency, REM latency, and sleep efficiency. There might also be some degree of night to night variability in parameters like periodic limb movement index. Alternative strategies for diagnosing obstructive sleep apnea include home overnight oximetry. This procedure has limited sensitivity, however, and may be positive only in severe cases. Consequently, if oximetry is noninformative in a child with suspected OSA, one might still need to resort to PSG. The Pediatric Sleep Questionnaire (PSQ) and the Sleep Disturbance Scale for Children (SDSC) may be applied for screening for sleep-disordered breathing [6, 7], but PSG is unfortunately still necessary to confirm the diagnosis.

Multiple Sleep Latency Test (MSLT)

In combination with the nocturnal polysomnogram, the MSLT forms the gold standard in the assessment of daytime sleepiness in both children and adults. This applies especially to the diagnosis of narcolepsy and idiopathic hypersomnia. The strengths of the test lie in its intuitive design (sleepy individuals are likely to fall asleep more quickly in the daytime than those who are not sleepy), its reliability, and the availability of normative data across various ages [8].

The lower age limit at which one can apply the MSLT seems to be 5–6 years [9]. Application of the MSLT in children younger than this age is difficult because physiological daytime napping is common in preschool-age children. To the extent possible, the total sleep time on the preceding night's PSG must be similar to the sleep duration at home. As sleep loss in the days prior to the MSLT may influence the test findings, the parents should be advised to keep a log of the patient's sleep–wake schedule for 1–2 weeks prior to the MSLT. Alternatively, wrist actigraphy for 1–2 weeks prior to the PSG and MSLT can be utilized to gauge sleep time and sleep schedules at home. Medications that can influence sleep, such as stimulants/antidepressants/benzodiazepines/antihistamines, should be discontinued at least 2 weeks prior to the test. Long-acting selective serotonin reuptake inhibitors like fluoxetine that suppress REM sleep may need to be stopped for 4–6 weeks prior to the PSG and MSLT. The decision to stop antidepressants for the purpose of obtaining valid PSG and MSLT should be carefully thought out after weighing the risks and benefits. A discussion with the prescribing physician is also indicated in this regard. The patient's general physical examination should include a Tanner staging of sexual development as normal values for the mean sleep latency in children vary according to individual stages (Table 5.2; [10]). The test consists of the provision of four or five daytime nap opportunities at two hourly intervals, e.g., 0900, 1100, 1300, 1500, and 1700 h, during which the EEG, chin EMG, and horizontal as well as vertical eye movements (using at least two channels) are monitored. The time constant for the electrooculogram should be long enough to allow for the recording of slow, rolling eye movements seen at the onset of N1 sleep (250 ms). Electrode impedances should be below 5 kΩ.

At the designated hour, usually starting 2 h after the final morning awakening from the PSG, the lights are turned off, and the patient is encouraged to relax, close eyes, and to try to fall asleep while the electrophysiologic parameters are being monitored. For each nap, the time from "lights out" to sleep onset is termed the sleep latency. The nap is continued for 15 min after sleep onset. Thus, theoretically, if the patient does not fall asleep in the nap till min 19, the test is continued for a total of 34 min (15 + 19) from the time of commencement of the nap recording. If the patient does not fall asleep by min 20, the nap opportunity is terminated, the lights are turned on, and the sleep latency is designated as 20 min. An identical protocol is followed during all four to five nap opportunities. The patient is kept awake in between the nap opportunities. The assistance of the parents is helpful in this regard. The mean sleep latency is the average of the sleep latency derived from all five naps. Normal values for the pediatric MSLT that have been adapted from a single night's polysomnogram are listed in Table 5.2. Mean sleep latencies for prepubertal children are higher than those of adults, approximating 16–18 min. The

Table 5.2 Reference values for the MSLT

Tanner stage	General corresponding age (years)	Mean sleep latency	Standard deviation
Stage 1	<10	18.8	1.8
Stage 2	10–12	18.3	2.1
Stage 3	11.5–13	16.5	2.8
Stage 4	13–14	15.5	3.3
Stage 5	>14	16.2	1.5
Older teenagers	>14	15.8	3.5

Data from Carskadon [10]

MSLT is however well suited for diagnosing narcolepsy, in which the mean sleep latency is invariably below 8 min [3]. Daytime sleep latencies for MSLT naps parallel the circadian drive for wakefulness, with increased sleep propensity in the afternoon (low sleep latency).

The MSLT also helps evaluate whether the transition from wakefulness into sleep is into REM or NREM sleep. A sleep-onset REM period (SOREMP) is defined by the occurrence of REM sleep within 15 min of sleep onset. About 80 % of patients with narcolepsy show two or more SOREMPs during the MSLT [11]. If the patient manifests a SOREMP on the polysomnogram obtained on the night prior to MSLT, one needs to document only one SOREMP on the latter study for making a diagnosis of narcolepsy [12]. False-negative results may occur in the early stages of childhood narcolepsy, when the patient may manifest daytime somnolence documented by reduced mean sleep latencies, but only 0–1 SOREMPs. Further, one must also recognize that otherwise healthy teens may at times show a SOREMP during the first nap of the MSLT.

There is level 1 evidence regarding the clinical utility of MSLT in the diagnosis of narcolepsy. With regard to hypersomnia disorders other than narcolepsy, such as idiopathic hypersomnia or Kleine–Levin syndrome, however, there is less available evidence. Nevertheless, the MSLT is still utilized in diagnosis of these disorders based on empiric, clinical rationale. In adults, the sensitivity of the MSLT in the diagnosis of narcolepsy in adults has been reported to be around ~61 % [13]. There was no major difference in the diagnostic sensitivity of the test between patients who manifested narcolepsy with cataplexy versus those having narcolepsy without cataplexy. The diagnostic specificity for narcolepsy in adults has been reported to be ~94 % [13] when two or more SOREMPs are present. In children, the diagnostic sensitivity of the MSLT for the diagnosis of narcolepsy is 79–100 % [3, 4].

Merits and Limitations of the MSLT

One advantage of the MSLT is that it has been reliably validated as a tool for assessing sleep propensity in several conditions such as sleep loss [8, 10] and sleep disruption [14] and the effects of hypnotics and alcohol [15, 16]. It measures the propensity for daytime sleepiness at multiple times of the day and provides numerical values which correlate with the level of sleepiness. A disadvantage is that it cannot accurately assess the effects of treatment, e.g., if there is a reliable increase in sleep latency after starting stimulant medication for narcolepsy treatment. Also, while one can control external variables like noise and light that impact sleep latency, the MSLT can in no way control for intrinsic variables that impact sleep latency such as anxiety or emotional disturbance. The issue of whether the MSLT in children should consist of four naps or five naps has not been adequately studied. Based on clinical experience, however, it is this author's opinion that a four-nap test is generally sufficient to diagnose narcolepsy.

Maintenance of Wakefulness Test (MWT)

The MWT is the mirror-image opposite of the MSLT. It measures the ability of the patient to stay awake in a darkened, quiet environment during the daytime [17]. Electrodes are applied for monitoring the EEG, eye movements, and chin EMG in a manner identical to the MSLT. The patient is provided five nap opportunities at two hourly intervals. The patient is advised to take the usual sleep-related medications in the morning, including stimulants. The MWT has been found useful in adult subjects in the assessment of effects of medications on sleepiness; for example, in the follow-up of patients with narcolepsy for quantifying the level of improvement following therapy with stimulant medications, or to determine the presence of a "carryover" effect of daytime sleepiness after nighttime hypnotic administration. In the management of children and adolescents with narcolepsy, the test may provide an estimate of the degree of residual sleepiness despite taking medications such as stimulants. Information derived from the MWT may help in adjustment of the total daily dose or of the time of administration of narcolepsy-related medications [18]. On other occasions, teens with chronic daytime sleepiness may wish to drive, for which this test may provide guidance. While the driving issue is best dealt with on a case by case basis, the clinician may utilize MWT data to help decide whether or not it will be safe for the patient to drive (author's opinion).

Actigraphy

This miniature device is about the size of a large wristwatch and can be conveniently strapped around the wrist. It consists of an acceleration sensor that translates physical motion into a numeric representation [19]. This numeric representation is sampled at regular intervals, e.g., every 0.1 s, and aggregated at a constant interval or epoch. Ambient illumination can also be recorded. The epoch length is usually 1 min. The stored movement data may be transferred to a computer for display, scoring, interpretation, and printing of results. By convention, the device is usually strapped to the non-dominant wrist. For deriving meaningful inferences about sleep–wake schedules, the duration of actigraph recordings has to be 1–2 weeks. Actigraphy is able to provide reliable data about average values of total time in bed, total sleep time, sleep efficiency, and sleep onset and offset times and if there has been excessive muscle activity during sleep.

Major indications for actigraphy include the investigation of insomnia and suspected circadian rhythm sleep disorders, e.g., delayed sleep phase syndrome. In patients with suspected narcolepsy, the actigraph recording can help ascertain whether there was adequate sleep at night prior to conducting PSG and MSLT. Actigraphy is also indicated for the investigation of sleep–wake problems of children with neurodevelopmental disorders such as autism and attention deficit hyperactivity disorders and to document treatment responses [20]. Conventional polysomnography may be difficult to obtain in this patient population due to lack of cooperation. Sadeh et al. [19] have found that the minute-by-minute agreement between actigraphic scoring and polysomnographic scoring was 90.2 % for normal adults and 89.9 % for children [21].

Utility and Limitations

Actigraphy is an excellent tool for the investigation of circadian rhythm disorders and insomnia. Advantages include its noninvasive nature and the ability to gather longitudinal information about sleep–wake function in the home environment over a 2–3-week period. It is relatively inexpensive when compared to nocturnal poly-somnography. Actigraphy is however unable to reliably differentiate REM from NREM sleep or assess sleep-disordered breathing. In-depth information about sleep architecture, e.g., percentage of time spent in various sleep stages or sleep electro-encephalographic events, also cannot be determined.

Dim Light Melatonin Onset (DLMO)

Melatonin is a major sleep-inducing and sleep-maintaining hormone that is pro-duced in the pineal gland following sympathetic neural activation by the suprachi-asmatic nucleus (SCN) of the hypothalamus. The SCN, in turn, is responsive to activation by light input from the retinohypothalamic pathway. There is generally good correlation between serum and salivary levels of melatonin. A rise in serum/salivary levels of melatonin usually occurs 2–3 h prior to sleep onset (dim light melatonin onset or DMLO) and signals sleep onset. DLMO is the most reliable measure of the timing of the circadian clock [22, 23]. The melatonin secretion rhythm is not affected by the rest–activity cycle, prior sleep, activity, or stress [24]. Melatonin has low levels during the daytime. Onset of darkness brings on a gradual rise in melatonin secretion. Typically, salivary or serum samples are collected every 30 min for 6 h prior to sleep onset. As melatonin secretion is very sensitive to per-turbation by ambient light exposure, the sample gathering is done in dim light (less than 30 lx). The samples are analyzed using radioimmunoassay techniques. The time of the clock at which there is a rise in melatonin levels by two standard devia-tions above the mean of three daytime values is termed DLMO [25]. The signifi-cance of DLMO is that it is the most reliable measure of activity of the SCN. A disadvantage of the DLMO testing process is that it requires considerable patient cooperation as well as involvement of sleep laboratory technical staff if the patient has a neurodevelopmental disability. DLMO is indicated in the investigation of cir-cadian rhythm disorders such as delayed sleep phase syndrome, advanced sleep phase syndrome, irregular sleep phase syndrome, and irregular sleep–wake rhythms. Disorders in which there is inversion of melatonin secretion, with low levels at night and higher secretion during the daytime, such as Smith–Magenis syndrome, may require round-the-clock sampling. Based upon longitudinal studies of DLMO, Carskadon et al. have lately raised an intriguing possibility of a decline in the pineal secretion of melatonin around puberty [26]. This might be one of the mechanisms underlying the sleep-onset phase delay that occurs in adolescents.

Sleep Survey Instruments

There are several excellent, clinically validated survey instruments that can be utilized in clinical practice and clinical sleep research. Only a few sleep survey instruments are reviewed here. Detailed reviews of the approximately 70 published survey instruments are available [27, 28]. Based upon the nature of patients in the practice, the sleep clinician should become familiar and comfortable with use of at least two to three survey instruments. In this era of rising healthcare costs where expensive and labor-intensive tools like PSG have limited in access, it is critical for the clinician to utilize survey instruments when possible. Assessment of treatment outcomes is also facilitated by the longitudinal use of sleep questionnaires.

The *Children's Sleep Habits Questionnaire* (CSHQ) is a 45-item validated questionnaire that asks parents to respond to questions about sleep–wake function of their child in the preceding 2 weeks. It is applicable to children between 4 and 10 years of age [29]. The eight domains of sleep disturbance that are addressed by CSHQ include bedtime resistance, sleep-onset delay, sleep duration, sleep anxiety, night awakenings, parasomnias, breathing disturbance, and daytime sleepiness. Responses are categorized as rarely, sometimes, or usually. Scores of 41 or greater correlate with a sleep disorder. The internal consistency of this questionnaire in a community sample of 4–10 year olds was 0.36–0.70, while the test–retest reliability over a 2-week period was 0.62–0.79 [29].

The *Sleep Disturbance Scale for Children* [7] is applicable to children 5–15 years of age. It is completed by the parent. Time consumed for survey completion is about 10 min. There are 27 items, with responses arranged on a 1–5 Likert scale. It is useful for evaluating insomnia, hypersomnia, parasomnias, and sleep-related respiratory disturbances. The questionnaire was developed after study of a large, predominantly urban, working, and middle-class Caucasian population from four public schools in Rome. It has excellent internal reliability (Cronbach's α 0.79 in a community sample and 0.71 in sleep disorder subjects). Test–retest reliability is also very good ($r = 0.71$).

The *Pediatric Sleep Questionnaire* [6] was developed for use in children ages 2–18 years. It's most commonly used 22-item sleep-disordered breathing subscale has sensitivity of 0.85 and specificity of 0.87 for sleep-disordered breathing. The scale is completed by the parent. The sleep-disordered breathing subscale takes 5–10 min for completion. Reference values for this scale are <0.33, and scores higher than this are generally associated with childhood obstructive sleep apnea.

The *Pediatric Daytime Sleepiness Scale* [30] is a self-report questionnaire, applicable to children 11–15 years of age. It was validated in a sample of 450, sixth to eighth grade students at a middle school, with 90% of the sample being white, reminder being a mix of other ethnicities. It has eight items that are scored on a 0–4 Likert scale, with scores higher than 16–18 indicative of sleepiness. It has good internal consistency (Cronbach's α 0.81)

Conclusions

Sleep laboratory tests yield accurate information and help guide management when they are integrated into the overall clinical assessment along with history and physical examination. Survey instruments are valuable in baseline and longitudinal assessment and in assessing impairments in the quality of life. Though there has been a shift toward unattended in-home polysomnography in adults, the indications, utility, and limitations of home sleep studies in children need study. The MSLT remains the gold standard test for study of daytime sleepiness. It is likely that with advances in the biomedical field, there will be further qualitative improvements in the assessment of sleep–wake function of children.

References

1. Iber C, Ancoli-Israel S, Chesson A, for the American Academy of Sleep Medicine, et al. The AASM manual for the scoring of sleep and associated events: rules, terminology, and technical specifications. 1st ed. Westchester: American Academy of Sleep Medicine; 2007.
2. Aurora RN, Zak RS, Karipoot A, et al. Practice parameters for the respiratory indications for polysomnography in children. Sleep. 2011;34:379–88.
3. Aurora RN, Lamm CI, Zak RS, et al. Practice parameters for the non-respiratory indications for polysomnography and multiple sleep latency testing for children. Sleep. 2012;35:1467–73.
4. Kotagal S, Nichols CD, Grigg-Damberger MM, et al. Non-respiratory indications for polysomnography and related procedures in children: an evidence based review. Sleep. 2012;35:1451–66.
5. Jasper HH. The ten twenty electrode system of the International Federation. Electroencepahlogr Clin Neurophysiol. 1958;10:371–5.
6. Chervin RD, Hedger K, Dillon JE, et al. Pediatric Sleep Questionnaire (PSQ): validity and reliability of scales for sleep disordered breathing, snoring, sleepiness and behavioral problems. Sleep Med. 2000;1:21–32.
7. Bruni O, Ottaviano S, Guidetti V, et al. The Sleep Disturbance Scale for Children (SDSC). Construction and validation of an instrument to evaluate sleep disturbances in childhood and adolescence. J Sleep Res. 1996;5:251–61.
8. Carskadon MA. Measuring daytime sleepiness. In: Kryger MH, Roth T, Dement WC, editors. Principles and practice of sleep medicine. 2nd ed. Philadelphia: Saunders; 1994. p. 961–83.
9. Kotagal S, Goulding PM. The laboratory assessment of daytime sleepiness in childhood. J Clin Neurophysiol. 1996;13:208–18.

10. Carskadon MA. The second decade. In: Guilleminault C, editor. Sleeping and waking disorders: indications and techniques. Menlo Park: Addison Wesley; 1982. p. 99–125.
11. Van den Hoed J, Kraemer H, Guilleminault C, et al. Disorders of excessive daytime somnolence: polygraphic and clinical data for 100 patients. Sleep. 1981;4:23–7.
12. Reiter J, Katz E, Scammell TE, et al. Usefulness of a nocturnal SOREMP for diagnosing narcolepsy with cataplexy in a pediatric population. Sleep. 2015;38:859–65.
13. Aldrich MS, Chervin RD, Malow BA. Sensitivity of the multiple sleep latency test (MSLT) for the diagnosis of narcolepsy. Neurology. 1995;45 suppl 4:A432.
14. Stepanski E, Lamphere J, Badia P, et al. Sleep fragmentation and daytime sleepiness. Sleep. 1984;7:18–26.
15. Lumley M, Roehrs T, Asker D, et al. Ethanol and caffeine effects on daytime sleepiness/alertness. Sleep. 1987;10:306–10.
16. Mamelak M, Buck L, Csima A, et al. Effects of flurazepam and zopiclone on the performance of chronic insomnia patients: a study of ethanol-drug interaction. Sleep. 1987;10:S79–87.
17. Mitler MM, Gujavarty KS, Brownman CP. Maintenance of wakefulness test: a polysomnographic technique for evaluating treatment in patients with excessive daytime somnolence. Electroencephalogr Clin Neurophysiol. 1982;53:648–61.
18. Zandieh S, Ramgopal S, Khatwa U, et al. The maintenance of wakefulness test in pediatric narcolepsy. Pediatr Neurol. 2013;48(6):443–6.
19. Sadeh A, Alster J, Urbach D, Lavie P. Actigraphically based automatic bedtime sleep-wake scoring: validity and clinical applications. J Amb Monitor. 1989;2:209–16.
20. Morgenthaler T, Alessi C, Friedman L, et al. Practice parameters for the use of actigraphy in the assessment of sleep and sleep disorders: an update for 2007. Sleep. 2007;30:519–29.
21. Sadeh A, Hauri PJ, Kripke D, Lavie P. The role of actigraphy in the evaluation of sleep disorders. Sleep. 1995;18:288–302.
22. Klerman EB, Gershengorn HB, Duffy JF, et al. Comparisons of the variability of three markers of the human circadian pacemaker. J Biol Rhythms. 2002;17:181–93.
23. Lewy AJ, Cutler NL, Sack RL. The endogenous melatonin profile as a marker for circadian phase position. J Biol Rhythms. 1999;14:227–36.
24. Lewy AJ, Sack RL. The dim light melatonin as a marker for circadian phase position. Chronobiol Int. 1989;6:93–102.
25. Kantermann T, Sung H, Burgess HJ. Comparing the morningness eveningness questionnaire and Munich chronotype questionnaire to the dim light melatonin onset. J Biol Rhythms. 2015;20:1–5.
26. Carskadon MA, Acebo C, Jenni OG. Regulation of adolescent sleep. Implications for behavior. Ann NY Acad Sci. 2004;1021:276–91.
27. Spruyt K, Gozal D. Pediatric sleep questionnaires as diagnostic or epidemiological tools: a review of currently available instruments. Sleep Med Rev. 2011;15:19–32.
28. Shahid A, Wilkinson K, Marcu S, Shapiro CM, editors. STOP, THAT and one hundred other sleep scales. New York: Springer; 2012. p. 1–333.
29. Owens JA, Spirito A, McGuinn M. The Children's Sleep Habits Questionnaire (CSHQ): psychometric properties of a survey instrument for school-aged children. Sleep. 2000;23:1043–51.
30. Drake C, Nickel C, Burduvalli E, et al. The Pediatric Daytime Sleepiness Scale (PDSS): sleep habits and school outcomes in middle school children. Sleep. 2003;26:455–8.

Chapter 6
Sleep Structure and Scoring from Infancy to Adolescence

Raffaele Ferri, Luana Novelli, and Oliviero Bruni

Abstract From birth to adolescence, substantial changes occur in sleep temporal organization, percentage of stages, and electroencephalographic patterns. A well-developed circadian rhythm is evident after 3 months of age, subsequently enriched by the appearance of an adult ultradian sleep cycle, after 9 months of age. In newborns, the NREM/REM alternation is included in a "polycyclic" sleep-wake pattern, as opposed to the "monocyclic" pattern, typical of adulthood/adolescence. While newborns sleep for about 60 % of the day, with increasing age the amount of daytime sleep shows a reduction and nighttime sleep becomes more stable and continuous, becoming somewhat consolidated starting from 12 months of life, when it lasts on average 12 h/night vs. 10 h of a 3-month-old baby. Sleep spindles appear as early as 4 weeks but are present in all subjects after 8 weeks of age; in infants and children, they are generally bilateral but asynchronous. K-complexes are well defined at 6 months of age, being most evident in the frontal areas. K-complex maturation progresses rapidly for the first 2 years of life. Slow-wave activity, the major feature of sleep, appears around 2 months of age, and its amplitude increases abruptly during the first years of life, peaking in childhood, and then declining across adolescence. After the manual developed by Anders et al. in 1971 for sleep scoring from birth to 4 months of age, the American Academy of Sleep Medicine more recently provided two sets of rules: one for scoring sleep in infants (<2 months) and another for scoring sleep in children. Finally, sleep microstructure can be assessed by the analysis of the cyclic alternating pattern (CAP) also in children;

R. Ferri, MD (✉)
Department of Neurology I.C, Sleep Research Centre, Oasi Institute for Research on Mental Retardation and Brain Aging (IRCCS), via C. Ruggero 73, 94018 Troina, Italy
e-mail: rferri@oasi.en.it

L. Novelli, PsyD
Department of Developmental Neurology and Psychiatry, Center for Pediatric Sleep Disorders, Sapienza University, Rome, Italy

O. Bruni, MD
Department of Developmental and Social Psychology, S. Andrea Hospital, Sapienza University, Rome, Italy

© Springer International Publishing Switzerland 2017
S. Nevšímalová, O. Bruni (eds.), *Sleep Disorders in Children*,
DOI 10.1007/978-3-319-28640-2_6

CAP rate shows a clear increasing trend with age, but the distribution of the different A subtypes (slow and fast) undergoes complex and different changes.

Keywords Sleep stage development • Sleep spindles • K-complexes • Slow-wave EEG activity • Sleep scoring • Active sleep • Quiet sleep • Cyclic alternating pattern

Introduction

Age and development are probably the most important key factors that regulate human sleep. From birth to adolescence, substantial changes occur in quality and quantity of sleep, its temporal organization, percentage of states of vigilance, and electroencephalographic (EEG) activity patterns. An important aspect is the fact that in infants, the features of the sleep EEG are determined not by chronological age (CA, number of days or weeks following birth) but by gestational age (GA, the time elapsed between the first day of the mother's last menstrual period and the day of delivery, expressed in completed weeks). Knowing an infant's GA is crucial for interpreting normality, immaturity, or abnormality of a sleep EEG. In fact, both brain and EEG develop and mature at a similar rate, independent of whether the infant is in utero or postdelivery [1].

A well-developed circadian rhythm is evident after 3 months of age, which is subsequently enriched by the appearance of an adult ultradian sleep cycle, after 9 months of age. Anders and Keener [2] described in newborns a NREM/REM alternation within a "polycyclic" sleep-wake pattern, as opposed to the "monocyclic" pattern, typical of adulthood/adolescence.

Easily measurable age-dependent changes are those concerning the sleep total amount and percentage distribution during the day. Newborns sleep for about 60 % of the day; with increasing age, the amount of daytime sleep shows a reduction and nighttime sleep becomes more stable and continuous [3]. The consolidation of nocturnal sleep starts to be evident from 12 months of life. At 12 months, a baby sleeps on average 12 h/night vs. 10 h of a 3-month-old baby [4].

Also the duration of sleep cycles changes with age, 60 min at 3 years vs. 120 min at 7 years, as well as the duration of total sleep, characterized by a progressive decrease from birth to elderly [4].

Key Sleep EEG Features During Infancy and Adolescence

Sleep Spindles

During the first 3 months of life, fundamental changes occur in the sleep EEG. Sleep spindles, a typical feature of stage 2 sleep, represent one of the EEG activities mostly influenced by age. Ellingson and Peters [5] reported that rolandic sleep spindle bursts appear in some subjects as early as 4 weeks post-term but are present in all after 8 weeks of age. Also, sleep spindles in infants and children have been reported to be generally bilateral but asynchronous [6]. Age-dependent changes also affect spindle duration and amount. Spindle density (number of spindles/min) reaches a peak between 4 and 9 months [7, 8]; subsequently, there is an evident increase that reaches a plateau at 5 years, persisting up to 16 years of age [9]. Jenni et al. [10] found, using spectral EEG analysis, a progressive increase in sigma activity from 3 to 9 months of age, confirming the age-dependent upward trend.

Rudimentary sleep spindles first appear at 43–48 weeks CA at the midline central (vertex) region. In infants, sleep spindles are often low-voltage 12–14 Hz, not the wider range of 11–16 Hz seen at later ages [11]. With respect to their scalp topographic location, Gibbs et al. [12] first reported the presence of two types of sleep spindles: slow (11–12 Hz) prevalent over the frontal regions and fast (14 Hz), peaking over the central and parietal scalp regions. The two types of spindle activities seem to show different courses of maturation. The peak frequency of the centroparietal spindles gradually increases with age, while frontal spindles decrease remarkably in power and become stable at about 13 years of age. The two types of spindles and the difference in their development may suggest the existence of different generators or a topographical difference during maturation in the thalamocortical network; the above authors suggested that frontal spindle activity could be a good indicator to evaluate CNS maturation in young children and adolescents.

K-Complexes

Another important phasic activity typical of sleep is the K-complex. Metcalf et al. [13] reported that K-complexes usually appear at 5 months post-term but are well defined by 6 months, being most evident in the frontal areas. K-complex maturation progresses rapidly for the first 2 years of life; then it slows down, although with increased variability, until the age of 5 years, progressing again toward a relative plateau in development at about 12 years of age [13]. At their first appearance, K-complexes are often characterized by low amplitude and long duration, while the faster negative component appears between 3 and 5 years of age and becomes more evident in adolescence [14]. From 3 to 9 years of age, K-complexes generally occur in rapid and repetitive runs, three to nine in 1–3 s, while from the adolescence their frequency decreases to 1/2–3 s [15]. K-complex frequency and amplitude decrease with age, in parallel with the decrease of spindle density and delta band power, and this fact can be attributed to the age-related changes of thalamocortical regulatory mechanisms [16].

Slow-Wave EEG Activity

Slow-wave activity (SWA) is probably the major feature of sleep and shows remarkable age-dependent changes. SWA appears around 2 months of age [10], and the amplitude of sleep slow waves increases abruptly during the first years of life [17], reaching a maximum in early childhood, and then declining markedly across adolescence [18–21]. This observation encouraged the hypothesis that during adolescence the human brain undergoes an extensive reorganization driven by synaptic elimination [22].

Jenni et al. [23] showed also that the nocturnal dynamics of sleep homeostasis are independent of the EEG derivation and remain stable across puberty; in fact, in both Tanner 4/5 and Tanner 1/2 adolescents, the decay rate of the sleep homeostatic process (reflected by the exponential decline of the 2 Hz EEG power band across the sleep episode) did not differ for derivations or groups. In this perspective, SWA may be considered to be a brain maturation index, and this finding might have several important clinical implication.

Sleep Staging

The manual developed by Anders et al. [24] in 1971 provides guidelines for sleep scoring from birth to 4 months of age, in normal full-term newborns. However, the increased knowledge of all the abovementioned age-dependent changes regarding the most important sleep activities has been central for the arrangement of more up-to-date criteria for sleep scoring, and the American Academy of Sleep Medicine [11] has more recently provided, in a new version of its scoring manual, two distinct sections: one concerning the criteria for scoring sleep in infants and another on the criteria of scoring sleep in children.

Sleep stage scoring is based on three basic measurements: the EEG, electrooculogram (EOG), and electromyogram (EMG). Also, especially in infants, heart rate, respiratory movements, airflow, and oxygen saturation are monitored and turn out to be essential for an appropriate sleep staging.

Anders Scoring Rules for Full-Term Newborns

Anders et al. [24] classified sleep from birth to 4 months of age into three states: active sleep (AS), quiet sleep (QS), and indeterminate sleep (IS); they further presumed that QS and AS were, respectively, antecedents of NREM and REM sleep. They recognized and defined also three states of wakefulness ("crying," "active awake," and "quiet awake").

Quiet sleep is characterized by minimal large or small muscle movements, and rhythmic breathing cycles, absence of eye movements; EEG shows typically slow waves and tracé alternant.

During active sleep, sucking motions, twitches, smiles, frowns, irregular breathing, and gross limb movements (converse to the typical REM sleep paralysis seen at later ages) are seen. Figure 6.1 shows examples of QS and AS in a 3-month-old infant.

Indeterminate sleep is the period of sleep that cannot be polysomnographically defined as either active or quiet sleep by predetermined criteria. EEG reveals low-voltage irregular activity or mixed activity.

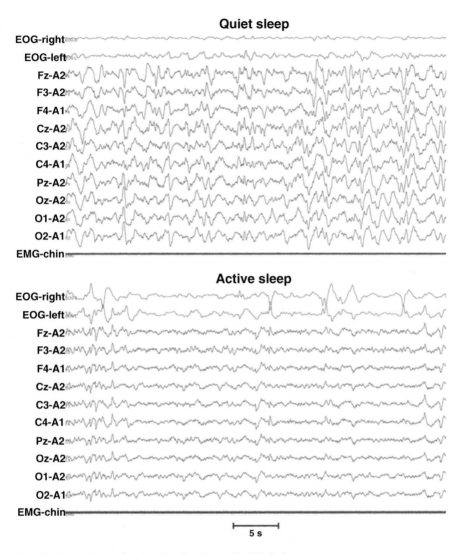

Fig. 6.1 Quiet sleep and active sleep in a 3-month-old infant

AASM Sleep Scoring Rules for Infants

The AASM manual recommends to apply these scoring rules in infants aged 0–2 months post-term (37–48 weeks CA). Sleep and wakefulness in infants 38–48 weeks CA are scored based on behavioral observation; regularity or irregularity of respiration; and EEG, EOG, and chin EMG patterns. We can distinguish four behavioral stages:

- Stage W (wakefulness)
- Stage N (NREM)

- Stage R (REM)
- Stage T (transitional)

Stage W can be scored if the following features are detected: eyes open for the major part of the epoch, vocalization (whimpering, crying, etc.) or actively feeding, sustained chin EMG tone with bursts of muscle activity, irregular respiration, and EEG background of continuous, symmetrical, irregular, low-to-medium amplitude mixed frequencies. EEG frequencies may include (a) irregular theta and delta activity, (b) diffuse irregular alpha and beta activity, (c) rhythmic theta activity, or (d) artifacts from body movements and eye movements.

Stage N (*NREM*) can be scored if four or more of the following features are present for more than half the length of the epoch: (a) eyes closed with no eye movements; (b) chin EMG tone present but lower than during W; (c) regular respiration; (d) tracé alternant (TA), high voltage slow (HVS), or sleep spindles; and (e) reduced movement relative to W. During this stage, sucking can occur.

Stage R (*REM*) can be scored if four or more of the following criteria are present: (a) low chin EMG; (b) eyes closed with at least one rapid eye movement; (c) irregular respiration; (d) mouthing, sucking, twitches, or brief head movements; and (e) continuous EEG pattern, including low voltage irregular (LVI), high voltage slow (HVS), and mixed (M) without sleep spindles.

Stage T (transitional) can be scored if an epoch contains either three NREM and two REM characteristics or two NREM and three REM characteristics. Most often, stage T occurs during transitions from stage W to stage R sleep, before awakening, and at sleep onset.

AASM Sleep Scoring Rules for Children

The AASM manual recommended applying the following scoring rules in children 2 months post-term or older.

- Stage W (wakefulness)
- Stage N1 (NREM 1)
- Stage N2 (NREM 2)
- Stage N3 (NREM 3)
- Stage N (NREM)
- Stage R (REM)

Stage W is characterized by age-appropriate posterior dominant rhythm over the occipital regions, eye blinks, rapid eye movements, and normal or high chin muscle tone. Posterior dominant rhythm (PDR) frequency that with age: 3.5–4.5 Hz at 3–4 months post-term, 5–6 Hz by 5–6 months, 7.5–9.5 Hz by 3 years of age, and alpha rhythm in older children.

The scoring rule for stage W is when more than 50 % of the epoch contains age-appropriate posterior dominant rhythm over the occipital region and/or if there is eye blinks (0.5–2 Hz), reading eye movements, or rapid eye movements associated with normal or high chin muscle tone.

Stage N1 is characterized by the presence of slow eye movements (SEM); low-amplitude, mixed-frequency activity (4–7 Hz); vertex sharp waves (sharply contoured waves with duration <0.5 s, maximal over the central region); hypnagogic hypersynchrony; and posterior dominant rhythm or high-amplitude, rhythmic 3–5 Hz activity. Stage N1 can be scored if the PDR is attenuated or replaced by low-amplitude, mixed-frequency activity for more than 50% of the epoch or if it is associated with theta activity (4–7 Hz) or with the other EEG patterns described above (SEMs, vertex waves, hypnagogic hypersynchrony, 3–5 Hz diffuse activity).

Stage N2 begins (in the absence of criteria for N3) if K-complexes unassociated with arousals and/or sleep spindles occur during the first half of one epoch or the last half of the previous epoch.

Stage N3 begins when ≥20% of an epoch consists of SWA, irrespective of age. Sleep spindles may persist in stage N3 sleep while eye movements are not typically seen. An example of this sleep stage in a 4-year-old infant can be seen in Fig. 6.2.

Stage R is characterized by the presence of rapid eye movements (REM), low chin EMG tone, sawtooth waves, transient muscle activity, and continuous, low-amplitude, mixed-frequency EEG activity. This EEG activity of stage R in infants and children looks like that of adults, although the dominant frequencies increase with age: 3 Hz activity at 7 weeks post-term, 4–5 Hz activity at 5 months, 4–6 Hz at 9 months, and 5–7 Hz theta activity at 1–5 years of age. By the age of 5–10 years, the low-amplitude, mixed-frequency activity in stage R is similar to that of adults [11].

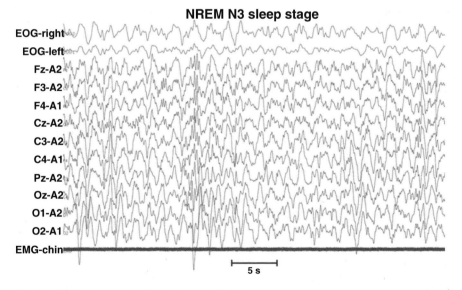

Fig. 6.2 NREM sleep stage N3 in a 4-year-old child

Stage N: Not all sleep waveforms are well developed by 2 months post-term; therefore, if all epochs of NREM sleep contain no recognizable sleep spindles, K-complexes, or high-amplitude 0.5–2 Hz slow-wave activity, score all epochs as stage N (NREM). However, NREM sleep can be scored as stage N1, N2, or N3 in most infants by age 5–6 months post-term and occasionally in infants as young as 4 months post-term.

Arousals: The rules for scoring arousals are similar to those of adults. During all sleep stages, it is characterized by an abrupt shift of EEG frequency including alpha, theta, and/or frequencies greater than 16 Hz (but not spindles) that lasts for at least 3 s, with at least 10 s of stable sleep preceding the change. In REM sleep, a concurrent increase in submental EMG lasting at least 1 s is required.

Cyclic Alternating Pattern (CAP)

CAP is an endogenous rhythm present in NREM sleep characterized by a periodic EEG activity with sequences of transient electrocortical activations (phase A of the cycle) that are distinct from the background EEG activity (phase B of the cycle). These sequences are repeated several times during the night and organized in a cyclic pattern interrupted by the presence of a stable sleep, without oscillations, called non-CAP (NCAP), longer than 60 s. CAP A phases have been subdivided into different subtypes: A1, A2, and A3, based on their frequency content [25, 26]. The A1 subtypes are composed prevalently by slow waves and the A3 subtype is generally composed of fast EEG activities, with subtype A2 presenting a combination of both.

In newborn and infants, CAP appears in a rudimentary form at 46–55 weeks CA, related to the emergence of an oscillating pattern of slow EEG activities, but the attainment of mature sleep EEG patterns is essential to score CAP. Miano et al. [27] suggested that two sleep EEG patterns are required to score CAP: (a) high-voltage slow activity (HVS) and rudimentary spindles and (b) SWS and spindles. In fact, CAP rate was 6.83 ± 3.58 S.D. in infants with the sleep EEG pattern (a) and increased to 12.9 ± 2.21 S.D. in children with pattern (b). The percentage of A1, A2, and A3 showed nonsignificant variations with age, but an increase of A1 index (number of events/hour) was observed in children with pattern (b). The duration of CAP events was similar in all age groups considered, and similarly, the arousal indexes were not statistically different [27].

In the preschool age, CAP rate clearly increases with highest values during SWS [28]. In comparison with infants and school-aged children, preschool subjects show a lower percentage of A1 and a corresponding increase in percentage of A2; this finding might represent an indirect marker of a more disturbed sleep or of the maturational processes of sleep [26].

The sleep structure in 6- to 10-year-old children is very stable and can be considered to be the "gold standard" for sleep quality because of its length, continuity, and restorative features [29]. Within this pattern of stable sleep architecture, CAP rate is higher than at younger ages and shows a progressive increase with the deepness of sleep, with the highest values during SWS [30]. In school-aged children, A1 subtypes are predominant (84.45 % of total) and occur mainly during SWS, followed by A3 (9.14 %) and A2 (6.44 %) subtypes. Similarly to preschool children and adults, CAP time structure shows the same periodicity of A1 subtypes, with a peak at around 25 s. The almost identical periodicity and time interval distribution of CAP A1 subtypes from infants to adults indicates that the periodicity of CAP components can be considered very stable during development [28, 31].

The way from preadolescence to adolescence is characterized by peculiar changes of the sleep EEG mainly represented by a decline of low EEG frequencies (theta and delta activities) in NREM [18]. These changes are convoyed by a great instability of sleep EEG that consequently affects CAP parameters. In fact, an important increase of CAP rate has been found in a group of peripubertal children (age 8–12 years; Tanner stage 2 and 3) who showed a CAP rate of 62.1 %; CAP A1 subtypes were the most numerous (85.5 %), whereas A2 were 9.1 % and A3 were 5 % [32]. Peripubertal and adolescents show the highest CAP rate among all life periods, if we exclude the elderly period [33] (Table 6.1).

CAP rate shows a clear increasing trend with age in the pediatric population, but the distribution of the different A subtypes shows a differential tendency with the percentage of A1 slightly declining in preschool children and then increasing, reaching the highest values during school age, and then decreasing again from school-aged children to adolescents (Fig. 6.3). On the contrary, A2 and A3 subtypes, apart from the preschool period, show a progressive increase from school age to elderly following the same trends of arousals [34]. The ratio between A1 and A2+A3 is highest in school-aged children, supporting the notion that sleep of these children is highly efficient and restorative. On the other hand, the increase of the percentage of A2 subtypes in preschoolers might represent the higher sleep instability of this age period. The A1 index (number of A1 subtypes per hour of NREM sleep) has a tendency to increase progressively until adolescence. This means that, although there is a decline of low EEG frequencies in this age period, the sleep process continues to produce the slow EEG oscillations needed for the restorative function of sleep and is probably related to the typical hormonal changes occurring during this phase of life.

Table 6.1 Age-related changes of the main CAP parameters during development

	1–4 months Miano et al. [27]	Preschool age Bruni et al. [28]	School age Bruni et al. [30]	Peripubertal Lopes et al. [32]	Adolescence Parrino et al. [33]
CAP rate%	12.9	25.93	33.43	62.1	43.4
A1 %	85.2	63.2	84.45	85.5	–
A2 %	10.3	21.5	6.44	9.1	–
A3 %	4.4	15.3	9.14	3.2	–
A1 index	19.8	24.8	39.54	–	45
A2 Index	2.8	6.5	2.66	–	12.4
A3 Index	0.5	4.0	3.30	–	5.7

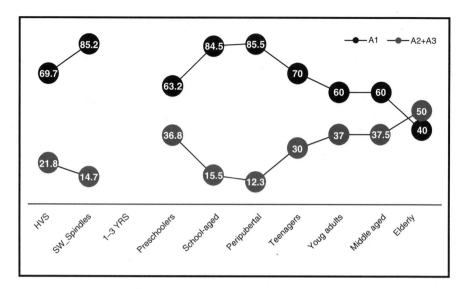

Fig. 6.3 Evolution of CAP A1 and A2+A3 subtypes during the life-span

Periodicity and interval distribution of CAP A1 subtypes are similar to those of school-aged children and adults, indicating that the periodicity of CAP components can be considered very stable during the whole life.

Conclusions

Cortical rhythms and functional networks change dramatically over infancy and childhood and provide a foundation upon which it is possible to understand better normal physiological brain development. These changes should be taken into account when approaching a sleep recording of an infant or a child since the variation of amplitude, frequency, and shape of the EEG waves should be fully considered in order to perform a correct scoring.

The power spectral analysis shows that the emergence of the peak in the NREM N2 sigma band corresponds with the development of sleep spindles, while lack of quantitative changes in the sigma band power after 3 months of age is consistent with the finding that sleep spindles are well developed by this age. The increase in the NREM N3 delta bandwidth may correspond with central brain maturation [35].

In relation to modifications of the EEG spectra, the main EEG patterns (vertex waves, spindles, K-complexes, slow-wave activity) undergo significant changes and follow a general pattern of maturation in which broadly distributed neuronal networks producing low-frequency oscillations increase in density, while networks characterized by high-frequency oscillations become sparser and highly clustered [36].

In conclusion, a correct scoring of sleep in infants and children cannot be performed without a deep knowledge of cortical maturation and of its changes at specific ages.

References

1. Grigg-Damberger M, Gozal D, Marcus CL, Quan SF, Rosen CL, Chervin RD, et al. The visual scoring of sleep and arousal in infants and children. J Clin Sleep Med. 2007;3(2):201–40.
2. Anders TF, Keener M. Developmental course of nighttime sleep-wake patterns in full-term and premature infants during the first year of life. I. Sleep. 1985;8(3):173–92.
3. McLaughlin C,V, Williams NA. Normal sleep in children and adolescents. Child Adolesc Psychiatr Clin N Am. 2009;18(4):799–811.
4. Iglowstein I, Jenni OG, Molinari L, Largo RH. Sleep duration from infancy to adolescence: reference values and generational trends. Pediatrics. 2003;111(2):302–7.
5. Ellingson RJ, Peters JF. Development of EEG and daytime sleep patterns in normal full-term infant during the first 3 months of life: longitudinal observations. Electroencephalogr Clin Neurophysiol. 1980;49(1–2):112–24.
6. Ellingson RJ, Peters JF. Development of EEG and daytime sleep patterns in low risk premature infants during the first year of life: longitudinal observations. Electroencephalogr Clin Neurophysiol. 1980;50(1–2):165–71.
7. Tanguay PE, Ornitz EM, Kaplan A, Bozzo ES. Evolution of sleep spindles in childhood. Electroencephalogr Clin Neurophysiol. 1975;38(2):175–81.
8. Shibagaki M, Kiyono S, Watanabe K. Spindle evolution in normal and mentally retarded children: a review. Sleep. 1982;5(1):47–57.
9. Scholle S, Zwacka G, Scholle HC. Sleep spindle evolution from infancy to adolescence. Clin Neurophysiol. 2007;118(7):1525–31.
10. Jenni OG, Borbely AA, Achermann P. Development of the nocturnal sleep electroencephalogram in human infants. Am J Physiol Regul Integr Comp Physiol. 2004;286(3):R528–38.
11. Berry RB, Brooks R, Gamaldo CE, Harding SM, Marcus CL, Vaughn BV. The AASM manual for the scoring of sleep and associated events: rules, terminology and technical specifications, Ver. 2.2. Darien: American Academy of Sleep Medicine; 2015.
12. Gibbs EL, Lorimer FM, Gibbs FA. Clinical correlates of exceedingly fast activity in the electroencephalogram. Dis Nerv Syst. 1950;11(11):323–6.
13. Metcalf DR, Mondale J, Butler FK. Ontogenesis of spontaneous K-complexes. Psychophysiology. 1971;8(3):340–7.
14. Sleep NE, EEG. In: Niedermeyer E, Lopes da Silva F, editors. Electroencephalography. Basic principles, clinical applications and related fields. Baltimore: Urban and Schwarzenburg; 1982. p. 175–81.
15. Kellaway P. Ontogenetic evolution of the electrical activity of the brain in man and animal. Acta Med Belg. 1957:141–54.
16. Halasz P. K-complex, a reactive EEG graphoelement of NREM sleep: an old chap in a new garment. Sleep Med Rev. 2005;9(5):391–412.
17. Feinberg I, Hibi S, Carlson VR. Changes in EEG amplitude during sleep with age. In: Nandy K, Sherwin I, editors. The aging brain and senile dementia. New York: Plenum Press; 1977. p. 86–98.
18. Campbell IG, Higgins LM, Trinidad JM, Richardson P, Feinberg I. The increase in longitudinally measured sleepiness across adolescence is related to the maturational decline in low-frequency EEG power. Sleep. 2007;30(12):1677–87.
19. Campbell IG, Feinberg I. Longitudinal trajectories of non-rapid eye movement delta and theta EEG as indicators of adolescent brain maturation. Proc Natl Acad Sci U S A. 2009;106(13): 5177–80.

20. Campbell IG, Darchia N, Khaw WY, Higgins LM, Feinberg I. Sleep EEG evidence of sex differences in adolescent brain maturation. Sleep. 2005;28(5):637–43.
21. Feinberg I, Higgins LM, Khaw WY, Campbell IG. The adolescent decline of NREM delta, an indicator of brain maturation, is linked to age and sex but not to pubertal stage. Am J Physiol Regul Integr Comp Physiol. 2006;291(6):R1724–9.
22. Feinberg I, Campbell IG. The onset of the adolescent delta power decline occurs after age 11 years: a comment on Tarokh and Carskadon. Sleep. 2010;33(6):737.
23. Jenni OG, Van RE, Carskadon MA. Regional differences of the sleep electroencephalogram in adolescents. J Sleep Res. 2005;14(2):141–7.
24. Anders T, Emde R, Parmelee A. A manual of standardized terminology, techniques and criteria for scoring of states of sleep and wakefulness in newborn infants. Los Angeles: UCLA Brain Information Service, NINDS Neurological Information Network; 1971.
25. Terzano MG, Parrino L, Smerieri A, Chervin R, Chokroverty S, Guilleminault C, et al. Atlas, rules, and recording techniques for the scoring of cyclic alternating pattern (CAP) in human sleep. Sleep Med. 2001;2:537–53.
26. Parrino L, Ferri R, Bruni O, Terzano MG. Cyclic alternating pattern (CAP): the marker of sleep instability. Sleep Med Rev. 2012;16(1):27–45.
27. Miano S, PiaVilla M, Blanco D, Zamora E, Rodriguez R, Ferri R, et al. Development of NREM sleep instability-continuity (cyclic alternating pattern) in healthy term infants aged 1 to 4 months. Sleep. 2009;32(1):83–90.
28. Bruni O, Ferri R, Miano S, Verrillo E, Vittori E, Farina B, et al. Sleep cyclic alternating pattern in normal preschool-aged children. Sleep. 2005;28(2):220–30.
29. Carskadon M, Keenan S, Dement WC. Nighttime sleep and daytime sleep tendency in preadolescents. In: Guilleminault C, editor. Sleep and its disorders in children. New York: Raven; 1987. p. 43–52.
30. Bruni O, Ferri R, Miano S, Verrillo E, Vittori E, Della MG, et al. Sleep cyclic alternating pattern in normal school-age children. Clin Neurophysiol. 2002;113(11):1806–14.
31. Bruni O, Novelli L, Miano S, Parrino L, Terzano MG, Ferri R. Cyclic alternating pattern: a window into pediatric sleep. Sleep Med. 2010;11(7):628–36.
32. Lopes MC, Rosa A, Roizenblatt S, Guilleminault C, Passarelli C, Tufik S, et al. Cyclic alternating pattern in peripubertal children. Sleep. 2005;28(2):215–9.
33. Parrino L, Boselli M, Spaggiari MC, Smerieri A, Terzano MG. Cyclic alternating pattern (CAP) in normal sleep: polysomnographic parameters in different age groups. Electroencephalogr Clin Neurophysiol. 1998;107(6):439–50.
34. Terzano MG, Parrino L, Rosa A, Palomba V, Smerieri A. CAP and arousals in the structural development of sleep: an integrative perspective. Sleep Med. 2002;3(3):221–9.
35. Sankupellay M, Wilson S, Heussler HS, Parsley C, Yuill M, Dakin C. Characteristics of sleep EEG power spectra in healthy infants in the first two years of life. Clin Neurophysiol. 2011;122(2):236–43.
36. Chu CJ, Leahy J, Pathmanathan J, Kramer MA, Cash SS. The maturation of cortical sleep rhythms and networks over early development. Clin Neurophysiol. 2014;125(7):1360–70.

Chapter 7
Algorithm for Differential Diagnosis of Sleep Disorders in Children

Stephen H. Sheldon

Abstract Process of solving clinical problems begins with a complaint or chief complaint. This statement begins a cascade of events that occurs very rapidly and, for the experienced clinician, almost instantaneously and unconsciously. Theories about potential underlying etiologies are entertained, and a "list" of possible diagnoses is created that guides all further clinical evaluation and inquiry. Following this key initial encounter with the patient and/or parents, questioning begins (history of the presenting problem). Questions are asked of the parents/patients *testing* each theory, based on symptoms of possible etiologies known to the clinician. Answers to these questions either support or refute a specific diagnosis. Questioning parents/patients continues until possible diagnoses are eliminated or maintained then ordered on a list of probable diagnoses. When no further questioning can either confirm or refute the presence of symptoms of particular diagnoses, the clinician then moves to reviewing various systems and obtaining other information that may have nothing to do with an initial hypothesis, but this questioning is required for completeness and because there are many sleep-related disorders with overlapping symptoms. Information regarding past medical history, family history, and social history is obtained as the clinician tests the original theories. There comes a point of diminishing returns when further questioning does not move the inquiry into the cause of the complaint further. A physical examination is then performed. Physical findings associated with those theories/etiologies are searched for, and their presence or absence either supports or refutes the theory respectively. Observations of experienced clinicians conducting a clinical evaluation have shown this process is repeated between patients, and data collected by the clinician from each patient is *not* accomplished in a regimented sequential manner as most history and physical forms and electronic medical records require. In fact, the process is quite rapid, and a comprehensive assessment of patients' complaints is accomplished in the first quarter of the clinical encounter.

S.H. Sheldon, DO, FAAP
Northwestern University Feinberg School of Medicine, Chicago, IL, USA

Sleep Medicine Center, Ann & Robert H. Lurie Children's Hospital of Chicago,
225 E. Chicago Avenue, Box 43, Chicago, IL 60611, USA
e-mail: ssheldon@luriechildrens.org; overa@luriechildrens.org;
chicgaosheldon@sbcglobal.net

Keywords Differential diagnosis • Clinical sleep assessment • Clinical problem-solving • Pediatric sleep diagnoses • Pediatric sleep assessment • Algorithm for diagnosis

Process of Solving Clinical Problems

Process of solving clinical problems begins with a complaint or chief complaint. This statement begins a cascade of events that occurs very rapidly and, for the experienced clinician, almost instantaneously and unconsciously [1]. Theories about potential underlying etiologies are entertained, and a "list" of possible diagnoses is created that guides all further clinical evaluation and inquiry. Following this key initial encounter with the patient and/or parents, questioning begins (history of the presenting problem). Questions are asked of the parents/patients *testing* each theory, based on symptoms of possible etiologies known to the clinician. Answers to these questions either support or refute a specific diagnosis. Questioning parents/patients continues until possible diagnoses are eliminated or maintained then ordered on a list of probable diagnoses. When no further questioning can either confirm or refute the presence of symptoms of particular diagnoses, the clinician then moves to reviewing various systems and obtaining other information that may have nothing to do with an initial hypothesis, but this questioning is required for completeness and because there are many sleep-related disorders with overlapping symptoms. Information regarding past medical history, family history, and social history is obtained as the clinician tests the original theories. There comes a point of diminishing returns when further questioning does not move the inquiry into the cause of the complaint further. A physical examination is then performed. Physical findings associated with those theories/etiologies are searched for, and their presence or absence either supports or refutes the theory respectively. Observations of experienced clinicians [1] conducting a clinical evaluations have shown this process is repeated between patients, and data collected by the clinician from each patient is *not* accomplished in a regimented sequential manner as most history and physical forms and electronic medical records require. In fact, the process is quite rapid, and a comprehensive assessment of patients' complaints is accomplished in the first quarter of the clinical encounter.

Following the history and physical examination, clinicians come to a point of closure, where no further clinical history or physical examination will contribute to defining the underlying diagnosis or refining those diagnoses that cannot be ruled out. What remains is termed a "differential diagnosis." Laboratory testing may or may not be required to further refine the differential diagnosis, and many sleep-related problems in childhood may be diagnosis on history and physical examination alone. When laboratory testing is required, the examinations ordered are based on the remaining differential diagnoses. Testing can then either confirm a main diagnosis and/or eliminate other diagnoses.

Underlying this process is structured approach to searching the history, and conducting a physical examination requires a wide knowledge base of presenting signs and symptoms of a large number of sleep-related disorders. The *International Classification of Sleep Disorders* – 3rd Edition [2] published by the American Academy of Sleep Medicine provides a comprehensive overview of signs, symptoms, and laboratory evaluation of sleep disorders in adults and several variations in children. Nonetheless, this comprehensive compilation of methods of diagnosis of sleep disorders is difficult to use in the clinical encounter and is structured to be used as a reference not a tool to guide the clinical encounter and clinical problem-solving when the clinician is with the patient in the examination room.

Screening tools and questionnaires are helpful, but cannot replace the clinician. Few are standardized and rarely provide the necessary diagnostic capability alone [3]. Sleep logs can help observations that might otherwise be overlooked or misinterpreted by sleepy parents. A 2-week sleep diary can provide the clinician quasi-objective information regarding parental interpretations of the child's sleep-wake schedule and can either confirm their original observations or provide a better assessment of habitual sleep habits and schedules. The *BEARS* screening tool created by Owens and Dalzell has a specific usefulness in the primary care setting and in the sleep clinic to help guide inquiry into the nightlife of children [4].

The following algorithms are based on questions developed and modified from the BEARS screening tool [4] and other suggested algorithms [5–7].

Bedtime

Inquiry Design:

1. What time does the child go to bed?
2. Does the child have problems falling to sleep?
3. How long does it take for the child to habitually fall to sleep?
4. What activities occur prior to bedtime?

Bedtime
Complaint: Problems Going to Bed/Problems Falling To Sleep (See Fig. 7.1)

Parent or caretaker reports the child has one or more of the following symptoms:

- Difficulty falling to sleep.
- Difficulty staying asleep.
- Early morning wakings, earlier than desired.
- Bedtime struggles at an age-appropriate time of the night.
- Parental/caretaker intervention required for easy transitioning to sleep.
- Daytime symptoms are present[*].
- There is adequate and appropriate environment and opportunity to sleep.
- Symptoms are present for more than 3 nights per week.

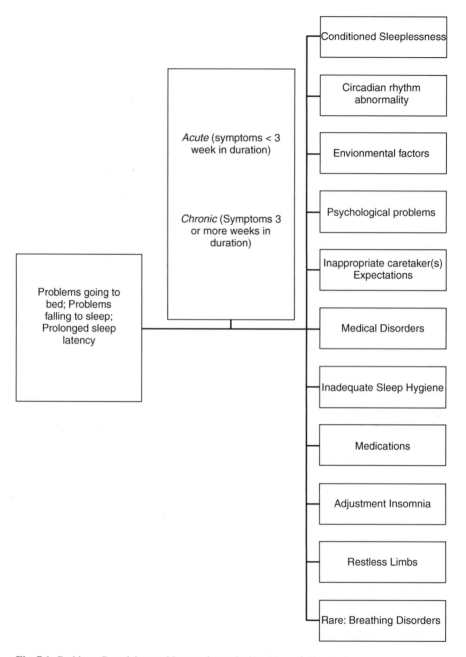

Fig. 7.1 Bedtime. Complaint: problems going to bed/problems falling to sleep

Acute Insomnia Disorder ⇦ ⇨ *Chronic Insomnia Disorder*

Symptoms have been present for less than 3 weeks   Symptoms have been present for more than 3 weeks.

*Symptoms might include one or more of the following: complaint of daytime fatigue; attention, concentration, or memory problems; school learning difficulties; socialization problems; mood difficulties; behavior problems; hyperactivity; impulsiveness; motor restlessness; fidgetiness; unusual aggression; difficulty with motivation; accidents; and parents are dissatisfied with the youngster's sleep.

Other Sleep Disorders (*see* Table 7.1)

Although Environmental Sleep Disorders was listed in ICSD-2 (REF), it is unclear whether this is a specific sleep-related disorder or part of the home environment, such that when the environment is different, sleep complaints resolve. This, however, is not the case for many children with problem on sleeplessness, where a physiological conditioning has created a biological problem that may be developmentally related.

Table 7.1 Other pediatric sleep disorders (May present with problem sleeplessness, problem sleepiness, or both)

Symptoms	Sleeps well somewhere and/or under certain circumstances	Daytime dysfunction	Excessive noise, light, temperature	Medications (even over the counter)	Other medical/ psychological problems
Diagnoses					
Conditioned sleeplessness	++[a]	+/−	−	−	−
Environmental factors	+	+/−	++	−	−
Psychological problems	+/−	+/−	+/−	+/−	++
Inappropriate caretaker's expectations	++[b]	+/−	−	−	−
Inadequate sleep hygiene	−	++[c]	+	+/−	+/−
Medications	−	+/−	−	++	+
Adjustment sleep disorder	−	+	−	−	+[d]
Medical disorders	−	+/−	−	++	+[e]

++ = Cardinal symptom(s), + = Typically present, +/− = May or may not be initially reported as present, − = Typically absent

[a]The child can sleep well when transitional objects and/or situations are present; they cannot transition well into sleep or fall back to sleep until these transitional objects and/or conditions are retrieved at night

[b]Parent's/caretaker's expectations of the child's sleep habits are significant inconsistent with normal sleep/wake habits and patterns for the child's chronological age

[c]Nighttime schedules and patterns are irregular and chaotic. Daytime schedules and patterns are also chaotic

[d]There may be situational stressors identified, including but not limited to holidays, travel, social stressors, and school pressures

[e]Signs and/or symptoms of other medical disorders may be present

Excessive Daytime Sleepiness (see Fig. 7.2)

Inquiry Design:
1. Does the child have difficulty waking in the morning?
    (Must differentiate whether the child "cannot wake up" or "does not want to wake up".)
2. Does the child experience unintentional sleep episodes or sleep attacks?
3. If the child is over 6 years of age, does he/she habitually nap?
4. Does the child fall, feel weak, become wobbly, or develop an unusual facial expression when laughing, giggling, or emotional?
5. Are there nightmares (particularly at wake-sleep transition)?
6. Does the child act out dreams?
7. Does bedtime and morning wake time significantly differ between school days and weekends?
8. Are there problems paying attention? Frequent daydreaming?
9. Are there school performance problems?
10. Does the child wake at night? How long? How many times?
11. Does the child walk or scream during sleep? Is there amnesia for the events?
12. What is the typical length of total sleep each 24 h?
13. Does the child have any acute or chronic medical illnesses or on any medication?
14. Are symptoms recurrent?
15. Does the child snore, pause, snort, gasp, choke, or cough during sleep?

Note: There is considerable overlap of symptoms and findings. Similar symptoms and comorbidities are common. See specific sections for differential diagnosis.

Excessive Daytime Sleepiness (Hypersomnias) (See Table 7.2)
The parent(s) and/or caretaker(s) report the child has one or more of the following symptoms:

Falling asleep at unusual times

> The child may fall to sleep while eating meals, talking on the telephone, playing a game, at a party, or on the playground.
> Note: Many children will fall to sleep as passengers in a car or watching television. Falling to sleep at unusual times means the child is consolidating sleep at a time that is not expected for this youngster's chronological and maturational age.

The child feels sleepy during the day.
Teachers or other observers report the child looks sleepy during the day.
Attention problems/concentration problems.
Hyperactivity/motor restlessness/fidgetiness.
Impulsiveness.
Learning difficulties in school.
Difficulty waking in the morning.

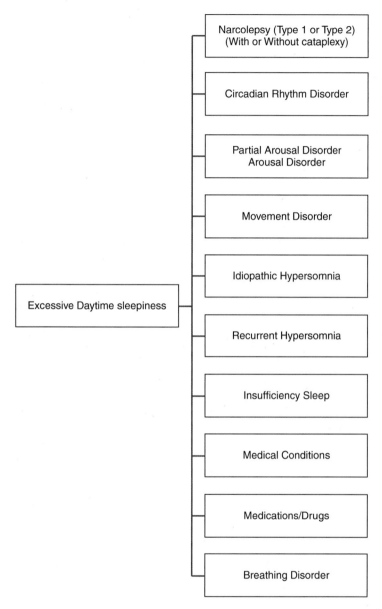

Fig. 7.2 Excessive daytime sleepiness

Awakening (See Fig. 7.3)

Inquiry Design:

1. Does the child wake at night? How many times? At what time?
2. How long does the child remain awake?
3. Does the youngster seem fully awake or is the child confused/disoriented?

Table 7.2 Excessive daytime sleepiness (hypersomnias)

Symptoms Diagnosis	Unintentional sleep episodes and/or sleep attacks	Habitual napping	Cataplexy	Hypnagogic hallucinations	Sleep paralysis	CSF hypocretin <110 pg/mL	Abnormal MSLT SOL <8 min and 2+ SOREMPS	Increased total sleep time	Recurrent symptoms	Other symptoms
Narcolepsy type 1	++	+	++	+/−	+/−	+	+[a]	+/−	−	[b]
Narcolepsy type 2	++	+	−	+/−	+/−	−	+[c]	+/−	−	[d]
Narcolepsy due to medical disorder	+	+	+/−	+/−	+/−	−	+	+/−	−	[e]
Hypersomnia due to medical disorder	+	+	−	−	−	−	+[f]	+	−	[g]
Idiopathic hypersomnia	+	+	−	−	−	−	+[h]	++	−	[i]
Kleine-Levin syndrome (recurrent hypersomnia)	+	+	−	−	−	−	+/−[j]	+	++	[k]

++ = Cardinal symptom(s), + = Typically present, +/− = May or may not be initially reported as present, − = Typically absent

[a]During childhood, if narcolepsy Type 1 is strongly considered and MSLT findings are not conclusive, repeat testing in 6 months to 1 year is recommended. MSLT findings that might suggest (but are not diagnostic of) the presence of excessive daytime sleepiness include shorter than expected mean sleep onset latency for age, consolidated sleep on three or more naps on five nap attempts, and frequent micro-sleep episodes on nap attempts. Symptoms that are not diagnostic of but may suggest excessive sleepiness include but are not limited to hyperactivity, attention span difficulties, learning difficulties, impulsivity, and behavior problems. These symptoms might alternate with sleepiness. Symptoms of cataplexy might be mistaken for *syncope*; hypnagogic hallucinations might be mistaken for nocturnal fears and/or nightmares; sleep paralysis might be mistaken for difficulty waking in the morning (resisting waking up rather than inability to move upon waking)

[b]REM sleep behavior disorder/REM sleep motor abnormalities might be present; nocturnal sleep, although normal in length, is considerably fragmented

[c]During childhood, if narcolepsy Type 1 is strongly considered and MSLT findings are not conclusive, repeat testing in 6 months to 1 year is recommended. MSLT findings that might suggest (but are not diagnostic of) the presence of excessive daytime sleepiness include shorter than expected mean sleep onset latency for age, consolidated sleep on three or more naps on five nap attempts, and frequent micro-sleep episodes on nap attempts. Symptoms that are not diagnostic of but may suggest excessive sleepiness include but are not limited to hyperactivity, attention span difficulties, motor restlessness, learning difficulties, impulsivity, and behavior problems. These symptoms might alternate with sleepiness

[d]Cataplexy is notably absent

[e]Para-neoplastic syndromes; Prader-Willi syndrome; myotonic dystrophy; head trauma

[f]Mean sleep latency may be short ($\leq$8 min), but $\leq$1 SOREMP is present

[g]Symptoms of associated medical disorder may be notable on history and/or physical examination

[h]Mean sleep latency may be short ($\leq$8 min), but $\leq$1 SOREMP is present

[i]Total sleep time is significantly greater than expected for age for each 24 h period

[j]MSLT may be significantly abnormal during episodes and normal during inter-episode periods

[k]Associated recurrent features might include hyperphagia and behavioral abnormalities (e.g., hypersexuality/sexually acting-out behavior)

4. Is there amnesia for the event?
5. Does the child report a dream?
6. Is there trouble falling back to sleep after the waking?
7. What is the sleeping environment like?
8. Are there lights on in the bedroom?
9. Does the child have "screen time" before bed?
10. Are there any acute or chronic illnesses?
11. Is the child taking any medication?

Note: There is considerable overlap of symptoms and findings. Similar symptoms and comorbidities are common.
See specific sections for differential diagnosis.

Awakenings During the Night (Parasomnias and Sleep-Related Movement Disorders)
Complaints/Symptoms
The patient exhibits and/or experiences one or more of the following symptoms:

- Falls to sleep easily but wakes frequently during the night.
- Walks, talks, or screams during sleep.
- There may or may not be difficulty falling back to sleep after waking at night.

Disorders of Arousal from NREM Sleep
The child exhibits the following general symptoms:

- Episodes of incomplete waking are noted.
- There has been inappropriate or lack of responsiveness to efforts to intervene or redirect the child during the spell.
- There is limited or no associated free memory during the spell.
- There is amnesia for the event.
- The event typically occurs during the first third to first half of the major sleep period.
- Complex behaviors may occur.
- Behaviors are not better explained by another sleep disorder, psychological problem, or medications/substances.

See Table 7.3 diagnosis and differential diagnostic findings.

Regularity (See Fig. 7.4)

Inquiry Design:

1. Has a regular sleep schedule been established?
2. Is the sleep schedule consistent from night to night?
3. What time does the child habitually get into bed?
4. What time does the child habitually wake in the morning?
5. Are there significant differences between bedtimes and wake times on weekdays, weekends, and/or holidays?

Fig. 7.3 Awakening

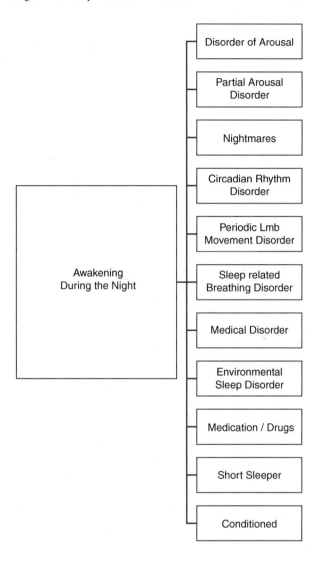

Note: There is considerable overlap of symptoms and findings. Similar symptoms and comorbidities are common.

See specific sections for differential diagnosis.

Regularity (Circadian Rhythm Sleep-Wake Disorders)
Complaints/Symptoms

The patient exhibits and/or experiences one or more of the following symptoms:

- A regular sleep/wake schedule has not been established.
- Bedtime is either inappropriate for the child's developmental level.
- Habitual time of morning sleep offset is inappropriate for the child's developmental level.

Table 7.3 Awakenings (arousals and/or partial arousals from sleep)

Symptoms	Recurrent episodes of partial and/or incomplete awakenings from sleep	Partial or complete amnesia for the event(s)	1st third to half of the sleep period (usually from N3 sleep)	Last third to half of the sleep period (usually from REM sleep)	Intense autonomic discharges and intense agitation	Exacerbated by fever or rebound from sleep deprivation	Displacement from the bed (leaves the bed during the spell)	Eats during the spell	Vivid dream recall	Occurs at sleep onset or sleep offset (while falling to sleep or just after waking)	Enuresis
Diagnosis											
Confusional arousals	++	+	+	−	−	+	−	−	−	−	−
Sleepwalking	++	+	+	−	−	+	++	−	−	−	+/−
Sleep terrors	++	+	+++	−	++	+	−	−	−	−	−
Sleep-related eating disorder	+	+/−	+/−	+/−	−	−	+	++[a]	−	−	−
REM sleep behavior disorder	+	−	−	+	+[b]	+/−	−	−	++	−	−
Recurrent isolated sleep paralysis	+/−	−	−	−	−	−	−	−	−	+	−
Nightmare sleep disorder	−	−	−	−	−	−	−[c]	−	++	+/−[d]	−
Sleep-related hallucinations	−	−	−	−	−	−	−	−	++[e]	+	−
Sleep enuresis (primary)	−	−	−	−	−	−	−	−	−	−	++[f]

Sleep enuresis (secondary)	−	−	−	−	−	−	−	−	−	−	++[g]
Parasomnias due to medical disorder[h]	−	−	−	−	−	−	−	−	−	−	−
Medication/ substance[i]	−	−	−	−	−	−	−	−	−	−	−

++ = Cardinal symptom(s), + = Typically present, +/− = May or may not be initially reported as present, − = Typically absent

[a] PICA may be present; injury surrounding preparing food or eating food is not uncommon

[b] The child appears and reports to be acting out dreams. Injury to self and/or others might occur

[c] The child might leave the bed to obtain caretaker comfort and may walk into parent room but awake. There is only mild agitation and autonomic discharge (if any). The child might act frightened and remain awake for an extended period of time

[d] If the nightmare occurs at sleep onset, it is more likely termed a hypnagogic hallucination; sleep latency might be prolonged and the child might complain of nocturnal fears

[e] Typically visual hallucinations occur

[f] The child is older than 5 years and has never had 6 months without a wet bed

[g] The child is older than 5 years and has had a 6 month dry interval with return of the symptom of bedwetting; although this may be behavioral, an organic etiology is much more likely when compared to primary sleep-related enuresis

[h] May be caused by an underlying neurological disorder; symptoms of the neurological abnormality may be present; seizure disorders may present as a parasomnia

[i] There is a temporal relationship between the onset of symptoms and ingestion of a medication or substance that can result in a parasomnia

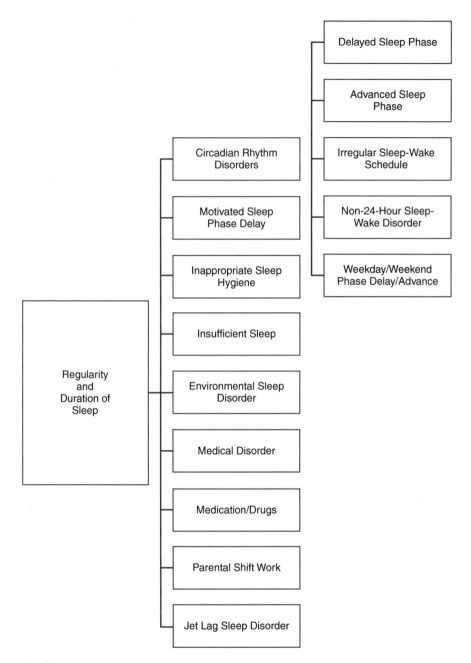

Fig. 7.4 Regularity

- There is significant difference between bedtime and morning time of sleep offset on school days when compared to weekends and/or holidays from school.

See Table 7.4 for diagnosis and differential diagnostic findings.

Snoring (See Fig. 7.5)

Inquiry Design:

1. Does the child snore three or more nights per week?
2. Is snoring or breathing associated with pauses, snorts, gasps, choking, or coughing?
3. Does the child breathe through his/her mouth at night? During the day?
4. Is sleep restless?
5. Does the child wake frequently at night?
6. Does the child wake in the morning with headaches?
7. Is the child excessively thirsty in the morning?
8. Does the child wet the bed at night? Primary enuresis? Secondary enuresis?
9. Are there reported witnessed apneas? Increased work of breathing? Paradoxical respiration?
10. Is there sleep-related diaphoresis?
11. Are there daytime symptoms of hyperactivity, attention problems, impulsivity, and/or learning difficulties?
12. Does hyperactivity and attention problems alternate with sleepiness?
13. Are the tonsils enlarged?
14. What is the child's Mallampati classification sitting and supine?

Note: There is considerable overlap of symptoms and findings. Similar symptoms and comorbidities are common.

See specific sections for differential diagnosis.

Snoring (Sleep-Related Breathing Disorders in Children)
Complaints/Symptoms

- Snoring for more than three nights per week
- Breathing punctuated by pauses, snorts, gasping, or choking
- Habitual mouth breathing
- Waking with morning headaches
- Sleep-related diaphoresis
- Inappropriate age-related secondary sleep enuresis
- Reported witnessed apneas
- Reported increased work of breathing
- Daytime sleepiness, inattention, hyperactivity
- Frequent nocturnal waking
- Sleep-related bruxism
- Habitual waking in the morning with a dry mouth

See Table 7.5 for diagnosis and differential diagnostic findings.

Table 7.4 Regularity (circadian rhythm disorders)

Symptoms Diagnosis	Difficulty falling to sleep at a desired time (complaint of insomnia)	Difficulty waking at a desired time	Wakes late when permitted to sleep ad lib	Complains of daytime sleepiness	Increased total sleep time	Asymptomatic periods	Irregularity of symptoms	Intermittent normal intervals	Other symptoms
Delayed sleep phase syndrome	++	+	+	+	−	−	−	−	a
Advanced sleep phase syndrome	−	−	−	−	−	−	−	−	b
Irregular sleep-wake cycle disorder	+	+	−	+	−	−	++	−	c
Non-24 h sleep-wake rhythm disorder/free-running disorder	+	+	−	+	+/−	+	+/−	++	d
Jet lag syndrome	+	+	+/−	+	−	−	+/−	−	e

++ = Cardinal symptom(s), + = Typically present, +/− = May or may not be initially reported as present, − = Typically absent

[a] Frequent napping may be present; poor school performance might occur. Weekend phase delay is common during adolescence; symptoms of delayed sleep phase are prominent during the beginning of the week only to improve later in the week

[b] Parents may complain of the child waking too early in the morning

[c] Chronic irregular sleep periods and wake periods throughout the 24 h period

[d] The child's "day" is longer than 24 h and may be common in sightless children

[e] Travel across two or more time zones is usually elicited on history; other somatic symptoms (particularly gastrointestinal) often occur

Fig. 7.5 Snoring

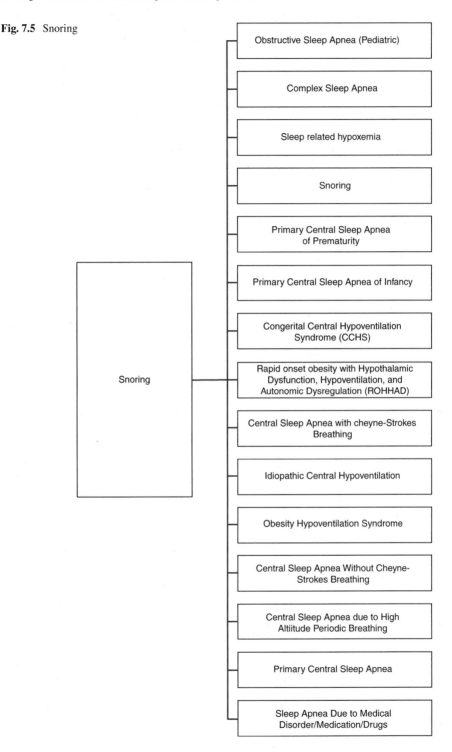

Table 7.5 Snoring (sleep-related respiratory disorders in children)

Symptoms	Snoring	Observed pauses, snorts, gasps	Increased work of breathing	PSG ≥5 obstructive apneas per hour of sleep	SpO2 falls >90% ≥5 min	EtCO₂ >50 mmHg for >25% of TST		Fragmented sleep	Excessive daytime sleepiness	Periodic breathing	PSG central apneas ≥5/h and/or CA ≥20 s	Autonomic dysfunction	Other symptoms
						Awake	Sleep						
Diagnosis													
Obstructive sleep apnea	++	+/-	+	++	[a]	-	+/-	+	+/-	-	-	-	[b]
Snoring	++	-	-	-	-	-	-	-	-	-	-	-	-
Obesity hypoventilation	++	+/-	+	+	+	++	++	+	+	-	-	-	[c]
Sleep-related hypoxemia	+/-	+/-	+/-	+/-	++	-	-	+	+/-	-	-	-	-
Complex sleep apnea	++	+/-	+	+	+	-	+/-	+/-	+/-	-	++	-	[d]
Hypoventilation due to medical disorder	+/-	+/-	+/-	+/-	+/-	+/-	++	+/-	+/-	-	+/-	+	[e]
Medication/substance	+/-	+/-	+/-	+/-	++	+/-	++	+/-	+/-	+/-	+/-	-	[f]
Primary CSA of prematurity	-	-	-	-	+/-	+/-	+/-	+/-	-	++	++	-	[g]
Primary CSA of infancy	-	-	-	-	+/-	+/-	+/-	+/-	-	++	++	-	[h]
Primary CSA	+	+	-	+/-	+/-	-	-	+	+	-	++	-	[i]
CSA with Cheyne-Stokes	+/-	+	-	-	+	+/-	+/-	+/-	+	++	+/-	-	[j]

Diagnosis

Symptoms Diagnosis	Snoring	Observed pauses, snorts, gasps	Increased work of breathing	SpO2 falls ≥3% from baseline	EtCO2 >50 mmHg for >25% of TST Awake	EtCO2 >50 mmHg for >25% of TST Sleep	Fragmented sleep	Excessive daytime sleepiness	Periodic breathing	Central apneas ≥5/h. and/or CA ≥20 s	Autonomic dysfunction	Other symptoms
CSA due to medical disorder WITHOUT Cheyne-Stokes	–	+	–	–	+/–	+/–	+/–	+/–	–	++	–	k
CSA due to medication or substance	–	+	+/–	+/–	+/–	+/–	+/–	+/–	–	++	–	l
Idiopathic central alveolar hypoventilation	–	–	–	+/–	–	++	+/–	+/–	–	–	–	m
Congenital central hypoventilation syndrome (CCHS)	+/–	+/–	+/–	+	++	++	+/–	+/–	+/–	+	+	n
Late-onset central hypoventilation with hypothalamic dysfunction (ROHHAD)	+/–	+/–	+/–	+	++	++	+	+/–	+/–	+/–	+	o

++ = Cardinal symptom(s), + = Typically present, +/– = May or may not be initially reported as present, – = Typically absent

a Oxygen desaturation of at least 3% from the baseline is required for identification of an obstructive apnea or hypopnea

b When there is less than 3% desaturation from the baseline, apneas, and hypopneas (and RERAS) may be also identified by arousals and/or awakenings following identification of flow limitation (see American Academy of Sleep Medicine [21])

c Body Mass Index (BMI) is greater than the 95th percentile for the patient's age and sex. Hypersomnia (excessive total sleep time in 24 h) and/or frequent extended naps can also be noted. Hypoventilation is primarily due to upper airway obstruction and obesity

d PAP therapy can relieve the obstructive component with the appearance or persistence of central respiratory pauses

e Upper airway is usually not involved, and the primary cause of the hypoventilation is due to lower airway disease, neuromuscular abnormalities, or chest wall weakness

f Identification of a medication or substance that affects respiration and/or ventilation is either reported or identified by a drug screen

g Gestational age is less than 37 weeks at the time of onset of symptoms

(continued)

Table 7.5 (continued)

[h]Gestational age is equal to or greater than 37 weeks at the time of onset of symptoms

[i]Patients and/or their parents may report the child is waking with shortness of breath

[j]A Cheyne-Stokes pattern of breathing is present. This may occur with CNS lesions. It may also occur in patients with myocardial failure

[k]CSA is present, but Cheyne-Stokes pattern of breathing is notably absent

[l]There is typically a history (or positive drug screening) of the patient taking a medication that suppresses the respiratory drive

[m]Primary neurological and/or pulmonary disease is absent; there may be an inadequate response to decreased oxygen and or elevated carbon dioxide

[n]PHOX2B gene mutation is present; other disorders of the autonomic nervous system are notable including but not limited to Hirschprung's disease, neural tumors, cardiac rate disturbances, blood pressure abnormalities, and/or ocular abnormalities

[o]Rapid onset of obesity (BMI >95th percentile for age and sex), hypothalamic dysfunction, hypoventilation, and autonomic dysregulation; PHOX2B gene mutation is notably absent

References

1. Barrows HS, Tamblyn RM. Problem-based learning: an approach to medical education. New York: Springer Publishing Company; 1980. p. 206.
2. American Academy of Sleep Medicine. International classification of sleep disorders. 3rd ed. Darien: American Academy of Sleep Medicine; 2014.
3. Spruyt K, Gozal D. Pediatric Sleep questionnaires as diagnostic or epidemiological tools: a review of currently available instruments. Sleep Med Rev. 2011;15(1):19–32.
4. Owens JA, Dalzell V. Use of the 'BEARS' sleep screening tool in a pediatric residents' clinic: a pilot study. Sleep Med. 2005;6:63–9.
5. Sheldon SH. Sleep history and differential diagnosis. In: Sheldon SH, Ferber R, Kryger MH, Gozal D, editors. Principles and practice of pediatric sleep medicine. 2nd ed. Philadelphia: Elsevier/Saunders; 2014. p. 67–71.
6. Sheldon SH, Spire JP, Levy HB. Pediatric sleep medicine differential diagnosis. In: Sheldon SH, Spire JP, Levy HB, editors. Pediatric sleep medicine. Philadelphia: W.B. Saunders/Harcourt Brace Jovanovich; 1992. p. 185–214.
7. Kryger MH. Differential diagnosis of pediatric sleep disorders. In: Sheldon SH, Ferber R, Kryger MH, editors. Principles and practice of pediatric sleep medicine. Philadelphia: Elsevier/Saunders; 2005. p. 17–25.

Part II
Sleep Disorders

Chapter 8
Sleep Disorders in Newborns and Infants

Rosemary S.C. Horne

Abstract During infancy, sleep is at a lifetime maximum, and the maturation of sleep is one of the most important physiological processes occurring during the first year of life, particularly the first 6 months. Sleep has a marked effect on cardiorespiratory control which is also rapidly maturing during infancy. Immaturity of cardiorespiratory control frequently leads to respiratory instability and prolonged pauses in breathing as manifest in apnea of prematurity and periodic breathing. During infancy, central apneas are common and obstructive apnea is rare. Although currently believed to be benign during this early period of development, there is growing evidence that they may be associated with developmental deficits in neurocognition. A failure of cardiorespiratory control mechanisms, together with an impaired arousal from sleep response, is believed to play an important role in the final event of the sudden infant death syndrome (SIDS). The "triple-risk model" describes SIDS as an event that results from the intersection of three overlapping factors: (1) a vulnerable infant, (2) a critical developmental period in homeostatic control, and (3) an exogenous stressor. In an attempt to understand how the triple-risk hypothesis is related to infant cardiorespiratory physiology, many researchers have examined how the known risk and protective factors for SIDS alter infant physiology and arousal, particularly during sleep. This review discusses the association between the three components of the triple-risk hypothesis and major risk factors for SIDS, such as prone sleeping and maternal smoking, together with three "protective" factors, and cardiovascular control and arousability from sleep in infants, and discusses their potential involvement in SIDS.

Keywords Pediatric obstructive sleep apnea • Periodic breathing • Apnea of prematurity • Sudden infant death syndrome • Sleeping position • Maternal smoking • Prematurity

R.S.C. Horne, PhD
The Ritchie Centre, Hudson Institute of Medical Research, Level 5, Monash Medical Centre, 246 Clayton Rd, Clayton, VIC 3168, Australia

Department of Paediatrics, Monash University, Melbourne, VIC, Australia
e-mail: rosemary.horne@monash.edu

© Springer International Publishing Switzerland 2017
S. Nevšímalová, O. Bruni (eds.), *Sleep Disorders in Children*,
DOI 10.1007/978-3-319-28640-2_8

Development of Sleep

The maturation of sleep is one of the most important physiological processes occurring during the first year of life and is particularly rapid during the first 6 months after birth [1]. Behavioral states are defined by physiological and behavioral variables that are stable over time and occur repeatedly in an individual infant and also across infants [2]. The emergence of sleep states is dependent on the central nervous system and is a good and reliable indicator of normal and abnormal development [3]. Sleep states and sleep architecture in infants are quite different to those in adults. In infants, sleep states are defined as active sleep (AS) and quiet sleep (QS), which are the precursors of adult rapid eye movement sleep (REM sleep) and non-rapid eye movement sleep (NREM sleep), respectively. QS is characterized by high-voltage low-amplitude electroencephalogram activity, the absence of eye movements, and regular heart rate and respiration. In contrast, AS is characterized by low-amplitude high-frequency electroencephalogram activity, eye movements, and irregular heart rate and respiration (Fig. 8.1). In addition a third state, that of indeterminate sleep (IS), is defined when criteria for AS and QS are not met. IS is usually considered a sign of immaturity and the incidence decreases with increasing postnatal age.

Rhythmic cyclical rest activity patterns can be observed in the human fetus from 28 weeks of gestation [4]. In infants born preterm, the infant sleep states cannot be distinguished in infants younger than 26 weeks of gestation [5]. By 28–30 weeks of gestation, AS can be recognized by the presence of eye movements, body movements, and irregular breathing and heart rate. At this gestational age, QS is

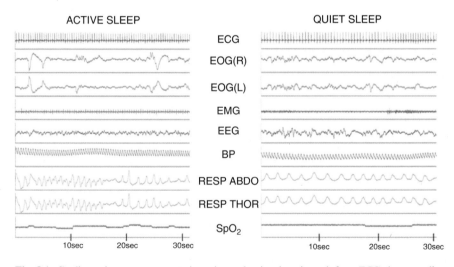

Fig. 8.1 Cardiorespiratory parameters in active and quiet sleep in an infant. *ECG* electrocardiograph, *EOG* electrooculograph, *EMG* electromyograph, *EEG* electroencephalograph, *BP* blood pressure, *RESP ABDO* abdominal respiratory effort, *RESP THOR* thoracic respiratory effort, *SpO2* oxygen saturation, *HR* heart rate. Note regular breathing and heart rate in quiet sleep compared to active sleep

difficult to identify as chin hypotonia is difficult to evaluate, and the majority of the sleep period is spent in AS. QS does not become clearly identifiable until about 36 weeks of gestational age [4]. The percentage of time spent in QS increases, and by term equal amounts of time are spent in both AS and QS with the two states alternating throughout each sleep period. The proportion of AS decreases across the first 6 months to make up approximately 25 % of total sleep time similar to that in adults [6]. In contrast, the proportion of QS increases with age to make up about 75 % of total sleep time by 6 months [6].

At term, infants sleep for about 16–17 h out of every 24 [4]. There is a gradual decrease in total sleep time with infants sleeping 14–15 h at 16 months of age and 13–14 h by 6–8 months of age. In the neonatal period, infants awaken every 2–6 h for feeding, regardless of the time of day, and stay awake for 1–2 h [7]. The major change in sleep/wake pattern occurs between 6 weeks and 3 months post term age [7]. During the first 6 months after term, consolidation and entrainment of sleep at night develops and sleep periods lengthen. At 3 weeks of age, the mean length of the longest sleep period has been reported to be 211.7 min, increasing to 358.0 min by 6 months of age [8]. The longest sleep period was randomly distributed between daytime and nighttime at 3 months but had moved to nighttime by 6 months [8].

Dramatic changes in the sleep electroencephalographic (EEG) patterns of infants occur during early infancy as the brain matures. The EEG patterns of QS and AS differ with a relatively continuous pattern in AS and a relatively discontinuous pattern in QS. A continuous pattern is defined by the presence of background activity throughout each 30 s epoch scored, and a discontinuous pattern is defined by the presence of higher amplitude EEG waves during <50 % of each epoch [9]. A semi-discontinuous EEG pattern of depressions and continuous delta activity during ≤70 % each epoch is called a *tracé alternant* pattern and can be identified at 32–34 weeks of gestational age [9]. This pattern is prominent in preterm infants but also occurs in infants born at term and disappears after 1 month after term equivalent age. Sleep spindles appear coincidentally with the disappearance of *tracé alternant* [10]. True continuous delta frequency does not appear until 8–12 weeks of age, and it is not until this age that adult criteria for determining the stages of NREM sleep can be used [11].

In summary, during infancy, sleep is at a lifetime maximum, and significant changes occur in the maturation of sleep which reflect maturation of the central nervous system. Sleep has a marked effect on cardiorespiratory control. Cardiorespiratory disturbances occur predominantly in AS sleep, so the predominance of AS in early infancy may increase the risk of cardiorespiratory disturbances during this period of development.

Apnea of Prematurity

One of the major problems facing preterm infants after birth is the immaturity of their cardiorespiratory system which often leads to repeated apneic events. Apnea of prematurity is defined as the cessation of breathing for >20 s, or if the breathing pause is shorter in duration, it is associated with bradycardia, cyanosis, marked pallor, or hypotonia [12]. Apnea of prematurity is extremely common, occurring in more than 85 % of infants born prior to 34 weeks of gestation. The incidence of apnea of prematurity is inversely related to gestational age: 3–5 % of term-born infants, 7 % of infants born at 34–35 weeks, 15 % of infants born at 32–33 weeks, 54 % of infants born at 30–31 weeks, and nearly 100 % of infants born less than 29 weeks experience episodes of apnea of prematurity [13, 14]. There are also marked changes in apnea frequency with postnatal age, with few events in the first week of life, then a progressive increase in weeks 2–3 which plateau in weeks 4–6, and then decrease in weeks 6–8 [15].

Frequently, the magnitude and frequency of the apneic events are underestimated due to the current clinical settings of pulse oximeter monitors, which often are set with long averaging times and to alarm at events longer than 20 s duration. In a study which used a 2 s averaging time and which counted apneas where oxygen saturation fell to $\leq 80\%$ for between 3 and 10 s, between 50 and 100 events/day were recorded [16]. It has recently been recommended that to take these frequent apneas which are associated with significant desaturation into account, that all events longer than 5 s should be recorded [17].

Studies have shown that excessive or persistent apnea and bradycardia are associated with long-term neurodevelopmental problems [18]. It is well known that obstructive sleep apnea in children and adults is associated with neurocognitive deficits, and the repetitive hypoxic events associated with this condition have been proposed as the primary mechanism. It is also possible that postnatal intermittent hypoxia can affect cardiovascular control beyond the neonatal period with studies in both rodent models [19] and human infants [20] demonstrating this.

Methylxanthines have been used since the 1970s for the treatment of apnea of prematurity and also to facilitate extubation and weaning off mechanical ventilation [21, 22]. Methylxanthines cross the blood-brain barrier [23], and their primary action is to antagonize the A_1/A_{2a} adenosine receptors in the CNS. Methylxanthines improve apnea of prematurity by increasing minute ventilation and improving both hypercapnic and hypoxic ventilatory drive [24, 25].

Today, caffeine is the most commonly used methylxanthine in neonatal units worldwide. Caffeine's universal acceptance followed the 2006 CAP (caffeine for apnea of prematurity) randomized control trial, which compared caffeine citrate (20 mg/kg loading dose of caffeine citrate followed by 5 mg/kg/day) with placebo in very low birth weight preterm infants. The study demonstrated both significant short-term benefits of reduced incidence of bronchopulmonary dysplasia, medically and surgically treated ductus arteriosus, and long-term benefits of improved rates of survival without neurodevelopmental delay and significantly reduced incidences of cerebral palsy at 18–21 months [26, 27]. Improved microstructural development of white matter has been demonstrated in a subsample of these children who underwent brain magnetic resonance imaging (MRI) at term equivalent age, a finding which may explain the improved neurodevelopmental outcomes [28]. However, when reassessed at 5 years of age, there was no longer any difference in rate of survival without disability between children treated with caffeine and those that were not [29].

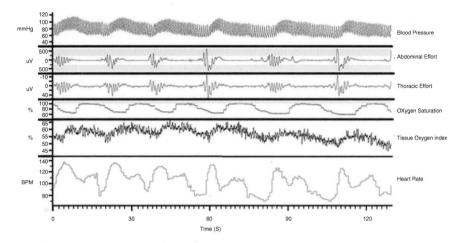

Fig. 8.2 Polysomnographic example of the effects of periodic breathing in an infant born at 27 weeks of gestational age and studied at 2–4 weeks corrected age after discharge home. Periodic breathing is associated with repetitive oxygen desaturations, marked falls in cerebral tissue oxygenation index as measured with near-infrared spectroscopy, and repetitive bradycardias which worsen over time. This infant spent 28 % of his total sleep time in periodic breathing

Apneas can occur in isolation or in a repetitive pattern termed periodic breathing. Repetitive short central apneas are termed periodic breathing (defined as three or more sequential central apneas each lasting ≥3 s) and are common in term babies in the first 2 weeks of life but significantly decrease with age [30]. In term babies, the frequency of periodic breathing is low, making up <1 % of total sleep time [30, 31]. Periodic breathing is significantly more prevalent in ex-preterm infants compared to term-born infants at term equivalent age [32]. Because of its high prevalence, and the fact that it is not usually associated with life-threatening hypoxia or bradycardia, the traditional view of periodic breathing is that it is simply due to immaturity of respiratory control and is benign [33]. However, recent studies have shown that periodic breathing can be associated with significant deficits in cerebral oxygenation [34] (Fig. 8.2), although any link to neurocognitive deficits has yet to be elucidated.

Sleep Apnea in Infants

Apneas are characterized as central, obstructive, or mixed. *Central* apneas are defined as a cessation of nasal and oral airflow in conjunction with an absence of respiratory effort. *Obstructive* apneas are defined as the cessation of nasal and oral airflow in the presence of continued respiratory effort against airway obstruction. Central apneas are common in infancy and can occur spontaneously but occur more frequently after a movement [35, 36]. Traditionally, they are considered benign as they are not associated with significant desaturation and occur in healthy infants [36]. The frequency of central apneas declines with age. In a study by Brockmann et al., the median number of events per hour declined from 5.5 (minimum 0.9; maximum 44.3) at 1 month of age to 4.1 (minimum 1.2; maximum 27.3) at 3 months [31]. The authors suggested these high rates of central apnea may be simply due to the fact that the current definitions for central apneas used for older children are not appropriate for young infants.

Obstructive apneas are reported to be rare in infancy [31, 37]. However, snoring is reported to be common, with prevalence rates ranging from 5.6 to 26 % [38–41]. These wide ranges in prevalence may have been due to confounders, with some studies including infants with colds and others studying different ethnicities. In a study of healthy predominantly Caucasian children aged 0–3 months, a prevalence of 9 % has been reported [42]. A significantly greater proportion of 2–3-month-old infants were reported to snore habitually than 0–1-month-old infants [42]. Cognitive ability at 6 months of age was found to be lower in those infants who began snoring frequently ($\geq$3 nights/week) within the first month of life [43].

In summary, central apnea is common in infants but obstructive apnea is rare. Both forms of apnea have been considered benign during infancy, but there is growing evidence that they may be associated with neurological deficits.

Sudden Infant Death Syndrome

Sudden infant death syndrome (SIDS) is defined as "the sudden and unexpected death of an infant under 1 year of age, with the onset of the lethal episode apparently occurring during sleep, that remains unexplained after a thorough investigation including performance of a complete autopsy and review of the circumstances of death" [44]. The incidence of SIDS was more than halved after public health campaigns publicized the known major risk factors of prone sleeping, maternal smoking, and overheating [45]. However, SIDS still remains the leading cause of unexpected death in infants in Western countries, contributing to almost 50 % of all postneonatal deaths [46, 47].

As SIDS is a diagnosis of exclusion, there has been considerable research into the underlying mechanisms which may underpin known risk factors. SIDS has long been believed to be multifactorial in origin. The triple-risk hypothesis [48] proposes that when a vulnerable infant, such as one born preterm or exposed to maternal smoking, is at a critical but unstable developmental period in homeostatic control and is exposed to an exogenous stressor, such as being placed prone to sleep, then SIDS may occur. The model proposes that infants will die of SIDS only if all three factors are present and that the vulnerability lies dormant until they enter the critical developmental period and are exposed to an exogenous stressor. SIDS usually occurs during sleep, and the peak incidence is between 2 and 4 months of age, when sleep patterns are rapidly maturing. The final pathway to SIDS is widely believed to involve immature cardiorespiratory control, in conjunction with a failure of arousal from sleep [45]. Support for this hypothesis comes from numerous physiological studies showing that the major risk factors for SIDS (prone sleeping, maternal smoking, prematurity, head covering) have significant effects on blood pressure and heart rate and their control [49] and impair arousal from sleep [50].

Vulnerable Infant

Neuropathologic findings from SIDS victims show significant deficits in brainstem and cerebellar structures involved in the regulation of respiratory drive, cardiovascular control, sleep/wake transition, and arousal from sleep [51–58]. Furthermore, genetic polymorphisms have been identified in SIDS victims which affect genes involved in autonomic function, neurotransmission, energy metabolism, and the response to infection [59–63].

Prenatal and/or postnatal exposure to cigarette smoke is one factor which increases infant vulnerability to SIDS [64, 65], with over 40 studies showing a positive association with risk ratios of between 0.7 and 4.85 [66–69]. This increased SIDS risk is likely to be due to the effects of nicotine exposure on autonomic control and arousal [58, 70–72]. In support of this idea, Duncan and colleagues [73] found that chronic exposure to nicotine in the prenatal baboon fetus altered serotonergic and nicotinic acetylcholine receptor binding in regions of the medulla, critical to cardiorespiratory control. Furthermore, they identified that these alterations were associated with abnormalities in fetal heart rate variability, indicating altered cardiovascular control [73]. Studies in infants exposed to maternal smoking have demonstrated altered heart rate and blood pressure control compared with control infants [74–80]. Maternal tobacco smoking also decreases both total arousability and the proportion of cortical arousals. Arousal impairment was observed for both spontaneous arousals from sleep and responses induced by various stimuli [81–87]. Few mothers change their smoking behavior postpartum [88]; therefore, it is difficult to ascertain whether these physiological effects are caused by prenatal or postnatal smoke exposure. Environmental smoke (in the same room) independently increases the risk of SIDS [89, 90]. Importantly, a recent study has shown that before discharge home from hospital, preterm infants of smoking mothers already exhibited disruptions in sleep patterns, prior to any postnatal smoke exposure [91]. Thus, there is considerable evidence from both animal and human studies suggesting that prenatal exposure to cigarette smoke has deleterious effects on the developing brain and cardiorespiratory system. It is suggested that these effects increase infant vulnerability to SIDS.

Maternal smoking may also be a confounding risk factor for SIDS due to its association with other risk factors, such as preterm birth and intrauterine growth restriction (IUGR) [92–95], which likely result from suboptimal intrauterine environments. Impaired heart rate control, manifest as shorter cardiac R-R intervals and higher resting sympathetic tone, has been reported in term-born IUGR infants when compared with infants of appropriate size for gestational age [96, 97]. Similarly, preterm infants demonstrated impaired autonomic control compared with term infants studied at or before term equivalent age, and this pattern was inversely related to gestational age at birth [98–103]. Longitudinal studies after term equivalent age have identified that preterm infants exhibited lower blood pressure, delayed blood pressure recovery following head-up tilting, and impaired baroreflex control of blood pressure and heart rate across the first 6 months corrected age, when compared with age-matched term infants [104–108]. Furthermore, maturation of baroreflex control of blood pressure during sleep is affected by gestational age at birth, with infants born very preterm (<32 weeks of gestation), having reduced increases in baroreflex sensitivity compared to both preterm and term infants [109]. Recently, studies have also identified that cerebral oxygenation is also lower in preterm compared to term infants across the first 6 months corrected age [110] and that cerebrovascular control after a head-up tilt is more variable [111], indicating immature or impaired control.

When compared with term infants at matched conceptional ages, preterm infants also exhibit decreased frequencies and durations of spontaneous arousals from sleep [112–114], together with decreased heart rate responses following arousal [115]. Furthermore, preterm infants exhibited longer arousal latencies after exposure to mild hypoxia (15 % inspired O_2), reaching significantly lower oxygen saturations than term infants [116]. Cardiorespiratory complications commonly associated with prematurity, apnea, and bradycardia have also been shown to suppress total arousability when these infants were compared to preterm infants with no history of apnea [117].

In summary, these alterations in cardiorespiratory control and arousability during sleep support the classification of prenatal smoke exposure and preterm birth as factors strongly linked with the idea of a preexisting vulnerability to SIDS. Such physiological disturbances may be further exacerbated during a critical developmental period within infancy and by exposure to exogenous stressors.

Critical Developmental Period

Approximately 90 % of SIDS deaths occur in infants aged less than 6 months [45, 118]. During this period, the central nervous system undergoes dramatic maturational changes which are reflected in extensive alterations to sleep architecture, electroencephalogram characteristics, and autonomic control. The 2–4-month period, in particular, has been described as a "developmental window of vulnerability" [119, 120] and coincides with the age where a distinct peak in SIDS incidence occurs [45, 118].

A number of other significant developmental factors may make an infant more vulnerable to a cardiorespiratory challenge during this critical developmental period. Studies in both preterm [105, 110] and term [121] infants have identified a nadir in basal blood pressure during sleep at 2–4 months of age, when compared to both earlier (2–4 weeks) and later (5–6 months) ages studied; a nadir in physiological anemia also occurs at this age. Blood pressure responses to a cardiovascular challenge (head-up tilting) are also impaired at 2–4 months compared to younger (2–4 weeks) and older (5–6 months) ages [122]. The maturational reduction in cerebral oxygenation is most marked between 2–4 weeks and 2–4 months of age, which may be due to limited or inadequate flow-metabolism coupling at this age [123]. Thus, the 2–4-month age represents a critical time period when the effects of low blood pressure could accentuate decrements in oxygen-carrying capacity and delivery to critical organs [124]. These studies suggest that there is a postnatal age effect on cardiovascular control, with critical maturational changes occurring when the risk of SIDS is greatest.

Infant arousal responses from sleep are also affected by postnatal age, although these maturational effects are sleep state dependent. Previous studies have demonstrated that in response to respiratory (mild hypoxia), tactile (nasal air-jet), and auditory stimulation, total arousability is reduced with increasing age during quiet sleep while remaining unchanged in active sleep [124–126]. Following the introduction of standard scoring criteria for subcortical activation and cortical arousal as separate entities, a recent study noted that spontaneous subcortical activations decreased with increasing postnatal age, while cortical arousals increased [127]. Conversely, another study analyzed both spontaneous and nasal air-jet-induced arousability during supine sleep and found no change in the percentage of cortical arousals (from total responses) throughout the first 6 months of life [128]. Interestingly, when the same infants slept in the prone position, an increased propensity of cortical arousal was identified at 2–3 months, the age when SIDS is most common [87, 128]. This increase in cortical arousals may reflect an innate protective response to ensure an appropriate level of arousal for restoring homeostasis, not only during a vulnerable period of development but also in the presence of an exogenous stressor (e.g., the prone sleeping position).

Exogenous Stressor(s)

An exogenous stressor constitutes the third aspect of the triple-risk model for SIDS. Epidemiological studies have identified numerous factors common to SIDS victims, such as the prone sleeping position, overheating, and recent infection, which may disrupt homeostasis [45, 59, 129, 130].

The prone sleeping position has long been considered the major risk factor for SIDS [94, 131–134], with some studies suggesting a causal relation between prone sleep and SIDS [135, 136]. Several physiological changes ensue when infants sleep prone, including increased peripheral skin temperature and increased baseline heart rate, together with decreased heart rate variability [121, 137–145]. In an effort to identify changes in autonomic cardiovascular control with sleeping position, studies examining heart rate responses to auditory and nasal air-jet stimuli have suggested an increase in sympathetic and a decrease in parasympathetic tone in the prone sleeping position [146, 147]. Furthermore, sympathetic effects on blood pressure and vasomotor tone are decreased in the prone sleeping position. Lower resting blood pressure and altered cardiovascular responses to head-up tilting have also been identified in term infants when sleeping in the prone position, compared with the supine position [121, 122]. Furthermore, cerebral oxygenation is reduced and cerebrovascular control impaired in the prone position in both term [123, 148] and preterm infants [110, 149]. In addition, prone sleeping infants exhibit reduced cardiac and respiratory responses when arousing from sleep, when compared to sleeping in the supine position [146, 147]. Previous studies of both term and pre-term infants have consistently identified increases in sleep time, with significant reductions in spontaneous arousability, associated with prone sleeping when com-pared with the supine position [150–153]. Furthermore, in other studies, the prone sleeping position depressed arousal responses provoked by postural change [137] and auditory [154] and somatosensory challenges [86, 138, 155]. It has been dem-onstrated that both spontaneous and induced arousal responses are similarly affected by sleep state and SIDS risk factors, suggesting that they are mediated through the same pathways [156]. Despite this well-documented decrease in total arousability, examining subcortical and cortical responses separately has produced conflicting results. Although one study reported a decreased frequency of sponta-neous cortical arousals in the prone position [153], more recent studies have found an increased proportion of cortical arousals (of total responses) in both nonsmoking and smoking exposed infants when sleeping prone [87, 128]. This apparent promo-tion of full cortical arousal, demonstrated for both spontaneous and stimulus-induced responses, may protectively compensate against the threat of altered autonomic control and the already blunted total arousability imposed by the prone position.

The prone sleeping position also potentiates the risk of overheating, by reducing the exposed surface area available for radiant heat loss and reducing respiratory heat loss when the infants face is covered [157]. Both physiological studies in healthy infants and theoretical model studies of heat balance have observed a decreased ability to lose heat when in the prone position [158–160]. Early studies observed decreased variation in behavior and respiratory pattern, increased heart rate, and increased peripheral skin temperature during prone compared with supine sleep [159]. These studies suggest that infants are less able to maintain adequate respira-tory and metabolic homoeostasis when sleeping prone.

Increased sweating occurs in SIDS victims, regardless of whether infants slept prone or supine; these cases were predominantly associated with a covered face [118, 161]. A history of profuse sweating in SIDS victims has been postulated to be a phenomenon representing an abnormality of function of the autonomic nervous system [162]. The involvement of thermal stress with SIDS is further supported by the finding of similar odds ratios for both too much and too little bedding [163] and the suggestion that future SIDS victims may have had atypical temperature regula-tion [164]. Infant arousability is also affected by body and room temperature; decreased sleep continuity and increased body movements have been associated with exposure to cooler temperatures [165], while infants sleeping in warmer environments (28 °C vs. 24 °C) exhibited increased arousal thresholds to auditory stimuli [166]. Furthermore, based on studies assessing blood pressure control in infants [139, 144], it has been suggested that in response to the increased peripheral skin temperature when infants sleep prone, thermoregulatory vasodilatation of the peripheral microvasculature occurs, resulting in a decrease in blood pressure and a reduction in vasomotor tone. Recent studies in preterm infants have shown that increased ambient temperature led to significant changes in autonomic control with elevated heart rates and lower heart rate variability compared to thermoneutral or cooler temperature [167].

Head covering has been identified as a major risk for SIDS with between 16 % and 28 % of SIDS infants found with their heads covered. Although a causal relationship with SIDS has not been established [168, 169], it appears likely that rebreathing and impaired arousal are involved. It has been suggested that the increased SIDS risk associated with head covering may result from hypoxia and hypercapnia via rebreathing of expired air [168, 170]. Head covering in healthy infants has profound effects on autonomic control during sleep [171]. Franco and colleagues [171] found that infants sleeping supine with their head covered by a bedsheet exhibited decreased parasympathetic activity, increased sympathetic activity, and increased body temperature when compared with head-free periods. In addition, arousal responses in active sleep were also depressed when the head was covered [172].

Bed-sharing or co-sleeping has also been reported to significantly increase the risk of SIDS, particularly when the mother smokes [118, 173–175] with more than 50 % of SIDS deaths occurring in this situation between 1997 and 2006 [176, 177]. There have been few studies investigating the physiology behind this risk factor. In infants from nonsmoking families who were studied on successive bed-sharing and solitary sleeping nights, bed-sharing was associated with increased awakenings and transient arousals during slow wave sleep compared to solitary nights [178]. In contrast, another study found that bed-sharing infants spent less time moving and were more likely to have their heads partially or fully covered by bedding than cot-sleeping infants [179]. Thus more studies are required to identify the exact physiological changes which occur during bed-sharing.

Other external stressors, such as infection, fever, and minor respiratory and gastrointestinal illnesses, commonly occur in the days to weeks preceding death of SIDS victims [180–182]. Although not identified as an independent risk factor for SIDS, minor infections have been associated with an increased likelihood of SIDS when combined with head covering or prone sleeping [183, 184]. In the prone sleeping position, minor infection, in combination with fever, could further exacerbate thermoregulatory effects on peripheral vasculature, which could increase the susceptibility of a hypotensive episode. Thus, hypotension, in combination with a decreased ability to arouse from sleep, which has been documented in term infants immediately following an infection [185], could potentially further impair an infant's ability to appropriately respond to a life-threatening challenge such as circulatory failure or an asphyxial insult.

SIDS "Protective" Factors and Autonomic Control

Some studies have suggested that infant care practices, such as breastfeeding, dummy/pacifier use, and swaddling (tight wrapping), decrease the risk of SIDS. These potentially protective factors for SIDS have all been associated with alterations to both cardiovascular autonomic control and arousal responses during sleep. However, results are often inconsistent, and supporting evidence is less extensive than for the risk factors discussed above; thus, these potentially preventative factors remain controversial among researchers.

Breastfeeding

Breastfeeding reduces the incidence of SIDS by approximately half (OR 0.52, 95 % CI: 0.46–0.60), even after multivariate analyses accounted for potentially confounding socioeconomic factors [180, 186, 187]. This apparent protection may be a biological effect, given that breastfeeding has been associated with a decreased incidence of diarrhea, vomiting, colds, and other infections; in addition, breast milk is rich in antibodies and many micronutrients [180, 188, 189]. Only one study has assessed the effects of breastfeeding on the cardiovascular system during sleep in term infants, and this study found that heart rate was significantly lower in breast-fed infants when compared with formula-fed infants [190]. Although little is known about the effects of breastfeeding vs. formula feeding on cardiovascular control in infants, physiological studies have demonstrated an apparent promotion of arousal from sleep associated with breastfeeding. One study found that breast-fed infants spent more time awake during the night, thus requiring more frequent parental visits [191]. Another study showed that healthy breast-fed infants aroused more readily from active sleep than formula-fed infants in response to nasal air-jet stimulation at 2–3 months postnatal age [192]. Although there is a general consensus that breastfeeding should be encouraged, the relationship between breastfeeding for SIDS prevention remains unclear.

Pacifier/Dummy Use

The finding that the use of a dummy/pacifier has a protective effect for SIDS has consistently emerged from epidemiological studies, with significant associations being described for both usage during the final sleep and "dummy ever used" (OR: 0.46. CI 0.36–0.59) [118, 193–198]. Studies have suggested that a likely mechanism for this protection against SIDS is increased heart rate variability which has been demonstrated during sucking periods [199, 200]. Conversely, dummy sucking has also been shown to have no effect on heart rate, heart rate variability, respiratory frequency, or oxygen saturation in term infants [201, 202]. In addition, dummy sucking has been shown to elicit increases in blood pressure in quietly awake or sleeping term infants [203]. Another potential mechanism for the protective nature of dummy use against SIDS is an enhanced arousability from sleep. However, results of the few studies which have been conducted are conflicting, with one study reporting decreased arousal thresholds to auditory stimulation observed in infants who regularly used a dummy, when compared with those who did not use a dummy [204]. In contrast, other studies have reported no effect of dummy use on either the frequency or duration of spontaneous arousals in sleeping infants, when studied both with and without a dummy in the mouth [205, 206]. It has also been hypothesized that sucking on a dummy during sleep may assist in maintaining airway patency, thus preventing a pharyngeal vacuum and the consequent sealing of the airway [207, 208]. Thus, the risk of oropharyngeal obstruction may be reduced due to the forward positioning of the tongue when sucking on a dummy [208]. Although epidemiological studies have provided strong support for dummy use to be protective for SIDS, the physiological mechanisms responsible for this protection remain uncertain.

Swaddling

Swaddling, or firm wrapping, is a traditional infant care practice which, according to an extensive historical review, has been used in some form or another by various cultures since medieval times [209]. Low incidences of SIDS in populations where swaddling is common have led to the proposal that swaddling may be protective [210, 211], and on this basis, a number of SIDS prevention organizations recommend it. Several studies have documented a "tranquil" behavioral state with longer sleep periods in swaddled infants; therefore, despite a disparity between studies on the risk for SIDS [174, 183, 212], swaddling has become increasingly popular as a soothing technique throughout the world [213, 214]. Swaddling is a common practice in infants throughout the first 6 months of life, during the period of increased SIDS risk. The duration of swaddling and the age of initiation of the practice vary widely. Currently, it is unclear if swaddling is protective against SIDS or is indeed a risk. In the United Kingdom during the mid-1990s, swaddling during the last sleep was more common among SIDS infants than age-matched controls (14 % vs. 9 %); furthermore, a more recent study showed that this difference has since become more marked (19 % vs. 6 %) [174].

Studies investigating the effect of swaddling on cardiovascular control are limited. Swaddling elicits a mild increase in respiratory frequency, most likely due to restricted tidal volumes imposed by the firm wrapping [215–217]. No significant effects have been documented on baseline heart rate, skin temperature, or oxygen saturation in term infants when swaddled during sleep [216, 218]. Studies which compared infants who were routinely swaddled to those who were unused to this practice found that sleep time and heart rate variability were only altered in those naïve-to-swaddling infants [219]. Several studies investigated the effects of swaddling in relation to infant arousability; however, divergent results have been published. The commonly observed decreases in spontaneous movements and startle responses with swaddling are in contrast to effects of other protective factors for

SIDS [209, 220]. One study reported that when infants were swaddled, fewer startle responses progressed to a full awakening, indicating an inhibition of the cortical arousal process [221]. More recent studies reported that swaddled infants exhibited increased arousal thresholds in response to nasal air-jet stimulation; furthermore, a decreased frequency of full cortical arousals was observed primarily in infants who were unaccustomed to being swaddled, at 3 months of age [216]. Spontaneous cortical arousals were also decreased in those infants unaccustomed to being swaddled, at 3 months of age [219]. These arousal differences between routinely swaddled and naïve-to-swaddling infants, only at this age of peak SIDS risk, may explain the contradictory findings of another group which found decreased auditory arousal thresholds in swaddled infants when compared to infants who were free to move [218]. The authors attributed these effects of swaddling on arousal to the greater autonomic changes found after auditory stimulation in swaddled conditions [222]. As with the other protective factors discussed above, the mechanisms whereby swaddling is protective for SIDS remain unclear, and further research is required.

Conclusions

In summary, the assessment of cardiovascular control and arousal processes during sleep is important in understanding sleep-related pathologies such as SIDS. In otherwise healthy infants, studies have demonstrated impairment of these physiological mechanisms in association with all three aspects of the triple-risk model, thus demonstrating the heterogeneous nature of SIDS. Altered cardiovascular and cerebrovascular control, in conjunction with a failure to arouse from sleep, could potentially impair an infant's ability to appropriately compensate for life-threatening challenges, such as prolonged hypotension or asphyxia during sleep. The concept of a close relationship between SIDS and autonomic dysfunction becomes more compelling with the demonstration of an apparent promotion of arousal from sleep by protective factors for SIDS. Despite successful public awareness campaigns dramatically reducing SIDS rates, this decline in SIDS incidence may have stabilized [223–226]. Thus, further research is imperative to elucidate the exact mechanisms involved in the final events of SIDS, allowing identification of "at-risk" infants in the future. The ability to identify these infants would have the potential to increase awareness of both parents and clinicians while minimizing the incidence of SIDS with close monitoring and early intervention.

References

1. Gaultier C. Cardiorespiratory adaptation during sleep in infants and children. Pediatr Pulmonol. 1995;19:105–17.
2. Prechtl HF. The behavioural states of the newborn infant (a review). Brain Res. 1974;76:185–212.

3. Curzi-Dascalova L, Challamel M-J. Neurophysiological basis of sleep development. In: Loughlin GM, Carroll JL, Marcus CL, editors. Sleep and breathing in children: a developmental approach. New York: Marcel Dekker; 2000.

4. Parmelee AH, Stern E. Development of states in infants. In: Clemente CD, Purpura DP, Mayer FE, editors. Sleep and the maturing nervous system. Academic Press New York. 1972;199–228.

5. Dreyfus-Brisac C. Sleep ontogenesis in early human prematurity from 24 to 27 weeks conceptual age. Dev Psychobiol. 1968;1:162–9.

6. de Weerd AW, van den Bossche RA. The development of sleep during the first months of life. Sleep Med Rev. 2003;7:179–91.

7. Coons SC, Guilleminault C. Development of sleep-wake patterns and non-rapid eye movement sleep stages during the first six months of life in normal infants. Pediatrics. 1982;69:793–8.

8. Coons S. Development of sleep and wakefulness during the first 6 months of life. New York: Raven Press; 1987.

9. Curzi-Dascalova L, Mirmiran M. Manual of methods for recording and analysing sleep-wakefulness states in preterm and full term infants. Paris: Les Edition INSERM; 1996.

10. Metcalf D. The ontogenesis of sleep-awake states from birth to 3 months. Electroencephalogr Clin Neurophysiol. 1970;28:421.

11. Grigg-Damberger M, Gozal D, Marcus CL, Quan SF, Rosen CL, Chervin RD, Wise M, Picchietti DL, Sheldon SH, Iber C. The visual scoring of sleep and arousal in infants and children. J Clin Sleep Med. 2007;3:201–40.

12. National Institutes of Health Consensus Development Conference on Infantile Apnea and Home Monitoring, Sept 29 to Oct 1, 1986. Pediatrics. 1987;79:292–9.

13. Henderson-Smart D. The effect of gestational age on the incidence and duration of recurrent apnoea in newborn babies. Aust Paediatr J. 1981;17:273–6.

14. Picone S, Bedetta M, Paolillo P. Caffeine citrate: when and for how long. A literature review. J Matern Fetal Neonatal Med. 2012;25 Suppl 3:11–4.

15. Martin RJ, di Fiore JM, Macfarlane PM, Wilson CG. Physiologic basis for intermittent hypoxic episodes in preterm infants. Adv Exp Med Biol. 2012;758:351–8.

16. di Fiore JM, Bloom JN, Orge F, Schutt A, Schluchter M, Cheruvu VK, Walsh M, Finer N, Martin RJ. A higher incidence of intermittent hypoxemic episodes is associated with severe retinopathy of prematurity. J Pediatr. 2010;157:69–73.

17. Elder DE, Whale J, Galletly D, Campbell AJ. Respiratory events in preterm infants prior to discharge: with and without clinically concerning apnoea. Sleep Breath. 2011;15:867–73.

18. Pillekamp F, Hermann C, Keller T, von Gontard A, Kribs A, Roth B. Factors influencing apnea and bradycardia of prematurity – implications for neurodevelopment. Neonatology. 2007;91:155–61.

19. Soukhova-O'Hare GK, Cheng ZJ, Roberts AM, Gozal D. Postnatal intermittent hypoxia alters baroreflex function in adult rats. Am J Physiol Heart Circ Physiol. 2006;290: H1157–64.

20. Cohen G, Lagercrantz H, Katz-Salamon M. Abnormal circulatory stress responses of preterm graduates. Pediatr Res. 2007;61:329–34.

21. Al-Saif S, Alvaro R, Manfreda J, Kwiatkowski K, Cates D, Qurashi M, Rigatto H. A randomized controlled trial of theophylline versus CO_2 inhalation for treating apnea of prematurity. J Pediatr. 2008;153:513–8.

22. Henderson-Smart DJ, Steer P. Methylxanthine treatment for apnea in preterm infants. Cochrane Database Syst Rev. 2001;(3):CD000140.

23. McCall AL, Millington WR, Wurtman RJ. Blood-brain barrier transport of caffeine: dose-related restriction of adenine transport. Life Sci. 1982;31:2709–15.

24. Montandon G, Kinkead R, Bairam A. Adenosinergic modulation of respiratory activity: developmental plasticity induced by perinatal caffeine administration. Respir Physiol Neurobiol. 2008;164:87–95.

25. Chardon K, Bach V, Telliez F, Cardot V, Tourneux P, Leke A, Libert JP. Effect of caffeine on peripheral chemoreceptor activity in premature neonates: interaction with sleep stages. J Appl Physiol. 2004;96:2161–6.

26. Schmidt B, Roberts RS, Davis P, Doyle LW, Barrington KJ, Ohlsson A, Solimano A, Tin W. Caffeine therapy for apnea of prematurity. NEJM. 2006;354:2112–21.
27. Schmidt B, Roberts RS, Davis P, Doyle LW, Barrington KJ, Ohlsson A, Solimano A, Tin W. Long-term effects of caffeine therapy for apnea of prematurity. NEJM. 2007;357: 1893–902.
28. Doyle LW, Cheong J, Hunt RW, Lee KJ, Thompson DK, Davis PG, Rees S, Anderson PJ, Inder TE. Caffeine and brain development in very preterm infants. Ann Neurol. 2010;68: 734–42.
29. Schmidt B, Anderson PJ, Doyle LW, Dewey D, Grunau RE, Asztalos EV, Davis PG, Tin W, Moddemann D, Solimano A, Ohlsson A, Barrington KJ, Roberts RS. Survival without disability to age 5 years after neonatal caffeine therapy for apnea of prematurity. JAMA. 2012;307:275–82.
30. Kelly DH, Stellwagen LM, Kaitz E, Shannon DC. Apnea and periodic breathing in normal full-term infants during the first twelve months. Pediatr Pulmonol. 1985;1:215–9.
31. Brockmann PE, Poets A, Poets CF. Reference values for respiratory events in overnight polygraphy from infants aged 1 and 3months. Sleep Med. 2013;14:1323–7.
32. Albani M, Bentele KH, Budde C, Schulte FJ. Infant sleep apnea profile: preterm vs. term infants. Eur J Pediatr. 1985;143:261–8.
33. Edwards BA, Sands SA, Berger PJ. Postnatal maturation of breathing stability and loop gain: the role of carotid chemoreceptor development. Respir Physiol Neurobiol. 2013;185: 144–55.
34. Decima PF, Fyfe KL, Odoi A, Wong FY, Horne RS. The longitudinal effects of persistent periodic breathing on cerebral oxygenation in preterm infants. Sleep Med. 2015;16:729–35.
35. Carskadon MA, Harvey K, Dement WC, Guilleminault C, Simmons FB, Anders TF. Respiration during sleep in children. West J Med. 1978;128:477–81.
36. Marcus CL, Omlin KJ, Basinki DJ, Bailey SL, Rachal AB, von Pechmann WS, Keens TG, Ward SL. Normal polysomnographic values for children and adolescents. Am Rev Respir Dis. 1992;146:1235–9.
37. Kato I, Scaillet S, Groswasser J, Montemitro E, Togari H, Lin J, Kahn A, Franco P. Spontaneous arousability in prone and supine position in healthy infants. Sleep. 2006;29: 785–90.
38. Gislason T, Benediktsdottir B. Snoring, apneic episodes, and nocturnal hypoxemia among children 6 months to 6 years old. An epidemiologic study of lower limit of prevalence. Chest. 1995;107:963–6.
39. Kelmanson IA. Snoring, noisy breathing in sleep and daytime behaviour in 2-4-month-old infants. Eur J Pediatr. 2000;159:734–9.
40. Mitchell EA, Thompson JM. Snoring in the first year of life. Acta Paediatr. 2003;92:425–9.
41. Montgomery-Downs HE, Gozal D. Sleep habits and risk factors for sleep-disordered breathing in infants and young toddlers in Louisville, Kentucky. Sleep Med. 2006;7:211–9.
42. Piteo AM, Lushington K, Roberts RM, van den Heuvel CJ, Nettelbeck T, Kohler MJ, Martin AJ, Kennedy JD. Prevalence of snoring and associated factors in infancy. Sleep Med. 2011;12:787–92.
43. Piteo AM, Kennedy JD, Roberts RM, Martin AJ, Nettelbeck T, Kohler MJ, Lushington K. Snoring and cognitive development in infancy. Sleep Med. 2011;12:981–7.
44. Krous HF, Beckwith JB, Byard RW, Rognum TO, Bajanowski T, Corey T, Cutz E, Hanzlick R, Keens TG, Mitchell EA, Krous HF, Beckwith JB, Byard RW, Rognum TO, Bajanowski T, Corey T, Cutz E, Hanzlick R, Keens TG, Mitchell EA. Sudden infant death syndrome and unclassified sudden infant deaths: a definitional and diagnostic approach. Pediatrics. 2004;114:234–8.
45. Moon RY, Horne RS, Hauck FR. Sudden infant death syndrome. Lancet. 2007;370: 1578–87.
46. Carpenter RG, Irgens LM, Blair PS, England PD, Fleming P, Huber J, Jorch G, Schreuder P. Sudden unexplained infant death in 20 regions in Europe: case control study. Lancet. 2004;363:185–91.

47. Byard RW, Krous HF. Sudden infant death syndrome: overview and update. Pediatr Dev Pathol. 2003;6:112–27.
48. Filiano JJ, Kinney H. A perspective on neuropathologic findings in victims of the sudden infant death syndrome: the triple risk model. Biol Neonate. 1994;65:194–7.
49. Horne RS, Witcombe NB, Yiallourou SR, Scaillet S, Thiriez G, Franco P. Cardiovascular control during sleep in infants: implications for sudden infant death syndrome. Sleep Med. 2010;11:615–21.
50. Franco P, Kato I, Richardson HL, Yang JS, Montemitro E, Horne RS. Arousal from sleep mechanisms in infants. Sleep Med. 2010;11:603–14.
51. Paterson DS, Trachtenberg FL, Thompson EG, Belliveau RA, Beggs AH, Darnall BA, Chadwick AE, Krous HF, Kinney HC. Multiple serotonergic brainstem abnormalities in sudden infant death syndrome. JAMA. 2006;286:2124–32.
52. Kinney HC, Cryan JB, Haynes RL, Paterson DS, Haas EA, Mena OJ, Minter M, Journey KW, Trachtenberg FL, Goldstein RD, Armstrong DD. Dentate gyrus abnormalities in sudden unexplained death in infants: morphological marker of underlying brain vulnerability. Acta Neuropathol. 2015;129:65–80.
53. Kinney HC, Filiano JJ, Sleeper LA, Mandell F, Valdes-Dapena M, White WF. Decreased muscarinic receptor binding in the arcuate nucleus in sudden infant death syndrome. Science. 1995;269:1446–50.
54. Panigrahy A, Filiano J, Sleeper LA, Mandell F, Valdes-Dapena M, Krous HF, Rava LA, Foley E, White WF, Kinney HC. Decreased serotonergic receptor binding in rhombic lip-derived regions of the medulla oblongata in the sudden infant death syndrome. J Neuropathol Exp Neurol. 2000;59:377–84.
55. Panigrahy A, Filiano JJ, Sleeper LA, Mandell F, Valdes-Dapena M, Krous HF, Rava LA, White WF, Kinney HC. Decreased kainate receptor binding in the arcuate nucleus of the sudden infant death syndrome. J Neuropathol Exp Neurol. 1997;56:1253–61.
56. Machaalani R, Say M, Waters KA. Serotinergic receptor 1A in the sudden infant death syndrome brainstem medulla and associations with clinical risk factors. Acta Neuropathol. 2009;117:257–65.
57. Machaalani R, Waters KA. Neuronal cell death in the sudden infant death syndrome brainstem and associations with risk factors. Brain. 2008;131:218–28.
58. Machaalani R, Waters KA. Neurochemical abnormalities in the brainstem of the Sudden Infant Death Syndrome (SIDS). Paediatr Respir Rev. 2014;15:293–300.
59. Kinney HC, Thach BT. The sudden infant death syndrome. N Engl J Med. 2009;361:795–805.
60. Lavezzi AM, Casale V, Oneda R, Weese-Mayer DE, Matturri L. Sudden infant death syndrome and sudden intrauterine unexplained death: correlation between hypoplasia of raphe nuclei and serotonin transporter gene promoter polymorphism. Pediatr Res. 2009;66:22–7.
61. Weese-Mayer DE, Ackerman MJ, Marazita ML, Berry-Kravis EM. Sudden infant death syndrome: review of implicated genetic factors. Am J Med Genet. 2007;143A:771–88.
62. Filonzi L, Magnani C, Lavezzi AM, Rindi G, Parmigiani S, Bevilacqua G, Matturri L, Marzano FN. Association of dopamine transporter and monoamine oxidase molecular polymorphisms with sudden infant death syndrome and stillbirth: new insights into the serotonin hypothesis. Neurogenetics. 2009;10:65–72.
63. Courts C, Madea B. Genetics of the sudden infant death syndrome. Forensic Sci Int. 2010;203:25–33.
64. Mitchell E, Scragg R, Stewart AW, Becroft DMO, Taylor B, Ford RPK, Hassell B, Barry DMJ, Allen EM, Roberts AP. Results from the first year of the New Zealand cot death study. NZ Med J. 1991;104:71–6.
65. Matturri L, Ottaviani G, Lavezzi AM. Maternal smoking and sudden infant death syndrome: epidemiological study related to pathology. Virchows Arch. 2006;449:697–706.
66. Anderson HR, Cook DG. Passive smoking and sudden infant death syndrome: review of the epidemiological evidence. Thorax. 1997;52:1003–9.

67. Blair PS, Bensley D, Smith I, Bacon C, Taylor B, Berry J. Smoking and the sudden infant death syndrome: results from 1993–5 case-control study for confidential inquiry into stillbirths and deaths in infancy. BMJ. 1996;313:195–8.

68. Dwyer T, Ponsonby A, Couper D. Tobacco smoke exposure at one month of age and subsequent risk of SIDS – a prospective study. Am J Epidemiol. 1999;149:593–602.

69. Haglund B. Cigarette smoking and sudden infant death syndrome: some salient points in the debate. Acta Paediatr Suppl. 1993;389:37–9.

70. Machaalani R, Ghazavi E, Hinton T, Waters KA, Hennessy A. Cigarette smoking during pregnancy regulates the expression of specific nicotinic acetylcholine receptor (nAChR) subunits in the human placenta. Toxicol Appl Pharmacol. 2014;276:204–12.

71. Machaalani R, Say M, Waters KA. Effects of cigarette smoke exposure on nicotinic acetylcholine receptor subunits alpha7 and beta2 in the sudden infant death syndrome (SIDS) brainstem. Toxicol Appl Pharmacol. 2011;257:396–404.

72. Lavezzi AM, Mecchia D, Matturri L. Neuropathology of the area postrema in sudden intrauterine and infant death syndromes related to tobacco smoke exposure. Auton Neurosci. 2012;166:29–34.

73. Duncan JR, Garland M, Myers MM, Fifer WP, Yang M, Kinney HC, Stark RI. Prenatal nicotine-exposure alters fetal autonomic activity and medullary neurotransmitter receptors: implications for sudden infant death syndrome. J Appl Physiol. 2009;107:1579–90.

74. Browne CA, Colditz PB, Dunster KR. Infant autonomic function is altered by maternal smoking during pregnancy. Early Hum Dev. 2000;59:209–18.

75. Dahlstrom A, Ebersjo C, Lundell B. Nicotine in breast milk influences heart rate variability in the infant. Acta Paediatr. 2008;97:1075–9.

76. Fifer WP, Fingers ST, Youngman M, Gomez-Gribben E, Myers MM. Effects of alcohol and smoking during pregnancy on infant autonomic control. Dev Psychobiol. 2009;51:234–42.

77. Cohen G, Vella S, Jeffery H, Lagercrantz H, Katz-Salamon M. Cardiovascular stress hyperreactivity in babies of smokers and in babies born preterm. Circulation. 2008;118:1848–53.

78. Thiriez G, Bouhaddi M, Mourot L, Nobili F, Fortrat JO, Menget A, Franco P, Rednard J. Heart rate variability in preterm infants and maternal smoking during pregnancy. Clin Auton Res. 2009;19:149–56.

79. Viskari-Lahdeoja S, Hytinantti T, Andersson S, Kirjavainen T. Heart rate and blood pressure control in infants exposed to maternal cigarette smoking. Acta Paediatr. 2008;97:1535–41.

80. Franco P, Chabanski S, Szliwowski H, Dramaix M, Kahn A. Influence of maternal smoking on autonomic nervous system in healthy infants. Pediatr Res. 2000;47:215–20.

81. Sawnani H, Jackson T, Murphy T, Beckerman R, Simakajornboon N. The effect of maternal smoking on respiratory and arousal patterns in preterm infants during sleep. Am J Respir Crit Care Med. 2004;169:733–8.

82. Tirosh E, Libon D, Bader D. The effect of maternal smoking during pregnancy on sleep respiratory and arousal patterns in neonates. J Perinatol. 1996;16:435–138.

83. Franco P, Groswasser J, Hassid S, Lanquart J, Scaillet S, Kahn A. Prenatal exposure to cigarette smoking is associated with a decrease in arousal in infants. J Pediatr. 1999;135:34–8.

84. Chang AB, Wilson SJ, Masters IB, Yuill M, Williams G, Hubbard M. Altered arousal response in infants exposed to cigarette smoke. Arch Dis Child. 2003;88:30–3.

85. Lewis KW, Bosque EM. Deficient hypoxia awakening response in infants of smoking mothers: possible relationship to sudden infant death syndrome. J Pediatr. 1995;127:691–9.

86. Horne RSC, Ferens D, Watts A-M, Vitkovic J, Andrew S, Cranage SM, Chau B, Greaves R, Adamson TM. Effects of maternal tobacco smoking, sleeping position and sleep state on arousal in healthy term infants. Arch Dis Child Fetal Neonatal Ed. 2002;87:F100–5.

87. Richardson HL, Walker AM, Horne RSC. Maternal smoking impairs arousal patterns in sleeping infants. Sleep. 2009;32:515–21.

88. Johansson A, Halling A, Hermansson G. Indoor and outdoor smoking. Impact on children's health. Eur J Public Health. 2003;13:61–6.

89. Schoendorf KC, Kiely JL. Relationship of sudden infant death syndrome to maternal smoking during and after pregnancy. Pediatrics. 1992;90:905–8.

90. Klonoff-Cohen HS, Edelstein SL, Lefkowitz ES, Srinivasan IP, Kaegi D, Chang JC, Wiley KJ. The effect of passive smoking and tobacco exposure through breast milk on sudden infant death syndrome. JAMA. 1995;273:795–8.

91. Stephan-Blanchard E, Telliez F, Leke A, Djeddi D, Bach V, Libert J, Chardon K. The influence of in utero exposure to smoking on sleep patterns in preterm neonates. Sleep. 2008;31:1683–9.

92. Andriessen P, Koolen AMP, Berendsen RCM, Wijn PFF, ten Broeke EDM, Oei SG, Blanco CE. Cardiovascular fluctuations and transfer function analysis in stable preterm infants. Pediatr Res. 2003;53:89–97.

93. Mitchell EA, Ford RPK, Stewart AW, Taylor BJ, Becroft DMO, Thompson JMD, Scragg R, Hassell IB, Barry DM, Allen EM, Roberts AP. Smoking and the sudden infant death syndrome. Pediatrics. 1993;91:893–6.

94. Brooke H, Gibson A, Tappin D, Brown H. Case control study of sudden infant death syndrome in Scotland, 1992–5. BMJ. 1997;314:1516–20.

95. Schellscheidt J, Oyen N, Jorch G. Interactions between maternal smoking and other perinatal risk factors for SIDS. Acta Paediatr. 1997;86:857–63.

96. Galland BC, Taylor B, Bolton DPG, Sayers RM. Heart rate variability and cardiac reflexes in small for gestational age infants. J Appl Physiol. 2006;100:933–9.

97. Spassov L, Curzi-Dascalova L, Clairambault J, Kauffmann F, Eiselt M, Medigue C, Periano P. Heart rate and heart rate variability during sleep in small-for-gestational age newborns. Pediatr Res. 1994;35:500–5.

98. Katona PG, Frasz A, Egbert J. Maturation of cardiac control in full-term and preterm infants during sleep. Early Hum Dev. 1980;4:145–59.

99. Eiselt M, Curzi-Dascalova L, Clairambault J, Kauffmann F, Medigue C, Peirano P. Heart rate variability in low-risk prematurely born infants reaching normal term: a comparison with full-term newborns. Early Hum Dev. 1993;32:183–95.

100. Eiselt M, Zwiener U, Witte H, Curzi-Dascalova L. Influence of prematurity and extrauterine development on the sleep state dependant heart rate patterns. Somnologie. 2002;6:116–23.

101. Patural H, Barthelemy JC, Pichot V, Mazzocchi C, Teyssier G, Damon G, Roche F. Birth prematurity determines prolonged autonomic nervous system immaturity. Clin Auton Res. 2004;14:391–5.

102. Patural H, Pichot V, Jaziri F, Teyssier G, Gaspoz JM, Roche F, Barthelemy JC. Autonomic cardiac control of very preterm newborns: a prolonged dysfunction. Early Hum Dev. 2008;84:681–7.

103. Longin E, Gerstner T, Schaible T, Lanz T, Konig S. Maturation of the autonomic nervous system: differences in heart rate variability in premature vs. term infants. J Perinat Med. 2006;34:303–8.

104. Witcombe NB, Yiallourou SR, Walker AM, Horne RSC. Delayed blood pressure recovery after head-up tilting during sleep in preterm infants. J Sleep Res. 2010;19:93–102.

105. Witcombe NB, Yiallourou SR, Walker AM, Horne RSC. Blood pressure and heart rate patterns during sleep are altered in preterm-born infants: implications for sudden infant death syndrome. Pediatrics. 2008;122:1242–8.

106. Witcombe NB, Yiallourou SR, Sands SA, Walker AM, Horne RS. Preterm birth alters the maturation of baroreflex sensitivity in sleeping infants. Pediatrics. 2012;129:e89–96.

107. Fyfe KL, Yiallourou SR, Wong FY, Odoi A, Walker AM, Horne RS. The effect of gestational age at birth on post-term maturation of heart rate variability. Sleep. 2015;38:1635.

108. Yiallourou SR, Witcombe NB, Sands SA, Walker AM, Horne RS. The development of autonomic cardiovascular control is altered by preterm birth. Early Hum Dev. 2013;89:145–52.

109. Fyfe KL, Yiallourou SR, Wong FY, Odoi A, Walker AM, Horne RS. Gestational age at birth affects maturation of baroreflex control. J Pediatr. 2015;166:559–65.

110. Fyfe KL, Yiallourou SR, Wong FY, Odoi A, Walker AM, Horne RS. Cerebral oxygenation in preterm infants. Pediatrics. 2014;134:435–45.

111. Fyfe K, Odoi A, Yiallourou SR, Wong F, Walker AM, Horne RS. Preterm infants exhibit greater variability in cerebrovascular control than term infants. Sleep. 2015;38:1411.
112. Horne RSC, Cranage SM, Chau B, Adamson TM. Effects of prematurity on arousal from sleep in the newborn infant. Pediatr Res. 2000;47:468–74.
113. Scher MS, Steppe DA, Dahl RE, Asthana S, Guthrie RD. Comparison of EEG sleep measures in healthy full-term and preterm infants at matched conceptional ages. Sleep. 1992;15:442–8.
114. Richardson HL, Horne RS. Arousal from sleep pathways are affected by the prone sleeping position and preterm birth: preterm birth, prone sleeping and arousal from sleep. Early Hum Dev. 2013;89:705–11.
115. Tuladhar R, Harding R, Adamson TM, Horne RSC. Comparison of postnatal development of heart rate responses to trigeminal stimulation in sleeping preterm and term infants. J Sleep Res. 2005;14:29–36.
116. Verbeek MMA, Richardson HL, Parslow PM, Walker AM, Harding R, Horne RSC. Arousal and ventilatory responses to mild hypoxia in sleeping preterm infants. J Sleep Res. 2008;17:344–53.
117. Horne RSC, Andrew S, Mitchell K, Sly DJ, Cranage SM, Chau B, Adamson TM. Apnoea of prematurity and arousal from sleep. Early Hum Dev. 2001;61:119–33.
118. Carpenter RG, Irgens LM, Blair PS, Fleming PJ, Huber J, Jorch G, Schreuder P. Sudden unexplained infant death in 20 regions in Europe: case control study. Lancet. 2004;363: 185–91.
119. Kohyama J. Sleep as a window on the developing brain. Curr Probl Pediatr. 1998;28:69–92.
120. Carroll JL. Developmental plasticity in respiratory control. J Appl Physiol. 2003;94:375–89.
121. Yiallourou SR, Walker AM, Horne RSC. Effects of sleeping position on development of infant cardiovascular control. Arch Dis Child. 2008;93:868–72.
122. Yiallourou SR, Walker AM, Horne RSC. Prone sleeping impairs circulatory control during sleep in healthy term infants; implications for sudden infant death syndrome. Sleep. 2008;31:1139–46.
123. Wong FY, Witcombe NB, Yiallourou SR, Yorkston S, Dymowski AR, Krishnan L, Walker AM, Horne RS. Cerebral oxygenation is depressed during sleep in healthy term infants when they sleep prone. Pediatrics. 2011;127:e558–65.
124. Parslow PM, Harding R, Cranage SM, Adamson TM, Horne RSC. Ventilatory responses preceding hypoxia-induced arousal in infants: effects of sleep-state. Respir Physiol Neurobiol. 2003;136:235–47.
125. Trinder J, Newman NM, Le Grande M, Whitworth F, Kay A, Pirkis J, Jordan K. Behavioural and EEG responses to auditory stimuli during sleep in newborn infants and in infants aged 3 months. Biol Psychol. 1990;90:213–27.
126. Parslow PM, Harding R, Cranage SM, Adamson TM, Horne RSC. Arousal responses to somatosensory and mild hypoxic stimuli are depressed during quiet sleep in healthy term infants. Sleep. 2003;26:739–44.
127. Montemitro E, Franco P, Scaillet S, Kato I, Groswasser J, Villa MP, Kahn A, Sastre J, Ecochard R, Thiriez G, Lin J. Maturation of spontaneous arousals in healthy infants. Sleep. 2008;31:47–54.
128. Richardson HL, Walker AM, Horne RSC. Sleep position alters arousal processes maximally at the high-risk age for sudden infant death syndrome. J Sleep Res. 2008;17:450–7.
129. Blackwell C, Moscovis S, Hall S, Burns C, Scott RJ. Exploring the risk factors for sudden infant deaths and their role in inflammatory responses to infection. Front Immunol. 2015;6:44.
130. Galland BC, Elder DE. Sudden unexpected death in infancy: biological mechanisms. Paediatr Respir Rev. 2014;15:287–92.
131. Oyen H, Markstead T, Skjaerven R, Irgens LM, Helweg-Larsen K, Alm B, Norvenius G, Wennergren G. Combined effects of sleeping position and the perinatal risk factors in sudden infant death syndrome: the Nordic epidemiological study. Pediatrics. 1997;100:613–21.
132. Mitchell EA. Sleeping position of infants and the sudden infant death syndrome. Acta Paediatr. 1993;389:26–30.

133. Ponsonby AL, Dwyer T. The Tasmanian SIDS case-control study: univariate and multivariate risk factor analysis. Paediatr Perinat Epidemiol. 1995;9:256–72.
134. Taylor JA, Krieger JW, Reay DT, David RL, Harruff R, Cheney LK. Prone sleeping position and sudden infant death syndrome in King County, Washington: a case control study. Pediatrics. 1996;128:626–30.
135. Beal SM, Finch CF. An overview of retrospective case-control studies investigating the relationship between prone sleeping position and SIDS. J Paediatr Child Health. 1991;27: 334–9.
136. Fleming PJ, Gilbert R, Azaz Y, Berry PJ, Rudd PT, Stewart A, Hall E. Interaction between bedding and sleeping position in the sudden infant death syndrome: a population based case-control study. BMJ. 1990;301:85–9.
137. Galland BC, Reeves H, Taylor B, Bolton DPG. Sleep position, autonomic function, and arousal. Arch Dis Child Fetal Neonatal Ed. 1998;78:189–94.
138. Horne R, Ferens D, Watts A, Vitkovic J, Lacey B, Andrew S, Cranage S, Chau B, Adamson T. The prone sleeping position impairs arousability in term infants. J Pediatr. 2001;138: 811–6.
139. Galland B, Taylor B, Bolton D, Sayers R. Vasoconstriction following spontaneous sighs and head-up tilts in infants sleeping prone and supine. Early Hum Dev. 2000;58:119–32.
140. Ariagno RL, Mirmiran M, Adams MM, Saporito AG, Dubin AM, Baldwin RB. Effect of position on sleep, heart rate variability, and QT interval in preterm infants at 1 and 3 months' corrected age. Pediatrics. 2003;111:622–5.
141. Sahni R, Schulz H, Kashyap S, Ohira-Kist K, Fifer WP, Myers MM. Postural differences in cardiac dynamics during quiet and active sleep in low birthweight infants. Acta Paediatr. 1999;88:1396–401.
142. Gabai N, Cohen A, Mahagney A, Bader D, Tirosh E. Arterial blood flow and autonomic function in full-term infants. Clin Physiol Funct Imaging. 2006;26:127–31.
143. Kahn A, Grosswasser J, Sottiaux M, Rebuffat E, Franco P, Dramaix M. Prone or supine body position and sleep characteristics in infants. Pediatrics. 1993;91:1112–5.
144. Chong A, Murphy N, Matthews T. Effect of prone sleeping on circulatory control in infants. Arch Dis Child. 2000;82:253–6.
145. Ammari A, Schulze KF, Ohira-Kist K, Kashyap S, Fifer WP, Myers MM, Sahni R. Effects of body position on thermal, cardiorespiratory and metabolic activity in low birth weight infants. Early Hum Dev. 2009;85:497–501.
146. Franco P, Grosswasser J, Sottiaux M, Broadfield E, Kahn A. Decreased cardiac responses to auditory stimulation during prone sleep. Pediatrics. 1996;97:174–8.
147. Tuladhar R, Harding R, Cranage SM, Adamson TM, Horne RSC. Effects of sleep position, sleep state and age on heart rate responses following provoked arousal in term infants. Early Hum Dev. 2003;71:157–69.
148. Wong F, Yiallourou SR, Odoi A, Browne P, Walker AM, Horne RS. Cerebrovascular control is altered in healthy term infants when they sleep prone. Sleep. 2013;36:1911–8.
149. Fyfe KL, Yiallourou SR, Wong FY, Horne RS. The development of cardiovascular and cerebral vascular control in preterm infants. Sleep Med Rev. 2014;18:299–310.
150. Ariagno R, van Liempt S, Mirmiran M. Fewer spontaneous arousals during prone sleep in preterm infants at 1 and 3 months corrected age. J Perinatol. 2006;26:306–12.
151. Goto K, Maeda T, Mirmiran M, Ariagno R. Effects of prone and supine position on sleep characteristics in preterm infants. Psychiatry Clin Neurosci. 1999;53:315–7.
152. Bhat RY, Hannam S, Pressler R, Rafferty GF, Peacock JL, Greenough A. Effect of prone and supine position on sleep, apneas, and arousal in preterm infants. Pediatrics. 2006;118: 101–7.
153. Kato I, Franco P, Groswasser J, Kelmanson I, Togari H, Kahn A. Frequency of obstructive and mixed sleep apneas in 1,023 infants. Sleep. 2000;23:487–92.
154. Franco P, Pardou A, Hassid S, Lurquin P, Groswasser J, Kahn A. Auditory arousal thresholds are higher when infants sleep in the prone position. J Pediatr. 1998;132:240–3.

155. Horne RSC, Bandopadhayay P, Vitkovic J, Cranage SM, Adamson TM. Effects of age and sleeping position on arousal from sleep in preterm infants. Sleep. 2002;25:746–50.

156. Richardson HL, Walker AM, Horne R. Stimulus type does not affect infant arousal response patterns. J Sleep Res. 2010;19:111–5.

157. Ponsonby A, Dwyer T, Gibbons LE, Cochrane JA, Jones ME, McCall MJ. Thermal environment and sudden infant death syndrome: case-control study. BMJ. 1992;304:279–91.

158. Tuffnell CS, Peterson SA, Wailoo MP. Prone sleeping infants have a reduced ability to lose heat. Early Hum Dev. 1995;43:109–16.

159. Skadberg BT, Markstead T. Behaviour and physiological responses during prone and supine sleep in early infancy. Arch Dis Child. 1997;76:320–4.

160. Bolton DPG, Nelson EAS, Taylor BJ, Weatherall IL. Thermal balance in infants. J Appl Physiol. 1996;80:2234–42.

161. L'Hoir MP, Engelberts AC, van Well GTJ, McClelland S, Westers P, Dandachli T, Mellenbergh GJ, Wolters WHG, Huber J. Risk and preventive factors for cot death in The Netherlands, a low-incidence country. Eur J Pediatr. 1998;157:681–8.

162. Kahn A, Wachholder A, Winkler M, Rebuffat E. Prospective study on the prevalence of sudden infant death and possible risk factors in Brussels: preliminary results (1987–1988). Eur J Pediatr. 1990;149:284–6.

163. Williams SM, Taylor BJ, Mitchell EA, Other Members of the National Cot Death Study Group. Sudden infant death syndrome: insulation from bedding and clothing and its effect modifiers. Int J Epidemiol. 1996;25:366–75.

164. Naeye RL, Ladis B, Drage JS. Sudden infant death syndrome: a prospective study. Am J Dis Child. 1976;130:1207–10.

165. Bach V, Bouferrache B, Kremp O, Maingourd Y, Libert JP. Regulation of sleep and body temperature in response to exposure to cool and warm environments in neonates. Pediatrics. 1994;93:789–96.

166. Franco P, Scaillet S, Valente F, Chabanski S, Groswasser J, Kahn A. Ambient temperature is associated with changes in infants' arousability from sleep. Sleep. 2001;24:325–9.

167. Stephan-Blanchard E, Chardon K, Leke A, Delanaud S, Bach V, Telliez F. Heart rate variability in sleeping preterm neonates exposed to cool and warm thermal conditions. PLoS One. 2013;8:e68211.

168. Blair PS, Mitchell EA, Heckstall-Smith EMA, Fleming PJ. Head covering a major modifiable risk factor for sudden infant death syndrome: a systematic review. Arch Dis Child. 2008;93:778–83.

169. Mitchell EA, Thompson JM, Becroft DM, Bajanowski T, Brinkmann B, Happe A, Jorch G, Blair PS, Sauerland C, Vennemann MM. Head covering and the risk for SIDS: findings from the New Zealand and German SIDS case-control studies. Pediatrics. 2008;121:e1478–83.

170. Paluszynska DA, Harris KA, Thach BT. Influence of sleep position experience on ability of prone-sleeping infants to escape from asphyxiating microenvironments by changing head position. Pediatrics. 2004;114:1634–9.

171. Franco P, Lipshut W, Valente F, Adams M, Grosswasser J, Kahn A. Cardiac autonomic characteristics in infants sleeping with their head covered by bedclothes. J Sleep Res. 2003;12:125–32.

172. Franco P, Lipshutz W, Valente F, Adams S, Scaillet S, Kahn A. Decreased arousals in infants who sleep with the face covered by bedclothes. Pediatrics. 2002;109:1112–7.

173. Carpenter R, McGarvey C, Mitchell EA, Tappin DM, Vennemann MM, Smuk M, Carpenter JR. Bed sharing when parents do not smoke: is there a risk of SIDS? An individual level analysis of five major case-control studies. BMJ Open. 2013 May 28;3(5). pii: e002299. doi: 10.1136/bmjopen-2012-002299.

174. Blair PS, Sidebotham P, Evason-Coombe C, Edmonds M, Heckstall-Smith EMA, Fleming P. Hazardous co-sleeping environments and risk factors amenable to change: case-control study of SIDS in south west England. BMJ. 2009;339:b3666.

175. Blair PS, Sidebotham P, Pease A, Fleming PJ. Bed-sharing in the absence of hazardous circumstances: is there a risk of sudden infant death syndrome? An analysis from two case-control studies conducted in the UK. PLoS One. 2014;9:e107799.

176. Escott AS, Elder ED, Zuccollo JM. Sudden unexpected infant death and bedsharing: referrals to the Wellington Coroner 1997–2006. N Z Med J. 2009;122:59–68.
177. Hauck FR, Signore C, Fein SB, Raju TNK. Infant sleeping arrangements and practices during the first year of life. Pediatrics. 2008;122:S113–20.
178. McKenna JJ, Mosko SS. Sleep and arousal synchrony and independence among mothers and infants sleeping apart and together (same bed): an experiment in evolutionary medicine. Acta Paediatr Suppl. 1994;397:94–102.
179. Baddock SA, Galland BC, Bolton DP, Williams SM, Taylor BJ. Differences in infant and parent behaviors during routine bed sharing compared with cot sleeping in the home setting. Pediatrics. 2006;117:1599–607.
180. Hoffman HJ, Damus K, Hillman L, Krongrad E. Risk factors for SIDS. Results of the National Institute of Child Health and Human Development SIDS Cooperative Epidemiological Study. Ann NY Acad Sci. 1988;533:13–30.
181. Leach CE, Blair PS, Fleming PJ, Smith IJ, Platt MW, Berry PJ, Golding J, Group., C. S. R. Epidemiology of SIDS and explained sudden infant deaths. Pediatrics. 1999;104:43–53.
182. Heininger U, Kleemann WJ, Cherry JD, Group., S. I. D. S. S. A controlled study of the relationship between bordetella pertussis infections and sudden unexplained deaths among German infants. Pediatrics. 2004;114:9–15.
183. Ponsonby A-L, Dwyer T, Gibbons LE, Cochrane JA, Wang Y-G. Factors potentiating the risk of sudden infant death syndrome associated with the prone position. N Engl J Med. 1993;329:377–82.
184. Hunt CE, Hauck FR. Sudden infant death syndrome. Can Med Assoc J. 2006;174:1861–9.
185. Horne RS, Osborne A, Vitkovic J, Lacey B, Andrew S, Chau B, Cranage SM, Adamson TM. Arousal from sleep in infants is impaired following an infection. Early Hum Dev. 2002;66:89–100.
186. Vennemann MM, Bajanowski T, Brinkmann B, Jorch G, Yucsesan K, Sauerland C, Mitchell EA, GeSID Study Group. Does breastfeeding reduce the risk of sudden infant death syndrome? Pediatrics. 2009;123:e406–10.
187. Hauck FR, Thompson JM, Tanabe KO, Moon RY, Vennemann MM. Breastfeeding and reduced risk of sudden infant death syndrome: a meta-analysis. Pediatrics. 2011;128:103–10.
188. Gordon AE, Saadi AT, Mackenzie DAC, Molony N, James VS, Weir DM, Busuttil A, Blackwell CC. The protective effect of breast feeding in relation to Sudden Infant Death Syndrome (SIDS): III. Detection of IgA antibodies in human milk that bind to bacterial toxins implicated in SIDS. FEMS Immunol Med Microbiol. 1999;25:175–82.
189. Mcvea KLSP, Turner PD, Peppler DK. The role of breastfeeding in sudden infant death syndrome. J Hum Lact. 2000;16:13–20.
190. Butte NF, Smith EO, Garza C. Heart rate of breast-fed and formula-fed infants. J Pediatr Gastroenterol Nutr. 1991;13:391–6.
191. Elias MF, Nicolson NA, Bora C, Johnston J. Sleep/wake patterns of breast-fed infants in the first 2 years of life. Pediatrics. 1986;77:322–9.
192. Horne R, Franco P, Adamson T, Grosswasser J, Kahn A. Influences of maternal cigarette smoking on infant arousability. Early Hum Dev. 2004;79:49–58.
193. Fleming PJ, Blair PS, Pollard K, Platt MW, Leach C, Smith I, Berry PJ, Golding J, CESDI SUDI Research Team. Pacifier use and sudden infant death syndrome: results from the CESDI/SUDI case control study. Arch Dis Child. 1999;81:112–6.
194. Hauck FR, Omojokun OO, Siadaty MS. Do pacifiers reduce the risk of sudden infant death syndrome? A meta-analysis. Pediatrics. 2005;116:e716–23.
195. Li D, Willinger M, Petiti DB, Odouli R, Liu L, Hoffman HJ. Use of a dummy (pacifier) during sleep and risk of Sudden Infant Death Syndrome (SIDS): population based case-control study. BMJ. 2006;332:18–22.
196. Mitchell EA, Blair PS, L'Hoir MP. Should pacifiers be recommended to prevent sudden infant death syndrome? Pediatrics. 2006;117:1755–8.

197. Vennemann MM, Bajanowski T, Brinkmann B, Jorch G, Sauerland C, Mitchell EA, Group, T. G. S. Sleep environment risk factors for sudden infant death syndrome: the German Sudden Infant Death Syndrome Study. Pediatrics. 2009;123:1162–70.

198. Horne RS, Hauck FR, Moon RY, L'Hoir MP, Blair PS, Physiology, Epidemiology Working Groups of the International Society for the, S., Prevention of, P. & Infant, D. Dummy (pacifier) use and sudden infant death syndrome: potential advantages and disadvantages. J Paediatr Child Health. 2014;50:170–4.

199. Franco P, Chabanski S, Scaillet S, Grosswasser J, Kahn A. Pacifier use modifies infant's cardiac autonomic controls during sleep. Early Hum Dev. 2004;77:99–108.

200. Yiallourou SR, Poole H, Prathivadi P, Odoi A, Wong FY, Horne RS. The effects of dummy/pacifier use on infant blood pressure and autonomic activity during sleep. Sleep Med. 2014;15:1508–16.

201. Lappi H, Valkonen-Korhonen M, Georgiadis S, Tarvainen MP, Tarkka IM, Karjalainen PA, Lehtonen J. Effects of nutritive and non-nutritive sucking on infant heart rate variability during the first 6 months of life. Infant Behav Dev. 2007;30:546–56.

202. Hanzer M, Zotter H, Sauseng W, Pichler G, Mueller W, Kerbl R. Non-nutritive sucking habits in sleeping infants. Neonatology. 2010;97:61–6.

203. Cohen M, Brown DR, Myers MM. Cardiovascular responses to pacifier experience and feeding in newborn infants. Dev Psychobiol. 2001;39:34–9.

204. Franco P, Scaillet S, Wermenbol V, Valente F, Groswasser J, Kahn A. The influence of a pacifier on infants' arousals from sleep. J Pediatr. 2000;136:775–9.

205. Hanzer M, Zotter H, Sauseng W, Pichler G, Pfurtscheller K, Mueller W, Kerbl R. Pacifier use does not alter the frequency or duration of spontaneous arousals in sleeping infants. Sleep Med. 2009;10:464–70.

206. Odoi A, Andrew S, Wong FY, Yiallourou SR, Horne RS. Pacifier use does not alter sleep and spontaneous arousal patterns in healthy term-born infants. Acta Paediatr. 2014;103:1244–50.

207. Tonkin SL, Lui D, Mcintosh CG, Rowley S, Knight DB, Gunn AJ. Effect of pacifier use on mandibular position in preterm infants. Acta Paediatr. 2007;96:1433–6.

208. Cozzi F, Albani R, Cardi E. A common pathophysiology for sudden cot death and sleep apnoea. "The vacuum-glossoptosis syndrome". Med Hypotheses. 1979;5:329–38.

209. Lipton EL, Steinschneider A, Richmond JB. Swaddling, a child care practice: historical, cultural, and experimental observations. Pediatrics. 1965;35:521–67.

210. van Sleuwen BE, L'Hoir MP, Engleberts AC, Westers P, Schulpen TWJ. Infant care practices related to cot death in Turkish and Moroccan families in the Netherlands. Arch Dis Child. 2003;88:784–8.

211. Beal SM, Porter C. Sudden infant death syndrome related to climate. Acta Paediatr Scand. 1991;80:278–87.

212. Wilson CA, Taylor BJ, Laing RM, Williams SM, Mitchell EA. Clothing and bedding and its relevance to sudden infant death syndrome: further results from the New Zealand Cot Death Study. J Paediatr Child Health. 1994;30:506–12.

213. Karp H. The happiest baby on the block. New York: Bantam; 2002.

214. van Sleuwen BE, Engelberts AC, Boere-Boonekamp MM, Kuis W, Schulpen TWJ, L'Hoir MP. Swaddling: a systematic review. Pediatrics. 2007;120:e1097–106.

215. Gerard CM, Harris KA, Thach BT. Physiologic studies on swaddling: an ancient child care practice, which may promote the supine position for infant sleep. J Pediatr. 2002;141:398–403.

216. Richardson HL, Walker AM, Horne RSC. Minimizing the risk of sudden infant death syndrome: to swaddle or not to swaddle? J Pediatr. 2009;155:475. ePub August 2009.

217. Narangerel G, Pollock J, Manaseki-Holland S, Henderson J. The effects of swaddling on oxygen saturation and respiratory rate of healthy infants in Mongolia. Acta Paediatr. 2007;96:261–5.

218. Franco P, Seret N, van Hees J, Scaillet S, Grosswasser J, Kahn A. Influence of swaddling on sleep and arousal characteristics of healthy infants. Pediatrics. 2005;115:1307–11.

219. Richardson HL, Walker AM, Horne RS. Influence of swaddling experience on spontaneous arousal patterns and autonomic control in sleeping infants. J Pediatr. 2010;157:85–91.
220. Chisholm JS. Swaddling, cradleboards and the development of children. Early Hum Dev. 1978;2:255–75.
221. Gerard CM, Harris KA, Thach BT. Spontaneous arousals in supine infants while swaddled and unswaddled during rapid eye movement and quiet sleep. Pediatrics. 2002;110:70–6.
222. Franco P, Scaillet S, Grosswasser J, Kahn A. Increased cardiac autonomic responses to auditory challenges in swaddled infants. Sleep. 2004;27:1527–32.
223. Leiter JC, Bohm I. Mechanisms of pathogenesis in the sudden infant death syndrome. Respir Physiol Neurobiol. 2007;159:127–38.
224. Chang RR, Keens TG, Rodriguez S, Chen AY. Sudden infant death syndrome: changing epidemiologic patterns in California 1989–2004. J Pediatr. 2008;153:498–502.
225. Hauck FR, Tanabe KO. International trends in sudden infant death syndrome: stabilization of rates requires further action. Pediatrics. 2008;122:660–6.
226. Fleming PJ, Blair PS, Pease A. Sudden unexpected death in infancy: aetiology, pathophysiology, epidemiology and prevention in 2015. Arch Dis Child. 2015;100:984.

Chapter 9
Pediatric Insomnia

Oliviero Bruni and Marco Angriman

Abstract Sleep disorders in children can compromise quality of life of both children and families, and chronic sleep deprivations are associated with poorer developmental outcome, overweight, and behavioral disturbances.

Assessment should follow medical approach and examining primary and secondary contributing factors and maladaptive behaviors related to sleep, and clinicians should incorporate questions about sleep into their routine health assessment of children, examining the sleep/wake schedule, abnormal movements or behavior during sleep, and daytime consequences of sleep deprivation.

Sleeping environment and bedtime routines should be examined to identify behavioral issues related to sleep.

Polysomnography is not routinely indicated for children with insomnia, but actigraphy can give an estimation of objective sleep parameters.

Treatment options include sleep hygiene, behavioral strategies, and pharmacological treatment for selected cases.

Keywords Pediatric insomnia • Diagnosis • Pharmacological treatment • Behavioral treatment

> **Box**
> That a child needs proper sleep and longer hours of sleep than an adult is such a well recognized fact among common-sense people that it seems strange it should be still necessary to preach it out to the public. *Nature March 18, 1909*

O. Bruni (✉)
Department of Developmental and Social Psychology, S. Andrea Hospital, Sapienza University, Via dei Marsi 78, Rome, Italy
e-mail: oliviero.bruni@uniroma1.it

M. Angriman
Department of Pediatrics, Child Neurology and Neurorehabilitation Unit, Central Hospital of Bolzano, Bohler Street 5, Bolzano 39100, Italy
e-mail: marco.angriman@gmail.com

© Springer International Publishing Switzerland 2017
S. Nevšímalová, O. Bruni (eds.), *Sleep Disorders in Children*,
DOI 10.1007/978-3-319-28640-2_9

Introduction

Sleep is one of the most discussed topics during a child visit [1].

Identification and treatment of sleep problems in children is important since a growing body of evidence suggests a link between sleep disorders and physical, cognitive, emotional, and social development.

Different epidemiological studies indicate that up to 50% of children experience a sleep problem [2–4], and about 4% have a formal sleep disorder diagnosis [5].

The presentation, natural history, and response to treatment of insomnia may differ considerably between adults and children, and even within the pediatric age group, the clinical manifestations of sleep problems may vary by age and developmental level.

Prevalence of Insomnia

About 20–30% of children under the age of 3 years were reported by parents as problematic for bedtime difficulties and frequent night wakings [6] that tend to persist in a large percentage of children [7].

There is a large data variability that is related to study methodology, definition of insomnia, and inclusion criteria (parental report of problematic sleep or strict definition of insomnia as more than three awakenings per night, and sleep latency higher than 30 minutes).

For parents of infants and toddlers, night awakenings are the most common sleep complaints, with 25–50% of children older than 6 months of age continuing to awaken during the night. Bedtime resistance is found in 10–15% of toddlers. A recent longitudinal study in the first year of life showed that about 10% of the infants were reported by parents as having a problematic sleep. Approximately 50% of infants had an average of 1–2 awakenings per night, while >2 awakenings were present in 9% at 3 months, 21% at 6 months, 26% at 9 months, and 17% at 12 months.

Infants with >2 nighttime awakenings slept more often in the parent bed than infants without awakenings, at 3 months and 9 months. From this study also emerges that parental perception of sleep problem at all ages significantly correlated with nocturnal awakenings and difficulties falling asleep [8].

Difficulties falling asleep and night wakings are also common in preschoolers (15–30%). In older children the main insomnia symptoms reported are sleep-onset difficulty (15%) and sleep-related anxiety (11%) [9].

The majority of adolescents sleep less than recommended on school nights and suffer from chronic sleep deprivation [10]; the tendency to delay sleep onset results in bedtimes that are too late to permit habitually sufficient nighttime sleep, and evening-time use of electronic devices such as computers, smart phones, televisions, or video games can delay bedtime or contrast melatonin secretion resulting in delayed sleep onset even after cessation of the activity; moreover, consumption of caffeinated beverages is another contributing factor that can disrupt sleep hygiene resulting in poor sleep quality [11–13].

The exact rate of insomnia among adolescents is uncertain [14]: 20–26 % of adolescents took more than 30 min to fall asleep [15].

A high prevalence of insomnia ranging from 23.8 to 18.5 to 13.6 % was found most pronounced in girls than boys [16].

A recent study showed that adolescent sleep generally declined over 20 years with the largest change occurred between 1991–1995 and 1996–2000 [17].

A clear approximately twofold increasing trend in insomnia symptoms and tiredness was found from the mid-1990s to the end of the 2000s, but after 2008, the increase seems to have stopped. Insomnia symptoms and tiredness were associated with lower school performance, and they were more prevalent among girls (11.9 and 18.4 %) compared to boys (6.9 and 9.0 %, respectively) [18].

Sleep patterns of adolescents between 16 and 19 years were characterized by late bedtimes, long sleep latency, and short sleep duration, contributing to a daily sleep deficiency of about 2 h on weekdays, including a sleep-phase shift to later bedtimes during weekends [15, 19].

Declines in self-reported adolescent sleep across the last 20 years are concerning since chronic insufficient sleep in adolescents has been associated with declines in school and occupational performances; decreased attention and altered regulation of impulses; the use of caffeine, alcohol, stimulant meds, cannabis, and other drugs; increased risk-taking behaviors; depression; suicide ideation; and somatic health and psychological problems [20].

In general, the total sleep duration of children and adolescents seems to be decreasing over time compared with previous generations [21], and the reason why children and adolescents are getting less sleep is in part related to changes of social habits.

Environmental and psychosocial factors such as the increased use of electronic media have a considerable influence on the amount of sleep obtained by children and adolescents.

The intrusion of technology in the sleep of children and adolescents is an emerging problem. It should be taken into account that mobile telephone technology has evolved at such a rate that children and adolescents now use their mobile telephone to access the internet, send and receive emails, engage in social networking, listen to music, and play games [22]. Among a range of technologies, interactive technological devices are most strongly associated with sleep complaints [23].

A recent research comparing preadolescents and adolescents sleep pattern in relation to the use of technology showed that adolescents reported more sleep problems, more eveningness, increase of Internet, social network and phone activities, while preadolescents were more involved in gaming console and TV. The transition from preadolescence to adolescence should be considered at high risk for the development of sleep problems and bad sleep habits. Therefore, it is extremely important to focus on the preadolescence period to inform about the risks related to the use of technology at bedtime in order to prevent sleep problems in adolescence [24, 25].

Apart from the environmental factors (i.e., technologies), some studies highlighted also the influence of cultural background, since prevalence of insomnia varied greatly in relation to the different countries: for example, sleep problems ranged from 10 % in Vietnam and Thailand to 25–30 % in the United States and Australia and even 75 % in China and Taiwan [26].

Specific pediatric populations have an increased incidence of insomnia, especially children with neurodevelopmental and chronic medical and psychiatric conditions [9, 27, 28].

Consequences of Insomnia

Several data from the literature indicates that pediatricians and parents should be aware of the consequences of insomnia in infants, children, and adolescents:

(a) Longitudinal studies have demonstrated that sleep problems often persist throughout childhood and adolescence [11, 12, 29–31].
(b) Inadequate sleep quality and quantity in children and adolescents is associated with negative functional outcomes, including sleepiness, inattention, and other cognitive and behavioral deficits [32], as well as psychiatric and health outcomes, such as obesity and metabolic consequences [33, 34].
(c) Insomnia and sleep disturbances increase the risk of depression, as well as suicide and self-harm behaviors [35–37].
(d) There is also a significant impact on families, with negative effects on daytime function and well-being, as well as elevated levels of family stress [38–43].

A recent meta-analysis of 11 longitudinal studies, comprising 24,821 participants, revealed that children and adolescents with short sleep duration had twice the risk of being overweight/obese, compared with subjects sleeping for long duration, providing evidence that short sleep duration in young subjects is significantly associated with future overweight/obesity [44].

Definition of Pediatric Insomnia

Pediatric insomnia represents a complex combination of biological, circadian, neurodevelopmental, environmental, and behavioral variables; insomnia is defined as a persistent difficulty with sleep initiation, duration, consolidation, or quality that occurs despite adequate opportunity and circumstances for sleep, and results in some form of daytime impairment [45].

According to the previous ICSD-2 [46], "pediatric insomnia" was defined as a "repeated difficulty with sleep initiation, duration, consolidation, or quality that occurs despite age-appropriate time and opportunity for sleep and results in daytime functional impairment for the child and/or family."

The diagnosis of behavioral insomnia of childhood (BIC) was introduced in 2005 in ICSD-2 as a unique diagnostic entity to emphasize sleep difficulties that result from inappropriate sleep associations or inadequate parental limit setting. The diagnosis of sleep-onset behavioral insomnia was characterized by reliance on maladaptive and inappropriate sleep associations such as rocking, watching television, falling asleep in the parents' bed, and so forth. The child is usually unable to fall asleep in the absence of these conditions at both bedtime and following nocturnal arousals. Inadequate parental limit setting can also result in a form of behavioral insomnia characterized by sleep-onset delay secondary to a child's refusing to go to bed or stalling.

The ICSD-3 [45] describes chronic insomnia disorder with no specific pediatric classification; as a consequence, a related unresolved issue is whether the current global classification promotes a generic approach to insomnia therapy that ultimately fails to benefit some insomnia subgroups. The ICSD-3 defines chronic insomnia as "a persistent difficulty with sleep initiation, duration, consolidation, or quality that occurs despite adequate opportunity and circumstances for sleep, and results in some form of daytime impairment"

The criteria include the report from patient or parents/caregivers of difficulty initiating or maintaining sleep, early morning awakenings, resistance to go to bed on appropriate schedule, and difficulty sleeping without parent or caregiver intervention.

The nighttime sleep difficulty determined fatigue/malaise; attention, concentration, or memory impairment; impaired social, family, occupational, or academic performance; mood disturbance/irritability; daytime sleepiness; behavioral problems; reduced motivation/energy/initiative; proneness for errors/accidents; and concerns about sleep. The sleep disturbance and associated daytime symptoms occur at least three times per week and should have been present for at least 3 months.

Based on the ICSD-3, there are several issues that should be considered when approaching an infant/child with insomnia [45]:

1. Parents may have unrealistic sleep expectations for their children and predispose them to insomnia by putting them in bed too early or assigning them too much time in bed each night.
2. Child insomnia is often comorbid with difficult temperament or other comorbid medical and psychiatric conditions.
3. There should be risk factors like difficult home situations, safety concerns, caregiver relationship, and domestic abuse that should be considered or excluded.
4. If the children had a current or past history of medical problems, parents may have difficulty setting limits, because of guilt, a sense that the child is "vulnerable," or concerns about doing psychological harm.
5. Environmental factors such as the child sharing a room with others and cramped living accommodations may contribute to negative sleep-onset associations or poor limit setting.
6. The psychological asset of the parents (especially depressive symptoms) should be always evaluated.

A debated issue is at what age the diagnosis of insomnia could be done: because children are not expected to sleep through the night with regularity until they are

3–6 months of age, 6 months is a reasonable age to first consider a diagnosis of chronic insomnia disorder, unless the sleeplessness is very marked at an earlier age.

The Diagnostic and Statistical Manual of Mental Disorders, 5th edition, DSM-5 [47] does not present any classification of sleep disorders specific for childhood; it includes sleep disorders defined according to criteria that are common for children and adults, although, in some instances, they specify developmental features of particular sleep disorders. The DSM-5 integrated pediatric and developmental criteria and also replaced "primary insomnia" with the diagnosis of "insomnia disorder," a switch to avoid the primary/secondary designation when this disorder co-occurs with other conditions and to reflect changes throughout the classification. Furthermore, it introduced a temporal criterion (more than three "bad nights" a week for the last 3 months). DSM-5 underscores the need for independent clinical attention of a sleep disorder regardless of mental or other medical problems that may be present.

The most apparent change in ICSD-3 is the collapse of all previous chronic insomnia diagnoses into a single *chronic insomnia disorder* diagnosis.

Based on duration of symptoms, three insomnia diagnostic categories are identifiable: chronic insomnia disorder, short-term insomnia disorder, and other insomnia disorder. These diagnoses apply to patients with and without comorbidities.

"Chronic insomnia disorder" is characterized by chronic sleep onset and/or sleep maintenance complaints with associated daytime impairment and is reserved for individuals whose sleep difficulties exceed minimal frequency and duration thresholds shown to be associated with clinically significant morbidity outcomes. "Short-term insomnia disorder" is characterized by sleep/wake difficulties that fail to meet the minimal frequency and duration criteria of chronic insomnia disorder. Nonetheless, short-term insomnia disorder is associated with clinically significant sleep dissatisfaction or waking impairment.

"Other insomnia disorders" category should be assigned to those rare cases that fail to meet criteria for short-term insomnia disorder, yet are thought to have sufficient symptoms of insomnia to warrant clinical attention.

The ICSD-3 integrates pediatric insomnia into the major clinical diagnosis of "chronic insomnia disorder" and includes parent/caregiver report of sleep disturbances and associated impairments in daytime function in the child and family. In this classification, however, the differentiation into two different categories of insomnia representing the main clinical manifestations is maintained: the sleep-onset association and the limit-setting disorder.

The "sleep-onset association type" is characterized by the child's inability or unwillingness to fall asleep or return to sleep in the absence of specific conditions (i.e., inappropriate associations), such as a parent rocking the child to sleep, watching television, feeding, and the presence of parents in the room; in the absence of these conditions, sleep onset is significantly delayed, and when the conditions associated with falling asleep are re-established, the child usually resumes sleep relatively quickly.

Because sleep-onset associations are highly prevalent in young children, the phenomenon is defined as a disorder only if (1) the associations are highly problematic or demanding (e.g., extended rocking, car rides); (2) sleep onset is significantly delayed or sleep is otherwise disrupted in the absence of the associated conditions; and (3) caregiver intervention is frequently required to aid the onset or resumption of sleep.

"Limit-setting" issues are characterized by bedtime stalling or bedtime refusal that is met with and reinforced by inadequate limit setting by a caregiver. Sleep problems occur when caregivers institute no or few limits or when limits are instituted inconsistently or in an unpredictable manner, such as when the parents allow the child to sleep in their bed when the child refuses to sleep.

Fear of sleeping alone, being in the dark, or having nightmares may lead some children to demand certain sleep-promoting conditions (the presence of parent in the bedroom) or to repeatedly delay their bedtimes.

Complications may result from the consequent sleep loss and include irritability, mood dysregulation, inattention, and poor school performance, together with increased family tensions with negative feelings toward the child, parental conflicts, and caregiver sleep loss.

Clinical Approach to Pediatric Insomnia

A thorough knowledge of normal sleep ranges and expected developmental changes is required; since children are not expected to sleep through the night with regularity until they are 3–6 months of age, 6 months is a reasonable age to first consider a diagnosis of insomnia disorder, unless the sleeplessness is very marked at an earlier age [45]. However, when sleep difficulties are persistent and pronounced in infants, underlying medical causes should be considered (like sleep-disordered breathing, gastroesophageal reflux, otitis, allergies, pain, etc.) [48].

The physician must be aware that medical insomnia can be aggravated in combination with behavioral insomnia due to the early alteration of sleep quality inducing wrong associations at bedtime: caregivers may eventually do whatever it takes for everyone to get to sleep, facilitating the development of negative sleep associations.

Multiple night awakenings, mainly in the first year of life, may suggest the presence of gastroesophageal reflux (GERD) or food allergies; diurnal hypersomnolence constitutes an important clinical sign, which suggests another possible diagnosis, such as metabolic or endocrinologic disorders [48].

Sleep-related GERD may present with nocturnal awakenings with a sour taste in the mouth or breath, burning discomfort in the chest, and increased nocturnal arousals leading to sleep fragmentation. Other associated symptoms include abdominal pain, regurgitation, cough, feeding problems, failure to thrive, and respiratory problems.

Many chronic pain conditions – including fibromyalgia, rheumatologic disorders, and other causes of musculoskeletal pain, functional abdominal pain, headaches and migraine, cancer, and spasticity-related pain in cerebral palsy – have been linked to both disturbed sleep and daytime fatigue in children and adolescents [49–53].

Assessment

The assessment of sleep and sleep disturbances in children is performed through subjective (i.e., information reported by the child and/or parents, questionnaires) or objective (i.e., measure of motor or neurophysiologic parameters) tools.

Clinical evaluation is the most important part of the process of assessment and diagnosis of insomnia in the pediatric patients.

An important first step is obtaining information regarding the typical/habitual sleep patterns and difficulties. A sleep history obtained from a frustrated, sleepy parent can be vague and inaccurate, with the parent focusing, at times, on the wrong details. For example, parents often describe the child's sleep pattern only for the most severe or most recent night or period. A more accurate description of the sleep patterns across time can be obtained from a 2-week sleep diary, log, or chart.

It is also important to assess daytime consequences of sleep disruption and comorbid conditions such as depression, anxiety, chronic medical conditions, and other primary sleep disorders.

Physical examination and laboratory assessment may be valuable as well, though they are not always necessary.

The physical examination depends on the medical history, the specifics of the sleep complaint, and the hypotheses generated during assessment, but some aspects are mandatory to evaluate especially if insomnia is comorbid with other sleep disorders: auxologic parameters (obesity or failure to thrive), neurologic examination, abnormal skull or facial features, oropharyngeal crowding, palatal abnormalities, and chest or spine abnormalities.

A number of screening tools have been developed to assist the child healthcare practitioner in assessing for sleep-related disorders and also for insomnia: a quick memory aid to assess sleep is known as BEARS, which provides a comprehensive screening tool usefulness in the primary care setting as well as in the sleep medicine center.

It consisted of different questions regarding *b*edtime, *e*xcessive daytime sleepiness, *a*wakenings at night, *r*egularity/duration, and *s*noring that could suggest a series of possible diagnoses [54].

Specific questionnaires can be very helpful both in clinical and research settings, to complete sleep history and focus the parents on specific aspects of her child sleep, for example, the Sleep Disturbance Scale for Children [55], the Brief Infant Sleep Questionnaire (BISQ) [56] or the Children's Sleep Habits Questionnaire [2, 3], or the Pediatric Sleep Questionnaire [57].

Tests including laboratory and radiographic procedures are not routinely indicated in chronic insomnia, and overnight polysomnography is helpful only to exclude other sleep disorders, such as obstructive sleep apnea, sleep-related movement disorders, or parasomnias.

According to American Academy of Sleep Medicine practice parameters [58], PSG is not indicated for the routine evaluation of insomnia, in the context of an insomnia complaint; it is appropriate if the clinical evaluation raises the suspicion of sleep-related breathing disorders and periodic limb movements.

Actigraphy, although not regarded as a replacement for polysomnography, represents a useful and cost-effective tool to assess pediatric insomnia and response to treatment. It is based on small wristwatch-like devices that monitor movements for extended periods of time. The raw activity scores (i.e., epochs) are translated to sleep/wake scores based on computerized scoring algorithms. There are different commercial devices in the market, and each device has its own measurement characteristics [59].

Actigraphy can be placed on the nondominant wrist, but may also be placed on the dominant wrist, the ankles, or the trunk; extended monitoring (5 days or longer) reduces the inherent measurement errors in actigraphy and increases reliability.

Sleep parameters most closely estimated by actigraphy include sleep duration, sleep efficiency, and waking time after initial sleep onset. A concomitantly maintained sleep log provides important supplemental data for accurate interpretation of actigraphy. Actigraphy-documented improvement in sleep may constitute a strong positive feedback for parents to constantly implement and apply behavioral strategies.

Finally, in adolescence it could be important also to evaluate the body clock type of the patient to exclude circadian rhythm disorders: (a) *Morning chronotypes*, also referred to as *larks* or *early risers*, prefer relatively early bed and wake-up times, and they describe their optimal mental and physical performance to be in the early part of the wake episode; (b) *evening chronotypes*, sometimes referred to as *owls* or *late sleepers*, prefer relatively late bed and wake-up times, and they describe their period of optimal mental and physical performance to be late in the wake episode. The hallmark of circadian rhythm disorders is that when the child is allowed to sleep at his or her desired schedule, sleep is normal and daytime sleepiness rapidly subsides.

Hypothesis on a Clinical Classification of Pediatric Insomnia

Although several studies have been published on the treatment of insomnia in infants and children, the translation of research findings to practice settings remains unclear for several reasons:

(a) Most treatment studies define sleep problems by symptoms and fail to classify using diagnostic criteria [60, 61].
(b) There is no indication on the appropriate treatment for specific insomnia subtypes [62].
(c) There is no clear evidence on frequency and duration of non-pharmacological and pharmacological treatment [41].
(d) There are no long-term follow-up studies either for non-pharmacological and pharmacological treatment.
(e) No specific instruments for assessing the severity of insomnia are available.

The generic classification insomnia in ICSD-3 and DSM-V incorporating adult and pediatric insomnia into a unique entity might be misleading for clinicians and might be difficult to define the exact type of insomnia and to find the correct patient-oriented treatment approach, either non-pharmacological or pharmacological.

In order to guide the decision on the best treatment approach of pediatric insomnia, we hypothesize a clinical categorization of childhood insomnia that might be conceptualized as follows [63–65]:

- Insomnia with motor hyperactivity
- Insomnia with prevalent middle-of-the-night awakenings
- Insomnia with multiple night awakenings and falling asleep difficulties

These three different types are the most commonly encountered in the pediatric sleep field and can be easily identified in the clinical practice. They might be related to different pathophysiological mechanisms:

(a) The *insomnia characterized by motor hyperactivity* (parental report of a child that kicks the legs or described as a "horse in the bed") is probably linked to a dopaminergic dysfunction since it could represent the early manifestations of the restless legs syndrome reported by Picchietti et al. [66]. In a recent study, it has been shown that symptoms of restless legs syndrome may already start in the first year of life and are related to low serum ferritin level. The authors showed that the most striking single symptom was awakening after 1–3 h of sleep followed by screaming, crying, kicking, and slapping the legs or by verbally expressing that the legs "hurt" with a seemingly comforting effect of massage and cycling movements performed by the parents [67]. Recently, we described the case of a toddler with severe insomnia, bedtime and nocturnal hyperactivity, and night awakenings associated with leg kicking and rubbing, highly suggestive of restless legs syndrome but presenting as severe insomnia responsive to gabapentin [64, 65].

(b) The *insomnia with prevalent middle-of-the-night awakenings* could resemble the insomnia of people with mood disorders, that is, mainly characterized by no falling asleep troubles but prolonged midnight awakening with difficulty returning to sleep. Recent studies have demonstrated a link between sleep difficulties in childhood and depression in mid-adolescence [68] and in adulthood [69] and an improvement of sleep quality with the administration of some antidepressants: 5HT2A receptor antagonists determined an increase of slow-wave sleep, a reduction of REM, and an improvement of sleep continuity [70].

(c) The *insomnia with multiple night awakenings and falling asleep difficulties* is often a symptom related to infants who present with milk allergy or gastro-esophageal reflux and therefore are highly suspected to be related to a histaminergic dysfunction. The histaminergic system in the brain is exclusively localized within the posterior hypothalamus with projection to almost all the major regions of the central nervous system. Administration of histamine or H1 receptor agonists induces wakefulness, whereas administration of H1 receptor antagonists promotes sleep. The first generation of antihistamines easily penetrates the blood-brain barrier and causes drowsiness and sedation. Several of these antihistamines, including the nonselective H1 receptor antagonists from the phenothiazine class and "over the counter" diphenhydramine, have positive effects on subjective and objective measures of nocturnal sleep in healthy human subjects [71].

This kind of categorization has important implications for treatment and could allow the clinicians to personalize pharmacological therapy, based on the hypothesized neurotransmitter dysfunction.

This approach is also based on the results of recent genetic studies suggesting that genetic factors play an important role on the development of insomnia of childhood. For example, heritability contributed for 30.8 % on nocturnal sleep duration, for 36.3 % on diurnal sleep duration, and for 35.3 % on night wakings [72]. Furthermore, the variance in consolidated nighttime sleep duration is largely influenced by genetic factors with a critical environmental time-window influence at around 18 months. A strong heritability (71 %) was observed for the short-persistent nighttime sleep duration trajectory [73].

In order to correctly categorize the specific type of insomnia, a careful family and personal history should be collected to evaluate the presence of symptoms/diseases that could be associated with the hypothesized classification of insomnia. LeBlanc et al. [74] point out that family history was the second strongest predictive factor in new cases of insomnia syndrome with the implication that there may be a familial predisposition and, in other words, a vulnerable phenotype. Further, there was a trend toward a higher familial incidence in those reporting earlier onset vs. those reporting a later onset. Furthermore, evidence suggests that the expression of 5HTTLPR, which affects synaptic serotonin levels, is critical in the development of the neonatal brain, and also the 5HTTLPR contributes to the onset of insomnia rather than the severity [75].

However, also several epigenetic mechanisms seem to be involved in the regulation of sleep and in the development of insomnia: stressful experiences during prenatal/early life development may contribute to changes in stress reactivity that may persist into adulthood through epigenetic mechanisms. If epigenetic mechanisms are potentially reversible via environmental or pharmacological interventions, it might be hypothesized that both cognitive behavioral treatment for insomnia and pharmacological interventions might influence epigenetic modification in insomnia [76].

From the previous studies, it is clear that a predisposition to insomnia seems to exist, driven by factors associated with response to stress at both a psychological and physiological level. Understanding vulnerability to insomnia will inform our understanding of the etiology of other disorders, specifically depression.

To summarize our hypothesis on the different types of insomnia reported above, we propose the following treatment approach:

(a) An infant who presents with no particular difficulties in falling asleep but prolonged middle-of-the-night awakenings and a family and clinical history of insomnia, parasomnias, headache/migraine, depression, and mood disorders probably underlies a serotonergic dysfunction and therefore should be treated with serotonergic drugs. Obviously selective serotonin reuptake inhibitors

(SSRI) are not indicated in infants and children, and therefore L-5-hydroxytryptophan could be the choice for this type of insomnia.

(b) An infant presenting with difficulty in falling asleep linked to restless legs or kicking legs and with nocturnal hyperactivity and a family and clinical history of restless legs syndrome or periodic limb movements during sleep, iron deficiency anemia, and growing pains might indicate a dopaminergic dysfunction and should be evaluated for anemia and eventually treated with iron.

(c) An infant showing multiple night awakenings and falling asleep difficulties with a clinical history of atopic dermatitis or milk allergy or gastroesophageal reflux and with a high presence of allergies in the family might reveal a histaminergic dysfunction. In this case obviously the treatment of choice should be the first generation of antihistamines with high affinity for the H1 receptor.

Treatment of Pediatric Insomnia

Prevention is the best treatment for behavioral insomnia of childhood, but unfortunately, most frequently parents request an evaluation when the disorder is chronic. Good sleep practices and behavioral interventions are the first recommended treatments for pediatric insomnia [27]. It is important to discuss parents' knowledge and beliefs as well as strategies they have used to help address their child's sleep problems. For example, in the case of multiple night awakenings, it assumes crucial importance to clarify age-appropriate sleep structure: although parents often perceive that their children with night wakings have more frequent arousals than do other children, arousals are a normal part of sleep architecture and are experienced equally by children with and without reported night waking. It is the child's signaling at times of waking – by crying, calling, or getting out of bed (because of difficulty returning to sleep independently) – that makes the parents aware of, and thus report as frequent, the night wakings [77].

Sleep Hygiene

Sleep hygiene plays an important role in virtually all sleep interventions and typically involves a combination of creating an environment that is conducive to sleep and engaging in healthy sleep habits. In terms of environment, the bedroom should be quiet and dark and have a cool temperature [78].

Scheduling regular, appropriate sleep and wake times allows an adequate sleep opportunity. In addition, the bedroom should be envisioned as a calming, relaxing sleep sanctuary. For this reason, televisions, video games, and other electronic devices should not be kept in the bedroom, and parents should not use the bedroom as a place to send the child when they are punished [79, 80].

The above strategies will work best when used in combination with healthy sleep hygiene habits. These include implementing a regular bedtime routine (e.g., bathe, get in pajamas, brush teeth, read a book, say goodnight) and a consistent sleep schedule, avoiding stimulating activities (e.g., watching television or playing video games) prior to bedtime, limiting caffeine (e.g., cola and chocolate) intake before bed, and engaging in daily physical activity [81].

As with infants and toddlers, parents play a crucial role in treating sleep problems in this age group. It is important that parents model and begin to teach their preschoolers about healthy sleep hygiene. With their parents' help, preschoolers can begin to play a more active role in choosing appropriate sleep hygiene options (e.g., choosing to read a book rather than watch television right before going to sleep). The earlier sleep hygiene habits are established, the better, as sleep habits developed in childhood shape sleep habits exhibited in adulthood.

Addressing nighttime fears in this age group can help reduce negative associations with sleep and may be another important aspect of intervention that should be considered. A common intervention for nighttime fears in children is for the parent to make the child feel safe and secure by co-sleeping (e.g., allowing the child to sleep in the parent's bed). Although this intervention offers short-term alleviation of symptoms, parents often find themselves co-sleeping for extended periods of time. This habit can be challenging to change and often results in the need for an intervention for co-sleeping.

Healthy sleep practices include daytime and nighttime sleep practices that positively impact sleep initiation/maintenance and sleep quantity and quality; it usually includes bedtime routine, consistent bedtime and wake time, a quiet, dark, and cool bedroom, avoidance of caffeinated products, and daily physical activity (Table 9.1). A critical aspect of sleep hygiene is the use of technology in the bedroom (computer, TV, cell phone, video games), which is clearly associated with decreased sleep quantity and quality in children [82].

Non-pharmacological Treatment

Behavioral treatment for bedtime problems and night wakings is claimed to be highly effective in improving child sleep [27]; no published studies have shown any adverse effects of behavioral interventions for bedtime problems and night waking

Table 9.1 Healthy sleep practices

Infants and children should be put to bed wide awake
Bedtime and wake time should remain as consistent as possible
Naps should be timed early enough in the afternoon so as to allow for adequate sleep pressure to accumulate by bedtime
Enhance morning light exposure and limit light exposure in the evening, including light from television, video games, and computer screens, to reinforce physiologic circadian and melatonin rhythm
Avoid chocolate, energy drinks, or caffeinated beverages in the evening

in young children, including interventions involving periods of crying in infants and toddlers [83, 84].

The American Academy of Sleep Medicine published recommendations for behavioral treatment of bedtime problems and night awakenings in infants and young children [60–62]; cardinal elements of a behavioral treatment plan for infant and young children are optimization of sleep hygiene, maintaining a regular sleep schedule, and structured bedtime routines appropriate for age, such as bathing, toothbrushing, or reading stories. Exposure to ambient light at bedtime and during the night should be minimized except for small night lights in cases of children with fear of the dark.

Recent studies showed parent education to be efficacious [85].

For more specific behavioral interventions, there is no evidence to suggest any one approach is more effective than another. Thus parents should be presented with different options and select an approach that matches the infant's temperament and family's preferences. With any strategy, it is important to problem solve with parents how to handle child distress (e.g., parent engages in a distracting activity during infant crying or contact with another supportive adult during the process). With all behavioral interventions, it is important to explain to parents that although the first night will be challenging, the second night will be worse, and that the parents must persist and remain consistent [27].

Treatment of insomnia for older children and adolescents is seldom successful unless all pertinent influences are addressed and the child is motivated enough to make the lifestyle and sleep schedule changes that are usually necessary to correct the problem [13]; consumption of caffeinated beverages should be reduced and any late-day intake should be eliminated. The use of electronic devices should be moved to alternative times and optimally replaced with a structured pre-bedtime routine incorporating less stimulating activities. Efforts should be made to keep bedtime and waking time on non-school days consistent with those on school days to eliminate irregularity of sleep schedule. Daytime napping should be eliminated.

Several behavioral techniques are available, and the clinician should propose to the family the most appropriate, based on parental preferences and child temperament [86]; consistent and sustained application of these interventions is usually necessary to achieve sustained clinical improvement in children with more severe forms of bedtime resistance and night waking.

Positive Routines

Positive routines involve the parents developing a set bedtime routine characterized by quiet activities that the child enjoys. Faded bedtime with response cost involves taking the child out of bed for prescribed periods of time when the child does not fall asleep. Bedtime is also delayed to ensure rapid sleep initiation and that appropriate cues for sleep onset are paired with positive parent-child interactions. Once the behavioral chain is well established and the child is falling asleep quickly, the bedtime is moved earlier by 15–30 min over successive nights until a preestablished bedtime goal is achieved.

Unmodified Extinction

Extinction has been found to be an effective intervention for sleep problems in infants and very young children [87].

In fact, most behavioral methods for treating sleep problems in these age groups incorporate principles of extinction. Extinction is based on the hypothesis that night wakings and attention-seeking behaviors are positively reinforced by parental attention and other behaviors. Thus, extinction involves parents helping their children to establish self-soothing skills (e.g., parents are told to put their infants to bed drowsy, but not asleep, which helps the child learn to settle to sleep on his/her own). The parent is not to respond to their child's attempts at reengaging the parent to provide external soothing techniques (e.g., feeding, rocking, singing). The goal is for the child to learn to self-soothe.

The biggest obstacle associated with extinction is lack of parental consistency. Parents must ignore their child's cries every night, no matter how long it lasts. Many parents are unable to ignore crying long enough for the procedure to be effective.

Tikotzky and Sadeh [87] reported that it can be helpful and encouraging to inform parents that research has not found that limiting parental involvement in order to promote self-soothing results in adverse effects on the infant's emotional well-being or on the parent-child relationship. The child is placed in bed while awake, left alone until asleep, and night wakings are ignored. The infant learns to self-soothe once realizing that nighttime crying does not result in parental attention.

If parents respond after a certain amount of time, the child will only learn to cry longer the next time. Parents are also instructed that post-extinction response bursts may occur. That is, often at some later date, there is a return of the original problematic behavior. Parents are instructed to avoid inadvertently reinforcing this inappropriate behavior following such an extinction burst. The common term used in the media and self-help books to describe unmodified extinction techniques is the "cry it out" approach.

As a variant to unmodified extinction, some studies have utilized *extinction with parental presence.* (The parent remains in the room during extinction, acting as a reassurance for the child but providing little interaction.) This procedure involves the parents staying in the child's room at bedtime but ignoring the child and his/her behavior. Some parents find this approach more acceptable and are able to be more consistent.

Graduated Extinction

For parents who are opposed to unmodified extinction, other variants of extinction, such as graduated extinction or parental presence extinction, may be a better intervention alternative. Graduated extinction involves parents ignoring disruptive bedtime behaviors for a predetermined period. If the child has not settled at the end of that time, the parent settles the child back in bed, but minimizes interaction with the child. Extinction with parental presence involves the parent lying down in a separate bed in the infant's room during settling and awakening. Parents feign sleep and do not attend to the infant directly. Parents follow this procedure for 1 week, after which they follow an unmodified extinction procedure. This technique has been found to reduce the extinction burst (increase in signaling behaviors) that is typically seen when using unmodified extinction. This involves ignoring negative behaviors (i.e., crying) for a given amount of time before checking on the child. The parent gradually increases the amount of time between crying and parental response. Parents provide reassurance through their presence for short durations and with minimal interaction.

Either parents can employ a fixed schedule (e.g., every 5 min), or they can wait progressively longer intervals (e.g., 5 min, 10 min, then 15 min) before checking on their child. With incremental graduated extinction, the intervals increase across successive checks within the same night or across successive nights. The checking procedure itself involves the parents comforting their child for a brief period, usually 15 s to a minute. The parents are instructed to minimize interactions during check-ins that may reinforce their child's attention-seeking behavior.

The goal of graduated extinction is to enable a child to develop "self-soothing" skills in order for the child to fall asleep independently without undesirable sleep associations (e.g., nursing, drinking from a bottle, rocking by parent). Once these skills are established, the child should be able to independently fall asleep at bedtime and return to sleep following normal nighttime arousals.

Scheduled Awakenings

Scheduled awakening entails establishing a baseline of the number and timing of spontaneous night wakings. Then a preemptive waking schedule wherein parents awaken their child approximately 15–30 min before typical spontaneous night waking is implemented. As the treatment progresses, the time between scheduled awakenings is increased until eventually there are no awakenings. When parents awaken the child, they are instructed to engage in their typical behaviors (e.g., feeding, rocking, soothing) as if the child had awakened spontaneously.

Scheduled awakenings appear to increase the duration of consolidated sleep, but the mechanisms behind why this intervention decreases nighttime awakenings are not well understood. Scheduled awakenings are a treatment option for frequent nighttime awakenings, but are not appropriate for problems with sleep initiation. Also, compared to extinction, it can be more complicated to carry out and may take several weeks rather than days before improvements are seen.

Bedtime Fading

Faded bedtime, often used in combination with sleep hygiene, involves determining a time at which it is likely the child will fall asleep within about 15 min of going to bed [88].

Once the child falls asleep at this time with little resistance, the bedtime is set earlier after a series of successful nights until the desired bedtime is achieved. Also, the child's wake time is set at the same time each day, and the child is not allowed to sleep outside the prescribed sleep times. A modified version of this technique, faded bedtime with response cost, involves bedtime fading, as described above. However, if the child does not fall asleep within a certain period of time, the child is removed from bed (response cost) to decrease the negative association between being in bed and awake and to increase the likelihood that the child will fall asleep. After a predetermined time (typically about 30 min during which time the child engages in a non-arousing activity), the child returns to bed. This procedure is repeated until the child falls asleep. Once successful at the target bedtime, an earlier bedtime is set as the goal. The aims of the treatment are in line with the goals of extinction: to increase appropriate behaviors and positive associations with sleep and to decrease arousal by helping the child to develop self-soothing skills and fall asleep independently. This technique involves delaying bedtime closer to the child's target bedtime. The goal of this treatment is for the child to develop a positive association between being in bed and falling asleep rapidly. Bedtimes can be gradually moved earlier.

Efficacy Studies on Behavioral Treatments

It should be taken into account that the long-term efficacy of behavioral treatment is not completely assessed: a systematic review, although acknowledging the efficacy in short term, reported finally that moderate-level evidence supports behavioral interventions for pediatric insomnia in young children and even low evidence in adolescents and in children with neurodevelopmental disabilities. This review showed that only four studies assessed sleep-onset latency, with a significant overall effect and small to medium effect size at posttreatment. Also the evaluation of the efficacy on the frequency of night wakings (seven studies), and on the night waking duration (four studies), resulted in a significant effect but with a small to medium effect size. Finally, a nonsignificant overall effect on night wakings was found at 3–12-month follow-up across five studies [89].

Following the results of this study, we should reconsider the claimed "efficacy" of behavioral interventions; more studies are needed to identify factors that may predict treatment success and to tailor behavioral interventions for young children based on child (e.g., temperament, age), parental, and environmental factors [86]. Finally, more longitudinal studies are needed to demonstrate whether treatment benefits for insomnia are maintained over time and to examine other functional outcomes (child mood, behavior, health, as well as parental mood, marital satisfaction, and family functioning).

Box: Behavioral Strategies for Insomnia of Childhood
1. Create solid and positive bedtime routines (e.g., songs, books, relaxing activities).
2. If possible, put the child in bed sleepy but not fully asleep.
3. Put in the child's bed only few familial objects he can use to sooth himself in the case of nocturnal awakenings (avoid plushes or dangerous objects).
4. Establish a constant "good-bye phrase," for example, "You can sleep alone here with your favorite toys."
5. Before leaving the child's room, give a plausible explanation ("mama will go to the kitchen to drink some water and then come back to you").
6. Speak to the child from the other room to reassure him.
7. If he begins to cry, let him cry for a brief period (5–10 s) before returning in the room.
8. Reassure the child, letting him in his bed and remain in the room until he has calmed down; reduce as much as possible the direct interaction with the child.
9. Leave the room repeating point 4.
10. If the child cries, return in the room and repeat point 7 awaiting a little more time (10–15 s).
11. Next night, repeat from point 1 to 10, increasing time of awaiting of 10 s.

For waiting times in case of nocturnal awakenings, follow those indications:

	1° awakening (s)	2° awakening (s)	3° awakening (s)
Day 1	10	15	20
Day 2	20	25	30
Day 3	30	35	40
Day 4	40	45	50
Day 5	50	55	60
Day 6	60	65	70
Day 7	70	75	80

Pharmacological Treatment

Children who do not respond to behavioral interventions could be candidates for pharmacological treatment of insomnia. Currently, there are no US Food and Drug Administration (FDA)-approved medications for the treatment of insomnia in children, and pharmacological treatment should always be considered in combination with behavioral treatment [26, 90].

Due to the lack of studies and of empirical evidence, different drugs have been traditionally used in pediatric insomnia and especially in children with special needs. Most used medications are sedating antihistamines (e.g., diphenhydramine and hydroxyzine), melatonin, benzodiazepines, α-2-receptor agonists (e.g., clonidine), pyrimidine derivatives (e.g., zaleplon and zolpidem), antipsychotics (e.g., risperidone and quetiapine), and sedating antidepressants (e.g., trazodone and mirtazapine) [90].

Clear, well-defined treatment goals must be established with the patient and family. Treatment goals should be realistic, clearly defined, and measurable, for example, it has to be clarified that the immediate goal of treatment will usually be to alleviate or improve, rather than to completely eliminate, sleep problems. Close communication with the family, including during frequent follow-up visits, is a key component of successful and safe management.

It should be taken into account that drugs could be initially useful for parent and child's relief, and in general it is better not to wait a long time to treat insomnia; it is better to implement a brief drug trial than act later on a chronic insomnia. Also when a drug has been administered, abrupt discontinuation should be avoided, and the treatment should be carefully monitored since there is a natural inclination of the parents to give the lowest dose [91]. Finally, it should be reminded that cognitive behavioral therapy should always be associated to drug treatment to ensure the best long-term efficacy [41].

It is of interest that about 50–60 % of pediatricians use drugs for insomnia in infants and children [92–95], but despite the widespread use of prescription therapies such as clonidine, antidepressants, mood stabilizers, and antihistamines, little data exist on their efficacy for the treatment of insomnia in children and adolescents [60, 61]. Few studies have evaluated pharmacologic interventions for childhood insomnia refractory to behavioral interventions, and even fewer have included children with neurodevelopmental or neuropsychiatric disorders.

Commonly, parents who ask for consultation for insomnia of the infant/child have already tried homeopathic, non-prescription, and off-label prescription agents, because of safety, economy, and evidence.

In the following paragraphs, different homeopathic, off-label prescription agents and drugs commonly used for insomnia are listed.

Tryptophan

Tryptophan is a precursor of serotonin and melatonin widely used in the 1980s for treatment of sleep disorders and headache prophylaxis. It does not have opioid-like effects and does not limit cognitive performance or inhibit arousal from sleep [96]. In the literature, several positive effects on sleep are reported: improvement of sleep latency [97–99].

The exact mechanism of action of the sedative effects of L-tryptophan is unknown, but the effect is not mediated by the conversion in serotonin.

5-Hydroxytryptophan (5-HTP)

5-HTP is the intermediate metabolite of the essential amino acid L-tryptophan (LT) in the biosynthesis of serotonin. 5-HTP is not found in the foods and eating foods with tryptophan slightly increases 5-HTP levels. It easily crosses the blood-brain barrier and effectively increases central nervous system (CNS) synthesis of serotonin. The effects of 5-HTP on sleep structure are conflicting: increase or decrease of REM and increase of SWS [100].

In 1989, the presence of a contaminant called Peak X was found in tryptophan supplements that could determine eosinophilia-myalgia syndrome (EMS); however, a recent study reported that there is no evidence to implement 5-HTP intake as a cause of any illness, especially the EMS or its related disorders [101].

Very limited data are available on the effects of 5-HTP on insomnia symptoms.

There is clear evidence of therapeutical effect for sleep terrors in children at dosage of 2 mg/kg [92, 93].

Antihistamines

Histamine is a wake-promoting neurotransmitter, and inactivation or suppression in various animal models has led to sedation and disrupted wakefulness patterns [102].

The first generations of antihistamines are lipid soluble and pass through the blood-brain barrier; they bind to H1 receptors in the CNS and have minimal effects on sleep architecture. They are often the more acceptable choice for many families, commonly well tolerated, and may acutely improve sleep and speed up behavioral programs.

These agents may worsen obstructive sleep apnea (OSA), and also may suppress rapid eye movement (REM) sleep [90].

Diphenhydramine is the most commonly used and is a competitive H1-histamine receptor blocker. Peak blood and tissue levels are achieved within 2 h of ingestion. The recommended dosage for adults is 25–50 mg, whereas in children the effective dose is between 0.5 mg/kg and 25 mg. A study showed a significant decrease in sleep latency time and number of awakenings [103], while other studies reported no more effectiveness than placebo [104, 105].

Very few studies have been conducted with other antihistamines in children with insomnia, reporting conflicting results. Trimeprazine was used in 22 children with night wakings showing a moderate improvement [106]; niaprazine showed a decrease of sleep-onset latency and an increase of sleep duration [107] even if compared with benzodiazepines [108].

The most common adverse reaction to antihistamines at therapeutic doses is impaired consciousness. The predominant features in an overdose are anticholinergic effects, including fever, blurred vision, dry mouth, constipation, urinary retention, tachycardia, dystonia, and confusion.

Melatonin

Melatonin (N-acetyl-5-methoxytryptamine) is a chronobiotic drug crucial for the regulation of the sleep/wake cycle. In older children and adults, its production and secretion begin in the evening and peak during the night between 2:00 and 4:00 AM; its production and release are inhibited by light. There is now a greater understanding that low doses (0.5 mg) can be effective for some children, with diminishing benefit with doses exceeding 6 mg, and unlike traditional hypnotics such as chloral hydrate and the benzodiazepines, melatonin does not affect sleep architecture [24].

In general MLT for treatment of chronic sleep-onset insomnia in children is effective in a dosage of 0.05 mg/kg given at least 1–2 h before desired bedtime [109].

Systematic reviews and meta-analyses of placebo-controlled, randomized controlled trials (RCTs) in children with neurodevelopmental disabilities, especially autism, have demonstrated that exogenous melatonin improves sleep, either by reducing the time taken to fall asleep (sleep-onset latency) or by increasing total sleep time (sleep maintenance and sleep efficiency), or both [110, 111].

Further, MLT at a dosage of 5 mg was effective in ADHD children with delayed sleep-phase syndrome (DSPS) and insomnia [112–115].

These effects have been also observed in typically developing children with delayed sleep-phase syndrome.

Melatonin is increasingly prescribed to many children using a wide range of doses, demonstrating efficacy in improving sleep quality, by reducing sleep-onset latency or slightly increasing total sleep time.

A large clinical trial confirmed the efficacy of melatonin in the treatment of sleep impairment in children with NDDs, using different doses, ranging from 0.5 to 12 mg; the main effects of melatonin were reduced sleep latency (from 102 to 55 min in 12 weeks) and increased total sleep time (40 min) [116].

Headaches, confusion, dizziness, cough, and rashes have been reported, but these are common symptoms in children and are likely to be coincidental or caused by impurities in the many imported and often unregulated formulations of melatonin. Previous reports of poor seizure control, poor asthma control, and adverse endocrinological problems during puberty have not been confirmed. The systematic reviews and meta-analyses of RCTs all suggest that there are no significant adverse side effects associated with the use of melatonin [24].

Further research is required to evaluate the metabolism of melatonin, the function of its receptors, and its value in specific neurodevelopmental disorders. Unanswered clinical questions include whether slow-release preparations are superior to immediate-release in increasing total sleep time, and whether a more rational and optimal prescription of melatonin might be achieved by measuring salivary melatonin before its use.

Iron

Iron is a cofactor for tyrosine hydroxylase, the enzyme responsible for catalyzing the conversion of the amino acid L-tyrosine to dopamine.

Iron deficiency anemia was reported to be associated with higher motor activity during sleep, shorter night sleep duration, and higher frequency of night waking [117], and supplemental iron was associated with longer sleep duration [118].

In some cases, night awakenings starting in the first year of life might be an early sign of restless legs syndrome [119, 120].

This kind of insomnia with motor hyperactivity and characterized by awakening after 1–3 h of sleep followed by screaming, crying, kicking, and slapping the legs or by verbally expressing that the legs "hurt" with a seemingly comforting effect of massage and cycling movements performed by the parents is reported to be related to low serum ferritin level [67].

Because iron deficiency is common in children, measuring the ferritin level is reasonable. Iron replacement should be initiated if ferritin levels are less than 50 mcg per L, and they should be rechecked in 3 months [121]; although the risk of iron overload is very low, parents should be asked for a personal and family history of hemochromatosis or unexplained liver disease.

Vitamin D

Clinical research on the relation between vitamin D and sleep is ongoing, and few studies have been published on the role of vitamin D metabolism and sleep disorders. Preliminary data suggest the possibility that altered vitamin D metabolism could play an important role in the presentation and severity of sleep disorders [122]. Vitamin D is related to dopamine metabolism; it could be useful to investigate vitamin levels in association with iron parameters in children with motor hyperactivity during sleep.

Clonidine

Clonidine is a central α_2 agonist that has been widely used in treating sleep disturbances (mainly sleep-onset delay) in children with ADHD [123].

Clonidine is rapidly absorbed and has onset of action within 1 h and peak effects in 2–4 h. Starting dose is usually 50 µg, increased in 50 µg increments.

Tolerance to the sedating effects may develop with sedative effects tending to decrease over time, thus necessitating gradual increases in dose and associated increased potential for adverse effects.

No randomized trials of clonidine specifically for children with insomnia exist, but the few studies showed a certain efficacy on sleep latency and night wakings. Side effects include hypotension, bradycardia, irritability, anticholinergic effects (e.g., dry mouth), and REM suppression [124].

Clonazepam

Benzodiazepines bind to the benzodiazepine subunit of the gamma aminobutyric acid (GABA) chloride receptor complex, facilitating the action of the inhibitory neurotransmitter GABA. These hypnotics have long been the first-choice treatment for insomnia in adults, but raise concerns about cognitive impairment, rebound insomnia, and the potential risk for dependence. These concerns, and little evidence-based data availability in the pediatric population, contribute to limit their use in children [125]. Possible side effects include daytime sedation, hypotonia, rebound insomnia on discontinuation, psychomotor/cognitive impairment, and impairment of respiratory function [126].

Zolpidem

It is a non-benzodiazepine receptor agonist (NBzRA) that binds preferentially to $GABA_A$ receptor complexes containing α_1 subunits; it has minimal effects on sleep architecture with a slight increase to slow-wave sleep [127].

There are very few studies conducted in children. A study on 6–11 years or 12–17 years children with ADHD and insomnia received treatment with zolpidem at 0.25 mg/kg per day (max 10 mg/day) vs. placebo. Mean change in latency to persistent sleep at week 4 did not differ between zolpidem and placebo groups. No next-day residual effects of treatment and no rebound phenomena occurred after treatment discontinuation. Most-frequent adverse events (>5 %) were dizziness, headache, and hallucinations [128]; also disinhibition and hallucinations have been reported [129].

Mirtazapine

Mirtazapine is an α_2-adrenergic, 5-HT receptor agonist with a high degree of sedation at low doses; this may result in residual daytime sleepiness [130]. It has been shown to decrease sleep-onset latency, increase sleep duration, and reduce wake after sleep onset (WASO), with relatively little effect on REM [131].

Trazodone

Trazodone is one of the most sedating antidepressants and the most widely studied of antidepressants in terms of sleep. It is a 5-HT$_{2A/C}$ antagonist and inhibits postsynaptic binding of serotonin and blocks histamine receptors. Trazodone suppresses REM sleep and increases slow-wave sleep; side effects are represented by morning hangover (common), hypotension, arrhythmias, and serotonin syndrome [132].

A resume of dosage, side effects, and indications is reported in Table 9.2.

Table 9.2 Selected medications for the treatment of insomnia

Medication	Dosage	Common adverse effects	Indications
Diphenhydramine	0.5 mg/kg	Sedation, anticholinergic effects	Primary insomnia with delayed sleep onset and/or frequent nocturnal awakenings
Hydroxyzine	1 mg/kg	Sedation, anticholinergic effects	Primary insomnia with delayed sleep onset and/or frequent nocturnal awakenings
Niaprazine	1 mg/kg	Sedation, anticholinergic effects	Primary insomnia with delayed sleep onset and/or frequent nocturnal awakenings
Melatonin	0.5–6 mg	Headache, nausea	Circadian rhythm disorders, primary insomnia with delayed sleep onset
Zolpidem	5–10 mg	Sedation, dizziness	Primary insomnia with delayed sleep onset
Trazodone	1 mg/kg	Sedation, anticholinergic effects, priapism	Primary insomnia; frequent nocturnal awakenings
Clonidine	0.05–0.1 mg	Sedation, cardiac arrhythmias	ADHD, disruptive behavior disorders
Gabapentin	3–5 mg/kg	Sedation, leukopenia	Restless legs syndrome, epilepsy, resistant sleep-onset insomnia
Clonazepam	0.25–0.5 mg	Sedation, dizziness	Epilepsy, restless legs syndrome, resistant sleep-onset insomnia, bruxism, rhythmic movement disorder
Mirtazapine	7.5–15 mg	Sedation, weight gain, xerostomia, may esacerbate restless legs syndrome	Sleep onset and sleep maintenance difficulties, Autism spectrum disorders insomnia in comorbidity with depression or anxiety

Conclusions

Insomnia in children has multifactorial origin and can cause impairment in quality of life of both patients and families.

The medical approach should follow the pathway of sleep medicine, examining medical and genetic contributing factors to find a patient-oriented treatment approach. Behavioral treatment strategies and pharmacological options are available. Despite the widespread use of pharmacological treatment, the lack of well-designed, controlled studies concerning the efficacy, tolerability, dosage, and safety profile of hypnotic medications in children raise the need of further research in this field of sleep medicine.

References

1. Olson LM, Inkelas M, Halfon N, Schuster MA, O'Connor KG, Mistry R. Overview of the content of health supervision for young children: reports from parents and pediatricians. Pediatrics. 2004;113(6 suppl):1907–16.
2. Owens JA, Spirito A, McGuinn M, Nobile C. Sleep habits and sleep disturbance in elementary school-aged children. J Dev Behav Pediatr. 2000;21(1):27–36.
3. Owens JA, Spirito A, McGuinn M. The Children's Sleep Habits Questionnaire (CSHQ): psychometric properties of a survey instrument for school-aged children. Sleep. 2000;23(8):1043–51.
4. Liu X, Liu L, Owens JA, Kaplan DL. Sleep patterns and sleep problems among schoolchildren in the United States and China. Pediatrics. 2005;115(1 suppl):241–9.
5. Meltzer LJ, Johnson C, Crosette J, Ramos M, Mindell JA. Prevalence of diagnosed sleep disorders in pediatric primary care practices. Pediatrics. 2010;125(6):e1410–8.
6. Sadeh A, Mindell JA, Luedtke K, et al. Sleep and sleep ecology in the first 3 years: a web-based study. J Sleep Res. 2009;18:60–73.
7. Kataria S, Swanson MS, Trevathan GE. Persistence of sleep disturbances in preschool children. J Pediatr. 1987;110:642–6.
8. Bruni O, Baumgartner E, Sette S, Ancona M, Caso G, Di Cosimo ME, Mannini A, Ometto M, Pasquini A, Ulliana A, Ferri R. Longitudinal study of sleep behavior in normal infants during the first year of life. J Clin Sleep Med. 2014;10(10):1119–27.
9. Owens JA, Mindell JA. Pediatric insomnia. Pediatr Clin North Am. 2011;58(3):555–69.
10. Owens J, Adolescent Sleep Working Group, Committee on Adolescence. Insufficient sleep in adolescents and young adults: an update on causes and consequences. Pediatrics. 2014;134(3):e921–32.
11. Roberts RE, Roberts CR, Chan W. Persistence and change in symptoms of insomnia among adolescents. Sleep. 2008;31(2):177–84.
12. Roberts RE, Roberts CR, Duong HT. Chronic insomnia and its negative consequences for health and functioning of adolescents: a 12-month prospective study. J Adolesc Health. 2008;42(3):294–302.
13. Hoban T. Sleep disorders in children. Contin (Minneap Minn). 2013;19(1):185–98.
14. Roane BM, Taylor DJ. Adolescent insomnia as a risk factor for early adult depression and substance abuse. Sleep. 2008;31(10):1351–6.
15. Gradisar M, Gardner G, Dohnt H. Recent worldwide sleep patterns and problems during adolescence: a review and meta-analysis of age, region, and sleep. Sleep Med. 2011;12(2):110–8.
16. Hysing M, Pallesen S, Stormark KM, Lundenvold AJ, Sivertsen B. Sleep patterns and insomnia among adolescents: a population-based study. J Sleep Res. 2013;22:549–56.

17. Keyes KM, Maslowsky J, Hamilton A, Schulenberg J. The great sleep recession: changes in sleep duration among US adolescents, 1991–2012. Pediatrics. 2015;135(3):460–8.
18. Kronholm E, Puusniekka R, Jokela J, Villberg J, Urrila AS, Paunio T, Välimaa R, Tynjälä J. Trends in self-reported sleep problems, tiredness and related school performance among Finnish adolescents from 1984 to 2011. J Sleep Res. 2015;24(1):3–10.
19. Crowley SJ, Acebo C, Carskadon MA. Sleep, circadian rhythms, and delayed phase in adolescence. Sleep Med. 2007;8(6):602–12.
20. Beebe DW, Ris MD, Kramer ME, Long E, Amin R. The association between sleep disordered breathing, academic grades, and cognitive and behavioral functioning among overweight subjects during middle to late childhood. Sleep. 2010;33(11):1447–56.
21. Matricciani L, Olds T, Petkov J. In search of lost sleep: secular trends in the sleep time of school-aged children and adolescents. Sleep Med Rev. 2012;16(3):203–11.
22. Cain N, Gradisar M. Electronic media use and sleep in school-aged children and adolescents: a review. Sleep Med. 2010;11:735–42.
23. Gradisar M, Wolfson AR, Harvey AG, Hale L, Rosenberg R, Czeisler CA. The sleep and technology use of Americans: findings from the National Sleep Foundation's 2011 sleep in America Poll. J Clin Sleep Med. 2013;9(12):1291–9.
24. Bruni O, Alonso-Alconada D, Besag F, Biran V, Braam W, Cortese S, Moavero R, Parisi P, Smits M, Van der Heijden K, Curatolo P. Current role of melatonin in pediatric neurology: clinical recommendations. Eur J Paediatr Neurol. 2015;19(2):122–33.
25. Bruni O, Sette S, Fontanesi L, Baiocco R, Laghi F, Baumgartner E. Technology use and sleep quality in preadolescence and adolescence. J Clin Sleep Med. 2015;11(12):1433–41.
26. Mindell JA, Sadeh A, Wiegand B, How TH, Goh DY. Cross-cultural differences in infant and toddler sleep. Sleep Med. 2010;11(3):274–80.
27. Angriman M, Caravale B, Novelli L, Ferri R, Bruni O. Sleep in children with neurodevelopmental disabilities. Neuropediatrics. 2015;46(3):199–210.
28. Honaker SM, Meltzer LJ. Bedtime problems and night wakings in young children: an update of the evidence. Paediatr Respir Rev. 2014;15(4):333–9.
29. Byars KC, Yolton K, Rausch J, Lanphear B, Beebe DW. Prevalence, patterns, and persistence of sleep problems in the first 3 years of life. Pediatrics. 2012;129(2):e276–84.
30. Jenni OG, Fuhrer HZ, Iglowstein I, Molinari L, Largo RH. A longitudinal study of bed sharing and sleep problems among Swiss children in the first 10 years of life. Pediatrics. 2005;115(1 Suppl):233–40.
31. Meltzer LJ, Plaufcan MR, Thomas JH, Mindell JA. Sleep problems and sleep disorders in pediatric primary care: treatment recommendations, persistence, and health care utilization. J Clin Sleep Med. 2014;10(4):421–6.
32. Beebe DW. Cognitive, behavioral, and functional consequences of inadequate sleep in children and adolescents. Pediatr Clin North Am. 2011;58(3):649–65.
33. Bell JF, Zimmerman FJ. Shortened nighttime sleep duration in early life and subsequent childhood obesity. Arch Pediatr Adolesc Med. 2010;164(9):840–5.
34. Magee L, Hale L. Longitudinal associations between sleep duration and subsequent weight gain: a systematic review. Sleep Med Rev. 2012;16(3):231–41.
35. Roberts RE, Roberts CR, Chen IG. Impact of insomnia on future functioning of adolescents. J Psychosom Res. 2002;53(1):561–9.
36. Singareddy R, Krishnamurthy VB, Vgontzas AN, Fernandez-Mendoza J, Calhoun SL, Shaffer ML, Bixler EO. Subjective and objective sleep and self-harm behaviors in young children: a general population study. Psychiatry Res. 2013;209(3):549–53.
37. Wong MM, Brower KJ, Zucker RA. Sleep problems, suicidal ideation, and self-harm behaviors in adolescence. J Psychiatr Res. 2011;45(4):505–11.
38. Hiscock H, Wake M. Randomised controlled trial of behavioural infant sleep intervention to improve infant sleep and maternal mood. BMJ. 2002;324(7345):1062–5.
39. Meltzer LJ, Mindell JA. Relationship between child sleep disturbances and maternal sleep, mood, and parenting stress: a pilot study. J Fam Psychol. 2007;21(1):67–73.

40. Thome M, Skuladottir A. Changes in sleep problems, parents' distress and impact of sleep problems from infancy to preschool age for referred and unreferred children. Scand J Caring Sci. 2005;19(2):86–94.
41. Hiscock H, Canterford L, Ukoumunne OC, Wake M. Adverse associations of sleep problems in Australian preschoolers: national population study. Pediatrics. 2007;119:86–93.
42. Owens JA, Fernando S, McGuinn M. Sleep disturbance and injury risk in young children. Behav Sleep Med. 2005;3:18–31.
43. Taveras EM, Rifas-Shiman SL, Oken E, Gunderson EP, Gillman MW. Short sleep duration in infancy and risk of childhood overweight. Arch Pediatr Adolesc Med. 2008;162:305–11.
44. Fatima Y, Doi SA, Mamun AA. Longitudinal impact of sleep on overweight and obesity in children and adolescents: a systematic review and bias-adjusted meta-analysis. Obes Rev. 2015;16(2):137–49.
45. American Academy of Sleep Medicine. International classification of sleep disorders, 3rd ed. Darien, IL, USA; 2014.
46. American Academy of Sleep Medicine. International classification of sleep disorders. 2nd ed. Westchester: Diagnostic and coding manual; 2005.
47. American Psychiatric Association. Diagnostic and statistical manual of mental disorders, 5th ed. (DSM-5). Washington; 2013.
48. Miano S, Peraita-Abrados R. Pediatric insomnia: clinical, diagnosis and treatment. Rev Neurol. 2014;58(1):35–42.
49. Perquin CW, Hazebroek-Kampschreur AAJM, Hunfeld JAM, et al. Pain in children and adolescents: a common experience. Pain. 2000;87(1):51–8.
50. Berrin SJ, Malcarne VL, Varni JW, et al. Pain, fatigue, and school functioning in children with cerebral palsy: a path-analytic model. J Pediatr Psychol. 2007;32(3):330–7.
51. Untley ED, Campo JV, Dahl RE, et al. Sleep characteristics of youth with functional abdominal pain and a healthy comparison group. J Pediatr Psychol. 2007;32(8):938–49.
52. Long AC, Krishnamurthy V, Palermo TM. Sleep disturbances in school-age children with chronic pain. J Pediatr Psychol. 2008;33(3):258–68.
53. Palermo TM, Wilson AC, Lewandowski AS, et al. Behavioral and psychosocial factors associated with insomnia in adolescents with chronic pain. Pain. 2011;152(1):89–94.
54. Mindell J, Owens J. A clinical guide to pediatric sleep. Philadelphia: Lipincott Williams & Wilkins; 2010.
55. Bruni O, Ottaviano S, Guidetti V, et al. The sleep disturbance scale for children (SDSC). Construction and validation of an instrument to evaluate sleep disturbance in childhood and adolescence. J Sleep Res. 1996;5:251–61.
56. Sadeh A. A brief screening questionnaire for infant sleep problems: validation and findings for an internet sample. Pediatrics. 2004;113(6):e570–7.
57. Chervin RD, Hedger K, Dillon JE, Pituch KJ. Pediatric Sleep Questionnaire (PSQ): validity and reliability of scales for sleep-disordered breathing, snoring, sleepiness, and behavioral problems. Sleep Med. 2000;1:21–32.
58. Kushida CA, Littner MR, Morganthaler T, et al. Practice parameters for the indications for polysomnography and related procedures: an update for 2005. Sleep. 2005;28:499–519.
59. Sadeh A. The role and validity of actigraphy in sleep medicine: un update. Sleep Med Rev. 2011;15(4):259–67.
60. Mindell JA, Emslie G, Blumer J, Genel M, Glaze D, Ivanenko A, Johnson K, Rosen C, Steinberg F, Roth T, Banas B. Pharmacologic management of insomnia in children and adolescents: consensus statement. Pediatrics. 2006;117(6):e1223–32.
61. Mindell JA, Kuhn B, Lewin DS, Meltzer LJ, Sadeh A, American Academy of Sleep Medicine. Behavioral treatment of bedtime problems and night wakings in infants and young children. Sleep. 2006;29(10):1263–76.
62. Morgenthaler T, Kramer M, Alessi C, Friedman L, Boehlecke B, Brown T, Coleman J, Kapur V, Lee-Chiong T, Owens J, Pancer J, Swick T, American Academy of Sleep Medicine.

Practice parameters for the psychological and behavioral treatment of insomnia: an update. An american academy of sleep medicine report. Sleep. 2006;29(11):1415–9.

63. Bruni O, Addessi E, Angriman M, Riccioni A, Dosi, Ferri R. Toward a clinical and therapeutic classification of insomnia of childhood. Sleep Med. 2013;S14:e18–92.

64. Bruni O, Angriman M. Pediatric insomnia: new insights in clinical assessment and treatment options. Arch Ital Biol. 2015;153(2–3):154–66.

65. Bruni O, Angriman M, Luchetti A, Ferri R. Leg kicking and rubbing as a highly suggestive sign of pediatric RLS. Sleep Med. 2015;16(12):1576–7.

66. Picchietti DL, Rajendran RR, Wilson MP, Picchietti MA. Pediatric restless legs syndrome and periodic limb movement disorder: parent-child pairs. Sleep Med. 2009;10(8): 925–31.

67. Tilma J, Tilma K, Norregaard O, Ostergaard JR. Early childhood-onset restless legs syndrome: symptoms and effect of oral iron treatment. Acta Paediatr. 2013;102:e221–6.

68. Gregory AM, Caspi A, Eley TC, Moffitt TE, O'Connor TG, Poulton R. Prospective longitudinal associations between persistent sleep problems in childhood and anxiety and depression disorders in adulthood. J Abnorm Child Psychol. 2005;33:157–63.

69. Greene G, Gregory AM, Fone D, White J. Childhood sleeping difficulties and depression in adulthood: the 1970 British Cohort Study. J Sleep Res. 2015;24:19–23.

70. Monti J. Serotonin control of sleep-wake behavior. Sleep Med Rev. 2011;15:269–81.

71. Thakkar MM. Histamine in the regulation of wakefulness. Sleep Med Rev. 2011;15:65–74.

72. Brescianini S, Volzone A, Fagnani C, Patriarca V, Grimaldi V, Lanni R, Serino L, Mastroiacovo P, Stazi MA. Genetic and environmental factors shape infant sleep patterns: a study of 18-month-old twins. Pediatrics. 2011;127(5):e1296–302.

73. Touchette E, Dionne G, Forget-Dubois N, Petit D, Pérusse D, Falissard B, Tremblay RE, Boivin M, Montplaisir JY. Genetic and environmental influences on daytime and nighttime sleep duration in early childhood. Pediatrics. 2013;131(6):e1874–80.

74. LeBlanc M, Mérette C, Savard J, Ivers H, Baillargeon L, Morin CM. Incidence and risk factors of insomnia in a population-based sample. Sleep. 2009;32(8):1027–37.

75. Harvey CJ, Gehrman P, Espie CA. Who is predisposed to insomnia: a review of familial aggregation, stress-reactivity, personality and coping style. Sleep Med Rev. 2014;18:237–47.

76. Palagini L, Biber K, Riemann D. The genetics of insomnia – evidence for epigenetic mechanisms? Sleep Med Rev. 2014;18(3):225–35.

77. Sadeh A. Assessment of intervention for infant night waking: parental reports and activity-based home monitoring. J Consult Clin Psychol. 1994;62:63–8.

78. Galland BC, Mitchell EA. Helping children sleep. Arch Dis Child. 2010;95(10):850–3.

79. Owens J, Maxim R, McGuinn M, Nobile C, Msall M, Alario A. Television-viewing habits and sleep disturbance in school children. Pediatrics. 1999;104(3):e27.

80. Davis KF, Parker KP, Montgomery GL. Sleep in infants and young children: part one: normal sleep. J Pediatr Health Care. 2004;18(2):65–71.

81. Driver HS, Taylor SR. Exercise and sleep. Sleep Med Rev. 2000;4(4):387–402.

82. Mindell JA, Meltzer LJ, Carskadon MA, Chervin RD. Developmental aspects of sleep hygiene: findings from the 2004 National Sleep Foundation Sleep in America Poll. Sleep Med. 2009;10(7):771–9.

83. Hiscock H, Bayer JK, Hampton A, Ukoumunne OC, Wake M. Long-term mother and child mental health effects of a population-based infant sleep intervention: cluster-randomized, controlled trial. Pediatrics. 2008;122:e621–7.

84. Price AM, Wake M, Ukoumunne OC, Hiscock H. Outcomes at six years of age for children with infant sleep problems: longitudinal community-based study. Sleep Med. 2012;13:991–8.

85. Adachi Y, Sato C, Nishino N, Ohryoji F, Hayama J, Yamagami T. A brief parental education for shaping sleep habits in 4-month-old infants. Clin Med Res. 2009;7:85–92.

86. Meltzer LJ. Clinical management of behavioral insomnia of childhood: treatment of bedtime problems and night wakings in young children. Behav Sleep Med. 2010;8(3):172–89.

87. Tikotzky L, Sadeh A. The role of cognitive–behavioral therapy in behavioral childhood insomnia. Sleep Med. 2010;11(7):686–91.

88. Taylor DJ, Roane BM. Treatment of insomnia in adults and children: a practice-friendly review of research. J Clin Psychol. 2010;66(11):1137–47.
89. Meltzer LJ, Mindell JA. Systematic review and meta-analysis of behavioral interventions for pediatric insomnia. J Pediatr Psychol. 2014;39:932–48.
90. Pelayo R, Yuen K. Pediatric sleep pharmacology. Child Adolesc Psychiatr Clin N Am. 2012;21(4):861–83.
91. Pelayo R, Dubik M. Pediatric sleep pharmacology. Semin Pediatr Neurol. 2008;15(2):79–90.
92. Bruni O, Ferri R, Miano S, Verrillo E. L-5-hydroxytryptophan treatment of sleep terrors in children. Eur J Pediatr. 2004;163(7):402–7.
93. Bruni O, Violani C, Luchetti A, Miano S, Verrillo E, Di Brina C, Valente D. The sleep knowledge of pediatricians and child neuropsychiatrists. Sleep Hypn. 2004;6(3):130–8.
94. Owens JA. Pharmacotherapy of pediatric insomnia. J Am Acad Child Adolesc Psychiatry. 2009;48(2):99–107.
95. Heussler H, Chan P, Price AM, Waters K, Davey MJ, Hiscock H. Pharmacological and non-pharmacological management of sleep disturbance in children: an Australian Paediatric Research Network survey. Sleep Med. 2013;14(2):189–94.
96. Lieberman HR, Corkin S, Spring BJ, Wurtman RJ, Growdon JH. The effects of dietary neurotransmitter precursors on human behavior. Am J Clin Nutr. 1985;42(2):366–70.
97. Körner E, Bertha G, Flooh E, Reinhart B, Wolf R, Lechner H. Sleep-inducing effect of L-tryptophan. Eur Neurol. 1986;25 Suppl 2:75–81.
98. Schneider-Helmert D, Spinweber CL. Evaluation of L-tryptophan for treatment of insomnia: a review. Psychopharmacology (Berl). 1986;89(1):1–7.
99. Hartmann E, Spinweber CL. Sleep induced by L-tryptophan. Effect of dosages within the normal dietary intake. J Nerv Ment Dis. 1979;167(8):497–9.
100. Meoli AL, Rosen C, Kristo D, et al. Oral nonprescription treatment for insomnia: an evaluation of products with limited evidence. J Clin Sleep Med. 2005;1(2):173–87.
101. Das YT, Bagchi M, Bagchi D, Preuss HG. Safety of 5-hydroxy-L-tryptophan. Toxicol Lett. 2004;150(1):111–22.
102. Mignot E, Taheri S, Nishino S. Sleeping with the hypothalamus: emerging therapeutic targets for sleep disorders. Nat Neurosci. 2002;5:1071–5.
103. Russo RM, Gururaj VJ, Allen JE. The effectiveness of diphenhydramine HCl in pediatric sleep disorders. J Clin Pharmacol. 1976;16(5–6):284–8.
104. Merenstein D, Diener-West M, Halbower AC, Krist A, Rubin HR. The trial of infant response to diphenhydramine: the TIRED study – a randomized, controlled, patient-oriented trial. Arch Pediatr Adolesc Med. 2006;160(7):707–12.
105. Gringras P. When to use drugs to help sleep. Arch Dis Child. 2008;93(11):976–81.
106. France KG, Blampied NM, Wilkinson P. A multiple-baseline, double-blind evaluation of the effects of trimeprazine tartrate on infant sleep disturbance. Exp Clin Psychopharmacol. 1999;7(4):502–13.
107. Ottaviano S, Giannotti F, Cortesi F. The effect of niaprazine on some common sleep disorders in children. A double-blind clinical trial by means of continuous home-video recorded sleep. Childs Nerv Syst. 1991;7(6):332–5.
108. Montanari G, Schiaulini P, Covre A, Steffan A, Furlanut M. Niaprazine vs chlordesmethyldiazepam in sleep disturbances in pediatric outpatients. Pharmacol Res. 1992;25 Suppl 1:83–4.
109. van Geijlswijk IM, van der Heijden KB, Egberts AC, Korzilius HP, Smits MG. Dose finding of melatonin for chronic idiopathic childhood sleep onset insomnia: an RCT. Psychopharmacology (Berl). 2010;212(3):379–91.
110. Phillips L, Appleton RE. Systematic review of melatonin treatment in children with neurodevelopmental disabilities and sleep impairment. Dev Med Child Neurol. 2004;46(11):771–5.
111. Braam W, Didden R, Maas AP, Korzilius H, Smits MG, Curfs LM. Melatonin decreases daytime challenging behaviour in persons with intellectual disability and chronic insomnia. J Intellect Disabil Res. 2010;54(1):52–9.
112. Van der Heijden KB, Smits MG, Van Someren EJ, Gunning WB. Idiopathic chronic sleep onset insomnia in attention-deficit/hyperactivity disorder: a circadian rhythm sleep disorder. Chronobiol Int. 2005;22(3):559–70.

113. Van der Heijden KB, Smits MG, Van Someren EJ, Ridderinkhof KR, Gunning WB. Effect of melatonin on sleep, behavior, and cognition in ADHD and chronic sleep-onset insomnia. J Am Acad Child Adolesc Psychiatry. 2007;46(2):233–41.
114. Smits MG, van Stel HF, van der Heijden K, Meijer AM, Coenen AM, Kerkhof GA. Melatonin improves health status and sleep in children with idiopathic chronic sleep-onset insomnia: a randomized placebo-controlled trial. J Am Acad Child Adolesc Psychiatry. 2003;42(11):1286–93.
115. Weiss MD, Wasdell MB, Bomben MM, Rea KJ, Freeman RD. Sleep hygiene and melatonin treatment for children and adolescents with ADHD and initial insomnia. J Am Acad Child Adolesc Psychiatry. 2006;45(5):512–9.
116. Appleton RE, Jones AP, Gamble C, et al. The use of Melatonin in children with neurodevelopmental disorders and impaired sleep: a randomised, double-blind, placebo-controlled, parallel study (MENDS). Health Technol Assess. 2012;16(40):i–239.
117. Kordas K, Siegel EH, Olney DK, Katz J, Tielsch JM, Chwaya HM, Kariger PK, Leclerq SC, Khatry SK, Stoltzfus RJ. Maternal reports of sleep in 6-18-month-old infants from Nepal and Zanzibar: association with iron deficiency anemia and stunting. Early Hum Dev. 2008;84(6):389–98.
118. Kordas K, Siegel EH, Olney DK, Katz J, Tielsch JM, Kariger PK, Khalfan SS, LeClerq SC, Khatry SK, Stoltzfus RJ. The effects of iron and/or zinc supplementation on maternal reports of sleep in infants from Nepal and Zanzibar. J Dev Behav Pediatr. 2009;30(2):131–9.
119. Kotagal S, Silber MH. Childhood-onset restless legs syndrome. Ann Neurol. 2004;56(6):803–7.
120. Picchietti DL, Stevens HE. Early manifestations of restless legs syndrome in childhood and adolescence. Sleep Med. 2008;9:770–81.
121. Kryger MH, Otake K, Foerster J. Low body stores of iron and restless legs syndrome: a correctable cause of insomnia in adolescents and teenagers. Sleep Med. 2002;3(2):127–32.
122. McCarty DE, Chesson Jr AL, Jain SK, Marino AA. The link between vitamin D metabolism and sleep medicine. Sleep Med Rev. 2014;18(4):311–9.
123. Prince JB, Wilens TE, Biederman J, et al. Clonidine for sleep disturbances associated with attention-deficit hyperactivity disorder: a systematic chart review of 62 cases. J Am Acad Child Adolesc Psychiatr. 1996;35(5):599–605.
124. Nguyen M, Tharani S, Rahmani M, Shapiro M. A review of the use of clonidine as a sleep aid in the child and adolescent population. Clin Pediatr (Phila). 2014;53(3):211–6.
125. Kotagal S. Treatment of dyssomnias and parasomnias in childhood. Curr Treat Options Neurol. 2012;14(6):630–49.
126. Owens JA, Babcock D, Blumer J, Chervin R, Ferber R, Goetting M, Glaze D, Ivanenko A, Mindell J, Rappley M, Rosen C, Sheldon S. The use of pharmacotherapy in the treatment of pediatric insomnia in primary care: rational approaches. A consensus meeting summary. J Clin Sleep Med. 2005;1(1):49–59.
127. Zisapel N. Drugs for insomnia. Expert Opin Emerg Drugs. 2012;17(3):299–317.
128. Blumer JL, Findling RL, Shih WJ, Soubrane C, Reed MD. Controlled clinical trial of zolpidem for the treatment of insomnia associated with attention-deficit/hyperactivity disorder in children 6 to 17 years of age. Pediatrics. 2009;123:e770–6.
129. Liskow B, Pikalov A. Zaleplon overdose associated with sleepwalking and complex behavior. J Am Acad Child Adolesc Psychiatr. 2004;43(8):927–8.
130. Younus M, Labellarte MJ. Insomnia in children: when are hypnotics indicated? Paediatr Drugs. 2002;4(6):391–403.
131. Wichniak A, Wierzbicka A, Jernajczyk W. Sleep and antidepressant treatment. Curr Pharm Des. 2012;18:5802–17.
132. Carrey N, Baath S. Trazodone for sleep in children. Child Adolesc Psychopharmacol News. 1996;1:10–1.

Chapter 10
Obstructive Sleep Apnea in Children: A Short Primer

Hui-Leng Tan, David Gozal, and Leila Kheirandish-Gozal

Abstract Since the modern description of obstructive sleep apnea (OSA) in the mid-1970s, this disease has rapidly emerged as a highly prevalent condition in children. Its major importance derives from the vast array of end-organ morbidities associated with pediatric OSA, as knowledge and understanding on such adverse consequences and their pathophysiological mechanisms have accrued over the last several decades. In parallel, a remarkable transition is currently underway to radically change the diagnostic and therapeutic approaches for OSA in children. This chapter will not only provide a succinct review of the clinical aspects of childhood OSA but also examine some of the newer directions that unavoidably will transition our practices from "one size fits all" to endotype- and phenotype-based precision approaches.

Keywords Sleep apnea • Adenotonsillar hypertrophy • Sleep fragmentation • Cognition • Cardiovascular • Metabolic • Inflammation • Children • Leukotriene • Corticosteroid

H.-L. Tan, MBBS
Department of Paediatric Respiratory Medicine, Royal Brompton Hospital, London, UK

D. Gozal, MD, MBA
Sections of Pediatric Sleep Medicine and Pediatric Pulmonology, Department of Pediatrics, Comer Children's Hospital, Pritzker School of Medicine, The University of Chicago, Chicago, IL, USA

L. Kheirandish-Gozal, MD, MSc (✉)
Sections of Pediatric Sleep Medicine and Pediatric Pulmonology, Biological Sciences Division, Department of Pediatrics, Comer Children's Hospital, Pritzker School of Medicine, The University of Chicago, 5841 S. Maryland Avenue, Office C-113 /MC2117, Chicago, IL 60637-1470, USA
e-mail: lgozal@peds.bsd.uchicago.edu

© Springer International Publishing Switzerland 2017
S. Nevšímalová, O. Bruni (eds.), *Sleep Disorders in Children*,
DOI 10.1007/978-3-319-28640-2_10

Introduction

Obstructive sleep-disordered breathing (SDB) is one of the most common disorders of sleep during childhood. It is defined as "a syndrome of upper airway dysfunction during sleep, characterized by snoring and/or increased respiratory effort that results from increased upper airway resistance and pharyngeal collapsibility" [1], and its phenotypic spectrum ranges from primary snoring through upper airway resistance syndrome to obstructive sleep apnea (OSA) and obstructive hypoventilation. Each of these disease severity categories is strictly defined with the following:

(a) *Primary snoring* comprising habitual snoring (>3 nights a week) without apneas, hypopneas, frequent arousals, or gas exchange abnormalities.
(b) *Upper airways resistance syndrome* being defined as habitual snoring, combined with increased respiratory effort and work of breathing resulting in arousals (i.e., sleep fragmentation), but no recognizable obstructive events or gas exchange abnormalities.
(c) *OSA* is the recurrent occurrence of either partial or complete obstruction of the upper airway during sleep (hypopneas, obstructive, or mixed apneas) with resultant disruption of normal oxygenation, ventilation, and sleep pattern.
(d) Lastly, *obstructive hypoventilation* is defined as snoring and abnormally elevated end-expiratory carbon dioxide partial pressure in the absence of recognizable obstructive events.

Obstructive sleep-disordered breathing in children was recognized back in the nineteenth century, as was the relief afforded by "nasopharyngeal scarifications." However, it was not until the mid-1970s that the first case series was described by Guilleminault et al. documenting the impact of OSA in eight children with symptoms of excessive daytime sleepiness, nighttime snoring, nocturnal enuresis, decreased school performance, morning headaches, mood and personality changes, weight problems, and pulmonary hypertension [2]. Nocturnal polygraphic recordings confirmed the diagnosis of OSA. Treatment with adenotonsillectomy or tracheostomy significantly improved their symptoms. As the early case series highlighted, the typical nocturnal symptoms of OSA include snoring, excessive sweating, restless sleep, mouth breathing, apneas, gasping, labored or paradoxical breathing, and hyperextension of the neck during sleep, along with night terrors or nightmares. Daytime symptoms in turn are usually more subtle and can include behavioral hyperactivity, difficulty concentrating and learning, conduct problems, morning headaches, excessive daytime sleepiness, and failure to thrive [3]. However, since the symptoms of OSA in children often are indistinct from other conditions, effective diagnosis is dependent upon either a high index of suspicion from experienced clinicians or requires the systematic implementation of explorative screening strategies in targeted populations.

Estimates of the true prevalence and incidence vary depending on the populations studied and the stringency of the diagnostic criteria used, but typically range between 1 and 5 % in the general pediatric population. However, the prevalence is appreciably increased in certain high-risk groups such as obese children or those with craniofacial syndromes. The peak prevalence occurs between 2 and 8 years of age [4–7].

The clinical relevance of OSA and to a certain extent in milder and of course more severe SDB categories resides in its impact on the neurocognitive, cardiovascular, and metabolic systems. In this chapter, we highlight the major concepts regarding the pathophysiology of OSA, its morbidity, diagnosis, and treatment.

Pathophysiology of OSA

The pathophysiological factors involved in OSA can be broadly divided into two major themes, those anatomical factors that result in reduced airway caliber and those that promote increased upper airway collapsibility. Examples of the former include adenotonsillar hypertrophy, micrognathia, and macroglossia; in turn, examples of the latter include the presence of upper airway inflammation and alterations in the neurological reflexes coordinating the upper airway musculature. In the majority of children, several factors will coexist to a greater or lesser degree, and there are usually a composite of complex pathophysiological processes which ultimately lead to upper airway dysfunction during sleep. Therefore, the situation clearly exists whereby children with "kissing tonsils" have no evidence of any SDB, even PS, while other children with relatively normal adenotonsillar and other upper airway lymphoid tissues will present severe OSA in their sleep studies. Thus, risk factors for OSA include craniofacial syndromes (e.g., Crouzon's syndrome, Apert's syndrome, Pierre Robin sequence, Treacher Collins syndrome), achondroplasia, micrognathia, mucopolysaccharidoses, macroglossia cerebral palsy, neuromuscular disorders, myelomeningocele, sickle cell disease, trisomy 21, allergic rhinitis, asthma, Afro-Caribbean ethnicity, and obesity [8].

Arens et al. have pioneered and extensively used MRI approaches to better understand the relative contributions of the various craniofacial structures and soft tissues in the context of SDB. These investigators compared the upper airway structures in otherwise healthy young children with OSA aged 3–7 years old with matched controls [9]. The volumetric measurements obtained revealed that in children with OSA, the tonsils and adenoids were significantly larger, as was the soft palate, with resultant smaller upper airway cross-sectional area and volumes. Schwab et al. performed a similar study in adolescents aged 12–16 years old, dividing them into three groups: obese adolescents with OSA, obese controls, and lean controls [10]. Surprisingly, results were similar to those found in the younger children, suggesting that adolescents with OSA have an anatomic risk profile more akin to that of children, rather than the one typically seen in adult OSA patients. In addition, obese adolescents with OSA had larger adenotonsillar tissues with concurrently smaller nasopharyngeal airways compared with the two control groups. Gender differences were also noted, whereby boys had larger tonsils and girls had larger adenoids. The new implementation of computational fluid dynamics to upper airway imaging [11–16] should yield very important insights in the near future regarding OSA heterogeneous endotypes and enable planning of their treatment with more individualized approaches [17, 18].

These findings, which have now been extensively confirmed across multiple studies, underpin the strategies for OSA management in childhood since they imply that either surgical removal or pharmacologically induced size reduction of upper airway lymphoid tissues should be the initial strategy for children including adolescents, rather than opt for immediate implementation of positive pressure therapy, which is the first-line therapy in adults. Indeed, not only do children with OSA usually present with enlarged adenoids and tonsils, they also have hypertrophy/hyperplasia of lymphoid tissues in other regions of the airway, such as the deep cervical lymph nodes [19] and lingual tonsils [20–23].

The mechanisms underlying follicular lymphoid proliferation and resultant hyperplasia in OSA children remain poorly understood. The in vitro culture of CD3, CD4, and CD8 cells derived from the tonsillar tissue of children with OSA showed higher proliferative rates compared with cells derived from the tonsillar tissue of children with recurrent tonsillitis [24, 25]. Pro-inflammatory cytokines TNF-α, IL-6, and IL-1α were more highly expressed in the OSA-derived tonsillar cells. It has been postulated that the recurrent vibration of the upper airway wall during snoring and/or respiratory viruses may promote localized inflammation [26–28]. Certainly exhaled breath condensate levels of leukotriene B4 (LTB4) and cysteinyl leukotrienes are higher in children with OSA [29], while induced sputum from children with OSA has increased neutrophilia compared with controls [30].

Prominent inferior nasal turbinates, deviation of the nasal septum, middle ear effusions, and opacification of the sinuses [31] have led some to hypothesize that OSA may in fact be a broader disorder affecting the airway as a whole, mediated by inflammatory processes, chronic or recurrent infectious processes, or a combination thereof [32].

However, other factors apart from anatomical ones must also play a role, since as mentioned above not all children with adenotonsillar hypertrophy have OSA and, conversely, some children without obvious anatomical risk factors have OSA. Indeed, the obstructive apnea-hypopnea index (AHI), the most frequently used measure of OSA severity, does not directly correlate with airway volume [9], and coefficients of correlation between AHI and adenotonsillar size are usually relatively weak, albeit statistically significant [33, 34]. This paradox has led to the concept of airway collapsibility as an important and critical determinant in OSA and has traditionally taken the approach that the upper airway should be modeled as a Starling resistor. The Starling resistor model posits that under conditions of flow limitation, the maximum inspiratory airflow is determined by the pressure changes upstream to a collapsible locus in the upper airway and is independent of the downstream pressure generated by the diaphragm. The pressure at which the upper airway collapses has been termed the critical closing pressure (P_{crit}) and is an objective measure of airway collapsibility. A study by Marcus and colleagues found that P_{crit} was 1 ± 3 cmH$_2$O in children with OSA compared with -20 ± 9 cmH$_2$O in primary snorers. These findings indicate that children with OSA essentially had demonstrably more collapsible upper airways during sleep. Interestingly, P_{crit} has been shown to become more negative, i.e., the airways become less collapsible, following treatment with adenotonsillectomy [35].

During wakefulness, however, active neural processes preserve upper airway patency and make it difficult to recognize such increased collapsibility. Gozal and Burnside used acoustic pharyngometry to study the upper airway dynamics before and after application of local anesthetic to the pharyngeal introitus in the awake child [36]. Upper airway collapsibility was determined from the percentage change in cross-sectional area (UAC) before and after topical anesthesia, and a change in UAC $\leq -30\%$ proved to be highly sensitive and specific in the identification of children with an AHI > 5/h TST.

Further evidence for airway collapsibility came from Carrera et al. who used the negative expiratory pressure (NEP) technique in awake children and showed that those children with OSA had upper airways that were more easily prone to collapse than controls [37]. This is mirrored by work in adult patients, whereby the degree of upper airway collapse when performing the Müller maneuver has been shown to correlate with AHI severity [38].

McGinley et al. aimed to identify surrogate markers of upper airway collapsibility by performing analyses of inspiratory flow patterns, attempting to derive flow limitation metrics from the nasal cannula flow-pressure signal during standard PSG recordings [39]. In REM sleep, children with OSA exhibited a higher %IFL (percentage of time with inspiratory flow-limited breathing) and lower $\%VI_{max}$ (maximal inspiratory airflow during flow-limited breaths), and these parameters improved following adenotonsillectomy. These findings are thought to be a reflection of decreased compensatory neuromuscular responses to upper airway obstruction in children with OSA during REM sleep. Limitations of this approach included the fact that quantitative changes in airflow can be markedly affected by mouth breathing and cannula displacement, such that the ability to detect these phenomena may be precluded during extensive periods of sleep among habitual mouth breathers. However, the concept is innovative, and further validation and exploration of its inherent value in relation to the clinical phenotypic variance of OSA should be of interest.

Obesity

With the current worldwide obesity epidemic, we are also seeing a change in the demographics of children with OSA. Previously, the archetypal presentation was a child aged between 2 and 8 years old with adenotonsillar hypertrophy and failure to thrive, whereas nowadays, the proportion of children with OSA who are obese is rapidly increasing and in many centers such as ours represents the majority of patients being referred for consultation. Indeed, obesity is undoubtedly one of the most significant risk factors for OSA in children [40]. Each 1 kg/m² increment in BMI above the 50th percentile is associated with a 12% increased risk of OSA [40].

These children often present at a slightly older age, and their clinical presentation more resembles that of the adult OSA phenotype with more prominent excessive daytime sleepiness symptoms [41]. While all the abovementioned pathophysiological mechanisms are still just as applicable in the context of obesity, there are some additional obesity-specific factors thought to be in play that deserve mention. As might be expected, when the upper airways of obese children with OSA were examined using MRI volumetric approaches, an increase in the size of the upper airway lymphoid tissues, parapharyngeal fat pads, and abdominal visceral fat was noted [42]. However, the size of the adenotonsillar tissues in obese children with OSA was smaller than in nonobese children with OSA who were gender, age, race, and obstructive AHI matched, while their Mallampati scores were higher. Overall, these findings indicated that the presence of obesity increases the risk for OSA not only via increased lymphadenoid tissue proliferation and hypertrophy but also by restricting the overall pharyngeal space [33]. Indeed, the percentage of obese children who have residual OSA post-adenotonsillectomy is significantly higher than in nonobese children [43].

The second additional burden as a consequence of obesity seems to be potential alterations in the functional mechanisms regulating upper airway patency resulting in increased collapsibility, with these changes stemming from the increase in fatty infiltrates within the neck and upper airway structures. Central obesity also reduces the functional residual capacity of the lungs due to abdominal visceral fat impinging on the chest cavity, limiting diaphragmatic descent, particularly when lying in the supine position [44]. Furthermore, thoracic fat weighing on the chest wall can lead to a decrease in the overall compliance of the respiratory system, which may contribute to hypoventilation, atelectasis, and ventilation-perfusion mismatch. The reduced lung volumes potentially decrease airway stiffness by reducing the tracheal tethering effect, further increasing the risk of upper airway collapse during sleep. When MRI scans were performed pre- and post-adenotonsillectomy in obese children with OSA, there was not only increased residual adenoidal tissue, but the volume of the tongue and soft palate were also greater after adenotonsillectomy [45]. The abovementioned factors may well underlie the relatively low success rate of adenotonsillectomy that has consistently been reported in obese children with OSA [43, 46–48].

An important guide to the impact of obesity on OSA in children is exemplified by the NANOS study, a cross-sectional, prospective multicenter study, which examined 248 obese children aged 3–14 years recruited from the community [49]. The study consisted of two phases, with phase 1 assessing the prevalence and risk factors for OSA, while phase 2 examined the treatment outcomes. The prevalence of OSA was high at 21.5 % when OSA was defined as an obstructive AHI ≥ 3/h TST, and this increased to 39.5 % when a respiratory disturbance index (RDI) ≥ 3/h TST was used [49]. Adenoidal and tonsillar hypertrophy still emerged as the most important risk factor for OSA. In phase 2, outcomes of 117 children from the original cohort were reported [50]. In group 1, the obese children without OSA, 21 % developed OSA on their follow-up sleep study (PSG). In group 2, obese children with mild OSA without adenotonsillar hypertrophy, managed with dietary modification to encourage weight loss, improvements in the sleep study parameters emerged, and half of this cohort no longer had evidence of OSA at follow-up. In group 3, the obese children with moderate/severe OSA with significant adenotonsillar hypertrophy who underwent AT, the severity of OSA improved post-AT, but 43.5 % still had residual OSA. Older age emerged as a significant risk factor for residual OSA, a finding that was consistent with findings from earlier studies [43, 45, 46, 48, 51–54]. The final group consisted of obese children with moderate/severe OSA who did not have adenotonsillar hypertrophy, and these patients were treated with CPAP. Overall, the authors concluded that at younger ages, the major determinant of OSA appears to be adenotonsillar hypertrophy, with BMI-adipose tissue mass apparently operating as an OSA enhancer, rather than as a causal contributor. However, in older children, obesity becomes a more prominent OSA contributor and appears to be an independent causal factor.

Such findings were overall not surprising, considering that OSA and obesity are both conditions in which low-grade systemic inflammation is present [55] and buttresses the potential for positive reinforcement and exacerbation. Kheirandish-Gozal et al. examined 100 obese children with OSA, measuring a panel of plasma inflammatory markers before and after treatment with adenotonsillectomy, and showed that when OSA was successfully treated, IL-6, IL-18, PAI-1, MCP-1, MMP-9, adropin, and leptin plasma levels decreased, whereas adiponectin levels increased [56]. These improvements were not seen in the 30 children whose postoperative OAHI remained >5/hTST, and leptin levels in fact increased, rather than decreased. This study would suggest that in obese children, not only does OSA amplify the underlying systemic inflammatory pathways that have been a priori activated by obesity, but more importantly, effective treatment of the OSA results in improvements in the overall inflammatory status. A recent study further provided confirmatory evidence that the personalized trajectory of an inflammatory marker such as high-sensitivity CRP in the context of adenotonsillectomy treatment of OSA provides a robust predictor of residual postoperative OSA [57]. Thus, future studies exploring panels of relevant and validated inflammatory biomarkers may provide opportunities for the establishment of robust surrogate reporters of OSA morbidity and also enable the identification of residual OSA after treatment.

A reciprocal interaction between obesity and OSA has also been suggested, whereby not only is obesity a major risk factor for OSA, but OSA may also contribute to the development of obesity. The excessive daytime sleepiness that can result from the presence of OSA likely reduces the commitment to and engagement in exercise and physical activity, and as such may reduce the overall energy expenditure [58]. Leptin, a key hormonal regulator of appetite and metabolism, promotes satiety and reduces food intake; in contrast, ghrelin is an appetite-stimulating hormone secreted in the gut. OSA can induce leptin resistance and increase ghrelin levels, both of which can potentiate obesogenic behaviors, in particular, the intake of high calorie comfort foods [58]. Thus, the end product of OSA, namely, reduced energy expenditure along with increased energy intake may promote the emergence of obesity, particularly when less severe hypoxemia is present, the latter potentially activating and fostering reduced activity of somatic growth pathways [59, 60].

OSA and Asthma

Given the interrelationship between obesity and OSA, it is perhaps unsurprising that a prominently pro-inflammatory disease such as asthma also appears to interact with OSA. Certainly, the prevalence of OSA in asthmatic children is higher than in non-asthmatic children and has been reported to increase with increasing asthma severity [61]. A history of poorly controlled asthma is associated with more severe OSA [62], and improved asthma control was demonstrated in a group of poorly controlled asthmatics following treatment of their OSA [63]. Asthma has also been identified as one of the risk factors for residual OSA post-AT [43]. It is worth noting that there was a high proportion of obese children in all of these cohorts, an observation that was anticipated, considering that obesity is an important risk factor for OSA, and that an epidemiological link has also been described between obesity and asthma, thereby suggesting an interplay between the three conditions [64].

The strongest evidence thus far for the presence of an association between OSA and asthma has been from work by Bhattacharjee et al. who examined this link by performing an electronic database analysis of 13,506 children with asthma in the US who underwent adenotonsillectomy, by examining their asthma control the year before and the year after surgery [65]. The authors found a 30 % reduction in asthma exacerbations, a 25 % decrease in the number of asthma-related emergency room visits, and a 36 % reduction in asthma-related hospital admissions after adenotonsillectomy. These findings contrasted with a 2 % reduction in asthma exacerbations seen in the 27,012 age-, sex-, and geographically matched control children with asthma who did not undergo adenotonsillectomy. Notwithstanding, the limitations emanating from database analyses must be acknowledged, more particularly the lack of information on obesity and ethnicity. However, the findings provide compelling real-life evidence that adenotonsillectomy is associated with improved asthma control, and many respiratory centers have already started screening for OSA in their difficult asthma programs. The mechanisms underlying this potential link between OSA and asthma are still poorly understood; however, one of the more attractive current hypotheses linking OSA and asthma is the united airway hypothesis [32]. There certainly appears to be biological plausibility that inflammation of the upper airway from OSA may exacerbate inflammation in the lower airways, with resultant deterioration in asthma control. Conversely, exhaled breath condensate containing inflammatory cytokines originating from the lower airways in poorly controlled asthmatics may initiate or contribute to the proliferation of upper airway lymphoid tissues and also promote upper airway collapsibility and thus OSA.

OSA and Inflammation

Much of the pathogenesis of OSA is thought to result from its activation and propagation of systemic inflammatory responses [66]. Microarray analyses of RNA from peripheral leukocytes of children with OSA have revealed the upregulation of gene clusters involved in inflammatory pathways [67]. Levels of the anti-inflammatory cytokine IL-10 have been reported to be reduced in children with OSA [68], whereas levels of pro-inflammatory cytokines, e.g., IL-6, IFN-γ, and TNF-α, have been reported to be increased [69–71], though not all studies have been uniformly consistent in these findings.

Increased high-sensitivity C-reactive protein (CRP) levels have also been demonstrated, correlating with OSA severity and evidence of decreased levels following treatment [72–75]. However, once again, not all children with OSA have raised CRP levels, and this may reflect the inherent genetic variations impact on phenotypic expression now being recognized in such factors as IL-6 and CRP [75, 76]. Indeed, it has been demonstrated that the promoter region of the FOXP3 gene which regulates the differentiation of lymphocytes into regulatory T lymphocytes (Tregs) exhibits severity-dependent increases in methylation in pediatric OSA [77]. Tregs play an important role in the suppression of inflammation. The concept that OSA can induce epigenetic changes, which then have downstream consequences on inflammation, was supported by the finding that numbers of Tregs in the peripheral blood and lymphoid tissue of children with OSA were decreased [78].

Environmental Modifiers

There is accumulating evidence that environmental modifiers contribute to the variance of phenotypic expression of OSA. Exposures to passive cigarette smoking have emerged as an independent risk factor for habitual snoring in preschool children with a dose-dependent relationship identified between urinary cotinine concentrations and frequency of snoring [79]. Environmental tobacco exposure has also been linked to increased severity of disease, with an associated 20 % increase in AHI [80]. Environmental air quality and low family social economic status have emerged as significant contributors, with the frequency of habitual snoring in school-aged children residing in neighborhoods with greatest air pollution reported as threefold higher than those who reside in neighborhoods with less air pollution [81, 82].

Morbidity of OSA

OSA can result in intermittent hypoxia, hypercapnia, swings in intrathoracic pressure, and sleep fragmentation. These physiological alterations trigger activation of inflammatory cascades and induction of oxidative stress as detailed, with resultant cellular injury, dysfunction, and even death. The resultant morbidities fall into the following main areas:

Neurocognitive and Behavioral Consequences

Considerable neurocognitive growth and development occurs during childhood. Therefore, any negative effects of OSA on behavior, attention, and learning can significantly negatively impact on the children's ability to fulfill their potential. One of the first papers to highlight the causative link between OSA and its negative impact on academic performance was a prospective study of 297 first-grade children whose school performance was in the lowest tenth percentile of their class [83]. Screening for OSA revealed a higher than expected prevalence of 18 %. More compellingly, the children with OSA who were treated showed significant improvements in their school grades in their subsequent academic year, whereas children with untreated OSA did not.

The association between OSA and neurocognitive and behavioral morbidity has received extensive attention in the last two decades [48, 84–95]. In the largest study to date that included both polysomnography (PSG) and cognitive testing, a community-based approach was implemented in 1010 children aged between 5 and 7 years [96]. These children were divided into four groups: controls who did not snore and had an AHI < 1/hrTST on PSG; primary snorers, i.e., children with habitual snoring (>3 nights/week) but normal sleep study (AHI < 1/hrTST); mild OSA (1 < AHI < 5/hrTST); and children who had moderate-to-severe OSA (AHI > 5/hrTST). There were significant differences in Differential Ability Scales verbal and nonverbal performance scores, Global Conceptual Ability scores, and NEPSY attention and executive-function subscores across the groups. A dose-response effect of OSA was seen, with performance of the children in the moderate-to-severe OSA group being significantly more impaired than the performance among the other three groups in these neurocognitive tests. An exception to this pattern was in the NEPSY Visual Attention subtest, where the group of primary snorers performed more poorly than the children with OSA.

Further evidence for the global neurocognitive impact of OSA comes from the findings that children with OSA require more learning opportunities and take longer to learn a pictorial-based short-term and long-term declarative memory test [97]. Preliminary functional MRI data show that children with OSA demonstrate greater neural recruitment of brain regions implicated in cognitive control, conflict monitoring, and attention in order to perform at the same level as children without OSA [98]. The findings complement electrophysiological data from EEG event-related potentials [99].

Some investigators have hypothesized that changes in regional cerebral blood flow during sleep as a result of OSA may also contribute to the degree of neurocognitive impairment. Children with mild OSA (AHI < 5/h) exhibit significantly raised middle cerebral artery blood flow velocities [100]. The situation is not straightforward, for example, both increased arousal indices and mean arterial pressure are strongly associated with OSA severity, and while increasing arousal indices are associated with decreased regional cerebral oxygenation, increasing mean arterial blood pressure is associated with increased regional brain oxygenation.

One research group has proposed a model to explain the sources of variability in cognitive function of children with sleep-disordered breathing. In this model, age, mean arterial pressure, oxygen saturation, and REM sleep have a positive effect on regional cerebral oxygen saturation during sleep, while male sex, arousal index, and NREM sleep are negative factors diminishing cerebral oxygenation [101]. Furthermore, the significantly higher degree of coexistence of endothelial dysfunction and neurocognitive impairment in children with OSA, an overlap whose likelihood is markedly greater than what might be predicted from random association alone [102], suggests that endothelial and cognitive dysfunction may either share similar pathophysiological mechanisms or even potential causative associations, i.e., endothelial dysfunction may lead to neurocognitive deficits.

Pediatric OSA can be associated with hyperactivity, attention and concentration deficits, and impulsivity [99, 103, 104]. These symptoms are remarkably similar to attention deficit hyperactivity disorder (ADHD), and clinicians should remember to consider OSA or even primary snoring, as one of the differential diagnoses when assessing a child for ADHD. A good example of such associations is reflected by the findings of the Tucson Children's Assessment of Sleep Apnea (TuCASA) study, a community-based observational cohort study of 6–12-year-old Caucasian and Hispanic children. While assessment of neurocognitive outcomes showed that OSA had a negative correlation between AHI and Full Scale IQ, Performance IQ, math achievement, and immediate recall [105], OSA was also clearly associated with behavioral morbidity. Thus, children in the upper 15 % respiratory disturbance index (RDI) had higher (i.e., worse) scores in the Aggressive, Attention Problems, Social Problems, Thought Problems, Total and Externalizing domains of the Child Behavior Checklist, as well as in the Oppositional, Cognitive Problems, Social Problems, Psychosomatic, ADHD Index on the Conners' Parent Rating Scale [106]. In Hong Kong, Lau et al. studied 23 children with OSA (mean obstructive AHI: 5.6/hrTST) and compared them with 22 matched controls. The children with OSA performed less well in both the basic storage and central executive components of working memory in the verbal domain than the controls [107]. The most prominent recent study to examine neurobehavioral outcomes as the primary outcome of interest was the CHildhood AdenoTonsillectomy (CHAT study) [108]. It was the first multicenter randomized controlled trial to compare adenotonsillectomy with watchful waiting in the management of pediatric OSA in school-aged children. No differences emerged between the two arms of the trial in the primary outcome – change in the attention and executive-function score in the Developmental Neuropsychological Assessment [48]. However, adenotonsillectomy resulted in significant improvements in symptoms, behavior, PSG parameters as well as parent-rated generic and OSA-specific quality-of-life measures [109]. It is important to note that due to ethical considerations, the children recruited only had mild OSA (median AHI 4.7/hTST) with no significant oxygen desaturations and were aged 5–9 years, and the follow-up period was relatively short at 7 months. Generalizations to children of other ages and severities of OSA are thus not possible. Furthermore, considering the overall findings indicating increased risk for cognitive deficits, but not the presence of universal deficits in pediatric OSA, the CHAT study may have been underpowered to identify small improvements in cognition when a large proportion of the children included was not cognitively affected. Therefore, sub-analyses of the changes in cognition among those with lower cognitive scores would be of interest and might confirm previous studies supporting improvements in cognitive measures.

As inferred from the above comments, it is important to emphasize that not all children with OSA exhibit cognitive or behavioral deficits. Genetic and environmental factors likely play a role in modifying the phenotypic expression of this morbidity [110]. Differences in systemic inflammatory responses as reflected by plasma CRP levels appear to differentiate children of similar OSA severity with and without cognitive deficits [111]. Furthermore, NADPH oxidase p22 subunit gene polymorphisms, IGF-1, and apoliprotein E allelic variants have all been identified as being potential modifiers of the risk for cognitive deficits in the context of OSA in children and account for discrepancies in the functional cognitive performance in children with OSA [112, 113].

Long-Term Neurobehavioral Follow-Up

This is still an area of some controversy with no clear consensus being reached. A subgroup of 43 children from the TuCASA study, when followed up 5 years later on, revealed no differences in the performance in the working memory, reaction time, and attention tests of the Sustained Working Memory Task between the OSA and control groups [114]. The OSA group did however show lower P300 evoked potential amplitudes, a marker used in the evaluation of an individual's neurocognitive processing of external stimuli, during the Simple Reaction Time and Multiplexing Tasks. Peak alpha power during the Multiplexing Task was also lower in the OSA group. In other words, the long-term impact of pediatric OSA may cause subtle long-term changes in executive function, which are not detectable with conventional functional neurocognitive testing but are evident on neuroelectrophysiologic testing. Long-term follow-up of behavioral indices in this cohort revealed that children with untreated OSA exhibit hyperactivity, have problems with attention, and display aggressive behaviors, lower social competencies, poorer communication, and diminished adaptive skills in adolescence [115].

More worryingly, an Australian study examining the long-term outcomes 3 years after the resolution of OSA in preschool children also found that behavioral functioning remained significantly worse in children who had been diagnosed with OSA compared with controls.

Cognitive function also decreased between baseline and follow-up, regardless of whether there had been resolution of the OSA [116]. Similarly, long-term follow-up of older school-aged children demonstrated no improvement in behavioral functioning; while there was improvement in performance IQ, there was no improvement in verbal IQ or overall academic outcomes [117]. These findings essentially confirm our initial observations that the presence of snoring in early childhood translates into reduced school performance at ages 13–14 years [118].

These studies somewhat challenge the current paradigm generated from shorter-term follow-up studies, which have generally shown improvements in neurobehavioral outcomes following OSA treatment [119, 120]. One possible explanation for these a priori discrepancies may be that in the short term, there is a "placebo-like" treatment effect, whereby the expectation of improvement with adenotonsillectomy may have biased parental responses when completing behavioral questionnaires, but since such "placebo" effect wears off with time, or since initial perceptions of behavior are a reflection of improved sleep, the re-emergence of the problems may occur at least in a subset of the patients. Alternatively, it is possible that an insult to a developing brain during a vulnerable period may result in long-term sequelae, particularly in children who are genetically at risk. Thus, some neurocognitive sequelae may only be partially reversible if OSA is left untreated for too long [118], highlighting the importance of early diagnosis and prompt effective treatment.

Cardiovascular System

Early case reports of pediatric OSA described consequences such as pulmonary hypertension and cor pulmonale [2, 121, 122]. Fortunately, with increased awareness and earlier diagnosis, the frequency of such cases has apparently lessened. It is still unclear however whether pulmonary hypertension will develop only in the most severe cases or whether the current techniques for noninvasive assessment of the pulmonary circulation in children are insufficiently sensitive to detect much milder involvement of the pulmonary vasculature. It is also uncertain whether exposures to chronic mild intermittent hypoxia may result in lesser recruitment of the pulmonary vascular network than sustained hypoxia of similar duration [123, 124]. These are important concepts to clarify, because potentially the occurrence of intermittent hypoxia and mobilization of the lung capillary endothelial network may promote long-term susceptibility to pulmonary hypertension even during adulthood [125].

Notwithstanding the development of pulmonary hypertension, there is increasing evidence that OSA can impose subclinical effects on the autonomic and cardiovascular systems, promoting disturbances in blood pressure regulation, left ventricular remodeling and endothelial dysfunction, all of which can lead to far reaching detrimental consequences if left unattended.

Of the three major cardiovascular morbidities, the effects of OSA on blood pressure are best explored to date. Marcus et al. found that children with OSA tend to have higher diastolic blood pressure during sleep compared with children with primary snoring [126]. The degree of increase in blood pressure during REM sleep has also been shown to correlate with the severity of OSA [127], which is perhaps to be expected considering OSA, in the majority of children, tends to occur during REM sleep and surges in arterial BP have been shown to occur after respiratory event termination [128]. Amin et al. studied slightly older children (mean age 10.8 ± 3.5 years) and found that children with OSA had evidence of blood pressure dysregulation: having significantly greater mean BP variability during both wakefulness and sleep, a higher night-to-day systolic BP, and reduction in nocturnal dipping of the mean BP when transitioning from wake to sleep [129]. In fact, these children had night-to-day systolic BP ratios that surpassed the established cutoff ratios of 0.899 for females and 0.9009 for males, which in adults is a risk factor for cardiovascular morbidity [130]. The research group subsequently reported that children with OSA exhibit increases in morning blood pressure surges, blood pressure load, and 24-h ambulatory blood pressures compared with healthy controls [131]. These differences were associated with left ventricular remodeling, and the effects were apparent even in children with mild OSA. Notably, even children who were just primary snorers were found to be at higher risk for elevations in systemic BP [132–134]. Walter et al. examined outcomes 3 years after the resolution of OSA in preschool children. Power spectral analysis of heart rate variability and measurement of urinary catecholamines were performed to assess autonomic function [135]. Overall, the resolution of OSA resulted in the normalization of previously increased heart rate variability to levels similar to controls. In contrast, children with residual OSA exhibited increased high-frequency HRV, suggesting significantly increased respiratory effort. Similar findings were observed even in children with primary snoring. A positive correlation between urinary catecholamines and low-frequency power in children with unresolved OSA was also noted, suggesting increased sympathetic activity in children with increasing severity of the OSA.

Although the left ventricular changes may merely reflect an adaptive response to higher blood pressures, the degree of the left-sided cardiac strain seen in OSA is reflected in the changes in brain natriuretic peptide (BNP) levels seen in OSA patients. This peptide is released by cardiac myocytes in response to cardiac wall distension, and overnight changes in BNP levels have been shown to be greater in children with moderate/severe OSA compared with mild OSA and controls [136]. This is thought to be most likely related to the increased and more frequent negative intrathoracic pressure swings seen in more severe OSA.

Endothelial dysfunction is believed to be a precursor to atherosclerosis. Assessment of endothelial function using various methodologies, such as flow-mediated dilation (FMD), pulse arterial tonometry (PAT), and laser-Doppler reperfusion kinetics [137–140] has revealed significant risk for impairments in endothelial function among children with OSA compared with controls. What is of concern is that although the majority of these children demonstrated resolution of endothelial dysfunction following treatment of their OSA [137], a subgroup did not show the anticipated improvements. They were noted to have a strong family history of early-onset cardiovascular disease, suggesting that the effects of OSA in a genetically susceptible subset of children may persist for unknown periods of time, potentially into adulthood. It should be stressed however that not every child with OSA manifests endothelial dysfunction [141]. Much research has focused on identifying the factors contributing to this phenotypic variation, both in the presence of endothelial dysfunction and the lack of resolution following OSA treatment. The severity of endothelial dysfunction is greater in obese children who have OSA, compared with either condition in isolation, once again, suggesting the convergence of the deleterious consequences of obesity and OSA [141].

The ability to recruit endothelial progenitors for endothelial repair [138, 142], numbers and function of T regulatory lymphocytes [143], epigenetic alterations in genes such as endothelial nitric oxide synthase, as well as polymorphisms in endothelin gene families are some of the factors recently identified as modifiers of the phenotypic variance in endothelial function [144, 145].

CRP, an acute phase reaction protein, is now recognized as a robust and independent predictor of cardiovascular morbidity and is extensively used to stratify risk for ischemic heart disease [146]. It has even been postulated that CRP may participate directly in atheromatous lesion formation through reduction of nitric oxide synthesis and induction of the expression of adhesion molecules on endothelial cells [147, 148]. It may be surmised that children with OSA in whom CRP levels are elevated may constitute a higher-risk group for the development of long-term cardiovascular complications. Indeed, markers of vascular injury and endothelial activation such as myeloid-related protein 8/14, plasma adhesion molecules, fatty-acid-binding protein, and circulating microparticles have all been shown to be elevated in children with OSA and are associated with the presence of endothelial dysfunction [149–152]. To what extent genetic and environmental factors confer protection or increase vulnerability and the identification of surrogate markers of endothelial dysfunction in the plasma are avenues of research currently being actively pursued [110, 153].

Metabolic System

Unlike in adult cohorts where OSA is an important risk factor for insulin resistance, diabetes, and dyslipidemia [154–160], this association in children is less clear-cut, with its effects moderated by such factors as age, ethnicity, pubertal status, degree of inflammatory response, and obesity. In postpubertal adolescents, strong associations have been demonstrated between OSA and the metabolic syndrome, as well as with individual metabolic parameters such as fasting insulin and HOMA [44, 161, 162]. Intermittent hypoxia and sleep fragmentation were also found to be associated with decreased insulin sensitivity in obese adolescent boys [163]. In younger children however, OSA was associated with reduced insulin sensitivity only when obesity was concurrently present [164, 165], and effective treatment of OSA improved insulin sensitivity in these children [166]. Any residual metabolic dysfunction appears to be associated with the degree of adiposity, rather than that of residual OSA severity [167]. These changes were seen in both obese and nonobese children, suggesting that OSA is causally involved in creating an adverse metabolic environment that is independent of obesity. Interestingly, when highly sensitive bioinformatics approaches and pathway analyses were employed to analyze transcriptomic microarrays in children with primary snoring, alterations in insulin homeostatic mechanisms emerged, suggesting that even mild perturbations in sleep may impose subclinical changes in peripheral tissue insulin receptor sensitivity [168]. OSA has also been associated with rises in LDL cholesterol with concomitant decreases in

HDL cholesterol in both obese and nonobese children [166, 169]. Significant improvements in lipid profile were observed after treatment of OSA.

Even as early as in childhood, evidence of end-organ morbidity in the form of fatty liver disease has been demonstrated in obese children with OSA [170–172]. OSA/nocturnal hypoxemia is present in up to 60 % of obese children with biopsy proven nonalcoholic fatty liver disease (NAFLD), and the severity of the OSA/duration of the hypoxemia was associated with biochemical and histological features of NAFLD severity, independent of BMI, abdominal adiposity, metabolic syndrome, and insulin resistance [173]. The percentage of time with oxygen saturation $\leq 90\%$ was also found to be associated with increased intrahepatic leukocytes, activated Kupffer cells, and circulating markers of hepatocyte apoptosis and fibrogenesis [174]. Treatment of OSA usually with adenotonsillectomy followed by CPAP in a large subset of these obese children resulted in improved liver serum aminotransferases in the vast majority [170].

The factors that may mediate these changes include Fas and FasL, which are part of the extrinsic apoptosis pathway, and their soluble forms are considered inhibitors of apoptosis because they effectively compete with the binding of FasL to Fas on the cell membrane. sCD163 is a marker of macrophage activation and has also been shown to be associated with hepatic steatosis and fibrosis in children with NAFLD. Alkhouri et al. showed that plasma levels of sFas and sFasL were lower in obese children with OSA compared with those who did not have OSA, and sCD163 levels were correlated with OSA severity [175]. There was a significant decrease in sCD163 levels after OSA treatment. These findings suggest the presence of higher levels of hepatic cellular apoptosis in OSA patients who are obese and that hepatocyte apoptosis and macrophage activation are possible mechanisms by which NAFLD develops in the context of OSA in obese children.

Animal models of OSA have expanded our understanding of the potential mechanisms mediating the metabolic dysfunction. Oxidative stress, elevated sympathetic activity, and inflammation have emerged as leading candidate pathways underlying disruption of homeostatic metabolic processes in several critical target organs such as the adipose tissue, pancreas, muscle, and liver (for in-depth review, see Gileles-Hillel et al.) [176].

Another potential mechanism may involve the impact of OSA on the gut microbiome. The influence of the gut microbiota in the modulation of nutrient absorption, control of appetite, and organ-specific changes that contribute to glucose homeostasis and hence its contribution to the pathogenesis of obesity and the metabolic syndrome has gained substantial attention in recent years. Little is yet known about changes to the gut microbiota in patients with OSA or the contribution of such changes to the metabolic consequences seen. However, initial data have revealed that OSA is associated with low-grade endotoxemia and impaired gut-barrier integrity. LPS-binding protein (LBP) is often used as a surrogate marker of underlying low-grade endotoxemia by LPS from the gut. Children with OSA have LBP plasma levels comparable to obese children without OSA, and both are significantly higher compared with healthy controls [177]. When both obesity and OSA were concurrently present, LBP levels were further augmented. LBP levels also correlated with HOMA. Similarly, in children with NAFLD and OSA, duration of $SaO_2 < 90\%$ independently predicted intestinal permeability, plasma LPS, and TLR-4 expression by hepatocytes, Kupffer cells, and hepatic stellate cells [178]. These findings suggest that OSA may promote liver injury by impairing intestinal barrier function and by promoting endotoxemia while also sensitizing the liver to endotoxin and pro-inflammatory stimuli.

Excessive Daytime Sleepiness

Although excessive daytime sleepiness (EDS) is described in pediatric OSA, it often is not as prominent a symptom as in adults with the condition, and indeed hyperactivity rather than EDS is more often reported by the parents. Melendres et al. showed by administering the Epworth sleepiness scale (ESS) score and the Conners Abbreviated Symptom Questionnaire in 180 children that children with OSA were both sleepier and more hyperactive than control subjects [179]. Only 28% of the children with OSA had ESS >10, and the mean ESS score of the OSA group was 8.1 ± 4.9, which is far lower than that typically described in adult OSA patients, though statistically higher than the ESS score of control subjects (5.3 ± 3.9). Interestingly, subgroup analysis of the ESS scores in children aged <5 years showed no significant differences between the OSA and control groups, and a possible explanation could be because this younger group often still nap during the day.

Objective measurements of EDS using the Multiple Sleep Latency Test have shown that children with OSA do have shortened sleep latencies compared with controls (20.0 ± 7.1 min vs 23.7 ± 3.0), but EDS is infrequent and tends to be seen in the more obese patients and in those with more severe OSA [180]. The magnitude of sleep latency reduction appears to be associated with measures of systemic inflammation, in particular, plasma TNF-α levels, which have been shown to be modulated by polymorphisms in the TNF-α gene [70, 181].

Healthcare Utilization

OSA has been reported to be a risk factor for community-acquired pneumonia in children aged <5 years [182]. It is also reported that children with OSA have increased healthcare utilization predominantly for respiratory infections and symptoms, compared with their peers [183, 184]. From their first year of life to time of diagnosis of OSA, children ultimately diagnosed with OSA had 40% more hospital visits, 20% more repeated visits, and higher prescriptions for respiratory system and antimicrobial medications [183]. While association does not necessarily equate to causation and the reasons for these findings still need to be elucidated, following adenotonsillectomy treatment of OSA, healthcare utilization was significantly reduced and total annual healthcare costs were reduced by as much as a third [185]. These findings have also been independently confirmed in another population-based cohort in Taiwan [186].

Nocturnal Enuresis

A high prevalence of nocturnal enuresis has been reported in children with OSA [187–189].

It has been postulated that enuresis may be due to the dampening effects of OSA on arousal responses to changes in bladder pressure or potentially associated with secretion of hormones involved in fluid regulation. BNP increases sodium and water excretion and also influences hormones in the renin-angiotensin pathway and vaso-pressin. Children with OSA have elevated morning BNP levels, and children with nocturnal enuresis have higher BNP levels compared with those without enuresis, at any degree of OSA severity, providing support to the hypothesis that sleep fragmentation and increased BNP secretion secondary to OSA may increase the risk of nocturnal enuresis [190].

A systematic review examining the association between sleep-disordered breathing and nocturnal enuresis in children identified 14 studies, in which a third of the 3550 children with OSA had a diagnosis of nocturnal enuresis [188]. Follow-up data was available in seven of the studies, demonstrating improvements in nocturnal enuresis post-adenotonsillectomy. However, several studies were weak in their experimental design and included skewed cohorts, such that randomized controlled trials are still needed to establish more definitive cause-effect relationships between pediatric OSA and nocturnal enuresis.

Somatic Growth

Failure to thrive (FTT) was identified in the first initial reports of pediatric OSA. Factors contributing to FTT include (a) increases in energy expenditure from increased work of breathing during sleep, (b) decreased caloric intake in children with large tonsils which are affecting swallowing, and (c) impairments of growth hormone secretion and tissue activity in children with OSA. Growth hormone secretory bursts occur during slow-wave sleep, and sleep fragmentation may impact the tightly regulated release of growth hormone [191]. Both insulin-like growth factor-1 (IGF-1) and IGF-binding protein 3 (IGFBP-3) concentrations have been reported to increase significantly posttreatment with adenotonsillectomy [192, 193]. Indeed in a study of 16 toddlers (6–36 months) pre- and post-adenotonsillectomy, there was a significant increase in BMI z-score and caloric intake with a corresponding decrease in hsCRP levels following surgery [60]. Multivariate analysis demonstrated that the improvement in somatic growth correlated with the improvement in systemic inflammation, rather than with changes in caloric intake.

Statistical modeling of anthropomorphic data from the CHAT study also showed that the BMI z-score increased more in the children who underwent adenotonsillectomy than in those who were randomly assigned to watchful waiting, even among the children who were already overweight at baseline [194]. The long-term effects of OSA on adipose tissue and weight are still unknown, but these findings highlight the importance of careful weight monitoring, nutritional counseling, and encouragement of physical activity after adenotonsillectomy for OSA.

Clinical Evaluation

When evaluating a child for OSA, both nocturnal and daytime symptoms should be elicited in the history. Physical examination should include assessment of tonsillar size, nasal patency, and other anatomical factors that may predispose to OSA such as relative size and position of the mandible. OSA-associated morbidities such as failure to thrive, hypertension, and neurocognitive deficits should also be elicited (summarized in Table 10.1).

Table 10.1 Summary of most recent AAP and ERS guidelines

AAP guidelines	ERS guidelines
In a child who snores and has signs or symptoms of OSA, clinicians should perform a more focused evaluation	Step 1,2,3 – identification of a child at risk of OSA, morbidity and conditions co-existing with OSA, recognition of factors predicting persistence of OSA
PSG is the gold standard diagnostic test for OSA	Step 4 – objective diagnosis and assessment of disease severity PSG or RP study
If PSG is not available, alternative diagnostic tests (such as nocturnal video recording, nocturnal oximetry, daytime nap PSG, or ambulatory PSG) or referral to a specialist for more extensive evaluation should be considered	If not available, alternatives include ambulatory PSG/RP, nocturnal oximetry, sleep clinical record, or pediatric sleep questionnaire

Adenotonsillectomy is the first-line treatment in children with OSA who have associated adenotonsillar hypertrophy. Other treatments can be considered if the child does not have adenotonsillar hypertrophy
Postoperatively, high-risk patients should be monitored as inpatients
CPAP is recommended if adenotonsillectomy is not performed or if there is residual OSA
Intranasal corticosteroids should be considered in children with mild OSA in whom AT is contraindicated or for mild residual OSA post-AT
Weight loss should be recommended in patients who are overweight/obese
	Step 5 – indications for treatment:
	  If AHI > 5/hrTST
	  If 1 > AHI > 5/hrTST, treatment may be warranted if any OSA-associated morbidities present
	  Treatment should be a priority in conditions such as craniofacial syndromes, trisomy 21, neuromuscular conditions, Prader-Willi syndrome, mucopolysaccharidoses, achondroplasia, Chiari malformation
	Step 6 – treatment interventions should be implemented in a stepwise manner addressing all abnormalities that predispose to OSA:
	  Weight loss in children who are overweight/obese
	  Medical therapy (nasal steroids/montelukast)
	  Adenotonsillectomy
	  Rapid maxillary expansion/orthodontic appliances
	CPAP/bilevel positive pressure ventilation
	Tracheostomy

(continued)

Table 10.1 (continued)

AAP guidelines	ERS guidelines
Patients should be reevaluated postoperatively to determine whether there is residual OSA and if further treatment is required Objective testing should be performed in patients who are high risk or have symptoms/signs of residual disease after therapy	Step 7 – recognition and management of residual OSA Reevaluation following intervention: If OSA symptoms persist or at risk of residual OSA, PSG $\geq$ 6 weeks after AT or $\geq$12 weeks after medical therapy PSG 12 months after rapid maxillary expansion, 6 months with an oral appliance PSG for initial titration of CPAP/NIV, then at least yearly Monitoring with PSG to guide tracheostomy decannulation When residual OSA is demonstrated, airway evaluation by drug-induced sleep endoscopy, nasopharyngoscopy, or MRI may help identify site/s of obstruction

Adapted from Refs. [1, 6]

Diagnosis

As already alluded to earlier in this chapter, clinical history and examination unfortunately have poor sensitivity and specificity for the diagnosis of OSA. Objective testing is therefore recommended for children with symptoms of OSA, and the American Academy of Pediatrics suggests that the gold standard investigation is a nocturnal, in-lab polysomnography (PSG) study [195]. A typical montage would include EEG, chin and anterior tibial EMG, bilateral electrooculogram, pulse oximetry and pulse waveform, nasal pressure transducer, oronasal airflow thermistor, end-tidal capnography, chest and abdominal respiratory inductance plethysmography, body position sensor, microphone, and videomonitoring. Pediatric scoring criteria should be used, and most sleep laboratories score according to the American Academy of Sleep Medicine (AASM) guidelines [196]. PSGs provide objective quantitative data regarding respiratory parameters and sleep patterns, thus allowing patients to be stratified into disease severities, while also enabling clinicians to tailor clinical management accordingly.

In countries where PSGs are not readily available, alternative options include:

(a) *Respiratory Polygraphy Studies* – These are essentially PSGs without the EEG, EMG, and EOG sensors, and they are the standard study performed in many countries in Europe. The experience however is limited and relatively higher technical failure rates are reported [197, 198].

(b) *Nocturnal Oximetry Studies* – Oximetry studies have a high specificity but low sensitivity for the diagnosis of pediatric OSA. A recent systematic review revealed that in otherwise healthy children with no symptoms of OSA, nocturnal SpO_2 drops <90%, greater than two clusters of desaturations events ($\geq$4%), and oxyhemoglobin desaturation index ($\geq 4\%$) >2.2/h are rare [199]. At least three clusters of desaturations and at least three SpO_2 drops below 90 % in a nocturnal oximetry recording of at least 6-h duration (McGill oximetry score >1) are suggestive of moderate-to-severe OSA (Fig. 10.1). An oxyhemoglobin desaturation index ($\geq 4\%$) >2/h combined with OSA symptoms also exhibits high positive predictive value for AHI >1/h. Children with normal oximetry, aged >3 years, and with no comorbidities have very low risk of major respiratory complications following adenotonsillectomy. Overnight oximetry can help in the prioritization of treatment and determining whether children need to be admitted overnight for observation following adenotonsillectomy. It has an important role in resource-poor countries where PSGs or RPs are not available. Improvements in oximetry-based approaches using neural networks suggest that this methodological approach can improve the accuracy of the diagnosis [200].

(c) *Sleep Clinical Record* – The sleep clinical record (SCR) is an instrument that has been developed to screen children for OSA and incorporates multidimensional data obtained from case history and physical examination [201]. A score

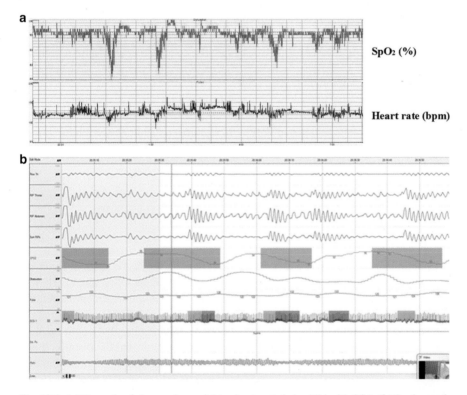

Fig. 10.1 (**a**) Example of abnormal overnight oximetry study in child with OSA. (**b**) 2-min epoch from a respiratory polygraphy study of the same patient performed the same night

of ≥ 6.5 is considered positive for OSA, with a reported sensitivity of 96.05 % and specificity of 67 %. Combining results from the SCR score and nocturnal oximetry has moderate success in predicting sleep-disordered breathing severity and is potentially useful in settings where resources are limited and PSG testing is not readily available [202].

In general and pragmatically speaking, while these investigations may not have the sensitivity and specificity of PSGs, provided clinicians recognize their limitations, the information they provide can still be highly valuable.

Home sleep apnea testing   There has been a lot of interest in home sleep apnea testing, and it is a direction that adult sleep medicine has readily adopted. Compared with in-lab PSGs, home sleep apnea testing has the potential to measure a more typical night's sleep as the child is sleeping at home, could be substantially less expensive, and more accessible to more children. Most of the interest in home sleep apnea testing has been in the use of home RPs. Unsurprisingly, the signal most at risk of disruption is the nasal flow signal, but overall, home RPs are feasible to perform, even in young preschool children [203, 204]. The probability of obtaining a successful study appears to be higher if the studies are set up by trained staff with the attendant logistic implications. Though results from the various published studies have been discordant [197], on the whole, the sensitivity and specificity of home RPs appear to be good for the diagnosis of moderate and severe OSA in children who have a high pretest probability of having the condition [205]. More research is required into how to further optimize the sensitivity and specificity of home sleep apnea testing in children with mild OSA.

CO_2 monitoring is important in children in whom there is concern regarding nocturnal hypoventilation, such as children with neuromuscular disease, underlying lung disease, or obesity hypoventilation. Not all home testing devices have a transcutaneous or end-tidal CO_2 channel, and therefore, home sleep apnea testing may not be suitable in these children.

Treatment

Most clinicians consider a PSG obstructive AHI ≤ 1/hrTST to be normal, $1 < OAHI \leq 5$/hrTST as mild OSA, $5 < OAHI \leq 10$/hrTST as moderate OSA, and OAHI >10/hrTST as severe OSA. Most sleep specialists would institute treatment in children with moderate/severe OSA, but there is considerable variability in current practice for the management of mild OSA. It is important to remember that treatment decisions should not only be guided by PSG results in isolation, and the overall clinical picture needs to be taken into consideration. Thus, symptom severity, examination findings, presence of risk factors, and associated disease morbidity need to be carefully evaluated and incorporated prior to the formulation and implementation of an individualized treatment plan.

Adenotonsillectomy

In contrast to adults with OSA, adenotonsillectomy is the recommended first-line treatment for pediatric OSA in children with adenotonsillar hypertrophy [195]. It is now clearly established that adenotonsillectomy results in improvements in the severity of OSA in the majority of children. While adenotonsillectomy is an effective treatment, recent studies have demonstrated that although the majority of children show marked improvements in their PSG parameters following surgery, a significant proportion do not achieve complete normalization of the PSG and have residual OSA [206].

Risk factors for significant residual postoperative OSA include obesity, severity of OSA presurgery, age (risk being higher in those aged >7 years), underlying asthma or allergic rhinitis, African-American ethnicity, and children who have primary genetic conditions leading to structural abnormalities, e.g., craniofacial anomalies/chromosomal defects, and those with neuromuscular diseases. In low-risk populations, the percentage of children with residual OSA is approximately 20–25 %, while in high-risk populations, it is significantly higher [43, 46]. Clinicians should be alert to this problem, and those children at high risk for residual OSA should be reevaluated post-adenotonsillectomy. However, even in low-risk patients, an open-minded approach should be implemented, with the recurrence of OSA symptoms warranting reevaluation.

While adenotonsillectomy is generally considered a safe procedure, as with all surgical procedures, there can be complications, the most common being respiratory compromise and secondary hemorrhage [207]. It is now apparent that children with OSA have an increased risk of respiratory complications after adenotonsillectomy when compared to children who are having adenotonsillectomy for other clinical indications (odds ratio 4.9). However, they appear less likely to have postoperative bleeding compared with children without OSA (odds ratio 0.41). A possible explanation is that recurrent tonsillitis, the other main indication for adenotonsillectomy, may be a risk factor for secondary hemorrhage, not that OSA is a protective factor. Of note, in the CHAT study, none of the PSG or demographic parameters were predictive of postoperative complications [208].

There has been a gradual shift in the past few years by some ENT surgeons toward performing tonsillotomies in preference to tonsillectomies because of the benefits of lower postoperative complication rates such as hemorrhage, less postsurgical pain, and shorter recovery time. A recent meta-analysis comparing tonsillectomy versus tonsillotomy for sleep-disordered breathing in children included ten studies and demonstrated that there was no significant difference in outcomes such as resolution of OSA symptoms, quality of life, and postoperative immune function [209]. However, the risk ratio of OSA recurrence was 3.33 times higher for tonsillotomy especially in younger children who appear to have a small risk of symptom-recurrence requiring repeat surgery within 2 years after tonsillotomy due to tonsillar regrowth [210]. The 2012 American Academy of Pediatrics guidelines suggest that data are currently insufficient to definitively recommend one surgical technique over the other [195]. However, children undergoing tonsillotomy should be monitored carefully long term to ensure that OSA symptoms do not recur, and families should be counseled about the possibility of OSA recurrence secondary to tonsillar regrowth. In a population-based study, the risk of recurrent surgical intervention was significantly higher when tonsillotomy was used [211].

A recent Cochrane systematic review to examine the evidence comparing adenotonsillectomy versus nonsurgical management of pediatric OSA identified only three prospective trials that met the inclusion criteria [212]. The previously mentioned CHAT study provided the highest-quality evidence and was the main basis for the recommendation that in healthy children with mild/moderate OSA, adenotonsillectomy was of benefit. It is still the duty of the physicians to carefully weigh the benefits and risks of adenotonsillectomy against watchful waiting, as it is possible the condition may recover spontaneously over time. Certainly one of the most striking findings of the CHAT study was that in the watchful waiting group, 42 % were found to have resolution of their OSA on follow-up PSG 7 months later [48]. This was particularly true in the children with milder disease (lower initial AHI) and with waist circumference <90 % percentile [213]. It should be pointed out that despite normalization of their PSG AHI, only 15 % of the 167 patients with a baseline PSQ > 0.33 experienced symptomatic resolution, and the independent predictors for symptom resolution included lower initial pediatric sleep questionnaire and snoring scores.

Positive Airway Pressure Therapy

In children who manifest residual OSA after adenotonsillectomy or in those who present minimally enlarged upper airway lymphadenoid tissues or opt not to undergo surgery, positive airway pressure therapy is recommended (provided nasal obstruction is not present). The aim is to maintain airway patency throughout the respiratory cycle, improve functional residual capacity (FRC), and thus decrease the work of breathing. This is usually delivered in the form of continuous positive airway pressure (CPAP), but in some children who require very high positive end-expiratory pressures or who also have nocturnal hypoventilation, for example, children with neuromuscular disease or obesity hypoventilation syndrome, bilevel PAP ventilation may be required (Fig. 10.2). While PAP is an effective therapy, achieving adequate adherence can be a major challenge in children.

When adherence and effectiveness were studied in a prospective multicenter study of children randomly assigned to 6 months of bilevel PAP ventilation or CPAP, a third of the subjects had already dropped out before 6 months [214]. There was no statistical difference between bilevel PAP ventilation and CPAP, both being highly efficacious, even though adherence, even in a research setting, was suboptimal with a mean nightly use of just 5.3 ± 2.5 (SD) hours. Nonetheless, achieving good adherence is not impossible, as evidenced by Ramirez et al. whose patients used PAP therapy for a mean of 8 h 17 min ± 2 h 30 min per night [215].

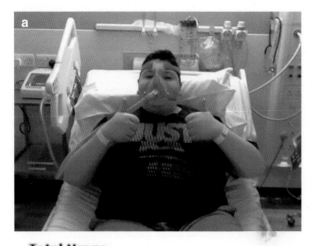

Total Usage

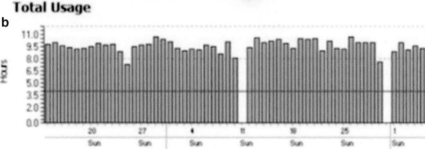

Fig. 10.2 (**a**) Children can take a little while to get used to PAP therapy, but once they get into a routine, they can feel symptomatically much better when they adhere to this therapy. (**b**) Example of adherence data from a child with OSA receiving CPAP therapy at home

This impressive outcome is most likely a reflection of the available resources, with the PAP therapy being initiated in a designated pediatric inpatient unit by experienced staff, very frequent home visits, and frequent inpatient follow-up sleep studies. However, even with suboptimal adherence (mean use just 170 ± 145 min/night), a study of 52 children found that there was still significant improvement after just 3 months of PAP therapy in several neurobehavioral domains, including attention deficits, sleepiness on the Epworth sleepiness scale, internalizing and total behavior symptom scores, and quality-of-life questionnaires [119].

PAP therapy does however require regular long-term follow-up in children as pressure requirements will change, and the interface will need to be upsized and adjusted, with the growth and development of the child. Side effects also need to be monitored, and these can include nasal bridge pressure sores from the mask, discomfort from air leak especially to the eyes, abdominal distension, and oronasal dryness. In the longer term, young children may develop flattening of the midface or maxillary retrusion from the effect of pressure of the mask on growing facial structures.

Medical Therapy

Most clinicians would now consider a trial of anti-inflammatory medication, namely, leukotriene receptor antagonists such as montelukast and intranasal steroids in children with mild OSA [216]. Tonsils from children with OSA have been shown to express increased levels of leukotriene receptors 1 and 2 compared with tonsils from children with recurrent tonsillitis [217]. Consequently, the application of leukotriene antagonists to an in vitro cell culture system of cells obtained from tonsillar tissues of children with OSA elicited dose-dependent reductions in cell proliferation and reductions in the secretion of the cytokines TNF-α, IL-6, and IL-12 [218]. In an initial open-label intervention study where children with mild OSA received 16 weeks of montelukast, significant reductions in adenoidal size and respiratory-related sleep disturbances were demonstrated [219]; these findings have subsequently been reproduced in a double-blind, randomized, placebo-controlled trial [220].

Similarly, the addition of steroids to this in vitro cell culture system resulted in decreased proliferative rates of the cells, increased apoptosis, and reduction in the secretion of the pro-inflammatory cytokines IL-6, IL-8, and TNF-α [221]. A randomized crossover trial of 6 weeks of treatment with intranasal budesonide in children with mild OSA showed improvements in the severity of OSA and reduction in the size of adenoidal tissues. Importantly, discontinuation of therapy for 8 weeks, in the group of children who started with the medication and then had a 2-week washout period followed by 6 weeks of placebo, did not promote the occurrence of rebound symptoms [222]. Intranasal fluticasone and mometasone have shown similar results [223, 224]. The use of both montelukast and nasal budesonide for 12 weeks in children who had residual mild residual OSA after adenotonsillectomy led to significant improvements in AHI, nadir oxygen saturation, and respiratory arousal index, whereas no significant changes occurred over this time period in the control subjects [225]. Recently, a large retrospective review of 752 children with mild OSA who received nasal steroids and montelukast showed an overall success rate of 80.5 % [226]. A subset of 445 patients had follow-up PSG and normalization of sleep parameters was seen in 62 %. Older children (aged > 7 years) and obese children were however less likely to respond favorably. Studies to determine optimal duration of treatment, optimal combinatorial approaches, longer-term outcomes, and optimal patient selection are critically needed.

Weight Loss

Weight loss should be encouraged in obese children with OSA, both as a therapy for their OSA and also for its beneficial effects on their overall health. In the NANOS study, the group of obese children with mild OSA without adenotonsillar hypertrophy who were managed with dietary modification to encourage weight loss demonstrated improvements in their respiratory parameters with 50 % showing OSA resolution at follow-up [50], while the weight loss required for such beneficial effects to be demonstrated was encouragingly small. A study in Belgium recruited 61 obese teenagers admitted to a weight loss camp where the children underwent a multimodality treatment program consisting of moderate dietary restriction, regular physical activity, as well as group and individual psychological support [227]. Sixty-two percent had OSA when they started the program, and after a median weight loss of 24 kg, repeat sleep screening revealed a significant improvement in the severity of OSA including the AHI, ODI, mean SpO_2, SpO_2 nadir, and time $SpO_2 < 90\%$, while the relative decrease in BMI z-score correlated with the change in AHI.

Rapid Maxillary Expansion

In rapid maxillary expansion (RME), a fixed appliance with an expansion screw anchored to opposing teeth is used to open the midpalatal suture, gradually increasing the transverse diameter of the hard palate over the course of several months. Data on RME are limited to small uncontrolled studies, but they suggest that it may have a role to play in carefully selected patients, such as children with OSA who have clinical signs of malocclusion (high, narrow palate associated with deep bite, retrusive bite, or crossbite) [228]. Results appear to be more promising when treatment is started at a younger age during the phase of late primary dentition or early mixed dentition [229]. In a pilot study of 31 children with OSA who had both narrow maxilla and moderately enlarged tonsils and OSA, half the children (group 1) had adenotonsillectomy performed followed by RME, and the other half (group 2) had RME, followed by adenotonsillectomy [230]. The AHI decreased after the first intervention, but it was only after the reciprocal intervention was performed that the AHI normalized. Complete resolution of OSA following just a single intervention alone (RME) occurred in only one child, and there were no significant differences as to which treatment was started first, as ultimately both treatments were needed in the vast majority of patients.

Myofunctional Reeducation

There has been recent interest in myofunctional reeducation to prevent the recurrence of OSA post-adenotonsillectomy or in the treatment of mild persistent OSA. Myofunctional reeducation involves teaching the patients oropharyngeal exercises aimed at improving labial seal and lip tone, facilitating nasal breathing rehabilitation, and improving tongue posture. These exercises need to be performed daily, with the aim of strengthening the tongue and orofacial muscles and realigning them in the correct position. In a retrospective review of 24 patients after adenotonsillectomy, 11 of whom had received myofunctional reeducation, those children who had not received myofunctional therapy developed recurrence of mild OSA symptomatically and on PSG, whereas those undergoing myofunctional reeducation had no recurrence [231]. Another study of 14 children who had residual OSA post-adenotonsillectomy demonstrated improvement in their AHI after treatment with oropharyngeal exercises for 2 months [232]. Morphofunctional evaluation also demonstrated improvements including reduction in oral breathing and increased labial seal and lip tone. One hypothesis is that residual OSA may be due to incomplete recovery of neuromuscular function after surgery, and myofunctional reeducation may help with this problem. However, studies so far have been small and uncontrolled, and therefore, larger prospective, multicenter controlled studies are required.

High-Flow Nasal Cannula Oxygen

A possible alternative to CPAP is high-flow nasal cannula oxygen (HFNC). This form of respiratory support has gained widespread use in the acute setting for the treatment of respiratory distress syndrome and bronchiolitis, and anecdotally appears to be better tolerated in infants than mask-based positive airway pressure. There has only been 1 study so far of 12 patients on HFNC for the treatment of OSA [233]. Results were promising, and the reduction in AHI was comparable to that of CPAP leading the authors to postulate that HFNC may be a gentler alternative to CPAP.

Newer Investigational Techniques

Drug-induced sleep endoscopy Drug-induced sleep endoscopy (DISE) is a technique whereby the upper airway is evaluated via a flexible fiber-optic endoscope inserted nasally during spontaneous breathing while the patient is under light sedation. The aim is to recreate the upper airway conditions during natural sleep, thus allowing the exact level of obstruction in the child to be identified and facilitating site-specific surgical therapy [234, 235]. It can be very useful in the assessment of children who have residual OSA after adenotonsillectomy, or in complex OSA cases, such as that seen in children with cerebral palsy, craniofacial syndromes, trisomy 21, etc. Common sites of obstruction include the tongue base, primarily due to lingual tonsillar hypertrophy, adenoid regrowth, inferior turbinate hypertrophy, and laryngomalacia.

Cine MRI Another technology potentially useful for the evaluation of children with complex upper airway obstruction is cine MRI. This approach provides high-resolution imaging of the dynamic airway without the need for ionizing radiation making it ideal for use in children. Cine MRI proponents advocate that this imaging modality allows for a better view of the airway in its entirety and enables observation of both the primary and secondary effects of obstruction. When Shott et al.

used cine MRI to evaluate the airways of 15 children with trisomy 21 who had persistent OSA following adenotonsillectomy, the cine MRI identified different areas and levels of obstruction including regrowth of adenoidal tissue, glossoptosis, soft palate collapse, hypopharyngeal collapse, and enlarged lingual tonsils, and treatment could thus be tailored to the individual patient [236, 237].

Guidelines

The most recent American and European guidelines for the diagnosis and management of pediatric OSA were published in 2012 and 2015, respectively. The American Academy of Pediatrics (AAP) focused on uncomplicated OSA, i.e., OSA associated with adenotonsillar hypertrophy or obesity in otherwise healthy children [6]. Upon reviewing the data from publications between 1999 and 2010, their main recommendations are summarized in Table 10.2.

In addition to the management of uncomplicated OSA, the European Respiratory Society guidelines also included recommendations regarding the management of obstructive sleep-disordered breathing in children with conditions such as craniofacial anomalies and neuromuscular disorders [1]. The variability in diagnostic facilities available in different European countries was also taken into consideration. Reviewing publications until 2014, a stepwise approach to the diagnosis and management of obstructive sleep-disordered breathing was suggested, and these are also summarized in Table 10.2.

Future Developments

PSGs are poorly predictive of OSA-associated morbidities: not every child fulfilling PSG criteria for OSA manifests end-organ morbidity, and conversely, some children with primary snoring already display sequelae despite a normal sleep study. As with many diseases, factors such as individual genetic susceptibility and environmental exposures/lifestyle will contribute to this phenotypic variance. Therefore, improving overall therapy requires individualization of evaluation and treatment and is dependent on patient-specific requirements. The development of potential biomarkers of susceptibility to and severity of OSA morbidity is therefore of critical importance. Proteomic interrogations coupled with the requisite bioinformatic analyses have revealed that OSA is associated with specific and consistent alterations in certain urinary proteins [238]. Increased levels of urinary catecholamines epinephrine and norepinephrine have been identified, and overnight increases in GABA and decreases in taurine and β-phenylethylamine (PEA) appear to differentiate children with OSA who have neurocognitive deficits from those without [239]. There is also emergent data that exosomal miRNAs may be a potential biomarker of cardiovascular risk in children with OSA [240].

Table 10.2 Pertinent symptoms and signs when evaluating a child for possible OSA

Clinical history
Are there any of the following symptoms?
During sleep
Snoring (is it loud? How frequently)
Heavy/loud/noisy breathing
Struggling to breath
Gasping
Mouth breathing
Witnessed apneas
Restless sleep
Frequent awakenings
Hyperextension of neck when asleep
Sleeps in sitting position
Excessive sweating when asleep
Cyanosis
What is the typical bedtime, wake time?
Is the child easy to wake in the mornings?
Does the child wake unrefreshed?
Nocturnal enuresis (especially if secondary)
Wake with morning headaches
Any other sleep symptoms, e.g., parasomnias or night terrors?
During wake
Nasal congestion
Mouth breathing when awake
Chronic rhinorrhea
Difficulty swallowing
Neurocognitive morbidity, e.g., academic impairment, excessive daytime sleepiness (consider questionnaire such as modified Epworth sleepiness scale), inattention, hyperactivity, behavioral problems
Are there any risk factors for OSA such as prematurity or family history of OSA?
Are there any other medical conditions, e.g., oromotor dysfunction, asthma, metabolic syndrome, recurrent otitis media, allergic rhinitis, recurrent chest infections, depression/ low self esteem, sickle cell disease, or previous cleft palate repair?
Is the child on any medications which can impact on sleep?
Physical examination
Tonsillar hypertrophy
Mandibular hypoplasia/micrognathia/retrognathia/midface deficiency/high-arched palate
Macroglossia
Pectus excavatum
Adenoidal facies
Examination of nose – nasal patency, any obvious causes of obstruction
Plot on growth chart
Calculate BMI percentile or z-score

Table 10.2 (continued)

Is there any evidence of other conditions commonly associated with OSA?
Neuromuscular conditions
Cerebral palsy
Achondroplasia
Mucopolysaccharidoses
Syndromes such as trisomy 21, Prader-Willi syndrome, craniofacial syndromes, etc.
Cardiovascular morbidity measure blood pressure, is there any evidence of pulmonary hypertension
Objective findings related to OSA
Parents now frequently take videos on their phone of events they are worried about which can provide useful information
Other investigations that can be considered or may already have been performed:
Lateral neck radiograph (adenoid: nasopharyngeal ratio)
Flexible nasoendoscopy
Cephalometry
Upper airway MRI or CT

The era of personalized medicine will require the development of coordinated combinatorial or multiplexed approaches, so that diagnosis and treatment can be tailored to the individual patient. In the future, algorithms that incorporate measures derived from the sleep study, from blood or urine tests, and from clinical elements obtained during history and physical examination may provide improved approaches to define those at risk of OSA, together with the timing and the nature of their required intervention. This unified approach is endorsed by an official American Thoracic Society statement on the importance of healthy sleep released in 2015 [241]. The research priorities are highlighted to include determining the molecular basis for OSA, using knowledge of these pathways to develop effective therapies, identifying the etiological role of OSA in the development of comorbidities, and determining the impact of OSA treatment on these comorbidities.

Financial Disclosures   DG is supported by the Herbert T. Abelson Chair in Pediatrics.

Conflicts of Interest Statement   The authors declare no conflicts of interest in relation to this work.

References

1. Kaditis AG, Alonso Alvarez ML, Boudewyns A, et al. Obstructive sleep disordered breathing in 2- to 18-year-old children: diagnosis and management. Eur Respir J. 2016;47:69–94.
2. Guilleminault C, Eldridge FL, Simmons FB, Dement WC. Sleep apnea in eight children. Pediatrics. 1976;58:23–30.
3. Kheirandish-Gozal L, Gozal D. Sleep disordered breathing in children. 1st ed. Berlin: Springer Science; 2012.

4. Bixler EO, Vgontzas AN, Lin HM, et al. Sleep disordered breathing in children in a general population sample: prevalence and risk factors. Sleep. 2009;32:731–6.
5. Li AM, So HK, Au CT, et al. Epidemiology of obstructive sleep apnoea syndrome in Chinese children: a two-phase community study. Thorax. 2010;65:991–7.
6. Marcus CL, Brooks LJ, Draper KA, et al. Diagnosis and management of childhood obstructive sleep apnea syndrome. Pediatrics. 2012;130:e714–55.
7. Rosen CL, Larkin EK, Kirchner HL, et al. Prevalence and risk factors for sleep-disordered breathing in 8- to 11-year-old children: association with race and prematurity. J Pediatr. 2003;142:383–9.
8. Tauman R, Gozal D. Obstructive sleep apnea syndrome in children. Expert Rev Respir Med. 2011;5:425–40.
9. Arens R, McDonough JM, Costarino AT, et al. Magnetic resonance imaging of the upper airway structure of children with obstructive sleep apnea syndrome. Am J Respir Crit Care Med. 2001;164:698–703.
10. Schwab RJ, Kim C, Bagchi S, et al. Understanding the anatomic basis for obstructive sleep apnea syndrome in adolescents. Am J Respir Crit Care Med. 2015;191:1295–309.
11. Slaats MA, Van HK, Van EA, et al. Upper airway imaging in pediatric obstructive sleep apnea syndrome. Sleep Med Rev. 2015;21:59–71.
12. Luo H, Sin S, McDonough JM, Isasi CR, Arens R, Wootton DM. Computational fluid dynamics endpoints for assessment of adenotonsillectomy outcome in obese children with obstructive sleep apnea syndrome. J Biomech. 2014;47:2498–503.
13. Wootton DM, Luo H, Persak SC, et al. Computational fluid dynamics endpoints to characterize obstructive sleep apnea syndrome in children. J Appl Physiol (1985). 2014;116:104–12.
14. Van HC, Vos W, Van HK, et al. Functional respiratory imaging as a tool to assess upper airway patency in children with obstructive sleep apnea. Sleep Med. 2013;14:433–9.
15. Persak SC, Sin S, McDonough JM, Arens R, Wootton DM. Noninvasive estimation of pharyngeal airway resistance and compliance in children based on volume-gated dynamic MRI and computational fluid dynamics. J Appl Physiol (1985). 2011;111:1819–27.
16. Mihaescu M, Murugappan S, Gutmark E, Donnelly LF, Kalra M. Computational modeling of upper airway before and after adenotonsillectomy for obstructive sleep apnea. Laryngoscope. 2008;118:360–2.
17. Deacon NL, Jen R, Li Y, Malhotra A. Treatment of obstructive sleep apnea. Prospects for personalized combined modality therapy. Ann Am Thorac Soc. 2016;13:101–8.
18. Owens RL, Edwards BA, Eckert DJ, et al. An integrative model of physiological traits can be used to predict obstructive sleep apnea and response to non positive airway pressure therapy. Sleep. 2015;38:961–70.
19. Parikh SR, Sadoughi B, Sin S, Willen S, Nandalike K, Arens R. Deep cervical lymph node hypertrophy: a new paradigm in the understanding of pediatric obstructive sleep apnea. Laryngoscope. 2013;123:2043–9.
20. Chan DK, Jan TA, Koltai PJ. Effect of obesity and medical comorbidities on outcomes after adjunct surgery for obstructive sleep apnea in cases of adenotonsillectomy failure. Arch Otolaryngol Head Neck Surg. 2012;138:891–6.
21. Friedman NR, Prager JD, Ruiz AG, Kezirian EJ. A pediatric grading scale for lingual tonsil hypertrophy. Otolaryngol Head Neck Surg. 2016;154:171–4.
22. Abdel-Aziz M, Ibrahim N, Ahmed A, El-Hamamsy M, Abdel-Khalik MI, El-Hoshy H. Lingual tonsils hypertrophy; a cause of obstructive sleep apnea in children after adenotonsillectomy: operative problems and management. Int J Pediatr Otorhinolaryngol. 2011;75:1127–31.
23. Fricke BL, Donnelly LF, Shott SR, et al. Comparison of lingual tonsil size as depicted on MR imaging between children with obstructive sleep apnea despite previous tonsillectomy and adenoidectomy and normal controls. Pediatr Radiol. 2006;36:518–23.
24. Kim J, Bhattacharjee R, Dayyat E, et al. Increased cellular proliferation and inflammatory cytokines in tonsils derived from children with obstructive sleep apnea. Pediatr Res. 2009;66:423–8.

25. Serpero LD, Kheirandish-Gozal L, Dayyat E, Goldman JL, Kim J, Gozal D. A mixed cell culture model for assessment of proliferation in tonsillar tissues from children with obstructive sleep apnea or recurrent tonsillitis. Laryngoscope. 2009;119:1005–10.
26. Goldbart AD, Mager E, Veling MC, et al. Neurotrophins and tonsillar hypertrophy in children with obstructive sleep apnea. Pediatr Res. 2007;62:489–94.
27. Snow A, Dayyat E, Montgomery-Downs HE, Kheirandish-Gozal L, Gozal D. Pediatric obstructive sleep apnea: a potential late consequence of respiratory syncytial virus bronchiolitis. Pediatr Pulmonol. 2009;44:1186–91.
28. Yeshuroon-Koffler K, Shemer-Avni Y, Keren-Naus A, Goldbart AD. Detection of common respiratory viruses in tonsillar tissue of children with obstructive sleep apnea. Pediatr Pulmonol. 2015;50:187–95.
29. Goldbart AD, Krishna J, Li RC, Serpero LD, Gozal D. Inflammatory mediators in exhaled breath condensate of children with obstructive sleep apnea syndrome. Chest. 2006;130:143–8.
30. Li AM, Hung E, Tsang T, et al. Induced sputum inflammatory measures correlate with disease severity in children with obstructive sleep apnoea. Thorax. 2007;62:75–9.
31. Arens R, Sin S, Willen S, et al. Rhino-sinus involvement in children with obstructive sleep apnea syndrome. Pediatr Pulmonol. 2010;45:993–8.
32. Gozal D. Pediatric OSA: a case for "United We Stand" in the way of a breath. Pediatr Pulmonol. 2010;45:1151–2.
33. Dayyat E, Kheirandish-Gozal L, Sans CO, Maarafeya MM, Gozal D. Obstructive sleep apnea in children: relative contributions of body mass index and adenotonsillar hypertrophy. Chest. 2009;136:137–44.
34. Li AM, Wong E, Kew J, Hui S, Fok TF. Use of tonsil size in the evaluation of obstructive sleep apnoea. Arch Dis Child. 2002;87:156–9.
35. Marcus CL, McColley SA, Carroll JL, Loughlin GM, Smith PL, Schwartz AR. Upper airway collapsibility in children with obstructive sleep apnea syndrome. J Appl Physiol. 1994;77:918–24.
36. Gozal D, Burnside MM. Increased upper airway collapsibility in children with obstructive sleep apnea during wakefulness. Am J Respir Crit Care Med. 2004;169:163–7.
37. Carrera HL, McDonough JM, Gallagher PR, et al. Upper airway collapsibility during wakefulness in children with sleep disordered breathing, as determined by the negative expiratory pressure technique. Sleep. 2011;34:717–24.
38. Thong JF, Pang KP. Clinical parameters in obstructive sleep apnea: are there any correlations? J Otolaryngol Head Neck Surg. 2008;37:894–900.
39. McGinley BM, Kirkness JP, Schneider H, Lenka A, Smith PL, Schwartz AR. Utilizing inspiratory airflows during standard polysomnography to assess pharyngeal function in children during sleep. Pediatr Pulmonol. 2015;51:431–8.
40. Redline S, Tishler PV, Schluchter M, Aylor J, Clark K, Graham G. Risk factors for sleep-disordered breathing in children. Associations with obesity, race, and respiratory problems. Am J Respir Crit Care Med. 1999;159:1527–32.
41. Gozal D, Kheirandish-Gozal L. Childhood obesity and sleep: relatives, partners, or both? – a critical perspective on the evidence. Ann N Y Acad Sci. 2012;1264:135–41.
42. Arens R, Sin S, Nandalike K, et al. Upper airway structure and body fat composition in obese children with obstructive sleep apnea syndrome. Am J Respir Crit Care Med. 2011;183:782–7.
43. Bhattacharjee R, Kheirandish-Gozal L, Spruyt K, et al. Adenotonsillectomy outcomes in treatment of obstructive sleep apnea in children: a multicenter retrospective study. Am J Respir Crit Care Med. 2010;182:676–83.
44. Canapari CA, Hoppin AG, Kinane TB, Thomas BJ, Torriani M, Katz ES. Relationship between sleep apnea, fat distribution, and insulin resistance in obese children. J Clin Sleep Med. 2011;7:268–73.
45. Nandalike K, Shifteh K, Sin S, et al. Adenotonsillectomy in obese children with obstructive sleep apnea syndrome: magnetic resonance imaging findings and considerations. Sleep. 2013;36:841–7.

46. Tauman R, Gulliver TE, Krishna J, et al. Persistence of obstructive sleep apnea syndrome in children after adenotonsillectomy. J Pediatr. 2006;149:803–8.
47. Mitchell RB, Boss EF. Pediatric obstructive sleep apnea in obese and normal-weight children: impact of adenotonsillectomy on quality-of-life and behavior. Dev Neuropsychol. 2009;34:650–61.
48. Marcus CL, Moore RH, Rosen CL, et al. A randomized trial of adenotonsillectomy for childhood sleep apnea. N Engl J Med. 2013;368:2366–76.
49. Alonso-Alvarez ML, Cordero-Guevara JA, Teran-Santos J, et al. Obstructive sleep apnea in obese community-dwelling children: the NANOS study. Sleep. 2014;37:943–9.
50. Alonso-Alvarez ML, Teran-Santos J, Navazo-Eguia AI, et al. Treatment outcomes of obstructive sleep apnoea in obese community-dwelling children: the NANOS study. Eur Respir J. 2015;46:717–27.
51. Lee CH, Hsu WC, Chang WH, Lin MT, Kang KT. Polysomnographic findings after adenotonsillectomy for obstructive sleep apnea in obese and non-obese children: a systemic review and meta-analysis. Clin Otolaryngol. 2015. doi: 10.1111/coa.12549.
52. Costa DJ, Mitchell R. Adenotonsillectomy for obstructive sleep apnea in obese children: a meta-analysis. Otolaryngol Head Neck Surg. 2009;140:455–60.
53. Apostolidou MT, Alexopoulos EI, Chaidas K, et al. Obesity and persisting sleep apnea after adenotonsillectomy in Greek children. Chest. 2008;134:1149–55.
54. Verhulst SL, De BJ, Van GL, De BW, Desager K. Adenotonsillectomy as first-line treatment for sleep-disordered breathing in obese children. Am J Respir Crit Care Med. 2008;177:1399.
55. Bhattacharjee R, Kim J, Kheirandish-Gozal L, Gozal D. Obesity and obstructive sleep apnea syndrome in children: a tale of inflammatory cascades. Pediatr Pulmonol. 2011;46:313–23.
56. Kheirandish-Gozal L, Gileles-Hillel A, Alonso-Alvarez ML, et al. Effects of adenotonsillectomy on plasma inflammatory biomarkers in obese children with obstructive sleep apnea: a community-based study. Int J Obes (Lond). 2015;39:1094–100.
57. Bhattacharjee R, Kheirandish-Gozal L, Kaditis AG, Verhulst SL, Gozal D. C-reactive protein as a potential biomarker of residual obstructive sleep apnea following adenotonsillectomy in children. Sleep. 2016;39:283–91.
58. Spruyt K, Sans CO, Serpero LD, Kheirandish-Gozal L, Gozal D. Dietary and physical activity patterns in children with obstructive sleep apnea. J Pediatr. 2010;156:724–30, 730.
59. Bonuck KA, Freeman K, Henderson J. Growth and growth biomarker changes after adenotonsillectomy: systematic review and meta-analysis. Arch Dis Child. 2009;94:83–91.
60. Nachalon Y, Lowenthal N, Greenberg-Dotan S, Goldbart AD. Inflammation and growth in young children with obstructive sleep apnea syndrome before and after adenotonsillectomy. Mediators Inflamm. 2014;2014:146893.
61. Goldstein NA, Aronin C, Kantrowitz B, et al. The prevalence of sleep-disordered breathing in children with asthma and its behavioral effects. Pediatr Pulmonol. 2015;50:1128–36.
62. Ramagopal M, Mehta A, Roberts DW, et al. Asthma as a predictor of obstructive sleep apnea in urban African-American children. J Asthma. 2009;46:895–9.
63. Kheirandish-Gozal L, Dayyat EA, Eid NS, Morton RL, Gozal D. Obstructive sleep apnea in poorly controlled asthmatic children: effect of adenotonsillectomy. Pediatr Pulmonol. 2011;46:913–8.
64. Kheirandish-Gozal L, Gozal D. Obesity, asthma, and sleep-disordered breathing. J Pediatr. 2012;160:713–4.
65. Bhattacharjee R, Choi BH, Gozal D, Mokhlesi B. Association of adenotonsillectomy with asthma outcomes in children: a longitudinal database analysis. PLoS Med. 2014;11:e1001753.
66. Gozal D. Sleep, sleep disorders and inflammation in children. Sleep Med. 2009;10 Suppl 1:S12–6.
67. Khalyfa A, Capdevila OS, Buazza MO, Serpero LD, Kheirandish-Gozal L, Gozal D. Genome-wide gene expression profiling in children with non-obese obstructive sleep apnea. Sleep Med. 2009;10:75–86.
68. Gozal D, Serpero LD, Sans CO, Kheirandish-Gozal L. Systemic inflammation in non-obese children with obstructive sleep apnea. Sleep Med. 2008;9:254–9.

69. Tauman R, O'Brien LM, Gozal D. Hypoxemia and obesity modulate plasma C-reactive protein and interleukin-6 levels in sleep-disordered breathing. Sleep Breath. 2007;11:77–84.
70. Gozal D, Serpero LD, Kheirandish-Gozal L, Capdevila OS, Khalyfa A, Tauman R. Sleep measures and morning plasma TNF-alpha levels in children with sleep-disordered breathing. Sleep. 2010;33:319–25.
71. Tam CS, Wong M, McBain R, Bailey S, Waters KA. Inflammatory measures in children with obstructive sleep apnoea. J Paediatr Child Health. 2006;42:277–82.
72. Kheirandish-Gozal L, Capdevila OS, Tauman R, Gozal D. Plasma C-reactive protein in non-obese children with obstructive sleep apnea before and after adenotonsillectomy. J Clin Sleep Med. 2006;2:301–4.
73. Gozal D, Kheirandish-Gozal L, Bhattacharjee R, Kim J. C-reactive protein and obstructive sleep apnea syndrome in children. Front Biosci (Elite Ed). 2012;4:2410–22.
74. Ingram DG, Matthews CK. Effect of adenotonsillectomy on c-reactive protein levels in children with obstructive sleep apnea: a meta-analysis. Sleep Med. 2013;14:172–6.
75. Li AM, Chan MH, Yin J, et al. C-reactive protein in children with obstructive sleep apnea and the effects of treatment. Pediatr Pulmonol. 2008;43:34–40.
76. Kaditis AG, Gozal D, Khalyfa A, Kheirandish-Gozal L, Capdevila OS, Gourgoulianis K, Alexopoulos EI, Chaidas K, Bhattacharjee R, Kim J, Rodopoulou P, Zintzaras E. Variants in C-reactive protein and IL-6 genes and susceptibility to obstructive sleep apnea in children: a candidate-gene association study in European American and Southeast European populations. Sleep Med. 2014;15:228–35.
77. Kim J, Bhattacharjee R, Khalyfa A, et al. DNA methylation in inflammatory genes among children with obstructive sleep apnea. Am J Respir Crit Care Med. 2012;185:330–8.
78. Tan HL, Gozal D, Wang Y, et al. Alterations in circulating T-cell lymphocyte populations in children with obstructive sleep apnea. Sleep. 2013;36:913–22.
79. Zhu Y, Au CT, Leung TF, Wing YK, Lam CW, Li AM. Effects of passive smoking on snoring in preschool children. J Pediatr. 2013;163:1158–62.e4.
80. Mitchell RB, Garetz S, Moore RH, et al. The use of clinical parameters to predict obstructive sleep apnea syndrome severity in children: the Childhood Adenotonsillectomy (CHAT) study randomized clinical trial. JAMA Otolaryngol Head Neck Surg. 2015;141:130–6.
81. Kheirandish-Gozal L, Ghalebandi M, Salehi M, Salarifar MH, Gozal D. Neighbourhood air quality and snoring in school-aged children. Eur Respir J. 2014;43:824–32.
82. Friberg D, Lundkvist K, Li X, Sundquist K. Parental poverty and occupation as risk factors for pediatric sleep-disordered breathing. Sleep Med. 2015;16:1169–75.
83. Gozal D. Sleep-disordered breathing and school performance in children. Pediatrics. 1998;102:616–20.
84. Chervin RD, Ruzicka DL, Hoban TF, et al. Esophageal pressures, polysomnography, and neurobehavioral outcomes of adenotonsillectomy in children. Chest. 2012;142:101–10.
85. Giordani B, Hodges EK, Guire KE, et al. Changes in neuropsychological and behavioral functioning in children with and without obstructive sleep apnea following Tonsillectomy. J Int Neuropsychol Soc. 2012;18:212–22.
86. Landau YE, Bar-Yishay O, Greenberg-Dotan S, Goldbart AD, Tarasiuk A, Tal A. Impaired behavioral and neurocognitive function in preschool children with obstructive sleep apnea. Pediatr Pulmonol. 2012;47:180–8.
87. Bourke R, Anderson V, Yang JS, et al. Cognitive and academic functions are impaired in children with all severities of sleep-disordered breathing. Sleep Med. 2011;12:489–96.
88. Garetz SL. Behavior, cognition, and quality of life after adenotonsillectomy for pediatric sleep-disordered breathing: summary of the literature. Otolaryngol Head Neck Surg. 2008;138:S19–26.
89. Wei JL, Bond J, Mayo MS, Smith HJ, Reese M, Weatherly RA. Improved behavior and sleep after adenotonsillectomy in children with sleep-disordered breathing: long-term follow-up. Arch Otolaryngol Head Neck Surg. 2009;135:642–6.
90. Wei JL, Mayo MS, Smith HJ, Reese M, Weatherly RA. Improved behavior and sleep after adenotonsillectomy in children with sleep-disordered breathing. Arch Otolaryngol Head Neck Surg. 2007;133:974–9.

91. Abman S, Jobe A, Chernick V, et al. Strategic plan for pediatric respiratory diseases research: an NHLBI working group report. Pediatr Pulmonol. 2009;44:2–13.

92. Gozal D, Kheirandish-Gozal L. Neurocognitive and behavioral morbidity in children with sleep disorders. Curr Opin Pulm Med. 2007;13:505–9.

93. Chervin RD, Ruzicka DL, Giordani BJ, et al. Sleep-disordered breathing, behavior, and cognition in children before and after adenotonsillectomy. Pediatrics. 2006;117:e769–78.

94. Montgomery-Downs HE, Crabtree VM, Gozal D. Cognition, sleep and respiration in at-risk children treated for obstructive sleep apnoea. Eur Respir J. 2005;25:336–42.

95. Friedman BC, Hendeles-Amitai A, Kozminsky E, et al. Adenotonsillectomy improves neurocognitive function in children with obstructive sleep apnea syndrome. Sleep. 2003;26:999–1005.

96. Hunter SJ, Gozal D, Smith DL, Philby MF, Kaylegian J, Kheirandish-Gozal L. Effect of sleep-disordered breathing severity on cognitive performance measures in a large community cohort of young school-aged children. Am J Respir Crit Care Med. 2016 [In Press].

97. Kheirandish-Gozal L, De Jong MR, Spruyt K, Chamuleau SA, Gozal D. Obstructive sleep apnoea is associated with impaired pictorial memory task acquisition and retention in children. Eur Respir J. 2010;36:164–9.

98. Kheirandish-Gozal L, Yoder K, Kulkarni R, Gozal D, Decety J. Preliminary functional MRI neural correlates of executive functioning and empathy in children with obstructive sleep apnea. Sleep. 2014;37:587–92.

99. Barnes ME, Gozal D, Molfese DL. Attention in children with obstructive sleep apnoea: an event-related potentials study. Sleep Med. 2012;13:368–77.

100. Hill CM, Hogan AM, Onugha N, et al. Increased cerebral blood flow velocity in children with mild sleep-disordered breathing: a possible association with abnormal neuropsychological function. Pediatrics. 2006;118:e1100–8.

101. Khadra MA, McConnell K, VanDyke R, et al. Determinants of regional cerebral oxygenation in children with sleep-disordered breathing. Am J Respir Crit Care Med. 2008;178:870–5.

102. Gozal D, Kheirandish-Gozal L, Bhattacharjee R, Spruyt K. Neurocognitive and endothelial dysfunction in children with obstructive sleep apnea. Pediatrics. 2010;126:e1161–7.

103. O'Brien LM, Mervis CB, Holbrook CR, et al. Neurobehavioral implications of habitual snoring in children. Pediatrics. 2004;114:44–9.

104. Barnes ME, Huss EA, Garrod KN, et al. Impairments in attention in occasionally snoring children: an event-related potential study. Dev Neuropsychol. 2009;34:629–49.

105. Kaemingk KL, Pasvogel AE, Goodwin JL, et al. Learning in children and sleep disordered breathing: findings of the Tucson Children's Assessment of Sleep Apnea (tuCASA) prospective cohort study. J Int Neuropsychol Soc. 2003;9:1016–26.

106. Mulvaney SA, Goodwin JL, Morgan WJ, Rosen GR, Quan SF, Kaemingk KL. Behavior problems associated with sleep disordered breathing in school-aged children – the Tucson children's assessment of sleep apnea study. J Pediatr Psychol. 2006;31:322–30.

107. Lau EY, Choi EW, Lai ES, et al. Working memory impairment and its associated sleep-related respiratory parameters in children with obstructive sleep apnea. Sleep Med. 2015;16:1109–15.

108. Redline S, Amin R, Beebe D, et al. The Childhood Adenotonsillectomy Trial (CHAT): rationale, design, and challenges of a randomized controlled trial evaluating a standard surgical procedure in a pediatric population. Sleep. 2011;34:1509–17.

109. Garetz SL, Mitchell RB, Parker PD, et al. Quality of life and obstructive sleep apnea symptoms after pediatric adenotonsillectomy. Pediatrics. 2015;135:e477–86.

110. Kheirandish-Gozal L, Gozal D. Genotype-phenotype interactions in pediatric obstructive sleep apnea. Respir Physiol Neurobiol. 2013;189:338–43.

111. Gozal D, Crabtree VM, Sans CO, Witcher LA, Kheirandish-Gozal L. C-reactive protein, obstructive sleep apnea, and cognitive dysfunction in school-aged children. Am J Respir Crit Care Med. 2007;176:188–93.

112. Gozal D, Sans CO, McLaughlin CV, Serpero LD, Witcher LA, Kheirandish-Gozal L. Plasma IGF-1 levels and cognitive dysfunction in children with obstructive sleep apnea. Sleep Med. 2009;10:167–73.

113. Gozal D, Capdevila OS, Kheirandish-Gozal L, Crabtree VM. APOE epsilon 4 allele, cognitive dysfunction, and obstructive sleep apnea in children. Neurology. 2007;69:243–9.
114. Quan SF, Archbold K, Gevins AS, Goodwin JL. Long-term neurophysiologic impact of childhood sleep disordered breathing on neurocognitive performance. Southwest J Pulm Crit Care. 2013;7:165–75.
115. Perfect MM, Archbold K, Goodwin JL, Levine-Donnerstein D, Quan SF. Risk of behavioral and adaptive functioning difficulties in youth with previous and current sleep disordered breathing. Sleep. 2013;36:517–525B.
116. Biggs SN, Walter LM, Jackman AR, et al. Long-term cognitive and behavioral outcomes following resolution of sleep disordered breathing in preschool children. PLoS One. 2015;10:e0139142.
117. Biggs SN, Vlahandonis A, Anderson V, et al. Long-term changes in neurocognition and behavior following treatment of sleep disordered breathing in school-aged children. Sleep. 2014;37:77–84.
118. Gozal D, Pope Jr DW. Snoring during early childhood and academic performance at ages thirteen to fourteen years. Pediatrics. 2001;107:1394–9.
119. Marcus CL, Radcliffe J, Konstantinopoulou S, et al. Effects of positive airway pressure therapy on neurobehavioral outcomes in children with obstructive sleep apnea. Am J Respir Crit Care Med. 2012;185:998–1003.
120. Mitchell RB, Kelly J. Behavioral changes in children with mild sleep-disordered breathing or obstructive sleep apnea after adenotonsillectomy. Laryngoscope. 2007;117:1685–8.
121. Serratto M, Harris VJ, Carr I. Upper airways obstruction. Presentation with systemic hypertension. Arch Dis Child. 1981;56:153–5.
122. Ross RD, Daniels SR, Loggie JM, Meyer RA, Ballard ET. Sleep apnea-associated hypertension and reversible left ventricular hypertrophy. J Pediatr. 1987;111:253–5.
123. Adegunsoye A, Ramachandran S. Etiopathogenetic mechanisms of pulmonary hypertension in sleep-related breathing disorders. Pulm Med. 2012;2012:273591.
124. Nisbet RE, Graves AS, Kleinhenz DJ, et al. The role of NADPH oxidase in chronic intermittent hypoxia-induced pulmonary hypertension in mice. Am J Respir Cell Mol Biol. 2009;40:601–9.
125. Abman SH, Ivy DD. Recent progress in understanding pediatric pulmonary hypertension. Curr Opin Pediatr. 2011;23:298–304.
126. Marcus CL, Greene MG, Carroll JL. Blood pressure in children with obstructive sleep apnea. Am J Respir Crit Care Med. 1998;157:1098–103.
127. Kohyama J, Ohinata JS, Hasegawa T. Blood pressure in sleep disordered breathing. Arch Dis Child. 2003;88:139–42.
128. Horne RS, Yang JS, Walter LM, et al. Elevated blood pressure during sleep and wake in children with sleep-disordered breathing. Pediatrics. 2011;128:e85–92.
129. Amin RS, Carroll JL, Jeffries JL, et al. Twenty-four-hour ambulatory blood pressure in children with sleep-disordered breathing. Am J Respir Crit Care Med. 2004;169:950–6.
130. Verdecchia P, Schillaci G, Borgioni C, et al. Altered circadian blood pressure profile and prognosis. Blood Press Monit. 1997;2:347–52.
131. Amin R, Somers VK, McConnell K, et al. Activity-adjusted 24-hour ambulatory blood pressure and cardiac remodeling in children with sleep disordered breathing. Hypertension. 2008;51:84–91.
132. Nisbet LC, Yiallourou SR, Walter LM, Horne RS. Blood pressure regulation, autonomic control and sleep disordered breathing in children. Sleep Med Rev. 2013. 18(2):179–89.
133. Li AM, Au CT, Ho C, Fok TF, Wing YK. Blood pressure is elevated in children with primary snoring. J Pediatr. 2009;155:362–8.
134. Kwok KL, Ng DK, Cheung YF. BP and arterial distensibility in children with primary snoring. Chest. 2003;123:1561–6.
135. Walter LM, Biggs SN, Nisbet LC, et al. Improved long-term autonomic function following resolution of sleep-disordered breathing in preschool-aged children. Sleep Breath. 2015. 20(1):309–19.

136. Goldbart AD, Levitas A, Greenberg-Dotan S, et al. B-type natriuretic peptide and cardio-vascular function in young children with obstructive sleep apnea. Chest. 2010; 138:528–35.
137. Gozal D, Kheirandish-Gozal L, Serpero LD, Sans CO, Dayyat E. Obstructive sleep apnea and endothelial function in school-aged nonobese children: effect of adenotonsillectomy. Circulation. 2007;116:2307–14.
138. Kheirandish-Gozal L, Bhattacharjee R, Kim J, Clair HB, Gozal D. Endothelial progenitor cells and vascular dysfunction in children with obstructive sleep apnea. Am J Respir Crit Care Med. 2010;182:92–7.
139. Kheirandish-Gozal L, Etzioni T, Bhattacharjee R, et al. Obstructive sleep apnea in children is associated with severity-dependent deterioration in overnight endothelial function. Sleep Med. 2013;14:526–31.
140. Dubern B, Aggoun Y, Boule M, Fauroux B, Bonnet D, Tounian P. Arterial alterations in severely obese children with obstructive sleep apnoea. Int J Pediatr Obes. 2010;5:230–6.
141. Bhattacharjee R, Kim J, Alotaibi WH, Kheirandish-Gozal L, Capdevila OS, Gozal D. Endothelial dysfunction in children without hypertension: potential contributions of obe-sity and obstructive sleep apnea. Chest. 2012;141:682–91.
142. Kheirandish-Gozal L, Farre R. The injury theory, endothelial progenitors, and sleep apnea. Am J Respir Crit Care Med. 2013;187:5–7.
143. Tan HL, Gozal D, Samiei A, et al. T regulatory lymphocytes and endothelial function in pediatric obstructive sleep apnea. PLoS One. 2013;8:e69710.
144. Chatsuriyawong S, Gozal D, Kheirandish-Gozal L, et al. Polymorphisms in nitric oxide syn-thase and endothelin genes among children with obstructive sleep apnea. BMC Med Genomics. 2013;6:29.
145. Kheirandish-Gozal L, Khalyfa A, Gozal D, Bhattacharjee R, Wang Y. Endothelial dysfunc-tion in children with obstructive sleep apnea is associated with epigenetic changes in the eNOS gene. Chest. 2013;143:971–7.
146. Pearson TA, Mensah GA, Alexander RW, et al. Markers of inflammation and cardiovascular disease: application to clinical and public health practice: a statement for healthcare profes-sionals from the Centers for Disease Control and Prevention and the American Heart Association. Circulation. 2003;107:499–511.
147. Pasceri V, Willerson JT, Yeh ET. Direct proinflammatory effect of C-reactive protein on human endothelial cells. Circulation. 2000;102:2165–8.
148. Pasceri V, Cheng JS, Willerson JT, Yeh ET. Modulation of C-reactive protein-mediated mono-cyte chemoattractant protein-1 induction in human endothelial cells by anti-atherosclerosis drugs. Circulation. 2001;103:2531–4.
149. O'Brien LM, Serpero LD, Tauman R, Gozal D. Plasma adhesion molecules in children with sleep-disordered breathing. Chest. 2006;129:947–53.
150. Kim J, Bhattacharjee R, Snow AB, Capdevila OS, Kheirandish-Gozal L, Gozal D. Myeloid-related protein 8/14 levels in children with obstructive sleep apnoea. Eur Respir J. 2010;35:843–50.
151. Kim J, Bhattacharjee R, Kheirandish-Gozal L, Spruyt K, Gozal D. Circulating microparticles in children with sleep disordered breathing. Chest. 2011;140:408–17.
152. Bhushan B, Khalyfa A, Spruyt K, et al. Fatty-acid binding protein 4 gene polymorphisms and plasma levels in children with obstructive sleep apnea. Sleep Med. 2011;12:666–71.
153. Gozal D, Kheirandish-Gozal L, Bhattacharjee R, Molero-Ramirez H, Tan HL, Bandla HP. Circulating adropin concentrations in pediatric obstructive sleep apnea: potential rele-vance to endothelial function. J Pediatr. 2013;163:1122–6.
154. Punjabi NM, Sorkin JD, Katzel LI, Goldberg AP, Schwartz AR, Smith PL. Sleep-disordered breathing and insulin resistance in middle-aged and overweight men. Am J Respir Crit Care Med. 2002;165:677–82.
155. Lam JC, Mak JC, Ip MS. Obesity, obstructive sleep apnoea and metabolic syndrome. Respirology. 2012;17:223–36.

156. Assoumou HG, Gaspoz JM, Sforza E, et al. Obstructive sleep apnea and the metabolic syndrome in an elderly healthy population: the SYNAPSE cohort. Sleep Breath. 2012;16:895–902.

157. Basoglu OK, Sarac F, Sarac S, Uluer H, Yilmaz C. Metabolic syndrome, insulin resistance, fibrinogen, homocysteine, leptin, and C-reactive protein in obese patients with obstructive sleep apnea syndrome. Ann Thorac Med. 2011;6:120–5.

158. Pillai A, Warren G, Gunathilake W, Idris I. Effects of sleep apnea severity on glycemic control in patients with type 2 diabetes prior to continuous positive airway pressure treatment. Diabetes Technol Ther. 2011;13:945–9.

159. Bhushan B, Misra A, Guleria R. Obstructive sleep apnea is independently associated with the metabolic syndrome in obese Asian Indians in northern India. Metab Syndr Relat Disord. 2010;8:431–5.

160. Ahmed QA. Metabolic complications of obstructive sleep apnea syndrome. Am J Med Sci. 2008;335:60–4.

161. Redline S, Storfer-Isser A, Rosen CL, et al. Association between metabolic syndrome and sleep-disordered breathing in adolescents. Am J Respir Crit Care Med. 2007;176:401–8.

162. Koren D, Levitt Katz LE, Brar PC, Gallagher PR, Berkowitz RI, Brooks LJ. Sleep architecture and glucose and insulin homeostasis in obese adolescents. Diabetes Care. 2011;34:2442–7.

163. Lesser DJ, Bhatia R, Tran WH, et al. Sleep fragmentation and intermittent hypoxemia are associated with decreased insulin sensitivity in obese adolescent Latino males. Pediatr Res. 2012;72:293–8.

164. Tauman R, O'Brien LM, Ivanenko A, Gozal D. Obesity rather than severity of sleep-disordered breathing as the major determinant of insulin resistance and altered lipidemia in snoring children. Pediatrics. 2005;116:e66–73.

165. Kaditis AG, Alexopoulos EI, Damani E, et al. Obstructive sleep-disordered breathing and fasting insulin levels in nonobese children. Pediatr Pulmonol. 2005;40:515–23.

166. Gozal D, Capdevila OS, Kheirandish-Gozal L. Metabolic alterations and systemic inflammation in obstructive sleep apnea among nonobese and obese prepubertal children. Am J Respir Crit Care Med. 2008;177:1142–9.

167. Koren D, Gozal D, Bhattacharjee R, Philby M, Kheirandish-Gozal L. Impact of adenotonsillectomy on insulin resistance and lipoprotein profile in nonobese and obese children. Chest. 2015. 149(4):999–1010.

168. Khalyfa A, Gharib SA, Kim J, et al. Peripheral blood leukocyte gene expression patterns and metabolic parameters in habitually snoring and non-snoring children with normal polysomnographic findings. Sleep. 2011;34:153–60.

169. Zong J, Liu Y, Huang Y, et al. Serum lipids alterations in adenoid hypertrophy or adenotonsillar hypertrophy children with sleep disordered breathing. Int J Pediatr Otorhinolaryngol. 2013;77:717–20.

170. Kheirandish-Gozal L, Sans CO, Kheirandish E, Gozal D. Elevated serum aminotransferase levels in children at risk for obstructive sleep apnea. Chest. 2008;133:92–9.

171. Verhulst SL, Jacobs S, Aerts L, et al. Sleep-disordered breathing: a new risk factor of suspected fatty liver disease in overweight children and adolescents? Sleep Breath. 2009;13:207–10.

172. Verhulst SL, Rooman R, Van GL, De BW, Desager K. Is sleep-disordered breathing an additional risk factor for the metabolic syndrome in obese children and adolescents? Int J Obes (Lond). 2009;33:8–13.

173. Sundaram SS, Sokol RJ, Capocelli KE, et al. Obstructive sleep apnea and hypoxemia are associated with advanced liver histology in pediatric nonalcoholic fatty liver disease. J Pediatr. 2014;164:699–706.

174. Nobili V, Cutrera R, Liccardo D, et al. Obstructive sleep apnea syndrome affects liver histology and inflammatory cell activation in pediatric nonalcoholic fatty liver disease, regardless of obesity/insulin resistance. Am J Respir Crit Care Med. 2014;189:66–76.

175. Alkhouri N, Kheirandish-Gozal L, Matloob A, et al. Evaluation of circulating markers of hepatic apoptosis and inflammation in obese children with and without obstructive sleep apnea. Sleep Med. 2015;16:1031–5.
176. Gileles-Hillel A, Kheirandish-Gozal L, Gozal D. Biological plausibility linking sleep apnoea and metabolic dysfunction. Nat Rev Endocrinol. 2016;12:290–8.
177. Kheirandish-Gozal L, Peris E, Wang Y, et al. Lipopolysaccharide-binding protein plasma levels in children: effects of obstructive sleep apnea and obesity. J Clin Endocrinol Metab. 2014;99:656–63.
178. Nobili V, Alisi A, Cutrera R, et al. Altered gut-liver axis and hepatic adiponectin expression in OSAS: novel mediators of liver injury in paediatric non-alcoholic fatty liver. Thorax. 2015;70:769–81.
179. Melendres MC, Lutz JM, Rubin ED, Marcus CL. Daytime sleepiness and hyperactivity in children with suspected sleep-disordered breathing. Pediatrics. 2004;114:768–75.
180. Gozal D, Wang M, Pope Jr DW. Objective sleepiness measures in pediatric obstructive sleep apnea. Pediatrics. 2001;108:693–7.
181. Khalyfa A, Serpero LD, Kheirandish-Gozal L, Capdevila OS, Gozal D. TNF-alpha gene polymorphisms and excessive daytime sleepiness in pediatric obstructive sleep apnea. J Pediatr. 2011;158:77–82.
182. Goldbart AD, Tal A, Givon-Lavi N, Bar-Ziv J, Dagan R, Greenberg D. Sleep-disordered breathing is a risk factor for community-acquired alveolar pneumonia in early childhood. Chest. 2012;141:1210–5.
183. Tarasiuk A, Greenberg-Dotan S, Simon-Tuval T, et al. Elevated morbidity and health care use in children with obstructive sleep apnea syndrome. Am J Respir Crit Care Med. 2007;175:55–61.
184. Reuveni H, Simon T, Tal A, Elhayany A, Tarasiuk A. Health care services utilization in children with obstructive sleep apnea syndrome. Pediatrics. 2002;110:68–72.
185. Tarasiuk A, Simon T, Tal A, Reuveni H. Adenotonsillectomy in children with obstructive sleep apnea syndrome reduces health care utilization. Pediatrics. 2004;113:351–6.
186. Tsou YA, Lin CC, Lai CH, et al. Does adenotonsillectomy really reduced clinic visits for pediatric upper respiratory tract infections? A national database study in Taiwan. Int J Pediatr Otorhinolaryngol. 2013;77:677–81.
187. Weider DJ, Hauri PJ. Nocturnal enuresis in children with upper airway obstruction. Int J Pediatr Otorhinolaryngol. 1985;9:173–82.
188. Jeyakumar A, Rahman SI, Armbrecht ES, Mitchell R. The association between sleep-disordered breathing and enuresis in children. Laryngoscope. 2012;122:1873–7.
189. Alexopoulos EI, Kostadima E, Pagonari I, Zintzaras E, Gourgoulianis K, Kaditis AG. Association between primary nocturnal enuresis and habitual snoring in children. Urology. 2006;68:406–9.
190. Sans CO, Crabtree VM, Kheirandish-Gozal L, Gozal D. Increased morning brain natriuretic peptide levels in children with nocturnal enuresis and sleep-disordered breathing: a community-based study. Pediatrics. 2008;121:e1208–14.
191. Born J, Muth S, Fehm HL. The significance of sleep onset and slow wave sleep for nocturnal release of growth hormone (GH) and cortisol. Psychoneuroendocrinology. 1988;13:233–43.
192. Nieminen P, Lopponen T, Tolonen U, Lanning P, Knip M, Lopponen H. Growth and biochemical markers of growth in children with snoring and obstructive sleep apnea. Pediatrics. 2002;109:e55.
193. Bar A, Tarasiuk A, Segev Y, Phillip M, Tal A. The effect of adenotonsillectomy on serum insulin-like growth factor-I and growth in children with obstructive sleep apnea syndrome. J Pediatr. 1999;135:76–80.
194. Katz ES, Moore RH, Rosen CL, et al. Growth after adenotonsillectomy for obstructive sleep apnea: an RCT. Pediatrics. 2014;134:282–9.
195. Marcus CL, Brooks LJ, Draper KA, et al. Diagnosis and management of childhood obstructive sleep apnea syndrome. Pediatrics. 2012;130:576–84.
196. Iber C, Chesson A, Quan S, for the American Academy of Sleep Medicine. The AASM manual for the scoring of sleep and associated events: rules, terminology and technical specifications. 2nd ed. Westchester: Darien, IL, USA; 2013.

197. Tan HL, Kheirandish-Gozal L, Gozal D. Pediatric home sleep apnea testing: slowly getting there! Chest. 2015;148:1382–95.
198. Gozal D, Kheirandish-Gozal L, Kaditis AG. Home sleep testing for the diagnosis of pediatric obstructive sleep apnea: the times they are a changing...! Curr Opin Pulm Med. 2015;21:563–8.
199. Kaditis A, Kheirandish-Gozal L, Gozal D. Pediatric OSAS: oximetry can provide answers when polysomnography is not available. Sleep Med Rev. 2015;27:96–105.
200. Alvarez D, Kheirandish-Gozal L, Gutierrez-Tobal GC, et al. Automated analysis of nocturnal oximetry as screening tool for childhood obstructive sleep apnea-hypopnea syndrome. Conf Proc IEEE Eng Med Biol Soc. 2015;2015:2800–3.
201. Villa MP, Paolino MC, Castaldo R, et al. Sleep clinical record: an aid to rapid and accurate diagnosis of paediatric sleep disordered breathing. Eur Respir J. 2013;41:1355–61.
202. Villa MP, Pietropaoli N, Supino MC, et al. Diagnosis of pediatric obstructive sleep apnea syndrome in settings with limited resources. JAMA Otolaryngol Head Neck Surg. 2015;141:990–6.
203. Jacob SV, Morielli A, Mograss MA, Ducharme FM, Schloss MD, Brouillette RT. Home testing for pediatric obstructive sleep apnea syndrome secondary to adenotonsillar hypertrophy. Pediatr Pulmonol. 1995;20:241–52.
204. Brockmann PE, Perez JL, Moya A. Feasibility of unattended home polysomnography in children with sleep-disordered breathing. Int J Pediatr Otorhinolaryngol. 2013;77:1960–4.
205. Alonso-Alvarez ML, Teran-Santos J, Ordax CE, et al. Reliability of home respiratory polygraphy for the diagnosis of sleep apnea in children. Chest. 2015;147:1020–8.
206. Tan HL, Kheirandish-Gozal L, Gozal D. Obstructive sleep apnea in children: update on the recognition, treatment and management of persistent disease. Expert Rev Respir Med. 2016 [In Press].
207. De Luca CG, Pacheco-Pereira C, Aydinoz S, et al. Adenotonsillectomy complications: a meta-analysis. Pediatrics. 2015;136:702–18.
208. Konstantinopoulou S, Gallagher P, Elden L, et al. Complications of adenotonsillectomy for obstructive sleep apnea in school-aged children. Int J Pediatr Otorhinolaryngol. 2015;79:240–5.
209. Wang H, Fu Y, Feng Y, Guan J, Yin S. Tonsillectomy versus tonsillotomy for sleep-disordered breathing in children: a meta analysis. PLoS One. 2015;10:e0121500.
210. Ericsson E, Graf J, Lundeborg-Hammarstrom I, Hultcrantz E. Tonsillotomy versus tonsillectomy on young children: 2 year post surgery follow-up. J Otolaryngol Head Neck Surg. 2014;43:26.
211. Odhagen E, Sunnergren O, Hemlin C, Hessen Soderman AC, Ericsson E, Stalfors J. Risk of reoperation after tonsillotomy versus tonsillectomy: a population-based cohort study. Eur Arch Otorhinolaryngol. 2016 [In Press].
212. Venekamp RP, Hearne BJ, Chandrasekharan D, Blackshaw H, Lim J, Schilder AG. Tonsillectomy or adenotonsillectomy versus non-surgical management for obstructive sleep-disordered breathing in children. Cochrane Database Syst Rev. 2015;(10):CD011165.
213. Chervin RD, Ellenberg SS, Hou X, et al. Prognosis for spontaneous resolution of OSA in children. Chest. 2015;148:1204–13.
214. Marcus CL, Rosen G, Ward SL, et al. Adherence to and effectiveness of positive airway pressure therapy in children with obstructive sleep apnea. Pediatrics. 2006;117:e442–51.
215. Ramirez A, Khirani S, Aloui S, et al. Continuous positive airway pressure and noninvasive ventilation adherence in children. Sleep Med. 2013;14:1290–4.
216. Kheirandish-Gozal L, Kim J, Goldbart AD, Gozal D. Novel pharmacological approaches for treatment of obstructive sleep apnea in children. Expert Opin Investig Drugs. 2013;22:71–85.
217. Goldbart AD, Goldman JL, Li RC, Brittian KR, Tauman R, Gozal D. Differential expression of cysteinyl leukotriene receptors 1 and 2 in tonsils of children with obstructive sleep apnea syndrome or recurrent infection. Chest. 2004;126:13–8.
218. Dayyat E, Serpero LD, Kheirandish-Gozal L, et al. Leukotriene pathways and in vitro adenotonsillar cell proliferation in children with obstructive sleep apnea. Chest. 2009;135:1142–9.
219. Goldbart AD, Goldman JL, Veling MC, Gozal D. Leukotriene modifier therapy for mild sleep-disordered breathing in children. Am J Respir Crit Care Med. 2005;172:364–70.

220. Goldbart AD, Greenberg-Dotan S, Tal A. Montelukast for children with obstructive sleep apnea: a double-blind, placebo-controlled study. Pediatrics. 2012;130:e575–80.

221. Kheirandish-Gozal L, Serpero LD, Dayyat E, et al. Corticosteroids suppress in vitro tonsillar proliferation in children with obstructive sleep apnoea. Eur Respir J. 2009;33:1077–84.

222. Kheirandish-Gozal L, Gozal D. Intranasal budesonide treatment for children with mild obstructive sleep apnea syndrome. Pediatrics. 2008;122:e149–55.

223. Brouillette RT, Manoukian JJ, Ducharme FM, et al. Efficacy of fluticasone nasal spray for pediatric obstructive sleep apnea. J Pediatr. 2001;138:838–44.

224. Chohan A, Lal A, Chohan K, Chakravarti A, Gomber S. Systematic review and meta-analysis of randomized controlled trials on the role of mometasone in adenoid hypertrophy in children. Int J Pediatr Otorhinolaryngol. 2015;79:1599–608.

225. Kheirandish L, Goldbart AD, Gozal D. Intranasal steroids and oral leukotriene modifier therapy in residual sleep-disordered breathing after tonsillectomy and adenoidectomy in children. Pediatrics. 2006;117:e61–6.

226. Kheirandish-Gozal L, Bhattacharjee R, Bandla HP, Gozal D. Antiinflammatory therapy outcomes for mild OSA in children. Chest. 2014;146:88–95.

227. Verhulst SL, Franckx H, Van GL, De BW, Desager K. The effect of weight loss on sleep-disordered breathing in obese teenagers. Obesity (Silver Spring). 2009;17:1178–83.

228. Villa MP, Malagola C, Pagani J, et al. Rapid maxillary expansion in children with obstructive sleep apnea syndrome: 12-month follow-up. Sleep Med. 2007;8:128–34.

229. Villa MP, Rizzoli A, Rabasco J, et al. Rapid maxillary expansion outcomes in treatment of obstructive sleep apnea in children. Sleep Med. 2015;16:709–16.

230. Guilleminault C, Monteyrol PJ, Huynh NT, Pirelli P, Quo S, Li K. Adeno-tonsillectomy and rapid maxillary distraction in pre-pubertal children, a pilot study. Sleep Breath. 2011;15:173–7.

231. Guilleminault C, Huang YS, Monteyrol PJ, Sato R, Quo S, Lin CH. Critical role of myofascial reeducation in pediatric sleep-disordered breathing. Sleep Med. 2013;14:518–25.

232. Villa MP, Brasili L, Ferretti A, et al. Oropharyngeal exercises to reduce symptoms of OSA after AT. Sleep Breath. 2015;19:281–9.

233. McGinley B, Halbower A, Schwartz AR, Smith PL, Patil SP, Schneider H. Effect of a high-flow open nasal cannula system on obstructive sleep apnea in children. Pediatrics. 2009;124:179–88.

234. Lin AC, Koltai PJ. Sleep endoscopy in the evaluation of pediatric obstructive sleep apnea. Int J Pediatr. 2012;2012:576719.

235. Truong MT, Woo VG, Koltai PJ. Sleep endoscopy as a diagnostic tool in pediatric obstructive sleep apnea. Int J Pediatr Otorhinolaryngol. 2012;76:722–7.

236. Shott SR, Donnelly LF. Cine magnetic resonance imaging: evaluation of persistent airway obstruction after tonsil and adenoidectomy in children with Down syndrome. Laryngoscope. 2004;114:1724–9.

237. Donnelly LF, Shott SR, LaRose CR, Chini BA, Amin RS. Causes of persistent obstructive sleep apnea despite previous tonsillectomy and adenoidectomy in children with down syndrome as depicted on static and dynamic cine MRI. AJR Am J Roentgenol. 2004;183:175–81.

238. Becker L, Kheirandish-Gozal L, Peris E, Schoenfelt KQ, Gozal D. Contextualised urinary biomarker analysis facilitates diagnosis of paediatric obstructive sleep apnoea. Sleep Med. 2014;15:541–9.

239. Kheirandish-Gozal L, McManus CJ, Kellermann GH, Samiei A, Gozal D. Urinary neurotransmitters are selectively altered in children with obstructive sleep apnea and predict cognitive morbidity. Chest. 2013;143:1576.

240. Khalyfa A, Kheirandish-Gozal L, Bhattacharjee R, Khalyfa AA, Gozal D. Circulating microRNAs as potential biomarkers of endothelial dysfunction in obese children. Chest. 2016;149:786–800.

241. Mukherjee S, Patel SR, Kales SN, et al. An Official American Thoracic Society statement: the importance of healthy sleep. recommendations and future priorities. Am J Respir Crit Care Med. 2015;191:1450–8.

Chapter 11
Sleep Disorders in Children: Simple Sleep-Related Movement Disorders

Pamela E. Hamilton-Stubbs and Arthur S. Walters

Abstract Simple sleep-related movement disorders are a group of conditions that must be differentiated from parasomnias which are more complex sleep-related movement disorders and appear goal directed but are outside the conscious awareness of the individual. Simple sleep-related movement disorders must also be distinguished from movement disorders that occur predominantly during wakefulness but may occur to a minor degree in sleep. A detailed medical history including the patient's age at onset of symptoms and a meticulous description of the movement help to differentiate these conditions. In some cases, polysomnography and video recording are essential diagnostic tools.

There is an expanding body of research identifying genes, chromosomes, and neurotransmitters in the pathophysiology of simple sleep-related movement disorders. Some of these disorders, such as isolated periodic limb movements in sleep, need not be treated at all unless they are associated with sleep disruption of the bed partner or are a presumptive cause of daytime fatigue when other causes of fatigue have been excluded. Others, including restless legs syndrome, leg cramps, and sleep-related bruxism, may require pharmacotherapy. Treatment of sleep-related movement disorders has evolved to include new collaborative roles for physicians, dentists, and other health professionals.

Keywords Restless legs syndrome • Periodic limb movement disorder • Leg cramps • Bruxism • Rhythmic movement disorder • Hypnagogic foot tremor • Alternating leg muscle activation (ALMA) • Excessive fragmentary myoclonus

P.E. Hamilton-Stubbs, BSN, MD
Dr. Hamilton-Stubbs' Sleep & Total Wellness Institute, LLC,
Richmond, VA 23222-2044, USA
e-mail: phstubbs@vcu.edu

A.S. Walters, MD (✉)
Division of Sleep Medicine, Vanderbilt University School of Medicine,
Medical Center North A-0118 1161 21st Ave South, Nashville, TN 37232-2551, USA
e-mail: Arthur.Walters@Vanderbilt.edu

© Springer International Publishing Switzerland 2017
S. Nevšímalová, O. Bruni (eds.), *Sleep Disorders in Children*,
DOI 10.1007/978-3-319-28640-2_11

Introduction

Simple sleep-related movement disorders are primarily monophasic, frequently stereotyped movements that occur predominantly around the sleep period and interrupt sleep [1]. The simple sleep-related movement disorders must be differentiated from more complex sleep-related movement disorders called the parasomnias that appear goal directed but are outside the conscious awareness of the individual and are therefore inappropriate. Examples of the parasomnias include the REM sleep behavior disorder and the non-REM parasomnias such as the disorders of partial arousal which include sleepwalking, sleep terrors, and confusional arousals. Other movement disorders which may disrupt sleep occur predominantly during the daytime with a minor component during sleep. Some of the movement disorders which are symptomatic primarily during the day but may also disrupt sleep include Tourette's syndrome and tics of other types, Huntington's disease and choreas of other types, Parkinson's disease and other forms of parkinsonism, myoclonus, dystonia, essential tremor, tardive dyskinesia, akathisia, ataxia, hemifacial spasm, and hemiballismus. These disorders sometimes are associated with changes in sleep architecture, increased wakefulness after sleep onset, or poor sleep efficiency. The focus of this chapter, however, revolves around the simple sleep-related movement disorders which are predominantly nocturnal and the relationship of such disorders to pediatric sleep. The parasomnias are covered in another chapter.

Although varying definitions of the disorders in this chapter exist, for purposes of simplicity, only definitions from the International Classification of Sleep Disorder third edition and the AASM polysomnographic scoring manual are included.

Restless Legs Syndrome (RLS)/Willis-Ekbom Disease (WED)

Restless legs syndrome (RLS)/Willis-Ekbom Disease (WED) is a neurological disorder initially described by Sir Thomas Willis [2]. In 1923, Oppenheim suggested RLS could be a genetic disorder [3]. Genome-wide association studies of restless legs syndrome identified common variants in genomic regions [4]. According to Rye, six candidate genes have been described although more have been added recently [5]. Rye also states, "two independent segregation analyses propose dominant inheritance influenced by a highly penetrant (90–100 %) single gene in families with symptom onset at a young age" [5].

The etiology of RLS is unknown. There is growing evidence of involvement of three areas: a genetic factor, involvement of the monoaminergic system, and intracerebral iron metabolism. Early onset RLS, defined as symptoms occurring before 45 years of age, has a familial pattern. Among children with RLS, 40–92 % are reported to have affected family members [1]. Improvement in symptoms with iron and dopaminergic agents suggests iron and/or monoaminergic systems as sites of pathology in RLS. There is a large body of literature showing comorbidity or RLS with ADHD and comorbidity with growing pains.

There is a growing body of research suggesting at least some involvement of peripheral microvascular circulation. Salminen et al. studied patients by monitoring oxygen levels in the lower extremities of patients treated with pramipexole both while off medication and when on medications as compared with controls. The authors found that the blood oxygen level increased when patients took pramipexole [6].

RLS most often affects the legs but can involve the arms, trunk, or face. Symptoms may lateralize or affect both limbs [7]. The most defining symptom is an almost irresistible urge to move the legs or involved body part. This urge to move is due to paresthesias which have been described as ranging from annoying sensations deep within the muscle to painful events. The paresthesias have a circadian pattern, occurring more frequently in the evening or night, but paresthesias have also been reported to occur during the day. Movement is associated with immediate, although sometimes temporary, relief or decrease in paresthesias [1].

Pediatric RLS was first described in the literature in 1994 [8]. Diagnostic criteria for pediatric onset RLS was introduced in 2003 and updated in 2010 and again in 2013 [9]. In 2013 the pediatric diagnostic criteria was updated to integrate diagnostic measures for children less than 12 years of age with those of adults and older children. The updated diagnostic criteria allows the use of descriptive terms and words commonly expressed by children, outlines specific considerations for the diagnosis of pediatric restless legs syndrome, and clarifies diagnostic criteria for probable and possible pediatric restless legs syndrome.

The updated diagnostic criteria for RLS (as previously) does not require leg sensations although they are usually present. The primary feature is the urge to move the legs with or without accompanying leg sensations. If sensations are present, they invariably involve the legs although the arms and sometimes other body parts can be added later in the clinical course. The current criteria from ICSD-3 for RLS are comprised of the following:

A. An urge to move the legs, usually accompanied by or thought to be caused by uncomfortable and unpleasant sensations in the legs. These symptoms must:

   1. Begin or worsen during periods of rest or inactivity such as lying down or sitting
   2. Be partially or totally relieved by movement, such as walking or stretching, as least as long as the activity continues
   3. Occur exclusively or predominantly in the evening or night rather than during the day

B. A new criterion that has been added is the need to exclude mimics of RLS which are disorders which may meet all of the above criteria but not be RLS and must therefore be distinguished from RLS by other historical features or a physical examination. Some of these mimics include leg cramps, positional discomfort, leg edema, venous stasis, myalgias, and habitual foot tapping.

C. In addition, symptoms must have clinical significance and cannot be better explained by other disorders, medication use, or substance use disorder [1]. Clinical significance has been defined as causing concern, distress, sleep disturbance, or impairment in mental, physical, social, occupational, educational, behavioral, or other important areas of functioning. The ICSD-3 also states that for certain research applications, such as genetic or epidemiological studies, it may be appropriate to omit this criterion. If so the ICSD-3 recommends that this should be clearly stated in the research report [1].

Because young children have difficulty describing symptoms in their own words, diagnosing RLS in children is challenging. The ICSD-3 clearly states that "for children, the description of these symptoms should be in the child's own words." Children at least 6 years of age and developmentally normal have been shown to adequately report symptoms of RLS. The use of pediatric prompts during the diagnostic interview may be helpful. Pediatric prompts should be straightforward interview questions phrased using words developmentally appropriate for the child. Additional special considerations are listed in Table 11.1 [1].

Periodic limb movements occurring with a frequency greater than 5 per hour in the child or a first-degree family member supports the diagnosis of RLS. The diagnosis of pediatric RLS is also supported if the child has a first-degree family member with RLS [1].

In children, an increase in symptoms during the evening or at night may not be reported. The majority of children with RLS, 66%, report daytime leg discomfort. One explanation is the number of hours children sit during the school day [1].

Restless legs syndrome affects 1.9% of children 8–11 years of age and 4% of children 12–17 years of age [10]. During early childhood, most children are thought to have mild symptoms that do not require medical care, and therefore RLS goes unreported [11]. Most people seeking medical treatment for RLS are adults, but 25% of adults diagnosed with RLS report the onset of symptoms between 10 and 20 years of age [9]. In addition, adult patients with RLS frequently report onset in childhood that remitted during adolescence only to return in adulthood often with recurrent onset in pregnancy. Among adults with RLS, many studies report a higher prevalence of RLS in women compared to men [12]. There is no significant gender difference among children.

Restless legs syndrome is associated with insomnia, impaired comprehension, impaired semantic/phonemic fluency, poor sleep quality, and decreased ability to sustain focused attention [9]. The neurocognitive deficits associated in short- and long-

Table 11.1 Special considerations when diagnosing RLS in pediatric patients

1. A description of the symptoms should be provided in the child's own words
2. Periodic limb movement disorder may develop before symptoms of RLS
3. The interviewer must be familiar with words typically used by children and adolescents to describe symptoms of RLS
4. Language and cognitive development determine the applicability of the RLS diagnostic criteria, rather than age
5. The interviewer must be mindful that adult specifiers for clinical course may not be applicable to the pediatric patient
6. Symptoms of RLS must be of clinical significance

Adapted from Picchietti et al. [9]

term memory, working memory, attention and executive functions, and semantic/phonemic fluency improve after 3 months of therapy with dopaminergic agents [13].

There is an overlap between RLS and attention deficit hyperactivity disorders (ADHD). Pullen et al. found 25 % of children with RLS met diagnostic criteria for ADHD [14]. Sleep deprivation does not solely explain the association between RLS and ADHD. Both disorders involve disruption in the dopaminergic system [15]. It has long been hypothesized that RLS involves dopamine dysfunction [16]. Most patients with RLS benefit from dopaminergic agents. It is also known that children with ADHD benefit from stimulants and these stimulants increase cerebral levels of dopamine [17]. Ernst et al. [18] studied dopaminergic pathways of children with ADHD. The researchers used dopamine tracers with positron emission tomography scans and documented decreased dopaminergic function in the brains of children with ADHD.

Children with RLS are more likely to suffer mood disorders than children who do not have RLS [19]. Pullen et al. studied 239 children with RLS. Sixty-four percent of children with RLS had one or more comorbid psychiatric disorders. Mood disturbances occurred in 29.1 %. Attention deficit hyperactivity disorder occurred in 25 %. Anxiety disorder occurred in 11.5 % and 10.9 % had behavioral disturbances. A gender difference was observed. Male children were more likely to have ADHD and disruptive behavior disorders. Female children had a higher incidence of mood disturbances and anxiety disorders [14].

A higher incidence of obstructive sleep apnea syndrome and parasomnias has been reported. Similar to adults, children with chronic renal disease have a high incidence of RLS. In adults, the incidence of RLS increases in the presence of type 2 diabetes and peripheral neuropathy. Children with these disorders may be at increased risk for developing RLS but scientific evidence has not been established.

The prevalence of growing pains among children is unknown, but a conservative estimate is that growing pains affect 4.7 % of children [20]. Halliwell et al. estimate that children with growing pains represent 7 % of office visits in a general pediatric medical practice [21]. Accurately differentiating growing pains from RLS is challenging [22]. One reason is the lack of universally accepted diagnostic criteria for diagnosing growing pains. Walters et al. reviewed the suggested diagnostic criteria for growing pains published by Evans et al. and Peterson [23–25]. Walters et al. documented an overlap in the symptoms of growing pains and RLS [20] (See Table 11.2). Halliwell et al. suggest important symptoms that differentiate the two disorders: growing pains are always described as painful, they do not affect the arms, and symptoms resolve around 12 years of age [21]. However, these distinctions do not help in cases of childhood RLS where isolated leg pain may occur in a not insignificant minority of children with RLS according to Picchietti et al. [9, 10]. The literature reviewed recently by Walters et al. [20] suggests that children with growing pains do not have symptoms made worse by rest, do not have a desire to move the legs to get relief by activity, nor do they get any relief by activity, whereas the exact opposite is true of RLS. However, these contentions have not been formally studied and could well be the basis of further investigational research [20].

Treatment of RLS involves non-pharmacologic and pharmacologic therapies. In all cases, non-pharmacologic therapies may help reduce or eliminate symptoms at

Table 11.2 Shared symptoms of RLS and growing pains (GP)

1. Pain occurs in the legs
2. Onset of symptoms starts between 3 and 12 years of age
3. The unpleasant sensations are worse in the evening or at night or only occur at night or in the evening
4. There are no significant limitations in activity or weight bearing
5. Pain usually affects the anterior thigh, calf, and posterior knee. The pain is felt in the muscles and not in the joints
6. The pain is intermittent with some pain-free days and nights
7. Physical examination is normal
8. Diagnostic tests such as erythrocyte sedimentation rate, radiograph, and bone scan are within normal values
9. Pain persists at least 3 months
10. There is no associated lack of well-being

Adapted from Walters et al. [20]

least temporarily. Non-pharmacologic treatments are considered first-line therapy and should be considered prior to initiation of prescription medications. When medically possible, consider discontinuing medications that trigger RLS symptoms: antihistamines, antidepressants, antiemetics, and antipsychotics [26]. Discontinuing commonly prescribed medications such as selective serotonin reuptake inhibitors (SSRI), metoclopramide, and diphenhydramine may improve RLS symptoms [27]. Abstinence from alcohol and caffeine may be helpful [28].

Massaging the legs may reduce discomfort. Massage increases dopamine levels and this may explain efficacy. Exercise is associated with decreased RLS symptoms. Avoid prolonged standing or sitting. Avoid artificial sweeteners, caffeine, and alcohol. Over-the-counter supplements and vitamins have been used to treat RLS in adults with variable results. Iron supplements have been found to reduce symptoms in children with low iron or low ferritin levels. Simakajornboon et al. induced the reduction of symptoms for a period of 1–2 years in children who were iron deficient. Children were administered 3 mg of elemental iron/kg/day for 3 months. Iron was then tapered over a period of 1 year [27]. Vitamin C enhances iron absorption [29]. Lee et al. found an association between low folate levels and RLS in pregnant women [30]. Folate (B9) synthesizes tetrahydrobiopterin. Sagheb et al. reported that a combination of vitamin C and vitamin E or either alone was found to decrease severity of RLS [31]. Melatonin may help induce sleep, but there is no evidence of decreased melatonin levels in patients with RLS [32]. There is no evidence supporting the use of homeopathic therapies as treatment for RLS [26].

The usefulness of magnesium is controversial. Horynyak et al. reported improvement in RLS symptoms in patients given 300 mg of elemental magnesium each evening for 4–6 weeks [33]. Walters et al. measured serum and CSF magnesium levels in patients with RLS and controls and found no statistically significant difference between the groups [34]. It is possible that magnesium may affect RLS symptoms at the muscular level because magnesium is associated with muscle relaxation and dilation of blood vessels [35]. Improved blood circulation is also thought to be the mechanism for the beneficial effects of exercise.

The pharmacologic choices for children are limited. Dopaminergic agents have documented effectiveness in treatment of adult RLS. But dopaminergic agents are not FDA approved for use in children with RLS. In a multicenter double-blind study, carbidopa/L-DOPA (25/100 CR) was found to effectively treat RLS/PLMs in children, and few side effects occurred [36]. Pramipexole and ropinirole are selective dopamine agonists and less likely to cause side effects such as augmentation compared to carbidopa/levodopa. Either pramipexole or ropinirole can be used to treat RLS in children. Start with the lowest available dose and titrate upward as needed weekly. In adults the maximum dose is 1.5 mg and may be effective at lower doses [29].

Clonidine has been reported to effectively treat RLS in children. Gabapentin and clonazepam have been shown to reduce symptoms, but clonazepam may increase symptoms of ADHD [27]. The Pediatric RLS Severity Scale offers a mechanism to document improvement of symptoms after treatment [37].

Periodic Limb Movements

Periodic limb movements (PLMs) are common but periodic limb movement disorder (PLMD) is not. PLMs are repetitive kicking movements in sleep usually of the legs, but have been reported to involve the arms. PLMD is defined as the presence of PLMS when there is accompanying fatigue or sleep disruption that can definitely be related to the PLMS. Even though PLMS are common in RLS (occur in up to 80% of adult RLS patients), PLMD cannot be diagnosed in the presence of any other sleep disorder such as RLS which might account for the sleep disruption and daytime fatigue. PLMD is usually a diagnosis of exclusion since PLMS are a very common finding on polysomnography done for unrelated purposes such as ruling out sleep apnea. Insomnia as a cause of sleep disruption and daytime fatigue is also common and may be coincidental to the PLMS. A good history will usually reveal that the insomnia is due to something other than the PLMS in which case a diagnosis of PLMD cannot be made. Similarly hypersomnia is not uncommonly seen in a sleep disorders practice. A good sleep history may also reveal that the fatigue or hypersomnia is due to sleep apnea, medications, and other medical or psychiatric problems rather than any accompanying PLMS. A multiple sleep latency test (MSLT) may reveal evidence of idiopathic hypersomnia or narcolepsy as a cause of the hypersomnia. Again, in these cases, if PLMS co-occur, the diagnosis of PLMD cannot be made. Although excessive sleepiness and sleep disturbance has been reported in the past, newer data do not find significantly elevated Epworth sleepiness scale scores or multiple sleep latency test (MSLT) values in subjects with PLMS [1].

Periodic limb movements are common in adults but rarely occur in children [38]. PLMs occur most often during sleep, but can occur during wakefulness as an accompaniment of RLS. Movements involve the stereotypic extension of the great toe frequently with simultaneous flexion of the ankle, knee, and hip. Movements last at least 0.5 s but not longer than 10 s. Arousals may precede, coincide with, or follow PLMs [1].

Periodic limb movement disorder requires the presence of periodic limb movements at a frequency of greater than 5 per hour in children and greater than 15 per hour in adults. Periodic limb movements must be associated with sleep disturbance or impairment of mental, physical, social, occupational, educational, behavioral, or other areas of important functioning [1]. The diagnosis of periodic limb movement disorder requires polysomnography or actigraphy. The polysomnogram montage should include surface electrodes on both legs and preferentially recorded on separate channels. The electrodes are placed longitudinally and symmetrically around the middle of the muscle 2–3 cm apart or one-third of the length of the anterior tibialis muscle, whichever is shorter. A periodic limb movement is defined as an 8 uV elevation above baseline in the EMG channel with a duration ≥ 0.5 s and ≤ 10 s. A series of four or more limb movements defined as ≥ 4 limb movements must be recorded. The limb movements must occur between 5 s and not longer than 90 s. The duration of each individual limb movement is anywhere from 0.5 to 10 s. In addition to occurring commonly in RLS, PLMS also occur commonly in obstructive sleep apnea, REM sleep behavior disorder, and narcolepsy and as a side effect to medications [39]. For aforementioned reasons, PLMD cannot be diagnosed in the presence of any of these conditions [1]. The etiology of PLMs is unknown but several hypotheses exist. One hypothesis implicates dopamine. According to Montplaisir et al., "there is a high occurrence of PLMs in RLS/WED, REM behavior disorder (RBD) and narcolepsy. Data suggest that these conditions are associated with impaired central dopaminergic transmission. Neuroleptics and gamma-hydroxybutyrate, medications that decrease dopamine, have been reported to trigger PLMs" [39].

The incidence of PLMs in children increases in the presence of obstructive sleep apnea syndrome. Hartzell et al. [40] quantified the frequency and severity of sleep disorders in a population of hypertensive pediatric patients. The researchers found 64 % of the children had obstructive sleep apnea and or PLMD [40]. Qubly et al. [41] studied 139 infants with obstructive sleep apnea and found 42 % also have periodic limb movements [41].

Asymptomatic periodic limb movements may be helpful in establishing a diagnosis of RLS/WED or narcolepsy in patients who do not clearly meet diagnostic criteria for RLS/WED or narcolepsy.

Treatment of periodic limb movement disorder is similar to the treatment of RLS. Asymptomatic periodic limb movements do not warrant treatment.

See Fig. 11.1 for examples of periodic limb movements in sleep.

→

Fig. 11.1 Periodic limb movements in sleep (PLMS) (three epochs at 30, 60, and 120 s). The burst duration of a single leg movement is ≥ 0.5 s and ≤ 10 s. Four or more limb movements in a row 5–90 s apart are needed for any of the movements to be counted as PLMS. In the first 30 s epoch, the two movements meet the burst duration and movement interval criteria for PLMS but would not be counted as PLMS unless there were at least four such movements 5–90 s apart. One would need to search the pages directly before and directly after to look for at least an additional two movements. PLMS can be discriminated from HFT and ALMA because the burst duration of PLMS is much longer (0.5–10 s), and the interval between PLMS is also much longer (5–90 s apart)

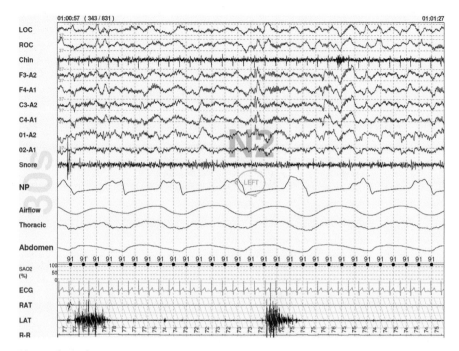

30 seconds epoch

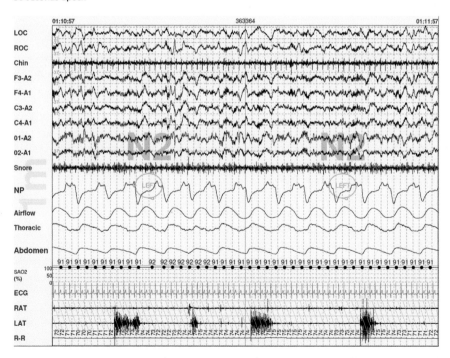

60 seconds epoch

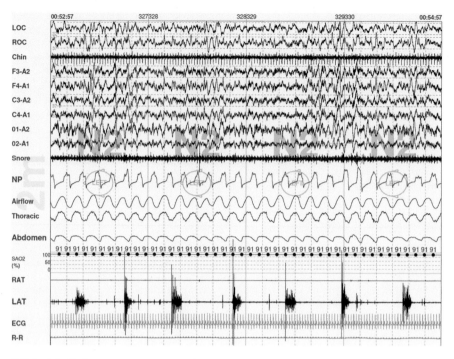

120 seconds epoch

Fig. 11.1 (continued)

Sleep-Related Rhythmic Movement Disorder

These commonly manifest in children as repetitive body rocking or repetitive head banging (jactatio capitis nocturna). Sleep-related rhythmic movements are also referred to as stereotypies [42]. Sleep-related rhythmic movements are only considered a disorder if the movements are associated with clinical symptoms. Sleep-related rhythmic movements involve large muscle groups in any part of the body but most commonly the head, torso, and legs. The movements are nonfunctional, repetitive, stereotyped behaviors that predominantly occur during sleep or at the transition from wakefulness to sleep. Movements may occur during quiet wakefulness [1].

Rhythmic movements are distinguished from tremors and other types of movements by a frequency of 0.5–2 Hz and duration of less than 15 min. Nevertheless, some reports exist of head banging lasting for 30 min to 1.5 h [43]. The movements are fixed in fashion, form, amplitude, and location. Movements stop with distraction [44].

The diagnostic criteria for sleep-related rhythmic movement disorders include all of the following: repetitive, stereotypic, and rhythmic motor behaviors of large muscle groups. Movements occur during times of sleepiness or around naps or bedtime and must interfere with sleep or impair daytime functioning or be associated with or have a high probability of associations with self-inflicted injury [1].

Although sleep-related rhythmic movements are common, sleep-related movement disorder which implies impairment of sleep, daytime function, or bodily injury is rare. Peak age of onset of the benign form of the condition occurs before a child's first birthday and decreases with increasing age. Almost 60 % of infants have sleep-related rhythmic movements, but the disorder occurs in only 5 % of children who have reached 5 years of age. Sleep-related rhythmic movements can persist into adulthood in normal adults, but more commonly persistence occurs in children with neurological or developmental disorders.

Each patient has his/her own pattern of stereotypic behavior. Although body rocking or rolling or head banging is the classic forms of the condition, the behaviors vary widely, and more than one type of movement may occur in the same patient. In younger children, the behaviors may also include sucking the thumb or arm flapping or hand washing movements characteristic of Rett's syndrome. Older children and young adults have behaviors such as nail biting, foot tapping, and hair twirling [45].

Sleep-related rhythmic movement disorders can be classified as primary or secondary. Primary sleep-related rhythmic movements occur in children who are developing normally and do not have behavioral or neurologic disorders. Secondary sleep-related rhythmic movements occur in the presence of signs or symptoms of behavioral or neurological diseases and commonly occur in children with degenerative disorders affecting the brain, pervasive developmental disorders such as autism spectrum disorders and Rett's syndrome. Secondary sleep-related rhythmic movements can be present in children who have Tourette's syndrome. Secondary sleep-related rhythmic movements may be associated with structural defects, autoimmune disorders, or an adverse drug reaction [46].

The etiology of sleep-related rhythmic movements is unknown. There are several theories. One popular hypothesis is that the movements are self-soothing behaviors. Sleep-related rhythmic movements appear to be related to the A phases of the cyclic alternating pattern (CAP cycle) [47].

Kohyama et al. studied the polysomnograms of two children with sleep-related rhythmic movements and retrospectively studied 31 additional children with sleep-related rhythmic movements who had been evaluated by polysomnography. Kohyama et al. found that the movements associated with head banging and head rolling rarely resulted in wakefulness. Both head banging and head rolling occurred in clusters. The frequency was increased during N1 and REM sleep. Kohyama et al. found that head banging was not limited to periods of sleep transitions. Head banging occurred during wakefulness but was not recorded during N3 and REM sleep [48].

In comparison, Mayer et al. found head rolling occurred during the transition to sleep and when transitioning to wakefulness. Mayer et al. also noted sleep-related rhythmic movements occurred during wakefulness, in all stages of sleep and was associated with arousals [42].

Treatment is not necessary unless SRMD is associated with sleep disturbance, bodily harm or could result in injury if not controlled. However, the main preventive measure is to make sure that the parent keeps the child in a safe sleeping environment to prevent injury. For violent forms of SRMD, protective measures such as wearing helmets are indicated. Behavioral therapy has been reported to decrease SRMD. Treatment with benzodiazepines, citalopram, and imipramine may be helpful [49].

See Fig. 11.2 for examples of rhythmic movement disorder.

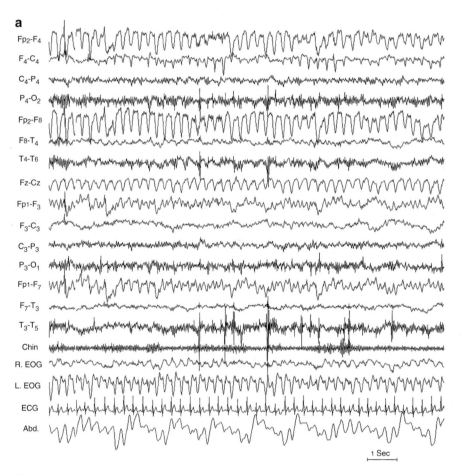

Fig. 11.2 Two examples of rhythmic movement disorder are provided. (**a**) In the first example of head banging in a 10-year-old male, artifact can be seen in the EEG and EOG. Here the patient is in a prone position putting his elbows on the bed. He forces his face on the pillow so the movement is of the entire head on the pillow. Although not in this case but in similar cases, movement can sometimes be seen on the chin EMG. (**b**) In the example of body rolling in an 18-year-old male, the patient is on the left side and there is rolling of the trunk from side to side. The artifact is prominent in the EEG and EOG, and there is some activation of the right tibialis anterior muscle as well

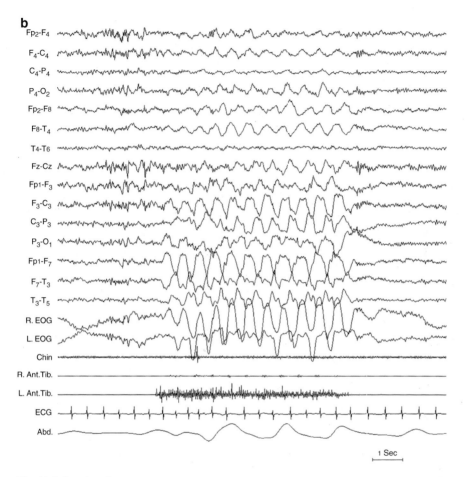

Fig. 11.2 (continued)

Sleep-Related Bruxism

Sleep-related bruxism involves contraction of masticatory muscles characterized by arousal from sleep associated with teeth grinding or clenching of the teeth. Diagnosis requires regular auditory tooth grinding during sleep in association with abnormal wear on the teeth and/or morning jaw muscle pain, jaw locking, or jaw muscle fatigue and/or temporal headache [1].

When sleep-related bruxism involves rhythmic activity of the masseter and temporalis muscles, the condition is called rhythmic masticatory muscle activity (RMMA). RMMA occurs in a cyclic pattern at 1Hz frequency. RMMA is thought to be the intensification of normal orofacial activity and is associated with phase A of the cyclic alternating pattern (CAP). RMMA occurs most often during NREM sleep with increased occurrence during N1 and N2 sleep and is associated with arousals and transitioning to wakefulness. Less common, sleep bruxism (SB) has been reported to occur during REM sleep.

There are three types of sleep-related bruxism. An episode of phasic RMMA is defined as a minimum of three EMG bursts with a duration of ≥ 0.2 s and <2 s. When the EMG burst is continuous for more than 2 s, the bruxism is considered tonic sleep-related bruxism which is characterized as teeth clenching. Mixed sleep-related bruxism is a combination of phasic and tonic activity. Severity of sleep-related bruxism is described by frequency of EMG burst. One event per hour is normal [50]. When a single episode comprised of three or more individual EMG bursts occur and is followed by more than 3 s of EMG silence, one starts counting new EMG bursts as part of a separate episode. There must be at least two episodes of audible grinding on video with audio as part of the overnight sleep study to meet polysomnographic criteria for a diagnosis of sleep-related bruxism [51].

In the general population, the prevalence of bruxism ranges from 6 to 20 % [52]. Sleep-related bruxism can start at any age. But onset of SRB most often occurs during childhood and decreases with increasing age [53]. Between the ages of 18 and 29, the prevalence of bruxism is 13 %. Among patients over 60 years of age, the prevalence of bruxism decreases to 3 %. Although SRB may resolve spontaneously, nearly 66 % of children with bruxism continue to have teeth grinding in adulthood [1].

The etiology of sleep-related bruxism is unknown. It is no longer accepted that bruxism is secondary to misalignment of teeth. Genetic factors may be involved. Among people with SRB, 20–50 % have a biological relative with a history of teeth grinding, and genetics may be a factor. A serotonin gene has been described in patients with bruxism [1]. One hypothesis is that sleep-related bruxism is secondary to an imbalance of neurochemicals and neurotransmitters such as dopamine and serotonin. Other possible explanations for sleep-related bruxism include sleep arousal mechanisms, sympathetic nervous system activation, and psychosocial factors.

Comorbidities associated with sleep-related bruxism include parasomnias, obstructive sleep apnea, periodic limb movements, epilepsy, Tourette's syndrome, allergies, Parkinson's disease, mental health disorders, and stress. Antipsychotics, neuroleptics, and antidepressants can trigger sleep-related bruxism. However, in the case of some of these disorders, the bruxism will be prominent in the day also. Bruxism must be differentiated from nocturnal facio-mandibular myoclonus which is characterized by rapid jerks of the jaw muscles or rapid tooth tapping. Facio-mandibular myoclonus, however, not infrequently accompanies sleep-related bruxism.

Evaluation requires a comprehensive medical history inclusive of symptoms suggestive of comorbid conditions or triggers. A detailed family medical history is necessary because a diagnosis of sleep-related bruxism in biological relatives suggests a genetic component. Twenty to 50 % of children with sleep-related bruxism have a family member with a history of tooth grinding or bruxism. Medications should be reviewed for side effects such as onset of bruxism.

A polysomnogram is not required for the diagnosis of sleep-related bruxism but helps to quantify the frequency. If bruxism occurs at a low frequency, bruxism may not be recorded on the polysomnogram due to night to night variability. The polysomnogram should include at least one channel over the masseter muscle and audio-visual recording.

Medical treatment should be coordinated with a dentist. The dentist is responsible for treatment and prevention of oral health complications. Treatment is divided into non-pharmacologic therapies and pharmacologic therapies.

Dietary change is one form of non-pharmacologic therapy. Lavigne et al. described the following major risk factors thought to exacerbate sleep-related bruxism: smoking, caffeine and heavy alcohol drinking, type A personality, anxiety, and sleep disorders such as snoring, sleep apnea or PLMS [50]. Dietary changes that eliminate caffeine, alcohol, and tobacco may decrease the frequency of bruxism. In the presence of medical conditions such as anxiety and sleep disorders, treating these conditions may decrease sleep-related bruxism.

In addition to dietary changes, other non-pharmacologic treatments include massage and occlusal devices.

Pharmacologic treatment is reserved for severe sleep-related bruxism. There is no FDA-approved medication for treatment of bruxism. In children, clonidine is frequently used off label as a sleep aid and may help reduce the frequency of bruxism. Other medications reported to help with symptoms include gabapentin, tiagabine, buspirone, topiramate, botulinum toxin, and benzodiazepines [54].

See Fig. 11.3 for an example of bruxism.

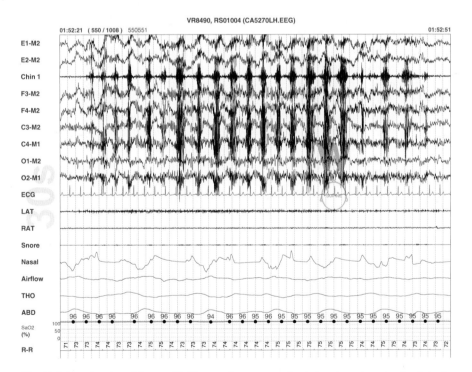

Fig. 11.3 Bruxism (one 30 s epoch). The epoch represents phasic bruxism. An episode of phasic bruxism is defined as a minimum of 3 EMG bursts with a duration of ≥0.2 s and <2 s. Note the bruxism on the chin EMG and note the artifact from the bruxism on the EEG channels. This is commonly seen

Comparison of Polysomnographic Findings in Sleep-Related Rhythmic Movement Disorder and Sleep-Related Bruxism

Compare Figs. 11.2a, b and 11.3. Bruxism and sleep-related rhythmic movement disorder may look very similar on polysomnography. If masseter EMG is added to the montage, bruxism will typically show activation of this muscle. If body rocking is a component of rhythmic movement disorder, then the leg muscles will often be activated. However, in some instances, movement artifact may obscure the origin of the EMG pattern in both disorders, and a recognizable EMG artifact reflected into the EEG of similar burst duration and frequency of 0.5–2 Hz may also occur in both disorders. In these circumstances, the accompanying audio and video may be necessary to discriminate the two conditions from one another.

Sleep-Related Leg Cramps

Sleep-related leg cramps, also known as rest cramps, charley horse, and nocturnal leg cramps, are abrupt spontaneous painful sensations of the legs or feet associated with strong muscle contractions that cause a characteristic hardening of the affected muscle [55]. The associated hardening of the muscle helps differentiate cramps from tetany. Sleep-related leg cramps arise during sleep but can occur during wakefulness. Calf muscles and plantar muscle of the feet are most commonly involved in sleep-related leg cramps. Cramps are most often unilateral but may be bilateral.

While nearly all adults over 50 years of age have experienced sleep-related leg cramps, the incidence of such leg cramps in children is age dependent. Leung et al. evaluated 2,527 children 3–18 years of age for nocturnal leg cramps. The researchers reported the overall incidence of sleep-related leg cramps in children was 7.3 %. When divided by age, the researchers found no reports of nocturnal leg cramps in children less than 8 years of age. By 12 years of age, the incidence of sleep-related leg cramps was nearly 25 %. The incidence of sleep-related leg cramps peaked at 16–18 years of age. The frequency of nocturnal leg cramps was one to four times per year [56].

In both pediatric and adult populations, sleep-related leg cramps can be a side effect of medications or occur in conditions such as McArdle's disease, endocrine disorders, electrolyte imbalances, and lead toxicity [55]. Chronic myelopathy, multiple sclerosis, peripheral neuropathy, akathisia, muscular pain-fasciculation syndrome, and disorders of calcium metabolism must also be considered [1]. Sleep-related leg cramps may occur in association with other sleep disorders, for example, Willis-Ekbom disease and periodic limb movement disorder. Pregnancy and strenuous exercise are normal conditions associated with increased occurrence of sleep-related leg cramps.

The pathophysiology of sleep-related leg cramps is unknown. Likewise, the site of origin of sleep-related leg cramps is not known. The origin may be multifactorial or dependent upon associated comorbidities [57]. There are several hypotheses. One hypothesis places origin at the motor unit. "During muscle cramps, the electromyogram records repetitive firing of motor unit action potentials. The number of motor units involved increases gradually then subsides when cramps cease" [57]. This hypothesis is bolstered by the absence of cramps in diseases of the muscle and an association of cramps in disease resulting in pathology of peripheral nerves, as well as diseases associated with loss of lower motor neurons. Another hypothesis suggests cramps are due to irritation of myofascial trigger points in calf and foot muscles.

Another hypothesis involves magnesium. Hypomagnesemia is associated with leg cramps [58]. Magnesium inhibits the release of acetylcholine and low levels of magnesium lead to muscle contraction [59]. But clinical documentation of hypomagnesemia is challenging. Magnesium is largely intracellular, and serum magnesium levels may not accurately reflect the body stores. In addition absorption of magnesium is complex requiring adequate amounts of selenium, parathyroid hormone, pyridoxine (B6), and vitamin D [59]. Deficiency in any of these decreases magnesium absorption. In addition, magnesium bioavailability decreases with increasing age. Issues of absorption were addressed by Garrison et al. To address concerns about absorption, researchers studied the effects of intravenous magnesium upon sleep-related leg cramps and did not find magnesium helpful [60].

The history and physical examination helps to differentiate cramps from tetany and dystonia. Routine testing of sodium, potassium, calcium, and magnesium levels is not indicated [61]. However, if the patient has conditions that could lead to electrolyte deficiencies, the deficit should be corrected. Spinal imaging to evaluate for nerve root entrapment and nerve conduction studies and EMG to identify motor neuron disease may be helpful. A review of medications and laboratory testing for associated endocrine and metabolic disorders may be indicated. On a polysomnogram, sleep-related cramps appear as nonrhythmic burst of EMG activity with no preceding evidence of physiologic changes [1].

Non-pharmacologic therapy is recommended as initial treatment and includes massage, application of heat, and stretching the muscle.

In the United States, there are no Food and Drug Administration (FDA)-approved pharmacologic treatments for sleep-related leg cramps. The off-label use of gabapentin and verapamil has been used with some measure of success.

Although quinine is commonly used by adults for treatment of sleep-related leg cramps, the FDA withdrew approval of quinine for treatment of sleep-related leg cramps due to severe adverse side effects including thrombocytopenia, hemolytic-uremic syndrome, and hepatitis [62–64].

Few authors have documented efficacy of magnesium in the treatment of nocturnal leg cramps. Sebo et al. completed a systematic review with meta-analysis using simulations and did not find objective evidence of usefulness of magnesium [65]. Adult patients with nocturnal leg cramps were administered 900 mg magnesium citrate twice a day for 1 month with no evidence of a decrease in leg cramps [66]. There is also debate as to which forms of magnesium should be administered with some authors favoring magnesium citrate and others favoring magnesium oxide. Nevertheless, because magnesium is inexpensive and relatively safe in patients with normal renal function, an empirical trial of magnesium can be given [67]. Magnesium is used as over-the-counter therapy but research demonstrates variable efficacy. The type of magnesium affects absorption. Saris et al. reported that only 4 % of a dose of magnesium oxide is absorbed [68]. Some researchers have observed some measure of success using magnesium citrate 300 mg per day. Patients should avoid caffeine, alcohol, high-fat diets, and dehydration, all dietary factors that increase elimination of magnesium [59].

There are no features on polysomnography that are specific for leg cramps, and a polysomnographic example of leg cramps is not provided.

Benign Sleep Myoclonus of Infancy

Benign sleep myoclonus of infancy (BSMI) is also termed benign neonatal sleep myoclonus. This non-epileptic condition occurs in neurologically normal children. Benign sleep myoclonus of infancy manifests as repetitive myoclonic jerks of the extremities, upper more so than lower, in a unilateral or symmetrical pattern. Myoclonic jerks may also involve the trunk or the entire body. The movements only occur during sleep. The incidence has been estimated at 3.7 per 10,000 live births, and more than 200 cases have been reported in the literature. Peak age of onset is birth to 1 month of age. In almost all children, BSMI resolves by 12 months of age with no sequelae [1].

Although an EEG may be ordered because of concerns about possible epilepsy, the EEG is normal but may show muscle artifact. Movements usually occur in clusters of four to five jerks per second, with a duration lasting 40–300 ms. Jerks are most often observed during quiet sleep but can occur during all stages of sleep. Jerks do not occur during wakefulness [69]. Wakefulness causes abrupt termination of movements. Rocking of the infant can precipitate myoclonus [1]. The etiology of BSMI is unknown.

BSMI must be differentiated from epilepsy, pyridoxine-dependency seizures, infantile spasms, PLMs, phasic REM muscle activity, and symptoms of neonatal drug withdrawal. BSMI must also be distinguished from benign myoclonus of early infancy. Symptoms of benign myoclonus of early infancy typically begin after 3 months of age and include myoclonic jerks, spasms, brief tonic contractions, and shuddering, all of which occur only during wakefulness [70].

In the absence of severe sleep disturbance, treatment of BSMI is not warranted. When treatment is indicated, clonazepam may be useful.

Benign sleep myoclonus of infancy does not have specific polysomnographic features, and a figure is not provided.

Hypnagogic Foot Tremor

Hypnagogic foot tremor is a common finding on polysomnography performed for other purposes. It manifests as oscillating movements of the whole foot or of the toes while falling asleep [71]. Tremors last between 10 and 15 s and have a frequency of 0.3–4 Hz with a burst duration of 250–1,000 ms [51]. It usually occurs repetitively in a single leg.

HFT affects both genders equally and has been reported in patients from 14 to 72 years of age. HFT is most commonly diagnosed in patients 40–65 years. Prevalence in children is unknown [52].

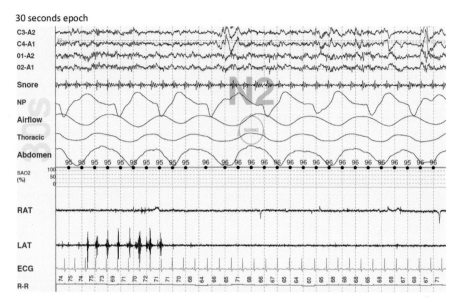

Fig. 11.4 Hypnagogic foot tremor (HFT) (one 30 s epoch). Tremors last between 10 and 15 s and have a frequency of 0.3–4 Hz with a burst duration of 250–1,000 ms. HFT is a commonly occurring benign condition. PLMS can be discriminated from HFT because the burst duration of PLMS is much longer (0.5–10 s), and the interval between PLMS is also much longer (5–90 s apart)

Since there is no known sequelae of this condition, treatment is unnecessary. It may cause minor disruption in the sleep of the bed partner.

See Fig. 11.4, for an example of hypnagogic foot tremor.

Alternating Leg Muscle Activation (ALMA)

"Alternating leg muscle activation (ALMA) describes brief activations of the anterior tibialis muscle in one leg followed by similar activation in the other leg during sleep or in association with an arousal" [72]. This may simply be a variant of hypnagogic foot tremor since it has a similar burst duration and frequency as HFT with the only exception being that the movements alternate from 1 ft to the other on a one-to-one basis. Again, it is found not uncommonly on polysomnography as an incidental finding. Similar to HFT it is to our current knowledge a benign disorder and may not require treatment. As with HFT, there may be some minor disruption of the bed partner's sleep.

The etiology of ALMA is unknown. Chervin et al. postulate ALMA is due to a spinal cord generator related to serotonin or dopamine because the researchers observed ALMA occurring in patients exposed to antidepressant medications [73]. Chervin's hypothesis is supported by the research of Cosentino et al. who documented by polysomnogram a reduction in wake after sleep onset (WASO) in patients with ALMA treated with dopaminergic agents [74].

Alternating leg muscle activation is thought to affect 1.1 % of the general population presenting to sleep disorders centers for polysomnography. It affects both genders but occurs more often in males. ALMA has been reported in patients ranging in age from 12 to 70 years of age. The peak age range of onset occurs between the ages of 35–55 years with a mean age of onset of 41 years. There is at least one reported case of ALMA responding to treatment with a dopamine agonist [1].

A polysomnogram is required to document ALMA. The polysomnogram recording of ALMA requires a minimum of four discrete and alternating EMG bursts of leg muscle activity between the frequency of 0.5–3 Hz. The usual duration of ALMA is 100–500 s [75].

Although HFT and ALMA are repetitive leg movements in sleep, they can be discriminated from periodic limb movements in sleep (PLMS) because the burst duration of PLMS is much longer (0.5–10 s) and the interval between PLMS is also much longer (5–90 s apart).

See Fig. 11.5 for an example of ALMA.

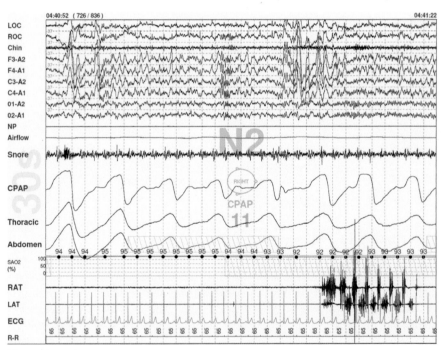

Fig. 11.5 Alternating leg muscle activation (ALMA) (one 30 s epoch). ALMA is similar to HFT except movements alternate from one foot to the other on a one-to-one basis. ALMA requires a minimum of four discrete and alternating EMG bursts of leg muscle activity between the frequency of 0.5 and 3 Hz. The usual duration of ALMA is 100–500 s. HFT and ALMA may represent benign variants of the same disorder. PLMS can be discriminated from ALMA because the burst duration of PLMS is much longer (0.5–10 s) and the interval between PLMS is also much longer (5–90 s apart)

Excessive Fragmentary Myoclonus (EFM)

EFM, also referred to as physiologic hypnic fragmentary myoclonus (PHM), is an NREM phenomenon characterized by small asynchronous, asymmetrical movements of the fingers, toes, or corners of the mouth. However, visible movements may be absent. EFM is often an incidental polysomnographic finding commonly occurring in the presence of other sleep disorders.

EFM is prominent in babies and infants [76]. EFM has been reported in children diagnosed with Niemann-Pick type C [1].

Polysomnographic criteria for scoring EFM includes a recording of at least 20 min of NREM with EMG burst usually of 150 msec duration and a minimum of 5 EMG potentials per minute of recording [51].

In adults, EFM has been associated with excessive daytime sleepiness. The condition is thought to be benign in children.

See Fig. 11.6 for a polysomnographic example of excessive fragmentary myoclonus.

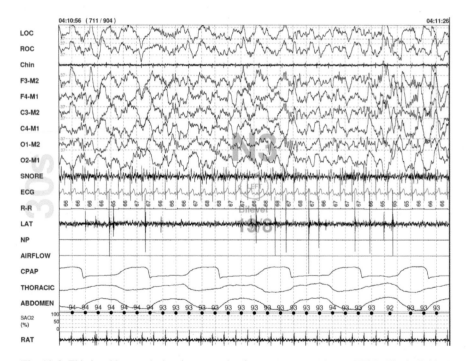

Fig. 11.6 This is a 30 s epoch showing excessive fragmentary myoclonus (EFM). The individual EMG muscle bursts are usually 150 ms in duration on average. EFM must be present for at least 20 min in NREM sleep with at least 5 EMG bursts/min. These tiny discharges are usually accompanied by small or no visible movement

Propriospinal Myoclonus at Sleep Onset

Propriospinal myoclonus at sleep onset involves sudden muscle jerks initially occurring in muscles of the abdomen and trunk followed by spreading to the proximal muscles of the limbs and neck. Symptoms usually occur during the transition from wakefulness to sleep and rarely during other phases of sleep [1].

Polysomnography documents brief EMG burst originating from spinal muscles and spreading caudally and rostrally. Jerks terminate during wakefulness and with the progression of sleep beyond N1.

Propriospinal myoclonus at sleep onset presents most often in adults and more frequently in men. We found one report of propriospinal myoclonus diagnosed in a 6-year-old girl who had sustained a back injury during the first year of life. Jerks were not limited to sleep onset [77].

Propriospinal myoclonus at sleep onset must be differentiated from PLMs, sleep starts, phasic REM twitches, EFM, and epileptic myoclonus [1].

There is no specific polysomnographic pattern for propriospinal myoclonus at sleep onset, and a figure is not provided.

Acknowledgments I thank God and my patients for the opportunity to practice Sleep Disorders Medicine, Dr. Walters for his mentorship, friendship and expertise, my husband Professor Jonathan Stubbs for his love and support in reviewing this manuscript and our daughter Amanda for her love and never ending encouragement .

Pamela Hamilton-Stubbs, BSN, M.D.

I would like to thank our two sleep fellows at Vanderbilt Dr. Huong Pham and Dr. Noel Vargas-Perez for locating the polysomnographic examples utilized in this manuscript. I would also like to thank Dr. Kanika Bagai of Vanderbilt and Dr. Federica Provini of the University of Bologna, Italy for providing polysomnographic examples.

Arthur S. Walters, M.D.

References

1. Sateia M, ed. Sleep related movement disorders. In: International classification of sleep disorders, 3rd ed. Darien: American Academy of Sleep Medicine; 2014. p. 282–320.
2. Teive H. Professor Karl-Axel Ekbom and restless legs syndrome. Parkinsonism Relat Disord. 2008;15(4):254–7.
3. Hamilton-Stubbs P, Walters A. Restless legs syndrome. In: Kompoliti K, Metman LV, editors. Encyclopedia of movement disorders, vol. 3. Oxford: Academic Press; 2010. p. 32–7.
4. Winkelmann J, Schormairb B, Lichtner P, Ripke S, Xiong L, Jalilzadeh S, et al. Genome-wide association study of restless legs syndrome identifies common variants in three genomic regions. Nat Genet. 2007;8:1000–6.
5. Rye D. The molecular genetics of restless. Sleep Med Clin. 2015;10:227–33.
6. Salmine A, Rimpilä V, Polo O. Peripheral hypoxia in restless legs syndrome (Willis-Ekbom disease). Neurology. 2014;82(21):1856–61.
7. Montplaisir J, Boucher S, Poirier G, Lavigne G, Lapierre O, Lesperance P. Clinical, polysomnographic, and genetic characteristics of restless legs syndrome: a study of 133 patients diagnosed with new standard criteria. Mov Disord. 1997;1:61–5.
8. Walters A, Picchietti DL, Ehrenberg BI, Wagner MI. Restless legs syndrome in childhood and adolescence. Pediatr Neurol. 1994;11:241–5.

9. Picchietti D, Bruni O, de Weerd A, Durmer J, Kotagal S, Owens J, Simakajornboon N. Pediatric restless legs syndrome diagnostic criteria: an update by the International Restless Legs Syndrome Study Group. Sleep Med. 2013;14:1253–9.

10. Picchietti D, Allen RP, Walters AS, Davidson JE, Myers A, Ferini-Strambi L. Restless legs syndrome: prevalence and impact in children and adolescents—the Peds REST study. Pediatrics. 2007;120:253–66.

11. Walters A, Hickey K, Maltzman J, Verrico T, Joseph D, Hening W, Wilson V, Chokroverty S. A questionnaire study of 138 patients with restless legs syndrome: the 'Night-Walkers' survey. Neurology. 1996;46:1,92–95.

12. Ohayon M, O'Hara R, Vitiello M. Epidemiology of restless legs syndrome: a synthesis of the literature. Sleep Med Rev. 2012;16(4):283–95.

13. Galbiati A, Marelli S, Giora D, Zucconi M, Oldani A, Ferini-Strambi L. Neurocognitive function in patients with idiopathic restless legs syndrome before and after treatment with dopamine-agonist. Int J Psychophysiol. 2015;95:304.

14. Pullen S, Wall C, Angstman E, Munitz G, Kotagal S. Psychiatric comorbidity in children and adolescents with restless legs syndrome: a retrospective study. J Clin Sleep Med. 2011;7(6):587–96.

15. Wagner M, Walters A, Fisher B. Symptoms of attention-deficit/hyperactivity disorder in adults with restless legs syndrome. Sleep. 2004;27:1499–504.

16. Trotti L, Bhadriraju S, Rye D. An update on the pathophysiology and genetics of restless legs syndrome. Curr Neurol Neurosci Rep. 2008;8:281–7.

17. Golmirzaei J, Mohboobi H, Yazdanparast M, Mushtag G, Kamal MA, Hamzeyi E. Psychopharmacology of attention-deficit hyperactivity disorder: effects and side effects. Curr Pharm Des. 2016;22(5):590–4.

18. Ernst M, Zametkin A, Matochik J, Pascualvaca D, Jons P, Cohen R. High midbrain [18F] DOPA accumulation in children with attention deficit hyperactivity disorder. Am J Psychiatry. 1999;156:1209–15.

19. Becker P, Sharon D. Mood disorders in restless legs syndrome (Willis-Ekbom disease). J Clin Psychiatr. 2014;75(7):e679–94.

20. Walters A, Gabelia D, Frauscher B. Restless legs syndrome (Willis-Ekbom disease) and growing pains: are they the same thing? A side-by-side comparison of the diagnostic criteria for both and recommendations for future research. Sleep Med. 2013;14:1247–52.

21. Halliwell P, Monsell F. Growing pains: a diagnosis of exclusion. Practitioner. 2001; 245(1625):620–3.

22. Rajaram S, Walters A, England S, Mehta D, Nizam F. Some children with growing pains may actually have restless legs syndrome. Sleep. 2004;27(4):767–73.

23. Evans A, Scutter S. Prevalence of "growing pains" in young children. J Pediatr. 2004;145:255–8.

24. Peterson HA. Leg aches. Pediatr Clin N Am. 1977;24:731–6.

25. Peterson HA. Growing pains. Pediatr Clin North Am. 1986;33:1365–72.

26. Sharon D. Nonpharmacologic management of restless legs syndrome (Willis-Ekbom Disease): myths or science. Sleep Med Clin. 2015;10:263–78.

27. Simakajornboon N, Kheirandish-Gozal L, Gozal D. Diagnosis and management of restless legs syndrome in children. Sleep Med Rev. 2009;13:149–56.

28. Hamilton-Stubbs, P, Walters A. Restless legs syndrome. In: Albanese A, Jankovic J, editors, Hyperkinetic movement disorders: differential diagnosis and treatment, 1st ed. Chichester: Wiley; 2012; p. 311–30.

29. Pelayo R, Yuen K. Pediatric sleep pharmacology. Child Adolesc Psychiatr Clin N Am. 2012;21:861–83.

30. Lee K, Zaffke M, Baratte-Beebe K. Restless legs syndrome and sleep disturbance during pregnancy: the role of folate and iron. J Womens Health Gend Based Med. 2001;10(4):335–41.

31. Sagheb M, Dormanesh B, Fallahzadeh M, et al. Efficacy of vitamins C, E, and their combination for treatment of restless legs syndrome in hemodialysis patients: a randomized, double-blind, placebo-controlled trial. Sleep Med. 2012;13:542–5.

32. Tribl G, Waldhauser F, Sycha T, Auff E, Zeitlhofer J. Unrinary 6-hydroxy-melatonin-sulfate excretion and circadian rhythm in patients with restless legs syndrome. J Pineal Res. 2003;35(4):295–6.

33. Hornyak M, Voderholze U, Hohagen E, et al. Magnesium therapy for periodic leg movements related insomnia and restless legs syndrome: an open pilot study. Sleep. 1998;2:502–5.
34. Walters A, Elin R, Cohen B, et al. Magnesium not likely to play a major role in the pathogenesis of restless legs syndrome: serum and cerebrospinal fluid studies. Sleep Med. 2007;8:186–7.
35. Fawcett W, Haxy E, Male D. Magnesium: physiology and pharmacology. Br J Anesth. 1999;83:302–20.
36. England S, Picchiett D, Couvadelli B, Fisher B, Siddiqui F, et al. L-Dopa improves restless legs syndrome and periodic limb movements in sleep but not attention-deficit-hyperactivity disorder in a double-blind trial in children. Sleep Med. 2011;12:471–7.
37. Arbuckle R, Abetz L, Durmer JS, Ivanenko A, Owens JA, Croenlein J, Bolton K, Moore A, Allen RP, Walters AS, Picchietti DL. Development of the pediatric restless legs syndrome severity scale (P-RLS-SS): a patient-reported outcome measure of pediatric RLS symptoms and impact. Sleep Med. 2010;11(9):897–906.
38. Hornyak M, Feige B, Riemann D, Voderholzer U. Periodic leg movements in sleep and period limb movement disorder: prevalence, clinical significance and treatment. Sleep Med Rev. 2009;10:169–77.
39. Montplaisir J, Michaud M, Denesle R, Gosselin A. Periodic leg movements are not more prevalent in insomnia or hypersomnia but are specifically associated with sleep disorders involving a dopaminergic impairment. Sleep Med. 2000;1:163–7.
40. Hartzell E, Avis K, Lozano d, Feig D. Obstructive sleep apnea and periodic limb movement disorder in a population of children with hypertension and/or nocturnal nondipping blood pressures. J Am Soc Hypertens. 2016;10(2):101–7.
41. Qubty F, Mrelashvili A, Kotagal S, Lloyg M. Comorbidities in infants with obstructive sleep apnea. J Clin Sleep Med. 2014;10(11):1213–6.
42. Mayer G, Wilde-Frenz J, Kurella B. Sleep related rhythmic movement disorder revisited. J Sleep Res. 2007;16:110–6.
43. Silber M. Sleep-related movement disorders. Continuum (Minneapolis, Minn). 2013;19(1):170.
44. Singer H. Motor control, habits, complex motor stereotypies, and Tourette syndrome. Ann N Y Acad Sci. 2013;1304(2013):22–31.
45. Singer H. Stereotypic movement disorders. In: Weiner W, Tolosa E, editors. Hyperkinetic Movement Disorders. Handbook of clinical neurology. Vol 100 Chapter 45 3rd series; 2011. Elsevier, Amsterdam. p. 632–8.
46. Edwards M. Stereotypies: a critical appraisal and suggestion of a clinically useful definition. Mov Disord. 2012;27(2):179–85.
47. Manni R, Terzaghi M, Sartori I, Veggiotti P, Parrino L. Rhythmic movement disorder and cyclic alternating pattern during sleep: a video-polysomnographic study in a 9 year old boy. Mov Disord. 2004;19(10):1186–90.
48. Kohyama J, Matsukura F, Kimura K, Tachibana N. Rhythmic movement disorder: polysomnographic study and summary of reported cases. Brain Dev. 2002;24:33–8.
49. Vetrugno R, Montagna P. Sleep-to-wake transition movement disorders. Sleep Med. 2011;12:S11–6.
50. Lavigne G, Khoury S, Abe S, Yamaguchi T, Raphael K. Bruxism physiology and pathology: an overview for clinicians. J Oral Rehabil. 2008;35:476–94.
51. Berry R, editor. The AASM manual for the scoring of sleep and associated events. VII movement rules hypnagogic foot tremor, alternating leg muscle activity, periodic limb movements. Darien: American Academy of Sleep Medicine; 2015.
52. Lavigne G, Montplaisir J. Restless legs syndrome and sleep bruxism: prevalence and association among Canadians. Sleep. 1994;17(8):739–43.
53. Insana S, Gozal D, McNeil D, Montgomery H. Community based study of sleep bruxism during early childhood. Sleep Med. 2013;14(2):183–8.
54. Meltzer L, Johnson C, Crosette J, Ramos M, Mindell J. Prevalence of diagnosed sleep disorders in pediatric primary care practices. Pediatrics. 2010;125(6):e1410–8.
55. Kanann N, Sawaya R. Clinically mysterious and painful-but manageable. Geriatrics. 2001;56(June):34–42.

56. Leung A, Wong B, Chan P, Cho H. Nocturnal leg cramps in children: incidence and clinical characteristics. J Natl Med Assoc. 1999;91:329–32.
57. Miller T, Layzer R. Muscle cramps. Muscle Nerve. 2005;32:431–42.
58. Sills S, Roffe C, Crome P, Jones P. Randomised, cross-over, placebo controlled trial of magnesium citrate in the treatment of persistent leg cramps. Med Sci Monit. 2002;8(5):CR326–30.
59. Johnson S. The multifaceted and widespread pathology of magnesium deficiency. Med Hypotheses. 2001;56(2):163–70.
60. Garrison S, Birmingham C, Koehler B, McCollom R, Khan K. The effect of magnesium infusion on rest cramps: randomized controlled trial. J Gerontol A Biol Sci Med Sci. 2011;66A(6):661–6.
61. Corliss J, Elbaum D, Long G, Villalba C. Patient information: nocturnal leg cramps. Uptodate; 2016.
62. Mohamed M, Hayes R. Quinine-induced severe thrombocytopenia: the importance of taking a detailed Drug history. BMJ Case Rep. 2013. pii: bcr2013200631. doi:10.1136/bcr-2013-200631.
63. Crum N, Gable P. Quinine-induced hemolytic-uremic syndrome. South Med J. 2000;93(7):726–8.
64. Katz B, Weetch M, Chopra S. Quinine-induced granulomatous hepatitis. Br Med J (Clin Res Ed). 1983;286(6361):264–5.
65. Sebo P, Cerutti B, Haller D. Effect of magnesium therapy on nocturnal leg cramps: a systematic review of randomized controlled trials with meta-analysis using simulations. Fam Pract. 2013;31(1):7–19.
66. Frusso R, Zárate M, Augustovski F, Rubinstein A. Magnesium for the treatment of nocturnal leg cramps a crossover randomized trial. J Fam Pract. 1999;48(11):868–71.
67. Allen R, Kirby K. Nocturnal leg cramps. Am Fam Physician. 2012;86(4):350–5.
68. Nils-Erik S, Mervaala E, Karppanen H, Khawaja J, Lewenstam A. Magnesium an update on physiological, clinical and analytical aspects. Clin Chim Acta. 2000;294:1–26.
69. Resnick R, Solomn M, Perotta L, Chambers H. Benign neonatal sleep myoclonus. Arch Neurol. 1986;43(3):266–8.
70. Bernardina B. Benign myoclonus of early infancy or Fejerman syndrome. Epilepsia. 2009;50:1289–300.
71. Wichniak A, Tracik F, Geisler P, Ebersbach G, Morrissey S, Zulley J. Rhythmic feet movements while asleep. Mov Disord. 2001;16(6):1164–70.
72. Merlino G, Gigli LG. Sleep-related movement disorders. Neurol Sci. 2012;33(3):491–513.
73. Chervin R, Consens F, Kutluay E. Alternating leg muscle activation during sleep and arousals: a new sleep related motor phenomenon? Mov Disord. 2003;18:551–9.
74. Cosentino FI, Iero I, Lanuzza B, Tripodi M, Ferri R. The neurophysiology of the alternating leg muscle activation (ALMA) during sleep: study of one patient before and after treatment with pramipexole. Sleep Med. 2006;7:63–71.
75. Berry RB, Brooks R, Gamaldo CE, Harding SM, Lloyd RM, Marcus CL, Vaughn BV for the American Academy of Sleep Medicine. Periodic limb movement disorder the AASM manual for the scoring of sleep and associated events: rules, terminology and technical specifications, version 2.2. 2015.
76. Barkoukis T, Matheson J, Ferber R, Doghramji. Movement disorders affecting sleep. In: Therapy in sleep medicine. Philadelphia: Elsevier Health Sciences; 2011.
77. Aydin Ö, Temucin C, Kayacik Ö, Türker H, Özyürek H. Propriospinal myoclonus in a child. J Child Neurol. 2009;25(7):912–5.

Chapter 12
Circadian Rhythm Disorders in Childhood

Silvia Miano

Abstract Chronobiology is a science that studies the physiology and pathology of circadian phenomena. In the last 50 years, numerous studies have been published on sleep changes during puberty and adolescence, which largely consist of delays in the timing of sleep. The most notable consequence of these shifts is a sleep debt due to a forced early wake-up during school days, despite no change in sleep requirements (around 9 h), and diurnal hypersomnolence. All these changes explain why teenagers are particularly vulnerable to delayed sleep phase syndrome, which is known to peak during adolescence (prevalence ranging from 7 % to 16 % compared with 0.15 % during adulthood). Advanced sleep phase disorder (ASPD), delayed sleep-wake phase disorder (DSWPD), irregular sleep-wake rhythm (ISWR), and the non-24-h sleep-wake syndrome or free-running disorder (non-entrained type) are referred to as "endogenous" circadian rhythm sleep disorders. The clinical features of each sleep circadian disorder are discussed together with the recommended treatment. Pediatric categories of subjects that are at risk of developing circadian disorders, such as those with a developmental disability, autism, attention-deficit hyperactivity disorders, and mood disorders, are investigated. Lastly, two case reports that provide examples of clinical practice are also presented.

Keywords Circadian sleep disorders • Sleep • Delayed sleep-wake phase disorder • Children • Adolescents • Melatonin • Light

S. Miano
Civic Hospital of Lugano, Neurocenter of Italian Switzerland, Sleep and Epilepsy Center, Lugano, Switzerland
e-mail: silvia.miano@eoc.ch; silvia.miano@gmail.com

© Springer International Publishing Switzerland 2017   253
S. Nevšímalová, O. Bruni (eds.), *Sleep Disorders in Children*,
DOI 10.1007/978-3-319-28640-2_12

Introduction

The Circadian Biology and Physiology

Chronobiology is a science that studies the physiology and pathology of circadian phenomena. The circadian system provides temporal organization of sleep-wake cycles, feeding, and reproduction. Many fundamental biological events are characterized by a regular interval and duration, with the cycle being referred to as circadian if they occur periodically 24 h, ultradian if the periods are shorter than 24 h, and infradian if longer. Evolution has selected species whose physiological rhythm corresponds approximately to the time it takes the Earth to rotate once. Circadian oscillations are genetically determined, their occurrence being controlled by endogenous and exogenous stimuli that act as an orchestra. The suprachiasmatic nucleus (SCN) is considered the endogenous master circadian pacemaker brain clock, which comprises a feed-forward circuit of similar cells that can auto-depolarize and that produce a coherent circadian rhythm output for the rest of the body, whereas the light-dark (LD) alternation is considered the most significant endogenous factor that influences circadian biological rhythms [1]. The majority of human cells display the same molecular clockwork and are synchronized to one another via redundant systemic signals that create an accurate correspondence with the environment. These cues originate mostly from the SCN either through autonomous nervous control of hormones, such as glucocorticoids, or through direct innervation of other brain regions. The SCN is synchronized with light via the retino-hypothalamic tract, the result being a flexible system of clocks, each of which has an intrinsic duration of about 1 day that is constantly readjusted to the timing of environmental light [2]. This synchronization is largely due to the light activation of retina photoreceptors, which are not linked to visual function. Light activation stimulates the retino-hypothalamic tract, which terminates in the SCN, as well as the genicolohypothalamic tract, which terminates in the thalamus. Retinal rod and cone cells are not required for photo-entrainment, but a subset of retinal cells containing a light-sensing pigment, melanopsin, which is involved in circadian photo-entrainment does exist [3].

Light is not the only exogenous entrainment of the circadian rhythm, though it is the strongest. Many social cues, and other biological factors such as food intake and locomotor activity, may influence and reset circadian physiological phenomena, especially in humans: the rhythmic control of the digestive function and detoxication can be synchronized with rhythmic food intake by sleep-wakefulness alternation and diurnal cardiac function control changes in energy needs on a systemic level, while mitochondrial cells optimize the regulation of circadian energy production on a cellular level [2]. The oscillatory property of SCN cells persists even when they are isolated from all exogenous factors, in both in vivo and in vitro experiments, maintaining their oscillatory capacity for approximately 24 h (free-running rhythm), which may be prolonged up to 25.5 h [4, 5]. The free-running period (τ) differs according to race, with African Americans displaying a shorter τ than

Caucasians [6]. When the free-running period is forced for an extended period of time, some circadian functions, such as body temperature, cortisol secretion, and REM sleep, become desynchronized, whereas others, such as food intake and loco-motor activity, do not, thereby suggesting that other endogenous pacemakers exist [1]. It should be borne in mind that the SNC is a very small hypothalamic nucleus that executes a single function, and if damaged, its function cannot be executed by any other tissue [7]. An orderly and reproducible spatiotemporal pattern of oscilla-tory gene expression that requires the integrity of the ventrolateral core region has been demonstrated in the SCN. When this core region is absent, the behavioral rhythm is abolished in vivo, although a low-amplitude rhythm can be detected in SCN slices in vitro [7]. These oscillatory genes are called "clock" genes and are a family of loci involved in circadian physiology and pathology, with a clear circadian rhythm of transcription [8]. Some cells within the SCN rhythmically express "clock" genes, whereas others express these genes upon exposure to light [8]. The clock genes are also considered tumor suppressor genes because they regulate cell divi-sion and cell differentiation by segregating DNA replication from periods of maxi-mum respiration and by optimizing the time available for the DNA repair process. The direct consequences of in vitro abolition of SCN is tumor growth that is two to three times faster, while mice without the circadian clock genes develop a range of pathologies, including diabetes, arthritis, and cancer [2]. Most of these circadian clock gene functions are unexpressed during embryogenetic life, possibly owing to the rapid rate of cell division, which disrupts the circadian regulation [2].

In humans sleep occurs during darkness, usually 2 h before the melatonin (MLT) peak and 4 h before the temperature nadir. The MLT and body temperature are com-monly used as markers of the master pacemaker, since it is impossible to measure SCN activity in vivo [1]. The MLT, which is produced by the pineal gland, controls circadian physiology, seasonal reproductive function, and stimulation of amphibian skin melanophores. Its role in regulating the immune system, gastrointestinal, ret-ina, antioxidant, and antiaging functions is still debated [1]. It is also involved in the early development of neurons and glia and in the ontogenetic establishment of diur-nal rhythms [9]. It regulates sleep states through the activation of two receptors: MT2 during NREM sleep and MT1 receptors during REM sleep [10]. The secretion of serum MLT concentrations starts at 3 months of age, reaches its highest nocturnal levels at 1–3 years of age, and steadily declines thereafter by 80 % to attain adult levels at puberty; levels remain stable during adulthood before decreasing in elderly age depending on a general increase in body size as opposed to decreasing pineal secretion (decreasing from 210 pg/ml in preschoolers to 130 pg/ml in school-aged children and to 50 pg/ml in young adults) [11, 12]. One study identified two patterns of early secretion in infants: one mature, with dim light melatonin onset (DLMO) in the evening, and one immature, with a flat distribution or rise in the morning, associ-ated with early sleep problems [13]. Another study demonstrated that MLT levels at 16 weeks of age are significantly lower in infants with abnormal development than in those with normal development at 3 and 6 months of age [14]. The synthesis of MLT involves the pathway of serotonin anabolism, which is acetylated by arylalkyl-amine (AANAT), and methylated to MLT by the acetylserotonin O-methyltransferase

(ASMT) enzyme. MLT has a short half-life, lasting approximately 30 min, and is first metabolized in the liver by cytochrome P450 1A2 (CYP1A2) and then degraded by cytochrome 450 in the liver, sulfonated, and secreted by the kidney in the urine [15]. Secretion of MLT, which occurs prevalently during the night, is controlled by the SCN and in particular by the retino-hypothalamic-pineal tracts. Output from the pineal gland includes MLT receptors in non-neuronal tissues (gut, ovaries and vessels, among others) and neuronal tissue, where their concentration is highest, with MLT2 in particular having been implicated in phase shift mechanisms and being widespread throughout retina and brain cells. MLT synthesis is strongly inhibited by light and dopamine, whereas MLT inhibits dopamine secretion [1]. A widely used technique to determine the circadian phase is the assessment of the secretory pattern of MLT, according to which circulating MLT is normally low during the daytime, increases abruptly close to bedtime, and once again drops to daytime levels close to wake-up time. Since light suppresses MLT secretion, it is measured in dim light conditions, when the dim light onset of MLT is usually identified (DLMO) [16]. Simultaneous salivary and plasma MLT concentrations have shown that the saliva concentration of MLT corresponds to 40 % of that in the plasma. Thus, if the plasma level threshold for MLT is 10 pg mL^{-1}, the saliva level threshold is considered to be 4 pg mL^{-1} [16].

Desynchronized and disorganized mammalian sleep persists after SCN ablation because another mechanism controls sleep: the homeostatic process S, which reflects sleep pressure, i.e., the buildup during wakefulness and dissipation during sleep [17]. Sleep propensity increases in a nonlinear fashion during the day; sleep deprivation increases sleep pressure, thereby inducing sleep even during the circadian window, which does not usually allow sleep, and overcoming the circadian drive. Both the circadian and homeostatic processes (the so-called C and S processes, respectively) interact to modulate the intensity and the possibility to sleep [1]. In addition, the thalamus synchronizes and transfers the summation of the oscillatory cortical signals via the intergeniculate leaflets to the hypothalamus. Here, the release of neuropeptide y results in several non-photic inputs that regulate sleep. The afferent and efferent projections of the SCN and of the intergeniculate leaflets are widespread [18]. Lastly, the SCN is a nonhomogeneous structure made up of various types of neurons, one of which responds to photic inputs, one to non-photic stimuli, and another to MLT feedback, whereas only some cells exhibit intrinsic rhythmicity [18].

Changes in the Circadian and Homeostatic Processes During Adolescence

Adolescents start going to bed later as they get older. In the last 50 years, numerous studies have been published on sleep changes that occur during puberty and adolescence, which largely consist of delays in the timing of sleep. The most notable consequence of these shifts is a sleep debt due to a forced early wake-up during school days, despite no change in sleep requirements (around 9 h), together with diurnal hypersomnolence. Studies from several countries have reported similar trends [19]. Adolescents consistently report going to bed later on weekend nights than on school nights and being forced to rise early during schooldays [19]. This shift has been attributed to either psychosocial exogenous factors, such as peer culture, family environment, academic demands, new jobs, and enjoying late-night activities (e.g., television or the Internet) or to changes in endogenous circadian clocks. The intrinsic circadian change, supported by data demonstrating a cross-cultural sleep phase delay during adolescence, may increase the capacity of adolescents to participate in evening activities, thereby reinforcing the changes in sleep timing. A National Sleep Foundation poll in the United States found that 45 % of adolescents report inadequate sleep [20]. A recent cross-sectional survey of adolescents in the United States conducted from 1991 to 2012 indicates that adolescent sleep generally declined over 20 years; the biggest change occurred in the years 1991–1995 and 1996–2000 [21].

Numerous papers have been published on this issue by Carskadon M. and co-workers during the so-called Stanford Summer Camps. The researchers hypothesize that human adolescence is associated with a physiological phase delay and a reduction in sleep pressure drive (around puberty) [22]. The authors found that the timing of MLT secretion was progressively shifted according to the pubertal stage, which is correlated with the circadian phase as defined by the timing of the MLT secretion: more mature children display a later MLT secretion offset phase [22]. A possible explanation for this finding is a longer τ during adolescence, which facilitates the delay in the circadian phase. Alternative explanations for the delayed sleep phase during puberty are an increased sensitivity and response to evening light and a reduced sensitivity to morning light [23]. One of the first studies conducted was designed to determine whether the typical daytime sleepiness reported by adolescents even occurs in the absence of sleep deprivation [24]. The authors found that total sleep time and REM sleep time during the night were stable across the Tanner stages, under controlled conditions in which sleep deprivation was absent (according to the pubertal development rating and secondary sexual characteristics) [26], while slow-wave sleep time declined, with a 40 % reduction from prepuberty to maturity, and daytime sleepiness increased [25]. Sleep timing, as explained above, is derived from the interaction between the circadian system and homeostatic process. The delay in pubertal sleep might also be caused by sleep pressure changes. The marker of sleep pressure changes is widely considered to be slow-wave activity (SWA, electroencephalogram, spectral power frequency range of 0.75–4.5 Hz), which is high during the first cycle of non-rapid eye movement (NREM) sleep, but declines progressively during the night in parallel with the drop in sleep pressure. A spectral analysis of a scalp sleep electroencephalogram (EEG) during adolescence conducted to compare the nocturnal dynamics of SWA in prepubertal and mature adolescents demonstrated a 40.1 % reduction in slow-wave sleep associated with a greater degree of sleep stage 2 NREM in mature adolescents compared with prepubertal adolescents. NREM sleep EEG power was lower in the frequency ranges <7 Hz, 11.8–12.6 Hz, and 16.2–16.8 Hz in mature adolescents. The dynamics of SWA were identical within the NREM sleep episodes and across the night in both developmental groups, indicating that the homeostatic recuperative drive during sleep remains unchanged across puberty and that the decline in slow-wave sleep during adolescence may reflect developmental changes within the brain rather than changes in sleep regulatory processes [25]. Similar results were obtained when regional sleep EEG power was analyzed in adolescents: the sleep-state-independent reduction in EEG power over almost the entire frequency range was greater in more mature though not in prepubertal adolescents, whereas the decay rate of the sleep homeostatic process did not differ between the two groups [27]. Another study demonstrated that, following 36 h of forced sleep deprivation, the buildup of homeostatic sleep pressure during wakefulness was slower in mature than in prepubertal adolescents, whereas the decline in the homeostatic process remained similar in both groups [28]. In addition, sleep tendency (assessed by measuring latency to sleep onset) was examined during extended waking in prepubertal and mature adolescents to determine whether sleep pressure was lower near bedtime in the latter group, with saliva samples of MTL also being obtained. The saliva sample DLMO was earlier in Tanner 1 group (mean clock time around 20:33 h) than in Tanner 5 group (mean clock time around 21:29 h), and sleep latencies were shorter in Tanner 1 group at 22:30 h, 00:30 h, and 02:30 h [29]. This study indicates that adolescents display a delayed circadian (or internal clock) phase, assessed according to daily endocrine rhythms, even several weeks following the introduction of regulated schedules that allow for sufficient sleep and are maintained under controlled laboratory conditions in which social influences are reduced to a minimum, and correlates with secondary-sex development [29]. Pubertal humans may have a blunted phase advance response to light exposure in the morning and an exaggerated phase delay response to light exposure in the evening [30]. Although girls start displaying a sleep delay 1 year earlier than boys, paralleling their younger pubertal onset [30], the magnitude of the delay is greater in boy than girls, as has been demonstrated by a large epidemiological study performed in Germany and Switzerland [31]. A recent review designed to analyze cross-culture differences found that Asian adolescents' bedtimes were later than those of peers from North America and Europe, while weekend sleep data were generally consistent worldwide, with bedtimes 2+ hours later. The magnitude of the school night-to-weekend discrepancy is associated to problematic outcomes, including impaired school performance and depressed mood. The authors noted a worldwide delayed sleep-wake behavior pattern that was consistent with symptoms of delayed sleep phase disorder, which may be exacerbated by cultural factors [32]. In addition, the delayed timing of sleep during human adolescence is likely to represent a developmental change shared by mammalian species [29]. All these changes explain why teenagers are particularly vulnerable to delayed sleep phase syndrome, which is known to peak during adolescence (a prevalence ranging from 7 to 16 % compared with 0.15 % during adulthood) [28]. The Carskadon laboratory developed a model of delayed sleep phase during adolescence that takes into account developmental changes in homeostatic drive and circadian timing: human adolescents become resistant to sleep pressure, allowing them to stay up later. At the same time, their circadian phase is delayed somewhat, which gives them the drive to stay awake later in the evening and to sleep later in the morning [33]. These findings should be borne in mind when measures need to be taken to avoid the negative effects of sleep deprivation on grades, the risk of car accidents, and mood [31]. A number of school districts have postponed middle and high school starting times in an attempt to reduce teenage sleep deprivation [34]. Teaching sleep and circadian principles in middle and high school health education is fundamental, instructing adolescents to minimize exposure to light at night and to reduce computer or TV usage immediately before bedtime, adding an outdoor morning activity into a teenage schedule [30] and reducing consumption of common beverages that contain caffeine in view of the long-lasting psychoactive effects of caffeine [35]. Consumption of common beverages that contain caffeine is known to have increased in childhood and adolescence. One recent cross-sectional study conducted on 4243 school-aged children found a twofold increased risk of sleep disturbances in school-aged and adolescent children who drank either coffee or soft drinks [36]. Children are very often unaware of the caffeine content in common drinks. Sodas are a common source of caffeine among adolescents and are associated with daytime sleepiness, insufficient sleep, and poorer sleep quality [36]. Environmental factors (such as decreased parental monitoring) and psychosocial factors (such as increased use of electronic media) exert a considerable influence on the amount of time adolescents sleep, despite reports in the press and information given by clinicians on the negative impact of electronic media on sleep [37]. Media use might impact sleep quality and quantity because it directly displaces not only sleep but even other activities related to good sleep hygiene (such as physical activity). Media use in the evenings may cause children to become physiologically aroused, making it more difficult for them to relax before they go to bed. In addition, evening exposure to bright light from television or computer screens, as well as electromagnetic radiation from mobile telephones, may suppress MLT secretion and consequently delay the circadian rhythm [37]. Almost all American adolescents (97%) were found to have at least one electronic media device in their bedroom, consisting of music players (90%), televisions (57%), video game consoles (43%), mobile (42%) or fixed-line telephones (34%), computers (28%), and Internet access (21%). Older adolescents had more media devices in their bedrooms than younger adolescents [37]. Television viewing among children and adolescents should be limited, especially in the evenings, with a recommended maximum of 2 h per day, and televisions should be kept out of bedrooms [38]. Children using electronic media as a sleep aid to relax at night have been reported to have later weekday bedtimes, experience fewer hours of sleep per week, and complain more of daytime sleepiness [39]. Time spent playing computer or electronic games should be restricted both during the day and in the evening for school-aged children and adolescents, with a viewing limit of 2 h per day, though a distinction may need to be made between violent and nonviolent games as playing nonviolent games in the evening appears to have positive effects on sleep [38].

Circadian Rhythm Sleep-Wake Disorders (CRSWDs)

The International Classification of Sleep Disorder – third edition [40] classifies CRSD as dyssomnias, with six subtypes: advanced sleep-wake phase disorder, delayed sleep phase disorder, irregular sleep-wake disorder, non-24-h sleep-wake rhythm disorder, jet lag disorder, and shift work disorder. The primary clinical characteristic of all CRSDs is an inability to fall asleep and wake at the desired time, caused by a problem with the internal biological clock (circadian timing system) and/or misalignment between the circadian timing system and the external 24-h environment, such as timing of patient's school, work, or social activities. A number of tools are available to assess sleep-wake patterns: sleep log and actigraphy are recommended to evaluate CRSWDs and should be conducted for at least 7 days, preferably for 14 days; circadian chronotype (Morningness-Eveningness Questionnaires) and physiological measures of endogenous circadian timing (salivary or plasma DLMO and urinary 6-sulfatoxymelatonin) are considered optional, though significant, additional tools when making a diagnosis. The most common presenting symptoms are difficulty in initiating and maintaining sleep and excessive sleepiness associated with significant impairments in important areas of functioning [40]. Advanced sleep-wake phase disorder (ASWPD), delayed sleep-wake phase disorder (DSWPD), irregular sleep-wake rhythm (ISWR), and the non-24-h sleep-wake syndrome or free-running disorder (non-entrained type, N24SWD) are considered the "endogenous" circadian rhythm sleep disorders, whereas jet lag disorder and shift work disorder are considered the "exogenous" circadian rhythm sleep disorders. The endogenous and exogenous factors in each disorder are, however, always combined to some extent [41]. Jet lag disorder and shift work disorder will not be discussed here because they are typical of adulthood and not adolescence. According to the practice parameters for the clinical evaluation and treatment of CRSWDs drawn up by the American Academy of Sleep Medicine [41], polysomnography is not routinely recommended to diagnose CRSWDs (standard), specific questionnaires such as the Morningness-Eveningness Questionnaire cannot be recommended because evidence pointing to their usefulness is insufficient, and circadian phase markers are indicated to diagnose non-24-h sleep-wake rhythm disorder (option), though not other circadian disorders because evidence of their usefulness is insufficient in this case as well. Actigraphy is recommended for the diagnosis of advanced and delayed sleep phase disorders (guidelines), as well as of non-24-h sleep-wake rhythm disorder and irregular sleep-wake rhythm (option), while sleep log or diary is recommended (guideline) to diagnose all endogenous circadian sleep disorders and actigraphy (guideline) to monitor the response to therapy in these disorders [41].

These following criteria must be met [40]:

1. Features:

    (a) DSWPD: significant delay in the phase of main sleep (habitual sleep-wake timing delayed ≥ 2 h, relative to conventional or socially acceptable timing, excessive morning sleep inertia, increased rates of psychiatric disturbances. An overlap with non-24-h sleep-wake disorder is possible).

(b) ASWPD: advance (early timing) in the phase of main sleep. Complaints of early morning or maintenance insomnia and excessive evening sleepiness, and chronic sleep debt.

(c) N24SWD: there is a history of insomnia, excessive daytime sleepiness, or both, which alternate with asymptomatic episodes, due to misalignment between the 24-h light-dark cycle and the endogenous sleep-wake circadian rhythm. The magnitude of the daily delay may range from <30 min (period is close to 24 h) to >1 h (period is longer than 25 h). The symptomatic episode will typically begin with a gradual increase in sleep latency and delayed sleep onset. Most individuals are totally blind. In sighted people, social and behavioral factors and psychiatric disorders play an important role. Occasionally, the disorder is associated with developmental intellectual disability or dementia. In sighted patients with N24SWD, the circadian period is about 25 h or longer; in totally blind patients, it is closer to 24 h and may rarely be shorter.

(d) ISWR: chronic or recurrent pattern of irregular sleep and wake episodes throughout the 24-h period, characterized by symptoms of insomnia during the scheduled sleep period, excessive sleepiness (napping) during the day, or both. The chronic or recurring sleep-wake pattern is temporally disorganized; sleep and wake episodes are variable throughout the 24-h cycle. It is more commonly observed in neurodegenerative disorders, such as dementia, and in children with developmental disorders. Total sleep time across the 24 h may be normal for age.

2. The symptoms are present for ≥3 months.
3. Sleep quality and duration improve when sleep schedule can be chosen.
4. Sleep log and actigraphy monitoring demonstrate a delay in the habitual sleep period. Both work/school days and days off must be included.
5. The sleep disturbance is not better explained by another current sleep, medical or neurological disorder, mental disorder, medication use, or substance use disorder.

Additional Pediatric Features of CRSWDs

Validated instruments are available for assessing phase preference in pediatric populations, including the Children's Chronotype Questionnaire (CCTQ) (parent report), the Morningness-Eveningness Scale for Children (self-report), and the Morningness-Eveningness Questionnaire for Children and Adolescents [40].

Delayed Sleep-Wake Phase Disorder

Weitzman and colleagues [42] first described delayed sleep phase insomnia, which is characterized by a cluster of features, including a chronic inability to fall asleep and wake at a desired clock time, and consequently locks patients into a sleep schedule that is out of phase with normal activities. Although it is prevalent above all among adolescents and young adults, onset in early childhood has been described, especially in familial cases. In younger children, DSWPD may present primarily as bedtime resistance, as caregivers attempt to establish bedtimes in conflict with the child's circadian time for sleep. A long history of repeated school absences, chronic tardiness, and/or school failure, rather than sleep complaints per se, is usually reported. Children and adolescents with DSWPD display higher rates of behavioral/emotional problems, including depression and suicidality, academic problems, and a higher likelihood of substance abuse. School avoidance, social maladjustment, and family dysfunction are contributing factors. Motivated DSWPD is a subtype belonging to adolescence, with little intrinsic motivation to successfully complete treatment to obtain a normal lifestyle, which is usually associated with a history of mood or anxiety disorder (school phobia and separation and social anxiety) or learning disorders. DSWPD is commonly associated with specific categories: mood disorders, severe obsessive-compulsive disorder, attention-deficit hyperactivity disorder, and autistic spectrum disorders [40]. Ill-defined medical issues may occasionally be a trigger or may complicate the course of DSWPD. This disorder is more common in the United States, a finding that may be due to the fact that school starting times in other countries, such as those in Europe, are later (08:00–08:30 h) and may thus be more suited to the delaying patterns of adolescence [19]. In adolescents and young adults, prevalence is of 7–16 %; 40 % of subjects have a family history, as an autosomal dominant trait. It is a chronic condition that may last into late life; the recurrence is high, despite appropriate treatments, with a higher risk of substance abuse disorder, increased risk of motor vehicle accidents, and chronic insomnia [40].

The endogenous circadian temperature length (τ) has been found to be longer in young adults with SDWPD than in good sleepers (>25 min). An abnormally long τ would generate a strong and continual tendency to delay the circadian system as well as the sleep-wake cycle and may account for the high relapse rate following treatment for this condition [43]. Moreover, suppression of MLT to light exposure in SDWPD is reported to be greater in adolescents than in controls, which suggests that hypersensitivity to evening light may be a precipitating or maintaining factor for the phase delay [44]. Another study demonstrated sleep deprivation and reduced sleep time in this disorder, thus suggesting such individuals have a scarce ability to compensate for lost sleep [45]. A recent paper confirmed that the timing of sleep in adolescents with SDWPD is delayed when compared with normal controls, though no group differences in sleep parameters emerged once sleep was initiated [46]. Recordings of sleep logs and actigraphy show sleep onset delayed until 1:00–6:00 am (may be earlier depending on age and developmental status), and wake time occurs in the late morning or afternoon. Unlike chronic insomnia disorder, sleep initiation and maintenance are improved when the patient is allowed to sleep on the preferred schedule; inadequate sleep hygiene and insufficient sleep syndrome must also be considered as differential diagnosis [40].

Advanced Sleep-Wake Phase Disorder

ASWPD has been reported in children with neurodevelopmental disorders, while in normal subjects, the typical onset is in elderly, with a prevalence of 1 %. Familial cases may be characterized by an earlier onset [40]. In particular, studies on children with autism spectrum disorders and Smith-Magenis syndrome have displayed marked alterations in MLT secretion profiles, which may become manifest as a phase advance characterized by very early morning waking. In some cases children develop this disorder because they are encouraged to wake up earlier than they wish to as a result of parental attention or by the opportunity they are offered to watch television or use other media upon waking [40]. Genetic analyses reveal a missense mutation in a casein kinase (CK1ε) binding region of a Period gene (hPer2). Recordings of sleep logs and actigraphy demonstrate an advance (typically ≥2 h) in the timing of circadian rhythms [40]. Poor sleep hygiene practices, particularly evening napping, and irregularity of the sleep-wake schedule, "free-running" (non-entrained) circadian rhythm, major depressive disorder that is a common cause of early awakening, must be considered as differential diagnosis [40].

Non-24-h Sleep-Wake Rhythm Disorder (N24SWD) and Irregular Sleep-Wake Rhythm Disorder (ISWRD)

N24SWD is extremely rare in normally developing or sighted children, but has been reported in children with intellectual disabilities and blindness. In congenitally blind children, onset can occur at birth or during infancy. Children with optic nerve hypoplasia due to a variety of causes, especially in children with a hypoplastic corpus callosum and comorbid severe intellectual and visual impairments, display N24SWD features. It has also been described in Rett syndrome and autism spectrum disorders. The underlying mechanism is postulated to be lack of entrainment to the 24-h day, with a failure to perceive and/or attend to social/environmental zeitgebers. Normal-sighted children or adolescents with N24SWD are likely to have psychiatric disorders that predispose them to social interaction avoidance. Children with chronic neurological conditions, such as blindness or neurodevelopmental disabilities, may have a more intractable pattern than children with more self-limited conditions [40]. Caregivers sometimes report that a child with ISWRD sleeps too much, too little, or at inappropriate times. The lack of prolonged consolidated sleep periods and the random distribution of sleep periods, with a marked day-to-day and week-to-week variability, are distinctive features that have a significant impact on caregivers. As occurs in N24SWD, children with developmental disorders, such as autism and Asperger syndrome, have an increased risk of ISWRD. Both non-24-h sleep-wake rhythm disorder and ISWRD are also common in children with Angelman syndrome or with Williams syndrome. In this regard, marked alterations in MLT secretion profiles due to polymorphisms in melatonin enzyme synthesis or variants in genes coding for melatonin receptors have been described in children and adults with autism spectrum disorders as well as in children with Smith-Magenis syndrome. Other postulated mechanisms include clock gene polymorphisms and decreased levels of entrainment by social/environmental zeitgebers. Traumatic brain injury and chronic fatigue syndrome may be other predisposing factors for both disorders. Brain tumor survivors, especially those in whom the hypothalamic-pituitary axis has been disrupted, may have an increased prevalence of circadian rhythm disorders, including ISWRD. The prevalence of ISWRD increases with advancing age, but it is likely that the age-related increase in neurodegenerative disorders, rather than aging per se, is responsible for this increase [40]. Recording of sleep log and actigraphy over prolonged periods (ideally ≥14 day in blind individuals) demonstrate the lack of a stable relationship between the timing of sleep and the 24-h day, in subjects with N24SWD. When sleep schedules follow the endogenous propensity, sleep onset and wake times are delayed each day. Sleep log and actigraphy reveal an irregular sleep-wake pattern, which is defined as having multiple sleep bouts (typically 2–4 h) during a 24-h period; the pattern may vary from day to day, among individuals with ISWRD.

Insufficient Sleep Syndrome

An inadequate amount of sleep time should always be taken into account when making a diagnosis of circadian sleep disorders, and the normative data for sleep duration should be borne in mind before diagnosing a DSWPD in all patients except long sleepers. Sleep duration recommendations were recently published by the National Sleep Foundation of the United States of America [47]. Chronic sleep loss is a characteristic of modern society, with large numbers of people stating that they are chronically sleeping significantly less, which in turn induces or exacerbates a sleep phase delay [48].

Insufficient sleep syndrome may be more frequent in adolescence, when the need to sleep is greater, but social pressure and a tendency to delay sleep often lead to chronic restricted sleep. The evening preference chronotype predisposes to insufficient sleep. It should be differentiated from delayed sleep phase disorder (in some complex cases in which there is an overlap by measuring circadian biological markers), from the effects of recreational drug use and from school avoidance behavior. Increased predisposition to substance abuse and accidents in teens may be consequent to insufficient sleep. Excessive diurnal somnolence or daytime lapses into sleep, or behavioral abnormalities attributable to sleepiness in prepubertal children, are common complaints. Sleep time, as established by history, sleep logs, or actigraphy, is usually shorter than that expected for age, though it tends to be markedly extended on weekend nights. In this disorder, the reduction in sleep duration is present most days for at least 3 months, and sleep paralysis and hypnagogic hallucinations may occur. Secondary symptoms such as irritability, concentration and attention deficits, reduced vigilance, distractibility, reduced motivation, anergia, dysphoria, fatigue, restlessness, uncoordination, malaise, and depression may, by becoming the patient's main focus, obscure the primary cause of the difficulties. The correct diagnosis of insufficient sleep syndrome may be particularly challenging in subjects who have a physiological need for unusually large amounts of sleep. Sleepiness and the other complaints can be successfully addressed in such patients by increasing total sleep time, whereas they cannot be in subjects with DSWPD [40].

Treatment of Circadian Rhythm Sleep-Wake Disorders (See Table 12.1)

The timing of treatment is crucial because unless therapy is started at the appropriate circadian time, the patients are likely to get worse. Morning exposure to light will facilitate entrainment in humans who have an intrinsic period that exceeds 24 h, whereas evening light exposure will entrain individuals with an intrinsic period that is shorter than 24 h [19]. The treatment options in clinical practice for circadian rhythm sleep disorders comprise bright light treatment and exogenous MLT administration. Although chronotherapy has been used, the data available documenting its efficacy are still insufficient [49]. Chronotherapy, which has proved to some extent successful in DSWPD, consists in delaying the sleep period by 2–3 h every day until the preferred target sleep time is achieved [40]. In order to administer the treatment correctly, it is essential to identify the circadian phase, i.e., the nadir of the core

Table 12.1 Recommendations for prescribing melatonin in children with circadian sleep disorder of sleep-onset insomnia

Time of administration in children	If used as chronobiotic, administer 2–3 h before dim light melatonin onset or administer melatonin 3–4 h before actual sleep-onset time
Dosage	Start with a low dose of 0.2–0.5-mg fast-release melatonin; increase by 0.2–0.5 mg every week until effect appears; if there is no response after 1 week, increase dose by 1 mg every week until effect appears. When 1 mg is effective: try lower dose; if there are sleep maintenance problems, start after melatonin treatment; melatonin dose is probably too high
	Maximum dose: <40 Kg, 3 mg; >40 Kg, 5 mg
Treatment duration	It should be no less than 1 month. It can be withdrawn just before puberty or shortly after puberty. Stop melatonin treatment once a year for 1 week (preferably in summer) after a normal sleep cycle has been established
When melatonin treatment is no longer effective:	Check timing of administration. In some cases dose reduction is warranted instead of dose escalation, because loss of efficacy of melatonin treatment is most likely caused by slow melatonin metabolism. Metabolism slower, oral contraceptives, cimetidine, fluvoxamine; metabolism faster, carbamazepine, esomeprazole, omeprazole
	Reconsider diagnosis: look for neuropsychiatric comorbidity. For very severe delayed sleep-wake rhythm, consider chronotherapy

Reproduced from Bruni et al. [51], with permission of Elsevier body temperature rhythm or the endogenous MLT rhythm. The core body temperature usually peaks in the late afternoon or evening and reaches its lowest point, i.e., nadir, in the early morning, with sleep normally ending approximately 2 h following the nadir. MLT secretion increases soon after the onset of darkness, peaks in the middle of the night, and gradually falls during the second half of the night [49]. The protocol followed to estimate the nadir of the core body temperature requires that the patient be placed in a semirecumbent position in a laboratory environment for a number of consecutive hours (often 26), with a light intensity of less than 50 lx; the patient receives a 100-kcal meal every hour [49]. The DLMO measurement is based on several samples of MLT (normally with a 30- or 60-min interval) of saliva, urine, or plasma. The level of illumination currently recommended for sampling is 10 lx [50]. While the samples are being collected, subjects should avoid drinks with artificial colorants, alcohol, or caffeine as well as teeth-brushing, lipstick/lip gloss, chewing gum, lemons, and bananas, as well as avoid eating, drinking, or using tobacco for 30 min prior to sampling [46]. In cases in which the sleep phase disorder is severely delayed or advanced, saliva should, if possible, be collected at later or earlier times or hourly for 24 h [51]. A simple way to assess the nadir is to instruct the patient to sleep until he/she wakes up spontaneously (i.e., without an alarm clock) – it is reasonable to assume that the nadir will be approximately 2 h before the subject awakens. The body temperature nadir usually coincides with the moment in which the greatest difficulty in staying awake is encountered, which is worth bearing in mind when the nadir in jet lag disorder and night workers needs to be calculated. Short wavelengths (blue light) have a stronger MLT-suppressing effect and a stronger phase-shifting effect on the human circadian rhythm. Light exposure before the nadir of the core body temperature rhythm causes a phase delay, whereas light administered after the nadir causes a phase advance. Bright light is typically administered by portable units yielding about 10,000 lx, with an exposure time of approximately 30–45 min per day being required to advance sleep, and units yielding about 4000 lx for 2 h being required to delay sleep. The patient is instructed to keep his gaze directed at the light source, but not continuously. Whenever outdoor light of a sufficient intensity is available, it is preferable to be outdoors than sit in front of a light box [49]. Some rare cases of mania as a side effect of phototherapy have been reported [52]. Compliance may be increased in some patients by using a light visor. Blue light-blocking glasses may be useful in adolescents as a countermeasure for alerting effects induced by light exposure through light-emitting diode screens [53], while a prototype light mask using narrow-band "green" light to deliver light through closed eyelids suppresses MLT by 40% through the closed eyelid without disrupting sleep [54]. In ASWPD, the subject should be exposed to bright light as close to bedtime as possible. The effects of bright light may not be as clear in ASWPD as in DSWPD because exposure to light in the former occurs many hours before the nadir, and waking up the patients in the middle of the night (i.e., just before the nadir) is normally not considered acceptable. In sighted individuals with a free-running disorder, exposure to bright light may be tried before administration of MLT, when the rhythm is in phase with the environment [49].

Exogenously administered MLT has phase-shifting properties, with the effect following a phase response curve (PRC) that is about 12 h out of phase with the PRC of light. MLT administered in the afternoon or early evening will phase advance the circadian rhythm, whereas when it is administered in the morning, it will phase delay the circadian rhythm, with maximal phase shifts occurring when melatonin is scheduled around dusk or dawn. The doses used in most studies range from 0.5 to 5 mg, though it is not clear whether the effects of MLT are dose-related [49]. The recommendations of a European consensus conference held in Rome in 2014 that was aimed at assessing the current role of melatonin in childhood sleep disturbances were recently published [51] (see Table 12.1, modified version of these recommendations). MLT displays its maximum phase-advancing effect 3–5 h before the DLMO, whereas when it is administered 2–3 h after the DLMO, it may have either no effect or a reversal effect in DSWPD [51]. There is no evidence that slow-release MLT is preferable to the fast-acting MLT [51]. Possible side effects include increased blood pressure, headache, dizziness, nausea, and drowsiness [55]. Bright light has been recommended as the first treatment approach to SDWPD; if the response is not satisfactory, MLT is added, usually 12 h before exposure to light [49]. MLT is administered 12 h after the last awakening in blind patients with free-running disorders. In conclusion, the most important practical points to bear in mind when treating CRSWDs are do not start bright light treatment for SDWPD in the early morning but wait until the patient wakes up spontaneously (without an alarm clock); bright light is subsequently administered 1 h earlier every day until entrainment. Appropriate timing of melatonin administration is approximately 12 h after bright light treatment [49].

Subjects with Neurodevelopmental Disorders Have Increased Risk of CRSWDs

Autism Spectrum Disorders (ASD)

Sleep problems are particularly common in children with ASD, with prevalence rates ranging from 50 to 80 % compared with 9–50 % in age-matched, normally developing children. Such problems tend to increase with age, rather than disappear [56, 57]. The most common sleep problem reported by caregivers is insomnia, whose pathogenesis is multifactorial and includes disruption of circadian rhythms and MLT dysregulation. It has recently been hypothesized that the increased use of media combined with the bright screen of the media devices may contribute to the alterations in MLT secretion in ASD [58]. An overresponse to sensory input at bedtime associated with increased precognitive arousal has been observed in such children [59]. Furthermore, the relationship between sleep problems and ASD is complex because circadian abnormalities and epilepsy are both strong, bidirectional contributors [60, 61]. The multifactorial factor that is implicated in ASD may explain the marked night-to-night variability of the sleep-wake cycle and the fragmented irregular sleep-wake patterns, including the inconsistent sleep onset and rise time, free-running sleep-wake rhythm, sleep onset delay, and early morning awakening [62, 63]. Significantly lower levels of nocturnal and daytime blood melatonin levels, as well as lower levels of its primary metabolite 6-sulfoxymelatonin, have been observed in many individuals with ASD when compared with normally developing controls [64, 65]. A disruption of the serotonin pathway, associated with high whole-blood serotonin levels and reduced plasma MLT, was also reported in one study on 278 ASD subjects [61]. Most of the studies that have investigated MLT-related genes in ASD focused on the ASMT gene, with reports indicating that a decreased expression of the ASMT transcript is correlated with decreased MLT blood levels in ASD patients and their relatives [65]. The few studies that analyzed genome-wide gene expression found 15 circadian rhythm regulatory or responsive genes that are differentially expressed in the most severe ASD subgroup though not in the mild or savant subgroups, thereby pointing to a link between circadian rhythm dysregulation and the severity of language impairment. In particular, the presence of the gene encoding AANAT was reported to be significantly reduced [66, 67]. Many polymorphisms within the CYP1A2 gene that alter MLT degradation and are predictive of slow metabolizing alleles have been implicated in the pathogenesis of ASD and sleep problems, accompanied by a loss of efficacy of MLT supplementation after 1 or 2 months [68]. It has been hypothesized that normal nocturnal blood values of MLT in some children with ASD may be caused by a combination of lower MLT production levels and the slow metabolic activity of CZP1A2 [68]. CRSWDs in children with ASD have been investigated above all by means of sleep questionnaires and actigraphic recordings (usually associated with sleep logs), while the detection of plasma, urine, or salivary MLT secretions continues to be used as a diagnostic tool for research purposes [56]. Basic principles of sleep hygiene, including the selection of an appropriate bedtime and establishment of a positive bedtime routine aimed at reducing emotional and/or behavioral stimulation at night and thus at minimizing television viewing and playing computer or video games, may represent an important means of improving sleep [58]. A parent group program of intervention may help to manage insomnia in ASD [69]. Supplemental MLT in ASD may go beyond the treatment of a deficiency state alone; for example, melatonin, which acts as a hypnotic when used independently of a deficiency state (in ASD children with normal endogenous MLT levels), also has antianxiolytic effects that may mitigate hyperarousal-related insomnia [68]. Moreover, some trials and meta-analysis studies in which MLT has been used to treat ASD highlighted the efficacy of MLT in this disorder (with varying dosages of up to 6 mg administered under both immediate- and controlled-release conditions, 5–6 h before the desired bedtime) [70, 71]. In one randomized placebo-controlled study, controlled-release melatonin treatment combined with behavioral interventions in 134 children with autism and long-lasting sleep problems proved to be highly effective [72].

Neurodevelopmental Disabilities (NDD)

The most common sleep disturbances in NDD are delayed sleep onset, frequent awakenings during sleep, lasting minutes or hours, and early morning awakenings. Day-night reversals, advanced sleep onset, and free-running sleep-wake rhythm disorders are much less common. Since individuals affected by NDD cannot sleep when sleep is desired, needed, or expected, most of the sleep disturbances belong to the diagnostic category of CRSWDs [73]. CRSWDs in children with NDD tend to be misunderstood and underdiagnosed. Light/darkness influences brain functions, including cognition, via pathways other than the monosynaptic retinal-hypothalamic tracts [74]. The prevalence of CRSWDs is increasing among normally developing and healthy children owing to a combination of lifestyle changes and increased exposure to light. This change also applies to children with NDD, 70% of whom are affected by CRSWDs, especially those with moderate-severe NDD, i.e., with bilateral and extensive brain lesions. Persistent early morning awakenings are common in children with NDD and fulfill the criteria of CRSWDs because such children are unable to sleep when sleep is desired, needed, or expected. Delayed sleep-onset disorders in children with severe NDD are associated with a marked variability in the timing of sleep onset and frequency of a delay, with the total sleep time per 24 h not being age appropriate, but frequently reduced [75]. A good response to melatonin administered at bedtime has been reported in such cases [76]. It is important to bear in mind that restless legs syndrome, with or without periodic limb movement, may also cause delayed sleep onset. The prevalence of this syndrome is likely to be underestimated because of the difficulties encountered in diagnosing it in children with NDD [73]. Free-running sleep-wake rhythms with no other sleep disturbances are generally observed in neurologically healthy children who have total ocular blindness, though this condition is rare because total ocular visual loss is now uncommon as a result of improved ophthalmological care. By contrast, children with loss of visual acuity due to occipital lobe visual impairment do not exhibit free-running sleep-wake disturbances because the monosynaptic retinal-hypothalamic pathways to the SCN remain intact. Since children with NDD have altered cortical connectivity, they may not be able to properly perceive the environmental cues required to develop the sleep-wake rhythm, which results in inadequate thalamic signals to the hypothalamus and, ultimately, in CRSWDs [73]. A recent EEG study on children with extensive brain damage and profound developmental disabilities showed that up to 100% of them had persistent, severely impaired sleep-wake patterns, though very few had ocular lesions, thus demonstrating that the cerebral structures play a major role in sleep-wake regulation [77]. Cerebral palsy (CP) is defined as a group of nonprogressive disorders of movement and posture resulting in activity limitations that occur in the developing fetal or infant brain and affect 1.5–2.5 children per 1000 live births. About 20–50% of children with CP have a cortical visual impairment, resulting in a free-running circadian rhythm [78]. Smith-Magenis syndrome (SMS) is a rare multisystemic disorder that occurs in 1:25,000 births. It is caused by a mutation or small deletion in a transcriptional regulator gene of the mammalian circadian clock, i.e., RAI1 (retinoic acid induced) on chromosome 17p11.258, and is characterized by intellectual disability of varying degrees, short stature, a deep hoarse voice, obesity, scoliosis, distinctive facies (deep, close-set eyes, midfacial hypoplasia, and broad, square-shaped face), and peripheral neuropathy [79]. Maladaptive and disruptive behavior is typical of this syndrome and is associated with 24-h sleep disorder. Actigraphic data have revealed a total sleep time that is 1 or 2 h shorter than that in normal healthy controls and fragmented sleep starting from as early as 6 months and persisting throughout school age [80]. Many studies have found that an alteration in the circadian clock gene action results in inverted endogenous melatonin secretion, which thus peaks during daytime, in the vast majority of children with SMS [81]. Oral acebutolol administered alone in the early morning and combined with MLT in the evening has been used in an attempt to improve the sleep-wake rhythm in patients with SMS [82]. Angelman syndrome (AS) is a neurodevelopmental disorder that is characterized by mental retardation, seizures, gait ataxia, speech impairment, epilepsy, craniofacial abnormalities, and easily provoked laughter and is due to abnormalities in chromosome 15q11–q13. The prevalence of sleep problems associated with this syndrome is usually very high, with up to 90 % subjects being affected [83]. Sleep problems mainly consist of difficulties in falling asleep and multiple awakenings. A lower level of MLT and a high prevalence of CRSWDs (irregular, free-running, and sleep phase delayed disorders) have been reported in AS, though open-label and placebo-controlled trials have shown that treatment with MLT supplementation yields a good response [84–86]. A possible explanation for this positive response is the lack of ubiquitin protein ligase E3A gene expression on the maternal chromosome 15q11–q13, which is reported in AS and is known to be implicated in the control and development of circadian rhythm [87]. This hypothesis is supported by another study in which a patient with Rett syndrome, an abnormality that affects the ubiquitin protein ligase E3A gene, N24SWD, markedly improved following MLT oral supplementation [88].

Although genetic and/or epigenetic abnormalities in sleep-wake circadian regulation may predispose children with NDD to CRSWDs, poor sleep hygiene, negative associations, and the lack of restrictions all contribute to the maintenance of sleep problems. The active collaboration of caregivers is essential to be able to adopt behavioral treatment strategies, such as creating a dark, quiet, non-stimulating environment and reducing the number of stimuli (such as electronic devices) [71]. A recent large clinical trial confirmed the efficacy of MLT as a means of treating sleep problems in children with NDDs, using doses ranging from 0.5 to 12 mg, which were found to reduce sleep latency and increase total sleep time [89].

Attention-Deficit Hyperactivity Disorders (ADHD)

About 25–50 % of children and adolescents with attention-deficit hyperactivity disorder (ADHD) experience sleep problems, with objective data based on actigraphic recordings demonstrating an increase in sleep-onset latency associated with a decreased amount of time spent asleep in such subjects [90]. According to the data in the literature, five sleep phenotypes may be identified in ADHD: a sleep phenotype characterized mainly by a hypoarousal state, resembling narcolepsy, which may be considered a "primary" form of ADHD; a second phenotype associated with a delayed sleep-onset latency and a higher risk of bipolar disorder; a third phenotype associated with sleep disordered breathing; a fourth phenotype related to restless legs syndrome and/or periodic limb movements, which may further extend the delays in the sleep phase disorder; and, lastly, a fifth phenotype related to epilepsy/or EEG interictal discharges [90]. We will discuss the second phenotype here. Sleep-onset delayed insomnia is the most common sleep disorder in children with ADHD. The onset of sleep delayed phase disorders may occur at as early as 3 years of age, with an accumulation of sleep deprivation over time. Children in this subgroup have a delayed DLMO associated with a significant delay in sleep latency when compared with ADHD children without insomnia [91]. Preliminary evidence from severe mood dysregulation-related disorders indicates that morning light therapy has a positive effect on depressive symptoms, circadian rhythms, inattention, and irritability [92]. It has been suggested that the core endophenotypic characteristic of pediatric bipolar sleep is a phase delayed circadian sleep-wake cycle rather than a reduced need for sleep per se (see below) [93]. Many studies have demonstrated the efficacy and safety of MLT in the treatment of insomnia in children with ADHD, with doses ranging between 3 and 6 mg [94]. MLT may, if required, be combined with light therapy, particularly in children that are at risk of developing bipolar disorder as the use of stimulants remains controversial in such subjects [90]. Stimulant medication does not appear to affect the core symptoms related to a lower vigilance state in children with sleep delayed insomnia. Furthermore, the use of stimulant medications may exacerbate insomnia in children with ADHD, thereby affecting circadian motor activity levels, as has been demonstrated by actigraphic analyses [95]. The authors of this review believe that the administration of long-acting medications may increase the risk of developing or worsening sleep-onset insomnia in children with ADHD [95]. A large placebo-controlled trial on ADHD studied the effects of 4-week MLT therapy on the sleep-onset latency and circadian phase, as assessed by means of the DLMO [96]. The results of that trial did not detect any improvement in ADHD symptoms or cognition at the end of the 4 weeks [96]. A follow-up study revealed that improvements in behavior and mood after long-term treatment (2–3 years) only occurred in those children still using melatonin, while discontinuation of MLT resulted in a relapse of sleep-onset insomnia [97]. In one study on adult ADHD patients [98], treatment with early morning bright light therapy improved ADHD symptoms after 3 weeks, with the positive effects appearing to occur more rapidly than following administration of MLT. Interestingly, the effects of both sensorimotor rhythm (SMR) and slow cortical potential (SCP) neurofeedback treatment of ADHD symptoms last longer than those induced by medication, possibly because they act by increasing sleep spindle density and normalizing sleep-onset insomnia, thereby resulting in vigilance stabilization. Although neurofeedback does not target the circadian phase delay directly, this effect is mediated by subcortical and cortical circuits that regulate sleep spindle production and sleep onset [99].

Mood Disorders

In view of the significant changes in sleep and circadian rhythms that occur during a person's lifespan, age may contribute to the heterogeneity in sleep-wake profiles linked to mood disorders. The severity of depressive symptoms is expected to be associated with a more pronounced phase delay during youth and later diagnosis of bipolar disorder, while a reduced sleep duration and consolidation and disorganization of circadian rhythms is expected in older age [100]. Indeed, it has been suggested that the restoration of normal circadian rhythms contributes to the remission of depression and prevention of relapses in young people with depressive symptoms. Actigraphic monitoring has been used to show that poor sleep is a hallmark of major depression during a stable depressive phase among young people (13–35 years old) [101]. A reduced need for sleep, together with elation, grandiosity, and racing thoughts, distinguishes mania and bipolar disorder from attention-deficit hyperactivity and other childhood psychiatric disorders. Children with manic bipolar I disorder typically experience a decreased need for sleep resembling that of adults, whereas many children who are bipolar, who exhibit part-day manic episodes (pediatric bipolar type IIA and type IIB), or who have chronic mixed conditions (pediatric bipolar type IIIA) do not [93]. Children with bipolar type IIA exhibit prominent diurnal cycles on most days (pediatric bipolar type IIA): initial morning depression and subsequent (typically late afternoon and/or evening) mania. They display disturbed sleep patterns, characterized by an evening acceleration and a significant delay in sleep onset, which may, or may not, be accompanied by a decreased need for sleep and difficulty in awakening for school; moreover, a decreased need for sleep has been observed in subjects with manic cycles lasting days (pediatric bipolar type I) or chronic mania [93]. It has been suggested that the main bipolar sleep defect is a heritable phase delay in the sleep-wake cycle resulting from mutations in SCN circadian clock genes, which interact with, but are independent of, evening or ongoing manic psychomotor accelerations [93]. Several clock genes, such as CRY1 and NPAS2, have been associated with affective disorders, with CLOCK and VIP being specifically linked to the mania-hypomania phenotype [102]. This hypothesis predicts (i) that most bipolar children and adolescents, whose afternoon and/or evening manic acceleration typically terminates overnight, with ultradian cycling (pediatric bipolar types IIA and IIB), will display delayed sleep onset but a low prevalence of decreased need for sleep; (ii) that the intrinsic sleep-onset phase delay, when coupled with bedtime and early morning manic psychomotor acceleration (hedonic or dysphoric), reduces the need for sleep; and (iii) that the reduced need for sleep is greatest among individuals whose manic cycles last longer than 1 day (pediatric bipolar type I) or among those with chronic mania (pediatric bipolar type IIIA). An increase in tobacco use was recently found among depressed young people with a delayed sleep phase and short sleep duration [103]. To sum up, sleep-onset phase delays and delayed sleep phase syndromes that occur during euthymic or depressed states may be trait markers of bipolar spectrum illness [93].

Case Reports

Case Report 1: SDWPD

A female adolescent aged 17.5 years came to the sleep disorder outpatient service of the Neurocenter of Italian Switzerland because she had been suffering from sleep-onset difficulties since she was 3 years old. Her bedtime had become increasingly delayed in the last 3 years (sleep time: from 01.30 am to 7 am), and she complained of excessive daytime sleepiness, requiring a 3-h nap, and of school difficulties. She also reported fear and strong nausea at bedtime and usually fell asleep at around 5 am. At weekends she tended to sleep for more than 12 h. She suffered from lypothymic attacks and dizziness during daytime, which made her feel more irritable. DSWPD was confirmed by means of the MLT salivary test (DLMO after 00.30 am) and actigraphic recording (see Fig. 12.1). She was placed on therapy with long-acting MLT 2 mg at 8 pm, which led to the complete disappearance of the anxiety, lipothymic attacks, and dizziness; restored healthy sleep, from 9:30 pm to 9 am; and eliminated the diurnal hypersomnolence or napping. She now feels happy.

Case Report 2: Sleep-Onset Insomnia (First Suspected Diagnosis of SDWPD)

A male 14-year-old adolescent came to the sleep disorder outpatient service of the Neurocenter of Italian Switzerland because he had been suffering from sleep-onset difficulties for many years. His sleep problems had got worse in the last months after he had started therapy with long-acting methylphenidate following a diagnosis of ADHD, learning disabilities, anxiety disorder, and suspected mood disorders (pediatric bipolar disorders type IIA). His anxiety increased in the afternoon and evening after the onset of treatment. He reported that his bedtime was 10.00 pm. Sleep onset occurred 30 min later, though sometimes even after midnight, and he woke up at 7.00 am. He said he had difficulties in waking up in the morning. He had a history of motor tics, tonsillitis, and respiratory allergy, as well as familiarity for somnambulism and ADHD. A video-polysomnographic recoding revealed a very mild mixed-sleep apnea disorder, some periodic leg movements during sleep, and

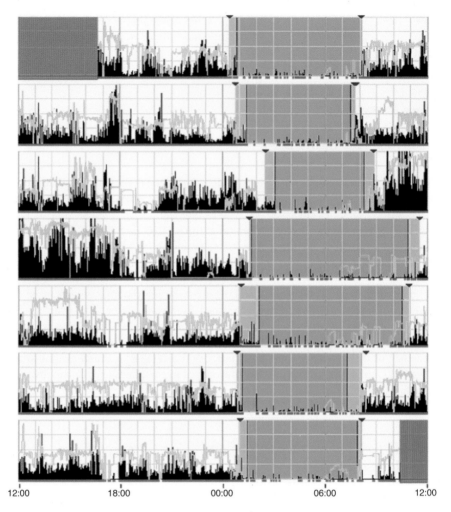

Fig. 12.1 Actigraphic recording of case report 2 (weekend fourth and fifth days)

increased sleep latency. A 1-week actigraphic recording demonstrated a tendency to fall asleep late (around 23:00 pm, with a mean sleep latency of one and a half hours), with no sleep fragmentations or diurnal nap (see Fig. 12.2). Blood examinations revealed a ferritin level of 54 mcgr/l. He was placed on therapy with long-acting MLT at 19.30, 2 mg, for 3 months, though with no benefit. The final diagnosis was sleep-onset insomnia with anxiety disorder exacerbated by stimulant therapy, which was subsequently replaced by a more appropriate therapy containing a mood stabilizer.

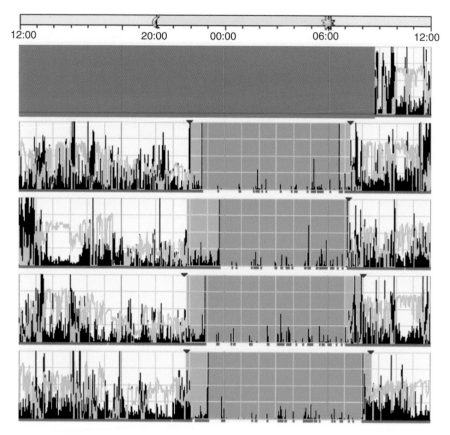

Fig. 12.2 An example of 4 days of actigraphic recording of case report 2

Conclusions

CRSWDs are an unrecognized cause of sleep loss in children that tend to persist over time unless adequately treated, particularly in view of ongoing changes in lifestyle and an increase in exposure to artificial light. The adverse effects of chronic sleep disorders on brain development in children often escape detection, with long-lasting sleep loss during critical developmental periods proving particularly harmful because it deprives young children of the environmental exposure required for healthy cognitive and motor development and consequently prevents them from achieving their full developmental potential. Persistent sleep difficulties may be associated with a number of health, economic, and emotional difficulties and raise the risk of suicide in sleep-deprived teenagers. Moreover, CRSWDs might contribute to the increased prevalence of cancer and cardiac and metabolic diseases that have been observed in recent times [2].

References

1. Manconi M, Ferini Strambi L. Circadian physiology. In: Ondo WG, editor. Restless legs syndrome. Diagnosis and treatment. New York: Informa Healthcare; 2007.
2. Brown SA. Circadian clock-mediated control of stem cell division and differentiation: beyond night and day. Development. 2014;141(16):3105–11.
3. Hattar S, Liao HW, Takao M, Berson DM, Yau KW. Melanopsin containing retinal ganglion cells: architecture, projections, and intrinsic photosensitivity. Science. 2002;295(5557):1065e70.
4. Inouye ST, Kawamura H. Persistence of circadian rhythmicity in a mammalian hypothalamic "island" containing the suprachiasmatic nucleus. Proc Natl Acad Sci U S A. 1979;76(11):5962–6.
5. Shibata S, Oomura Y, Kita H, Hattori K. Circadian rhythmic changes of neuronal activity in the suprachiasmatic nucleus of the rat hypothalamic slice. Brain Res. 1982;247(1):154–8.
6. Eastman CI, Molina TA, Dziepak ME, Smith MR. Blacks (African Americans) have shorter free-running circadian periods than whites (Caucasian Americans). Chronobiol Int. 2012;29(8):1072–7.
7. Yan L, Karatsoreos I, Lesauter J, Welsh DK, Kay S, Foley D, Silver R. Exploring spatiotemporal organization of SCN circuits. Cold Spring Harb Symp Quant Biol. 2007;72:527–41.
8. Antle MC, Silver R. Orchestrating time: arrangements of the brain circadian clock. Trends Neurosci. 2005;28(3):145–51.
9. Niles LP, Armstrong KJ, Rincon Castro LM, et al. Neural stem cells express melatonin receptors and neurotrophic factors: colocalization of the MT1 receptor with neuronal and glial markers. BMC Neurosci. 2004;5:41.
10. Comai S, Ochoa-Sanchez R, Gobbi G. Sleep wake characterization of double MT(1)/MT(2) receptor knockout mice and comparison with MT(1) and MT(2) receptor knockout mice. Behav Brain Res. 2013;243:231e8.
11. Waldhauser F, Ehrhart B, Förster E. Clinical aspects of the melatonin action: impact of development, aging, and puberty, involvement of melatonin in psychiatric disease and importance of neuroimmunoendocrine interactions. Experientia. 1993;49(8):671–81.
12. Griefahn B, Brode P, Blaszkewicz M, Remer T. Melatonin production during childhood and adolescence: a longitudinal study on the excretion of urinary 6-hydroxymelatonin sulfate. J Pineal Res. 2003;34:26e31.
13. Sadeh A. Sleep and melatonin in infants: a preliminary study. Sleep. 1997;20:185e91.
14. Tauman R, Zisapel N, Laudon M, Nehama H, Sivan Y. Melatonin production in infants. Pediatr Neurol. 2002;26:379e82.
15. Waldhauser F, Waldhauser M, Lieberman HR, Deng MH, Lynch HJ, Wurtman RJ. Bioavailability of oral melatonin in humans. Neuroendocrinology. 1984;39(4):307–13.
16. Lewy AJ, Cutler NL, Sack RL. The endogenous melatonin profile as a marker for circadian phase position. J Biol Rhythms. 1999;14(3):227–36.
17. Borbély AA. A two process model of sleep regulation. Hum Neurobiol. 1982;1(3):195–204.
18. Zee PC, Manthena P. The brain's master circadian clock: implications and opportunities for therapy of sleep disorders. Sleep Med Rev. 2007;11:59e70.
19. Crowley SJ, Acebo C, Carskadon MA. Sleep, circadian rhythms, and delayed phase in adolescence. Sleep Med. 2007;8(6):602–12.
20. National Sleep Foundation Sleep and Teens Task Force. Adolescent sleep needs and patterns: research report and resource guide. Washington, DC: National Sleep Foundation; 2000. p. 1–26.
21. Keyes KM, Maslowsky J, Hamilton A, Schulenberg J. The great sleep recession: changes in sleep duration among US adolescents, 1991–2012. Pediatrics. 2015;135(3):460–8.
22. Carskadon MA, Acebo C, Richardson GS, Tate BA, Seifer R. An approach to studying circadian rhythms of adolescent humans. J Biol Rhythms. 1997;12(3):278–89.
23. Carskadon MA, Labyak SE, Acebo C, Seifer R. Intrinsic circadian period of adolescent humans measured in conditions of forced desynchrony. Neurosci Lett. 1999;260(2):129–32.

24. Carskadon MA, Harvey K, Duke P, Anders TF, Litt IF, Dement WC. Pubertal changes in daytime sleepiness. Sleep. 1980;2(4):453–60.
25. Jenni OG, Carskadon MA. Spectral analysis of the sleep electroencephalogram during adolescence. Sleep. 2004;27(4):774–83.
26. Tanner J. Growth at adolescence. Oxford: Blackwell; 1962.
27. Jenni OG, van Reen E, Carskadon MA. Regional differences of the sleep electroencephalogram in adolescents. J Sleep Res. 2005;14(2):141–7.
28. Jenni OG, Achermann P, Carskadon MA. Homeostatic sleep regulation in adolescents. Sleep. 2005;28(11):1446–54.
29. Crowley SJ, Acebo C, Fallone G, Carskadon MA. Estimating dim light melatonin onset (DLMO) phase in adolescents using summer or school-year sleep/wake schedules. Sleep. 2006;29(12):1632–41.
30. Hagenauer MH, Perryman JI, Lee TM, Carskadon MA. Adolescent changes in the homeostatic and circadian regulation of sleep. Dev Neurosci. 2009;31(4):276–84.
31. Roenneberg T, Kuehnle T, Pramstaller PP, Ricken J, Havel M, Guth A, Merrow M. A marker for the end of adolescence. Curr Biol. 2004;14(24):R1038–9.
32. Gradisar M, Gardner G, Dohnt H. Recent worldwide sleep patterns and problems during adolescence: a review and meta-analysis of age, region, and sleep. Sleep Med. 2011;12(2):110–8. doi:10.1016/j.sleep.2010.11.008. Epub 2011 Jan 22.
33. Carskadon MA. Maturation of processes regulating sleep in adolescents. In: Marcus CL, Carroll JL, Donnelly DF, Loughlin GM, editors. Sleep in children: developmental changes in sleep patterns, vol. 2. 2nd ed. New York: Informa Healthcare; 2008. p. 95–109.
34. Wahlstrom KL. Accommodating the sleep patterns of adolescents within current educational structures: an uncharted path. In: Carskadon MA, editor. Adolescent sleep patterns: biological, social, and psychological influences. Cambridge: Cambridge University Press; 2002. p. 172–97.
35. Thakre TP, Deoras K, Griffin C, Vemana A, Podmore P, Krishna J. Caffeine awareness in children: insights from a Pilot Study. J Clin Sleep Med. 2015;11(7):741–6.
36. Orbeta RL, Overpeck MD, Ramcharran D, Kogan MD, Ledsky R. High caffeine intake in adolescents: associations with difficulty sleeping and feeling tired in the morning. J Adolesc Health. 2006;38:451–3.
37. National Sleep Foundation. Sleep in America poll. Washington, DC: National Sleep Foundation; 2006.
38. Cain N, Gradisar M. Electronic media use and sleep in school-aged children and adolescents: a review. Sleep Med. 2010;11(8):735–42.
39. Eggermont S, Van den Bulck J. Nodding off or switching off? The use of popular media as a sleep aid in secondary-school children. J Paediatr Child Health. 2006;42(7–8):428–33.
40. American Academy of Sleep Medicine. International classification of sleep disorders-ICSD. 3rd ed. Darine, IL: American Academy of Sleep Medicine: 2014.
41. Morgenthaler TI, Lee-Chiong T, Alessi C, Friedman L, Aurora RN, Boehlecke B, Brown T, Chesson Jr AL, Kapur V, Maganti R, Owens J, Pancer J, Swick TJ, Zak R. Standards of practice committee of the American academy of sleep medicine. Practice parameters for the clinical evaluation and treatment of circadian rhythm sleep disorders. An American academy of sleep medicine report. Sleep. 2007;30(11):1445–59.
42. Weitzman ED, Czeisler CA, Coleman RM, Spielman AJ, Zimmerman JC, Dement WC. Delayed sleep phase syndrome: a chronobiological disorder with sleep-onset insomnia. Arch Gen Psychiatry. 1981;38:737–46.
43. Micic G, de Bruyn A, Lovato N, Wright H, Gradisar M, Ferguson S, Burgess HJ, Lack L. The endogenous circadian temperature period length (tau) in delayed sleep phase disorder compared to good sleepers. J Sleep Res. 2013;22(6):617–24.
44. Aoki H, Ozeki Y, Yamada N. Hypersensitivity of melatonin suppression in response to light in patients with delayed sleep phase syndrome. Chronobiol Int. 2001;18(2):263–71.
45. Uchiyama M, Okawa M, Shibui K, Liu X, Hayakawa T, Kamei Y, et al. Poor compensatory function for sleep loss as a pathogenic factor in patients with delayed sleep phase syndrome. Sleep. 2000;23(4):553–8.

46. Saxvig IW, Wilhelmsen-Langeland A, Pallesen S, Vedaa O, Nordhus IH, Sørensen E, Bjorvatn B. Objective measures of sleep and dim light melatonin onset in adolescents and young adults with delayed sleep phase disorder compared to healthy controls. J Sleep Res. 2013;22(4):365–72.
47. Hirshkowitz M, et al. National Sleep Foundation's sleep time duration recommendations: methodology and results summary. Sleep Health. 2015;1:40–3.
48. Rogers NL, Dinges DF. Interaction of chronic sleep restriction and circadian system in humans. J Sleep Res. 2008;17(4):406–11.
49. Bjorvatn B, Pallesen S. A practical approach to circadian rhythm sleep disorders. Sleep Med Rev. 2009;13(1):47–60.
50. Pandi-Perumal SR, Smits M, Spence W, Srinivasan V, Cardinali DP, Lowe AD, et al. Dim light melatonin onset (DLMO): a tool for the analysis of circadian phase in human sleep and chronobiological disorders. Prog Neuropsychopharmacol Biol Psychiatry. 2007;31(1):1e11.
51. Bruni O, Alonso-Alconada D, Besag F, Biran V, Braam W, Cortese S, Moavero R, Parisi P, Smits M, Van der Heijden K, Curatolo P. Current role of melatonin in pediatric neurology: clinical recommendations. Eur J Paediatr Neurol. 2015;19(2):122–33.
52. Chan PK, Lam RW, Perry KF. Mania precipitated by light therapy for patients with SAD. J Clin Psychiatry. 1994;55(10):454.
53. Van der Lely S, Frey S, Garbazza C, Wirz-Justice A, Jenni OG, Steiner R, Wolf S, Cajochen C, Bromundt V, Schmidt C. Blue blocker glasses as a countermeasure for alerting effects of evening light-emitting diode screen exposure in male teenagers. J Adolesc Health. 2015;56(1):113–9.
54. Figueiro MG, Rea MS. Preliminary evidence that light through the eyelids can suppress melatonin and phase shift dim light melatonin onset. BMC Res Notes. 2012;5:221.
55. Buscemi N, Vandermeer B, Hooton N, Pandya R, Tjosvold L, Hartling L, et al. Efficacy and safety of exogenous melatonin for secondary sleep disorders and sleep disorders accompanying sleep restriction: meta-analysis. BMJ. 2006;332(7538):385e93.
56. Miano S, Ferri R. Epidemiology and management of insomnia in children with autistic spectrum disorders. Paediatr Drugs. 2010;12:75–84.
57. Kotagal S, Broomall E. Sleep in children with autism spectrum disorders. Pediatr Neurol. 2012;47:242–51.
58. Engelhardt CR, et al. Media use and sleep among boys with autism spectrum disorders. ADHD Typical Dev Pediatr. 2013;132:1081–9.
59. Richdale AL, et al. The role of insomnia, pre-sleep arousal and psychopathology symptoms in daytime impairment in ASD adolescents with high-functioning autism spectrum disorder. Sleep Med. 2014;15:1082–8.
60. Accardo JA, Malow BA. Sleep, epilepsy, and autism. Epilepsy Behav. 2014. pii: S1525–5050(14)00533-2.
61. Pagan C, et al. The serotonin-N acetylserotonin-melatonin pathway as a biomarker for autism spectrum disorders. Transl Psychiatry 2014;4:e479.
62. Giannotti F, et al. Sleep in children with autism with and without developmental regression. J Sleep Res. 2011;20:338–47.
63. Anders, et al. Six month sleep-wake organization in pre-school-afe children with developmental delay and typical development. Behav Sleep Med. 2011;829:92–106.
64. Kulman G, Lissoni P, Rovelli F, Roselli MG, Brivio F, Sequeri P. Evidence of pineal endocrine hypofunction in autistic children. Neuro Endocrinol Lett. 2000;21:31–4.
65. Melke J, Goubran BH, Chaste P, Betancur C, Nygren G, Anckarsater H, Rastam M, Stahlberg O, Gillberg IC, Delorme R, et al. Abnormal melatonin synthesis in autism spectrum disorders. Mol Psychiatry. 2008;13:90–8.
66. Hu VW, Sarachana T, Kim KS, Nguyen A, Kulkarni S, Steinberg ME, Luu T, Lai Y, Lee NH. Gene expression profiling differentiates autism case-controls and phenotypic variants of autism spectrum disorders: evidence for circadian rhythm dysfunction in severe autism. Autism Res. 2009;2:78–97.

67. Hu VW, Steinberg ME. Novel clustering of items from the autism diagnostic interview-revised to define phenotypes within autism spectrum disorders. Autism Res. 2009;2:67–77.
68. Veatch OJ, Goldman SE, Adkins KW, Malow BA. Melatonin in children with autism spectrum disorders: how does the evidence fit together? J Nat Sci. 2015;1(7):e125.
69. Stuttard L, et al. A preliminary investigation into the effectiveness of a group-delivered sleep management for parents of children with intellectual disabilities. J Infect Dis. 2015;19:342–55.
70. Reading R. Melatonin in autism spectrum disorders: a systematic review and metanalysis. Child Care Health Dev. 2012;38:301–2.
71. Angriman M, Caravale B, Novelli L, Ferri R, Bruni O. Sleep in children with neurodevelopmental disabilities. Neuropediatrics. 2015;46(3):199–210.
72. Cortesi F, Giannotti F, Sebastiani T, Panunzi S, Valente D. Controlled-release melatonin, singly and combined with cognitive behavioural therapy, for persistent insomnia in children with autism spectrum disorders: a randomized placebo-controlled trial. J Sleep Res. 2012;21(6):700–9.
73. Jan JE, Bax MC, Owens JA, Ipsiroglu OS, Wasdell MB. Neurophysiology of circadian rhythm sleep disorders of children with neurodevelopmental disabilities. Eur J Paediatr Neurol. 2012;16(5):403–12.
74. Jan JE, O'Donnell ME. Use of melatonin in the treatment of paediatric sleep disorders. J Pineal Res. 1996;21:193e9.
75. Wasdell MB, Jan JE, Bomben MM, Freeman RD, Rietveld WJ, Tai J, et al. A randomized, placebo-controlled trial of controlled release melatonin treatment of delayed sleep phase syndrome and impaired sleep maintenance in children with neurodevelopmental disabilities. J Pineal Res. 2008;44:57e64.
76. Smits MG, Nagtegaal EE, Van DerHeijden K, Coenen AML, Kerkhof GA. Melatonin for chronic sleep onset insomnia in children: a randomized placebo-controlled trial. J Child Neurol. 2001;16:86e92.
77. Jan JE, Ribary U, Wong PK, Reiter R, Bax M, Wasdell MB. Cerebral modulation of circadian sleep-wake rhythms. J Clin Neurophysiol. 2011;28:165e9.
78. Simard-Tremblay E, Constantin E, Gruber R, Brouillette RT, Shevell M. Sleep in children with cerebral palsy: a review. J Child Neurol. 2011;26(10):1303–10.
79. Williams SR, Zies D, Mullegama SV, Grotewiel MS, Elsea SH. Smith-Magenis syndrome results in disruption of CLOCK gene transcription and reveals an integral role for RAI1 in the maintenance of circadian rhythmicity. Am J Hum Genet. 2012;90(6):941–9.
80. Gropman AL, Duncan WC, Smith AC. Neurologic and developmental features of the Smith-Magenis syndrome (del 17p11.2). Pediatr Neurol. 2006;34(5):337–50.
81. Nováková M, Nevsímalová S, Príhodová I, Sládek M, Sumová A. Alteration of the circadian clock in children with Smith-Magenis syndrome. J Clin Endocrinol Metab. 2012;97(2):E312–8.
82. Carpizo R, Martínez A, Mediavilla D, González M, Abad A, Sánchez-Barceló EJ. Smith-Magenis syndrome: a case report of improved sleep after treatment with beta1-adrenergic antagonists and melatonin. J Pediatr. 2006;149(3):409–11.
83. Clayton-Smith J. Clinical research on Angelman syndrome in the United Kingdom: observations on 82 affected individuals. Am J Med Genet. 1993;46:12–5.
84. Zhdanova IV, Wurtman RJ, Wagstaff J. Effects of a low dose of melatonin on sleep in children with Angelman syndrome. J Pediatr Endocrinol Metab. 1999;12:57–67.
85. Braam W, Didden R, Smits MG, Curfs LM. Melatonin for chronic insomnia in Angelman syndrome: a randomized placebo-controlled trial. J Child Neurol. 2008;23:649–54.
86. Takaesu Y, Komada Y, Inoue Y. Melatonin profile and its relation to circadian rhythm sleep disorders in Angelman syndrome patients. Sleep Med. 2012;13(9):1164–70.
87. Lehman NL. The ubiquitin proteasome system in neuropathology. Acta Neuropathol. 2009;118:329–47.
88. Miyamoto A, Oki J, Takahashi S, Okuno A. Serum melatonin kinetics and long-term melatonin treatment for sleep disorders in Rett syndrome. Brain Dev. 1999;21:59–62.

89. Appleton RE, Jones AP, Gamble C, et al. The use of Melatonin in children with neurodevelopmental disorders and impaired sleep: a randomised, double-blind, placebo-controlled, parallel study (MENDS). Health Technol Assess. 2012;16(40):i–239.

90. Miano S, Parisi P, Villa MP. The sleep phenotypes of attention deficit hyperactivity disorder: the role of arousal during sleep and implications for treatment. Med Hypotheses. 2012;79(2):147–53.

91. Van der Heijden KB, Smits MG, Van Someren EJ, Gunning WB. Idiopathic chronic sleep onset insomnia in attention-deficit/hyperactivity disorder: a circadian rhythm sleep disorder. Chronobiol Int. 2005;22:559–70.

92. Heiler S, Legenbauer T, Bogen T, Jensch T, Holtmann M. Severe mood dysregulation: in the "light" of circadian functioning. Med Hypotheses. 2011;77:692–5.

93. Staton D. The impairment of pediatric bipolar sleep: hypotheses regarding a core defect and phenotype-specific sleep disturbances. J Affect Disord. 2008;108:199–206.

94. Bendz LM, Scates AC. Melatonin treatment for insomnia in pediatric patients with attention-deficit/hyperactivity disorder. Ann Pharmacother. 2010;44:185–91.

95. Ironside S, Davidson F, Corkum P. Circadian motor activity affected by stimulant medication in children with attention-deficit/hyperactivity disorder. J Sleep Res. 2010;19(4):546–51.

96. Van der Heijden KB, Smits MG, Van Someren EJ, Ridderinkhof KR, Gunning WB. Effect of melatonin on sleep, behavior, and cognition in ADHD and chronic sleep-onset insomnia. J Am Acad Child Adolesc Psychiatry. 2007;46:233–41.

97. Hoebert M, van der Heijden KB, van Geijlswijk IM, Smits MG. Long-term follow-up of melatonin treatment in children with ADHD and chronic sleep onset insomnia. J Pineal Res. 2009;47:1–7.

98. Rybak YE, McNeely HE, Mackenzie BE, Jain UR, Levitan RD. An open trial of light therapy in adult attention-deficit/hyperactivity disorder. J Clin Psychiatry. 2006;67:1527–35.

99. Arns M, Kenemans JL. Neurofeedback in ADHD and insomnia: vigilance stabilization through sleep spindles and circadian networks. Neurosci Biobehav Rev. 2014;44:183–94.

100. Robillard R, Naismith SL, Smith KL, Rogers NL, White D, Terpening Z, Ip TK, Hermens DF, Whitwell B, Scott EM, Hickie IB. Sleep-wake cycle in young and older persons with a lifetime history of mood disorders. PLoS One. 2014;9(2):e87763.

101. Robillard R, Naismith SL, Rogers NL, Ip TK, Hermens DF, Scott EM, Hickie IB. Delayed sleep phase in young people with unipolar or bipolar affective disorders. J Affect Disord. 2013;145(2):260–3.

102. Soria V, Martinez-Amoros E, Escaramis G, Valero J, Perez-Egea R, Garcia C, Gutierrez-Zotes A, Puigdemont D, Bayes M, Crespo JM, Martorell L, Vilella E, Labad A, Vallejo J, Perez V, Menchon JM, Estivill X, Gratacos M, Urreta-vizcaya M. Differential association of circadian genes with mood disorders: CRY1 and NPAS2 are associated with unipolar major depression and CLOCK and VIP with bipolar disorder. Neuropsychopharmacology. 2010;35:1279–89.

103. Glozier N, O'Dea B, McGorry PD, Pantelis C, Amminger GP, Hermens DF, Purcell R, Scott E, Hickie IB. Delayed sleep onset in depressed young people. BMC Psychiatry. 2014;14:33.

Chapter 13
Disorders Associated with Increased Sleepiness

Soňa Nevšímalová

Abstract Sleepiness presents as increased likelihood of falling asleep during the day; however, in young children, behavioral problems such as irritability and impulsiveness can prevail. Consequence of excessive daytime sleepiness includes cognitive impairment accompanied by inattentiveness, academic difficulties, and mood changes. The most frequent causes of increased sleepiness are insufficient nocturnal sleep in obstructive sleep apnea, periodic leg movements, and restless legs syndrome (RLS). Alteration of circadian rhythms, predominantly sleep delay associated with chronic sleep loss, has a substantial role in increased daytime sleepiness in adolescence. The main topics of this chapter are disorders connected with central hypersomnolence. Narcolepsy type 1 is characterized by excessive daytime sleepiness and signs of REM-sleep dissociation, the most specific of which is cataplexy. It is connected with hypocretin deficiency in the cerebrospinal fluid. Narcolepsy type 2 has no cataplexy, and hypocretin level is usually normal. Childhood narcolepsy, particularly in young children, has some specific features. Sleep attacks may last several hours, and cataplexy may affect mainly muscles of the face. Idiopathic hypersomnia occurs rather rarely and starts usually in adolescence similarly to narcolepsy. Nocturnal sleep may be excessively long with difficult waking up and long-lasting daily naps. Multiple sleep latency test without sleep-onset REM periods (SOREMs) differentiates this disease from narcolepsy. Kleine-Levin syndrome is characterized by relapsing-remitting episodes of severe hypersomnolence, usually in association with cognitive, psychiatric, and behavioral disturbances. Secondary hypersomnolence includes cases due to medical disorders, such as brain injury, genetic disorders, and brain tumors, or due to psychiatric disorder or medication and other substance abuses.

Keywords Excessive daytime sleepiness • Insufficient and fragmented nocturnal sleep • Narcolepsy • Idiopathic hypersomnia • Kleine-Levin syndrome • Secondary hypersomnolence

S. Nevšímalová
Department of Neurology, Charles University and General Teaching Hospital,
Katerinska 30, Prague, Czech Republic
e-mail: sona.nevsimalova@lf1.cuni.cz

© Springer International Publishing Switzerland 2017
S. Nevšímalová, O. Bruni (eds.), *Sleep Disorders in Children*,
DOI 10.1007/978-3-319-28640-2_13

Introduction

In young children, recognition of increased sleepiness can by complicated by the occurrence of daytime naps in normal children. However, these generally cease by the age of 3–4 years. In addition, in young children, sleepiness may take the form of an increased rather than decreased activity mistakenly diagnosed as features of attention-deficit/hyperactivity disorder (ADHD) [1–3]. Excessive daytime sleepiness (EDS) in preschool and school children is characterized by recurrent episodes of sleepiness or prolonged nighttime sleep that affects the child's everyday life. However, in older children, EDS can be frequently misidentified as laziness, inattentiveness, boredom, and learning disability [1, 4].

Clues helping to recognize childhood daytime sleepiness may be sleeping longer hours than expected for age, daytime naps longer than normal for age, being sleepy when other children of the same age are active and alert, and/or sleeping more than previously [5].

The prevalence of daytime sleepiness increases with advancing age. In school children and adolescents, it is reported to be 17–47 % [6, 7] and in high school children even as much as 68 % [8]. The main causes of EDS are insufficient nighttime sleep, fragmented nighttime sleep, and increased need of sleep [9]. Sleep deprivation (reduced sleep quantity) is the most common cause of hypersomnolence at all ages followed by sleep fragmentation (reduced sleep quality). Disorders that increase sleep drive (hypersomnias of central origin) are relatively rare causes of EDS.

According to Hirshkowitz et al. [10], the length of nighttime sleep duration for preschool children (3–5 years) should be 10–14 h, for school children (6–13 years) 9–11 h, and for teenagers (14–17 years) 8–10 h. However, in present days, most of the children, particularly from those of the school age, reduce this length due to different causes (including school duties, free time activities, games and communications on electronic media, etc.) and co-responsibility for behaviorally induced insufficient sleep syndrome accompanied by increased daytime sleepiness [11, 12]. In adolescence, delayed sleep-wake phase disorder also plays an important role in sleep restriction.

Similarly as insufficient sleep, also fragmented sleep may induce increased daytime sleepiness, which is associated with problematic behavior, impaired learning, and/or negative mood [13, 14]. Sleep disorder breathing (SDB) carries the highest risk for daytime sleepiness followed by periodic leg movement disorder (PLMD) and restless legs syndrome (RLS). Children with SDB ranging from primary snoring to obstructive sleep apnea (OSA) syndrome represent 10–25 % of children between 3 and 12 years. Increased daytime sleepiness can be one of the leading daytime symptoms. Perez-Chada et al. [15] found in SDB children that EDS, measured by Pediatric Daytime Sleepiness Scale (PDSS), was significantly associated with academic failure. Sleep fragmentation with increased arousals leads during obstructive sleep apnea to more inattention in the daytime, while acute intermittent hypoxemia during these episodes leads to more memory deficits. Beside executive dysfunction, other affected domains are expressive language skills, visual perception, and working memory [9]. Increased daytime sleepiness may accompany frequent periodic leg movements, and in some cases, RLS can be accompanied by EDS, too.

Chapter 5 is focused on sleep laboratory tests and includes the assessment of EDS in children; hence, this part is mentioned only marginally. Appropriate subjective screening tools include sleep logs and clinical sleeping scales: (1) Pediatric Daytime Sleepiness Scale (PDSS) for young children and (2) Epworth Sleepiness Scale (ESS) and Stanford Sleepiness Scale (SSS) for older ones. Sleep questionnaires can further help in identifying and quantifying the degree of sleepiness. Nocturnal polysomnography verifies normal sleep and excludes EDS as a consequence of sleep disorder with insufficient or fragmented sleep. An objective method for sleepiness degree estimation is multiple sleep latency test (MSLT); however, no standardization data are available for children younger than 6 years. Therefore, actigraphy and/or 24-h polygraphic monitoring can be a helpful method to detect EDS in younger children [16].

The aim of this chapter is a survey of diseases characterized by central disorders of hypersomnolence. Most of these diseases start usually in adolescence and have a chronic course with a great impact on physical and mental health from childhood till adulthood. They cover four main clinical entities: (1) narcolepsy, (2) idiopathic hypersomnia, and (3) Kleine-Levin syndrome; (4) secondary cases of central disorders of hypersomnolence include cases due to brain injury, suprasellar tumors, medical disorders, medication, and/or addictive drug abuse.

Narcolepsy

Narcolepsy in children is a serious disorder marked by a chronic course and lifelong handicap in school performance, by free time activity limitation and by behavior and personality changes with a major influence on the quality of life. The total prevalence of narcolepsy ranges from 0.02 % to 0.18 % [17, 18]; data on the incidence and prevalence of pediatric narcolepsy are not available. Both genders seem to be affected at equal rates. The disease may start at any age but most frequently during the adolescence [19]. A large prospective study identified only 5 % of the cases as prepubertal [20].

The symptoms in childhood narcolepsy can differ from those in adults and lead to misinterpretations and misdiagnosis. The diagnosis in adults is often delayed more than 10 years [21], and many patients remain undiagnosed. In children, the complaint is diagnosed earlier, mostly within 2 years of the disease onset [22]. A major increase in incidence of childhood narcolepsy after H1N1 vaccination with Pandemrix together with a widespread media campaign helped to bring increased awareness and the diagnosis closer to the disease onset [23–29].

The occurrence of cataplexy in childhood narcolepsy varies between 60 and 75 % [30, 31], and sleepiness alone can precede cataplexy for months up to years.

The best predictor of cataplexy developing later in life is hypocretin deficiency [32]. Therefore, the International Classification of Sleep Disorders – ICSD-3 [3] distinguishes between two basic forms of narcolepsy: narcolepsy type 1 (with hypocretin deficiency and cataplexy) and narcolepsy type 2 (without hypocretin deficiency and without cataplexy).

Narcolepsy Type 1

According to ICSD-3 [3], the following diagnostic criteria must be met:

A. The patient has daily periods of irrepressible need to sleep or daytime lapses into sleep occurring for at least 3 months.
B. The presence of one or both of the following:

1. Cataplexy and a mean sleep latency of ≤8 min and two or more sleep-onset REM periods (SOREMPs) on an MSLT. A SOREMP (within 15 min of sleep onset) on the preceding nocturnal polysomnogram may replace one of the SOREMP on the MSLT.
2. Cerebrospinal fluid (CSF) hypocretin-1 (hcrt-1) concentration, measured by immunoreactivity, is either ≤110 pg/mL or <1/3 of mean values obtained in normal subjects with the same standardized assay.

In young children, narcolepsy may sometimes present as excessively long night sleep or as resumption of previously discontinued daytime napping [3]. In some cases, the diagnosis of narcolepsy type 1 can be difficult. Increased daytime sleepiness may sometimes be the only clinical feature for years; the sleep episodes become increasingly long, lasting up to hours; confusional arousals with features of sleep drunkenness may be present. Cataplexy may develop with a delay. In addition, lumbar puncture necessary for hcrt-1 estimation is invasive procedure, and to obtain parent's consent cannot be easy in some cases.

Clinical Features of Pediatric Cases

- Excessive daytime sleepiness
  Excessive daytime sleepiness is usually the first symptom of narcolepsy [33]. Sleep attacks in children are, as a rule, of longer duration than in adults. The children may be sleepy during lessons at school, upon return to home in the afternoon, and their naps may last up to 2–3 h without being restorative [19, 34]. Sometimes, confusional arousals with features of sleep drunkenness may be present. Owing to inattentiveness due to persistent sleepiness, they can have school problems including poor educational progress and impaired

social integration. In young children, restlessness and motor hyperactivity can sometimes overcome the drowsiness and give rise to behavioral problems [1, 35, 36].

- Cataplexy
Cataplexy is an attack of sudden muscle tone loss, evoked by emotion, most frequently by laughter (Fig. 13.1). The consciousness is always conserved, and loss of muscle tone affects both extremities symmetrically. However, cataplexy, particularly in young children, has some specific features, too. Serra et al. [21] observed in 33 % of their patients typical features of "cataplectic facies" with repetitive mouth opening, tongue protrusion, and drooping eyelids appearing close to disease onset. The muscle weakness, typical for cataplectic attack, arise in the facial region and then spreading to the trunk, arms, and lower limbs, and finally lead to falls. However, in some cases, the muscle weakness affects only a part of the body (head, shoulder, arms, knees); it does not lead to a cataplectic fall down but to what is called a partial attack. The duration of a single cataplectic episode can be only several seconds, be prolonged, or consist of multiple repetitive attacks lasting up to several minutes. Plazzi et al. [37] found that children with narcolepsy-cataplexy displayed a

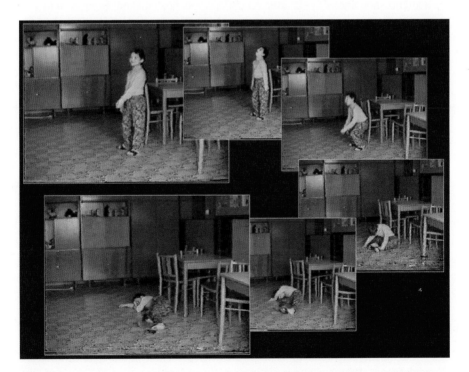

Fig. 13.1 A cataplectic attack illustrated on video sequences of a 9-year-old boy with narcolepsy-cataplexy. Note a rostro-caudal progression of weakness beginning on the mimic muscles and neck and spreading on the further body parts

complex array of "negative" (hypotonia) and "active" phenomena (ranging from perioral movements to dyskinetic-dystonic movements or stereotypes) of motor disturbances. These complex movements may disappear later in the course of the disease [38]. These phenomena in narcoleptic children may result from a recent streptococcal infection [39, 40], similar to involuntary movements evoked by streptococcal infection in children – Pediatric Autoimmune Neuropsychiatric Disorders (PANDAS).

• Associated features

Hypnagogic hallucination during falling asleep and/or hypnopompic hallucination during awakening arise as dreamlike experience occurring at the wake-sleep transition. They can be visual, auditory, and/or tactile and appear in one third up to one half of narcoleptic cases [21, 33, 41]. Visual hallucinations are more frequent and have in children usually only simple forms (colored circles, images of people or animals), rarely with an emotion content.

Sleep paralysis is an attack of temporary inability to move voluntary muscles. It is stressful, accompanied by heart rate and breathing irregularities. Sleep paralysis occurs again at sleep-wake transition and can be accompanied by hypnagogic or hypnopompic hallucinations. The episode usually lasts seconds to minutes and end spontaneously. If affected child is touched, shaken, or spoken to by a parent, sleep paralysis can be interrupted [1]. The occurrence is a little less frequent than hypnagogic/hypnopompic hallucinations [21, 33].

Disrupted nocturnal sleep with frequent awakenings, vivid dreams, and frightening nightmare annoys a majority of children with narcolepsy [21, 42]. In some cases, even REM behavior disorder can be one of the first symptoms of childhood narcolepsy [43]. However, some patients need longer sleep during the night [44], and their awakening is difficult with symptoms of sleep inertia (confusional arousal, sleep drunkenness). Similarly to morning sleep inertia, automatic behavior during the day affects up to one third of narcoleptic children. Being abnormally drowsy, they spent some time at an unpleasantly low level of alertness with movement or speech automatisms that can imitate states of cloaked consciousness, even partial epilepsy seizure [16].

Obesity frequently coexists in childhood narcolepsy (sometimes accompanied by nocturnal eating disorder), and the tendency toward increased weight gain is manifested early in the onset of the disease and connected with the appearance of cataplexy [45, 46]. It occurs despite lower caloric intake and does not appear to be due to inactivity or to medication [47, 48]. Precocious puberty can arise in children with narcolepsy type 1 in close temporal association with obesity, reflecting a broadly based hypothalamic dysfunction [49, 50].

Personality and behavior changes are often present in narcoleptic children and adolescents. They become more introverted and prone to feelings of inferiority, sorrowfulness, emotional lability, or sometimes irritability or even aggressiveness. Higher rates of behavioral problems, and particularly depression, take share in their decreased quality of life [51].

Diagnostic Evaluation

According to ICSD-3 [3], the main diagnostic criteria are hcrt-1 estimation and nocturnal polysomnography (PSG) followed by MSLT test.

Undetectable hcrt-1 level in CSF and/or lower level than 110 pg/mL are the most valuable diagnostic markers. A declining level of CSF hcrt-1 is usually closely related to appearance of cataplexy [52, 53]. An undetectable hcrt-1 level can be also one of the factors predicting the later appearance of cataplexy [32], in those children diagnosed only with isolated excessive daytime sleepiness. Human leukocyte antigen (HLA) typing can be a helpful method there. The presence of the DQB1*06:02 haplotype may add to the diagnostic probability of narcolepsy type 1, though DQB1*06:02 negativity does not exclude it [54].

The ICSD-3 [3] strongly recommended that the PSG and MSLT be preceded by at least 1 week of actigraphic recording with a sleep log. Particularly in children, actigraphy accompanied by sleep log are very useful methods illustrating the amount of daytime and nocturnal sleep (Fig. 13.2). Due to longer duration of sleep attacks in childhood narcolepsy, the examination can have a predictive value in the diagnosis. In younger children, sleep log should be completed by their parents. Both methods help to rule out sleep-wake cycle irregularity caused by poor sleep hygiene or sleep delay phase in older children [16].

Nocturnal PSG preceding MSLT illustrates a sufficiently long nighttime sleep and eliminates other causes of excessive daytime sleepiness such as sleep-disordered breathing and/or periodic limb movements. However, their presence does not rule out the presence of narcolepsy as they can coexist in a significant minority of narcoleptics [55–57]. PSG with extended EEG channels help exclude parasomnias as a cause of fragmented nocturnal sleep. In addition, SOREMP in nocturnal PSG increases significantly a probability of narcolepsy.

The MSLT is used as a standard diagnostic method in children older than 6 years, and two or more episodes of SOREMPs together with mean sleep latency ≤8 min are pathological [3]. Most MSLT studies of narcoleptic children give countenance to these criteria showing mean sleep latency to be short, even shorter than in adults, and the highest amount of SOREMPs just at the onset of the disease [20, 58, 59]. Aran et al. [60] collected, however, a cohort of 51 children with the onset both before and after puberty and found a significantly higher MSLT latency in prepubertal than in postpubertal pediatric patients. In rare cases, particularly in those with a later development of cataplexy, the MSLT criteria may not be met in the early clinical stage of the disease [52]. It can last months or even longer to develop a convincing presence of SOREMPs; MSLT then should be repeated.

In toddlers and young preschool children, continuous 24-h ambulatory PSG monitoring can serve as a practical diagnostic method. It can confirm daytime sleep-onset REM periods (SOREMPs) accompanied by sleep episodes as well as detect cataplexy [61]. It can also supply useful information in older children [62].

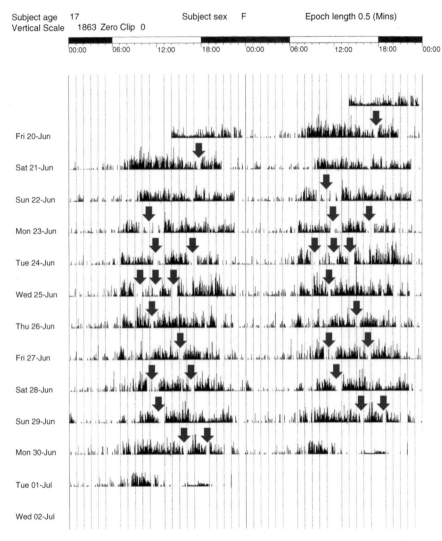

Fig. 13.2 Actigraphic recording of a 17-year-old girl with narcolepsy-cataplexy. Arrowheads indicate irregular daily naps lasting from 20 min up to more than 1 h

Predisposing and Precipitating Factors

Narcolepsy type 1 is supposed to be an autoimmune disease [63]. Several studies have described seasonal patterns in the onset of narcolepsy, which may point to a specific environmental trigger leading to the degeneration and loss of cells producing hypocretin. An increase in antibodies against beta-hemolytic streptococcus, which were strongest around onset of narcolepsy and decreased with disease duration, suggest that streptococcal infections may constitute an environmental trigger in genetically predisposed (HLA- DQB1*06:02 positive) subjects [39]. Similarly, Han et al. [24] showed a seasonal onset of narcolepsy with viral upper airway infection. A high increase in the occurrence of new cases of childhood narcolepsy type 1, occurring in a close connection with vaccination against H1N1 associated with influenza [23–29], support this hypothesis, too. Recently, a close connection between different comorbid immunopathological diseases and narcolepsy type 1 was described [64].

Genetic factors take a role in the narcolepsy type 1 predisposition. The risk of narcolepsy type 1 in the first-degree relatives of affected individuals is approximately 1–2 %. When compared to the population prevalence, this indicates a 10–40-fold increase in risk [3, 65]. So far, only a single case of narcolepsy type 1 has been described in association with a prehypocretin mutation [66].

Narcolepsy Type 2

According to ICSD-3 [3], the following diagnostic criteria must be met:

A. The patient has daily periods of irrepressible need to sleep or daytime lapses into sleep occurring for at least 3 months.
B. A mean sleep latency of ≤8 min and two or more sleep-onset REM periods (SOREMPs) are found on an MSLT. A SOREMP (within 15 min of sleep onset) on the preceding nocturnal polysomnogram may replace one of the SOREMP on the MSLT.
C. Cataplexy is absent.
D. Either CSF hcrt-1 concentration has not been measured or CSF hcrt-1 concentration measured by immunoreactivity is either >110 pg/mL or >1/3 of mean values obtained in normal subjects with the same standardized assay.
E. The hypersomnolence and/or MSLT findings are not better explained by other causes such as insufficient sleep, obstructive sleep apnea, delayed sleep phase disorder, or effect of medication or substances or their withdrawal.

If cataplexy develops later, or if CSF hcrt-1 concentration is below the recommended level, then the disorder should be reclassified as narcolepsy type 1. In all pediatric cases, the possibility of future development of cataplexy should be considered. In childhood, narcolepsy accompanied by cataplexy represents approximately two thirds of all cases of narcolepsy [16]; in adulthood this proportion increases up to 75–85 % of narcoleptic population [3].

With the exception of cataplexy, all associated features such as hypnagogic/hypnopompic hallucination and sleep paralysis can be present similarly as in narcolepsy type 1. These symptoms are very difficult to recognize in young patients. Frequent symptoms are sleep inertia during awakening; however, nocturnal sleep seems to be less impaired and fragmented. Body mass index (BMI) is lower than in narcolepsy type 1 [30]. In comparison with normal population, the frequency of HLA- DQB1*06:02 haplotype is increased; almost one half of narcolepsy type 2 patients are HLA- DQB1*06:02 positive.

The diagnosis of narcolepsy type 2 in childhood can be difficult. Normative data are not available for the MSLT in children younger than 6 years, and in peripubertal children and adolescents, the diagnosis is often challenging owing to physiologically increased need of sleep in this period. The most common causes of short sleep latencies, often with multiple SOREMPs on the MSLT, are chronic sleep deprivation and delayed sleep phase syndrome. Behavioral problems may be associated with the onset of the disorder including inattentiveness, lack of energy, insufficient nocturnal sleep, bizarre hallucinations, or a combination thereof can lead to a psychiatric misdiagnosis of schizophrenia or depression [3].

The pathophysiology of narcolepsy type 2 is unknown; the disease is probably heterogeneous and need further investigation.

Treatment and Managements of Pediatric Cases of Narcolepsy Types 1 and 2

There is no specific treatment for narcolepsy in children as distinct from adults, non-pharmacological and pharmacological means are applied in both. Children and their parents should be informed about the lifelong nature of the disease and about the need for long-term treatment. It is important to start the treatment in school age children as early as possible to avoid problems of poor achievement. Stimulant and anticataplectic medication represent only one component of the therapeutic program, and any drug therapy must take into account possible adverse effects.

The most effective non-pharmacological treatment for daytime sleepiness is regular sleep-wake schedules and planned naps. At least two planned daytime naps at lunchtime and during the afternoon (between four and five) are recommended in prepubertal and pubertal children [67]. Children should be encouraged to participate in after-school and sports activities; similarly, a well-designed exercise program can have a stimulating effect. Monitoring for emotional problems and particularly depression is also important.

Pharmacological treatment in children is not easy to manage. Almost all effective drugs used in adults, and having a positive effect on childhood symptoms, too [67], are off label according to the European Medicines Agency (EMA) and US Food and Drug Administration (FDA) rules. The only exceptions are methylphenidate and atomoxetine, used in pediatric conditions such as ADHD, and, therefore, some directions for dosage in children are available [68]. However, clinical experience suggests that modafinil decreasing EDS symptoms is an effective and safe treatment for pediatric narcolepsy comparable to adult patients [69, 70]. Similarly, sodium oxybate used in childhood cases of narcolepsy with cataplexy is safe and well tolerated. Its efficacy significantly decreases a number of cataplectic attacks and their severity, decreases daytime sleepiness, and improves nocturnal sleep [71, 72]. Table 13.1 summarizes treatment experience with the choice of drugs and their dosage given to children with narcolepsy according to their age.

Table 13.1 Treatment experience of drugs given to children to decrease sleepiness and cataplexy

Sleepiness	Cataplexy
Repeated naps during the day	Sodium oxybate (2–8 g)[a]
The whole age spectrum	The whole age spectrum
Modafinil (100–400 mg)[a]	Venlafaxine (75–150 mg)[a]
School children and adolescents	School children and adolescents
Armodafinil (50–400 mg)[a]	Fluoxetine (10–40 mg)[a]
School children and adolescents	School children and adolescents
Methylphenidate (10–30 mg)	Clomipramine (25–75) mg[a]
School children and adolescents	School children and adolescents
Atomoxetine (10–25 mg)	Imipramine (25–75 mg)[a]
School children and adolescents	School children and adolescents
Sodium oxybate (2–8 g)[a]	
The whole age spectrum	

[a]Off-label medication used in children according to EMA (European Medicines Agency) and FDA (US Food and Drug Administration) rules

Idiopathic Hypersomnia

Idiopathic hypersomnia (IH) is a rare disorder (the exact prevalence is not known) characterized by chronic non-imperative sleepiness in association with long unrefreshing daytime naps. Most of cases present difficulties reaching full alertness after awakening, even after napping with symptoms of sleep drunkenness (sleep inertia) [73].

According to ICSD [3], four diagnostic criteria must be met:

A. The patient has daily periods of irrepressible need to sleep or daytime lapses into sleep occurring for at least 3 months.
B. Cataplexy is absent.
C. An MSLT performed according to standard techniques shows fewer than two sleep-onset REM periods.
D. The presence of at least one of the following:

  1. The MSLT shows a mean sleep latency of ≤8 min.
  2. A total 24-h sleep time is ≥660 min (typically 12–14 h) on 24-h polysomnographic monitoring (performed after correction of chronic sleep deprivation) or by wrist actigraphy in association with a sleep log (average over at least 7 days with unrestricted sleep).

E. Insufficient sleep syndrome is ruled out.
F. The hypersomnolence and/or MSLT findings are not better explained by another sleep disorder, other medical or psychiatric disorders, or use of drugs or medications.

ICSD-2 [74] distinguished IH into two categories: IH with long sleep time (more than 10 h) and IH without long sleep time (less than 10 h). While IH with long sleep time is a homogeneous clinical entity with a great deal of genetic predisposition, IH without long sleep time is much more heterogeneous [75]. A recent findings using cluster analysis [76] shows that IH without long sleep time is close to narcolepsy type 2.

Nocturnal sleep demonstrates a high efficiency, and sleep drunkenness is present in one up to two thirds of IH cases. It is defined as prolonged difficulty waking up with repeated returns to sleep, automatic behavior, and confusion lasting usually 15 up to 30 min, rarely more than 1 h. Affected subjects do not hear alarm clock, they must be very heavily and repeatedly awakened by their parents or bed partners, or they used some specific alarms mechanisms. Cerebellar symptoms and decreased tendon reflexes are found if patients are neurologically examined during this state [77].

The disease develops usually during adolescence or young adulthood (the mean age of onset is between 16 and 21 years). CSF hcrt-1 level is normal, and no HLA predisposition has been found [3, 78, 79]. A dysfunction of the autonomic nervous system may be present as an associated symptom. It includes orthostatic disturbances (even faintness), headaches, temperature dysregulations, and peripheral vascular complaints (including Raynaud syndrome). Nevsimalova et al. [80] described in IH patients prolonged melatonin secretion with delayed peaks of both circadian hormones – melatonin as well as cortisol.

The IH diagnosis can be facilitated by a specific PSG protocol recommended by Billiard [75, 81, 82]. The first night of PSG examination is followed by a standard MSLT that continues with 24-h lasting PSG monitoring and freedom to sleep "ad libitum." Figure 13.3 illustrates this protocol in a young woman with IH, whose younger brother, father, and cousin were affected according to medical history, too (Fig. 13.4). In spite of a strong genetic predisposition, found in the literature in many cases [83, 84], no convincing molecular genetic background has been found [85].

Differential diagnosis is difficult, particularly in children and adolescents. A physiologically increased need of sleep should be adapted to the ICDD-3 [3] criteria. Hypersomnolence due to delayed sleep phase disorder, obstructive sleep apnea,

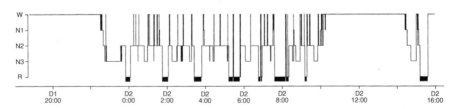

Fig. 13.3 A young 24-year-old woman suffering from idiopathic hypersomnia from childhood. Multiple sleep latency test (MSLT – not shown), registered after the first night of polysomnography (PSG), showed a shortened mean sleep latency of 5.2 min without sleep-onset REM periods (SOREMPs). PSG following the MSLT through the second day for 21 h demonstrated seven nocturnal cycles of NREM-REM sleep and one afternoon sleep cycle. The total sleep duration during the second day of PSG registration was 12 h and 12 min

Fig. 13.4 A family tree of the 24-year-old woman with idiopathic hypersomnia. Arrowhead indicates our proband; her young brother, father, and cousin suffering from the same complaints, however, refused to be examined in our Sleep Lab

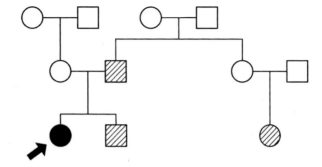

insufficient sleep syndrome, and abuse of drugs should be excluded. The prolonged attacks of daytime sleepiness in children, frequently accompanied by sleep drunkenness, is sometimes difficult to differentiate from narcolepsy. Difficulties in diagnosis can be, e.g., illustrated by an interesting patient of ours. A 10-year-old boy with increase daytime sleepiness was PSG examined, and his MSLT showed the borderline mean sleep latency without any SOREMPs. Two years later, typical cataplectic attacks appeared, the MSLT was repeated, mean sleep latency became shorter, and SOREMPs appeared. Therefore, the diagnosis was changed to narcolepsy type 1. We have to consider reclassification of the diagnosis in all children and adolescent cases when clinical picture is changing. An interface with behavioral and mood disturbances, included in psychiatric disorders, should be taken in account in the differential diagnosis, too [4].

IH management is more difficult than in narcolepsy; no data are available for children or adolescents. EMA withdrew the indication of modafinil for the treatment of IH in 2010 for insufficient data. However, Lavault et al. [86], as well as Mayer et al. [87] demonstrated in adult patients that modafinil has an excellent benefit/risk ratio in IH, similar to its effect on narcolepsy. The number of reported naps and duration of daytime sleepiness decreased significantly. Total sleep time of nocturnal sleep was slightly reduced, and the sleep diaries showed increases in feeling refreshed in the morning. Adverse events were mild to moderate. The two studies concluded that modafinil is an effective and safe medication in the treatment of IH patients. The recommended dosage was similar to that of medication used in narcolepsy. As regards the children and adolescents, treatment with methylphenidate and atomoxetine (used in ADHD) may be prescribed; however, treatment with modafinil is "off label," similarly to narcolepsy.

Kleine-Levin Syndrome

Kleine-Levin syndrome (KLS), known also as recurrent hypersomnia or periodic hypersomnolence, is a rare sleep disorder with the prevalence 1–2 cases per million [3], more frequently found in the Jewish population. The main features are intermittent periods of hypersomnolence accompanied by behavioral and cognitive disturbances, hyperphagia and in some cases hypersexuality [88]. According to ICSD-3 [3], four diagnostic criteria must be met:

A. The patient experiences at least two recurrent episodes of excessive sleepiness and sleep duration, each persisting for 2 days to 5 weeks.
B. Episodes recur usually more than once a year and at least once every 18 months.
C. The patient must demonstrate at least one of the following during episodes:

   1. Cognitive dysfunction
   2. Altered perception
   3. Eating disorder (hyperphagia or anorexia)
   4. Disinhibited behavior (such as hypersexuality)

D. The hypersomnolence and related symptoms are not better explained by another sleep disorder; other medical, neurologic, or psychiatric disorders (especially bipolar disorder); or the use of drugs or medications.

The usual age at onset is adolescence with males predominating (sex ratio 2:1). The first episode is often triggered by a flu-like illness or an infection of the upper airway and reoccurs in 1 or several months. The more frequent episodes are usually marked by shorter duration. A typical episode lasts approximately 10 days, during which patients may sleep as long as 16–20 h per day, waking or getting up only to eat and void. They remain rousable but are irritable if prevent from sleeping. Cognitive changes including difficulties speaking and reading, together with a specific feeling of derealization, and eating disturbance accompany almost all episodes. Overweight difference, caused by compulsive eating, can reach up to several kilograms. During the episode, about half of the patients experience depressed mood and hypersexuality [3, 89, 90]. The attacks cause school absenteeism; children have usually anterograde amnesia on the state. The functioning between episodes is normal.

If disease starts during childhood and adolescence, it typically resolves after a median of 14 years; in adult onset cases, the course may be more prolonged. The cause of this mysterious disappearance is not known. The earliest age of onset according to ICSD-3 [3] can be illustrated by the case of a 4-year-old boy with KLS [91]. However, almost 30 years ago, we described [92] a very interesting girl with periodic hypersomnia started in the infant age. She was repeatedly hospitalized for loss of consciousness of unknown etiology in an acute pediatric unit. The episodes lasted several days. EEG examination during one of these episodes showed quite normal sleep phenomena. The girl was therefore referred to our department, where recurrent hypersomnia was diagnosed. A longitudinal follow-up showed decreasing frequency and severity of these attacks of hypersomnolence. During puberty, these usually accompanied only some flu-like infection, and by 18 years of age, they completely disappeared.

EEG changes showing general deceleration of background activity and accompanied by paroxysmal high-voltage episodes of generalized and synchronous delta or theta waves were often described during the episodes. Sleep efficiency is poor, and nonspecific changes in sleep cycles together with changes in proportion of slow-wave and REM sleep were observed [93]. Figure 13.5 illustrates PSG monitoring of the second part of a KLS episode, when an 11-year-old girl was brought by parents to our department after more than 1 day lasting attack at home. Her first episode was provoked by an inflammation resembling encephalitis.

The KLS etiology is unknown; however, viral and autoimmune causative factors were suggested, promoted by often reported flu-like symptoms at the onset, as the most frequent precipitating factors. A rare KLS case preceded by encephalitis was reported [94]. In another case [95], even association with streptococcal infection (PANDAS) and KLS was described as pointing to an autoimmune etiology of both diseases. Huang et al. [96] found that an immunoresponsive HLA-DQB1, DQB1*0602 was detected in significantly higher quantities in patients with KLS than in controls. Dauvilliers et al. [97] presented an interesting role of hypothalamic dysfunction in the etiology of the attacks. The authors described the mean CSF hcrt-1 level in KLS during the asymptomatic periods as normal. However, in one patient, CSF samples were available during both symptomatic and asymptomatic periods. The results showed a twofold decrease in hcrt-1 level during one of the hypersomnia episodes when compared with the asymptomatic period.

Differences between attacks and asymptomatic periods have been documented also with several neuroimaging methods. Single-photon emission com-

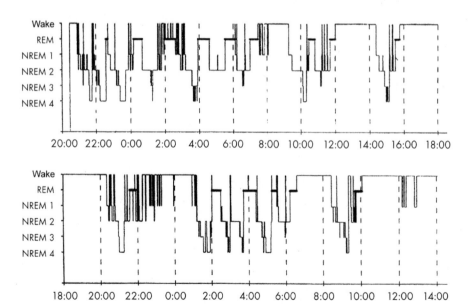

Fig. 13.5 An 11-year-old girl with Kleine-Levin syndrome. Polysomnography (PSG) illustrates the second part of her attack of sleepiness. The girl was brought to our sleep lab by her parents from home (almost 400 km away) for being sleepy for more than 1 day. The first monitored day sleep cycles include mostly interrupted superficial NREM sleep with an increased amount of REM sleep (nine irregular cycles), the second day illustrates six irregular cycles with increased percentage of REM sleep and blowing sleepiness away

puted tomography (SPECT) showed that depersonalization and derealization during symptomatic periods strongly correlated with the hypoperfusion of the right and left parietotemporal junctions and that defects in the dorsomedial prefrontal cortex may cause apathy. Persistent hypoperfusion in the diencephalic and the associative cortical area during asymptomatic periods is a marker of the disease, suggestive of an effort to compensate these deficient circuitries [98]. Similarly, functional brain imaging studies during episodes are frequently abnormal, showing hypometabolism in the thalamus, hypothalamus, mesial temporal lobe, and frontal lobe. Some of these abnormalities persist during asymptomatic periods in half of the patients. Hypoperfusion of both thalami is a consistent finding during the symptomatic period. It almost completely disappears during the asymptomatic period in most of the cases [99]. The longer the duration of this syndrome, the more extended the hypoperfusion regions during the asymptomatic period.

Menstrual-related KLS, a rare form of KLS, is also known as menstrual-related hypersomnia. Billiard et al. [100] collected in their meta-analytic review 339 cases of recurrent hypersomnia; 239 were cases of typical KLS, 54 cases of KLS without compulsive eating, 27 cases were recurrent hypersomnia with a different comorbidity, and 18 cases with menstrual-related hypersomnia were rated as a variant of recurrent hypersomnia.

Management of KLS is difficult. There is no conclusive treatment during the episode as well as during interepisodic period. Only lithium had a higher reported response rate (in 41 %) for stopping relapses when compared to medical abstention. Further medication such as carbamazepin, gabapentin, and other antiepileptics had a worse effect [90, 101–103]. Exceptionally, even sodium oxybate can be offered as an alternative option for KLS treatment [104].

Secondary Increased Sleepiness of Central Origin

Secondary central hypersomnolence occurs in children most frequently as a cause of medical disorder like (1) brain injury (posttraumatic etiology), in (2) association with different genetic disorders, and (3) secondary to brain tumors – most frequently in the suprasellar region. (4) Cases of some other etiologies such as medication, substance abuse, and of psychiatric origin should be considered in the differential diagnosis, too.

According to ICSD-3 [3], the following criteria must be met:

(A) The patient has daily periods of irrepressible need to sleep or daytime lapses into sleep occurring for at least 3 months.
(B) The daytime sleepiness occurs as a consequence of a significant underlying medical or neurological condition.
(C) If an MSLT is performed, the mean sleep latency is ≤8 min, and fewer than two SOREMPs are observed.

Posttraumatic Hypersomnia

Increased sleepiness appears to be common after traumatic brain injury (TBI). According to ICSD-3 [3], up to 28 % of all patients have EDS as a consequence of sever traumatic brain lesion. Osorio et al. [105] evaluated a multicentric study in the first 6 months after TBI in adolescent. They found that 51 % of adolescents with moderate to severe TBI showed significant daytime somnolence. Their daytime sleepiness correlated with TBI severity and predicted executive functioning difficulties in everyday circumstances. Greater sleep disturbance was described even after a mild TBI in younger school children [106]. Stores and Stores [107] suggest that TBI followed by sleep disorders in children is seriously neglected. Children with more frequent injuries had significantly more sleep problems in general, particularly sleep-related anxiety [108]. Besides daytime sleepiness, also shortened nocturnal sleep was reported [109]. On the other hand, it is a well-known fact that daytime sleepiness and short night sleep duration are two major reasons in children for further accidental injury [110].

Genetic Disorders Associated with Primary Central Nervous System (CNS) Somnolence

Genetic disorders associated with primary CNS somnolence were described in the Chapter 16, focused on "sleep in neurological and neurodevelopmental diseases." Daytime sleepiness may be a symptom of different chromosomal abnormalities and microdeletion syndromes like Smith-Magenis, Prader-Willi, fragile X, or Moebius syndrome. EDS and predominantly cataplexy can be a symptom of neurometabolic disorders such as Niemann-Pick type C disease [111]. Myotonic dystrophy as an example of neuromuscular diseases with triplet genetic component and increased daytime sleepiness was included in the chapter, too.

Secondary Hypersomnia due to Brain Tumors

Several studies showed that children treated for CNS tumors have increased somnolence, significantly increased fatigue and worsening daily functioning. The sleep symptoms did not appear to be directly related to the specific therapy the child received, nor to the presence of residual tumor. The primary determinant of the sleep symptoms lies rather in the area of the damaged brain. Particularly an affection of the hypothalamic/pituitary region will develop EDS regardless of whether the damage resulted from a tumor surgery, hydrocephalus, or radiation aimed at the whole brain or was localized in the suprasellar area [4, 11–114]. Craniopharyngiomas are the best studied tumor in childhood. Although it is histologically a benign tumor arising from remnants of Rathke's pouch in the hypothalamic-pituitary region, the prognosis is not good. The two common treatment approaches include primary total resection or limited resection followed by radiotherapy. However, severe late treatment complications decrease the quality of life for many long-time survivors. The most frequent complaints are endocrine deficiency including obesity and visual complications followed by neurological complications and significant school problems [115]. Increased daytime sleepiness is referred in approximately 30 % of craniopharyngioma patients [115, 116], sometimes with the conventional PSG criteria for secondary narcolepsy [117, 118]. Melatonin substitution is recommended on daytime sleepiness in childhood craniopharyngioma patients [118, 119].

Other Causes of Secondary CNS Hypersomnolence

Central hypersomnolence can be a consequence of any endocrine disorder – e.g., hypothyroidism. Every sleepy child needs to have screening for thyroid function to rule out subclinical hypothyroidism, especially in obese children with sleep-disordered breathing [120]. Also metabolic encephalopathy (of, e.g., hepatic origin), chronic renal, adrenal, or pancreatic insufficiency, can cause increased sleepiness [3]. A high dosage of anticonvulsants in epileptic children and/or antihistamines in children with allergy is the most frequent cause of hypersomnia due to sedating medication [120, 121]. Daytime sleepiness can occur in adolescents particularly with abuse of alcohol, marijuana, and other addictive substances. Hypersomnia associated with psychiatric conditions includes mainly mood disorders. Hypersomnolence occurs in 10–20 % of children with major depression, sometimes in combination with insomnia. Children and adolescents with depression generally manifest more pronounced symptoms, such as anhedonia and weight loss. Less frequently increased sleepiness can be associated with conversion or undifferentiated somatoform disorder, accidentally with other mental disorders such as schizoaffective disorder, adjustment disorder, or personality disorders [3].

Conclusion

Increased sleepiness in children and adolescents is a common feature. In toddlers and preschool children, it can be masked by irritability, inattentiveness, emotional lability, and hyperactive behavior. One of the most frequent causes of EDS is poor sleep hygiene with chronic sleep deprivation. However, other sleep disorders with interrupted nocturnal sleep such as sleep apnea syndrome and periodic leg movements should be ruled out. Therefore, nocturnal PSG followed by MSLT is a gold standard examination for increased sleepiness in children over 6 years. A course of actigraphic monitoring is a useful screening method excluding poor hygiene and sleep delayed phase, particularly in adolescents. Central disorders of hypersomnolence like narcolepsy are serious and long-lasting diseases that markedly influence quality of life. The management is difficult; almost all effective treatment is for children "off label." Therefore, controlled multicentric clinical trials are needed to verify effective treatment. Another important relation is a close connection between sleepiness and mood which is bidirectional. Sleepiness and fatigue can be a symptom of depression, while on the contrary, sleepiness frequently leads to changes of mood and behavior. A close cooperation between child neurologist, psychiatrist, and psychologist is needed, accompanied by understanding from teachers and special educationalists. Daytime sleepiness is an important symptom of impaired health during childhood and adolescence; hence, a comprehensive management is desirable.

References

1. Stores G, Montgomery P, Wiggs L. The psychosocial problems of children with narcolepsy and those with excessive daytime sleepiness of uncertain origin. Pediatrics. 2006;118:1116–23.
2. Walters AS, Silvestri R, Zucconi M, et al. Review of the possible relationship and hypothetical links between attention deficit hyperactivity disorder (ADHD) and simple sleep related movement disorders, parasomnias, hypersomnias and circadian rhythm disorders. J Clin Sleep Med. 2008;4:591–600.
3. American Academy of Sleep Medicine. International classification of sleep disorders-ICSD, 3rd ed. Westchester: American Academy of Sleep Medicine; 2014.
4. Kotagal S. Hypersomnia in children: interface with psychiatric disorders. Child Adolesc Psychiatr Clin N Am. 2009;18:967–77.
5. Kothare SV, Kaleyias J. The clinical and laboratory assessment of the sleepy child. Semin Pediatr Neurol. 2008;15:61–9.
6. Saarenpaa OS, Laippala P, Koivikko M. Subjective sleepiness in children. Fam Pract. 2000;17:129–33.
7. Gaina A, Sekine M, Hamanishi S, et al. Daytime sleepiness and associated factors in Japanese school children. J Pediatr. 2007;151:518–22.
8. Gibson ES, Powles AC, Thabane I, et al. Sleepiness is serious in adolescence: two surveys of 3235 Canadian students. BMC Public Health. 2006;6:116.
9. Kothare SV, Kaleyias J. Sleepiness in children. In: Thorpy MJ, Billiard M, editors. Sleepiness: causes, consequences and treatment. Cambridge: Cambridge University; 2011;262–76.
10. Hirshkowitz M, Whiton K, Albert SM, et al. National sleep foundation´s sleep time duration recommendations: methodology and results summary. Sleep Health. 2015;1:40–3.
11. Kohyma J. A newly proposed disease condition produced by light exposure during night: asynchronization. Brain Dev. 2009;31:255–73.
12. Gradisar M, Gardner G, Dohnt H. Recent worldwide sleep patterns and problems during adolescence: a review and meta-analysis of age, region, and sleep. Sleep Med. 2011;12:110–8.
13. O'Brien LM. The neurocognitive effects of sleep disruption in children and adolescents. Child Adolesc Psychiatr Clin N Am. 2009;18:813–23.
14. Calhoun SL, Fernandez-Mendoza J, Vgontzas AN, et al. Learning, attention/hyperactivity, and conduct problems as sequelae of excessive daytime sleepiness in a general population study of young children. Sleep. 2012;35:627–32.
15. Perez-Chada D, Perez-Lloret S, Videla AJ, et al. Sleep disordered breathing and daytime sleepiness are associated with poor academic performance in teenagers. A study using the Pediatric Daytime Sleepiness Scale (PDSS). Sleep. 2007;30:1698–703.

16. Nevsimalova S. The diagnosis and treatment of pediatric narcolepsy. Cur Neurol Neurosci Rep. 2014;14:469–78.
17. Silber MH, Krahn LE, Olson E, Pankratz VS. The epidemiology of narcolepsy in Olmsted County, Minnesota: a population-based study. Sleep. 2002;25:197–202.
18. Longstreth Jr WT, Koepsell TD, Ton TG, et al. The epidemiology of narcolepsy. Sleep. 2007;30:13–26.
19. Nevsimalova S, Buskova J, Kemlink D, et al. Does age at the onset of narcolepsy influence the course and severity of the disease? Sleep Med. 2009;10:967–72.
20. Guilleminault C, Pelayo R. Narcolepsy in prepubertal children. Ann Neurol. 1998;43:135–42.
21. Serra L, Montagna P, Mignot E, et al. Cataplexy features in childhood narcolepsy. Mov Dis. 2008;23:858–65.
22. Einen MA, Aran A, Mignot E, Nishino S. Pre-versus post-pubertal narcolepsy in children. Sleep. 2009;32(Suppl):A249–50.
23. Dauvilliers Y, Montplaisir J, Cochen V, Desautels A, Einen M, Lin L, et al. Post-H1NH1 narcolepsy-cataplexy. Sleep. 2010;33:1428–30.
24. Han F, Lin L, Warby SC, et al. Narcolepsy onset is seasonal and increased following the 2009 H1N1 pandemic in China. Ann Neurol. 2011;70:410–7.
25. Partinen M, Saarenpää-Heikkilä O, Ilveskoski I, et al. Increased incidence and clinical picture of childhood narcolepsy following the 2009 H1N1 pandemic vaccination campaign in Finland. PLoS One. 2012;7:e33723.
26. Nohynek H, Jokinen J, Partinen M, et al. AS03 adjuvanted AH1N1 vaccine associated with an abrupt increase in the incidence of childhood narcolepsy in Finland. PLoS One. 2012;7:e33536.
27. Szakács A, Darin N, Hallböök T. Increased childhood incidence of narcolepsy in western Sweden after H1N1 influenza vaccination. Neurology. 2013;80:1315–21.
28. Heier MS, Gautvik KM, Wannag E, et al. Incidence of narcolepsy in Norwegian children and adolescents after vaccination against H1N1 influenza A. Sleep Med. 2013;14:867–71.
29. Nevsimalova S. Childhood narcolepsy and H1N1 vaccination: stirring up a sleeping menance? Sleep Med. 2014;15:159–60.
30. Nevsimalova S, Jara C, Prihodova I, et al. Clinical features of childhood narcolepsy. Can cataplexy be foretold? Eur J Paed Neuro. 2011;15:320–5.
31. Vendrame M, Havaligi N, Matedeen-Ali C, et al. Narcolepsy in children: a single-center clinical experience. Pediatr Neurol. 2008;38:314–20.
32. Andlauer O, Moore H, Rico T, et al. Predictors of hypocretin (orexin) deficiency in narcolepsy without cataplexy. Sleep. 2012;35:1247–55.
33. Peterson PC, Husain AM. Pediatric narcolepsy. Brain Dev. 2008;30:609–23.
34. Challamel MJ. Hypersomnia in children. In: Billiard M, editor. Sleep-physiology, investigation and medicine. New York: Kluwer Academic/Plenum Publishers; 2003. p. 457–68.
35. Wise MS. Child Narcolepsy. 1998;50 Suppl 1:S37–42.
36. Nevsimalova S. Narcolepsy in childhood. Sleep Med Rev. 2009;13:169–80.
37. Plazzi G, Pizza F, Palaia V, et al. Complex movement disorders at disease onset in childhood narcolepsy with cataplexy. Brain. 2011;134:3480–92.
38. Pizza F, Franceschini C, Peltola H, et al. Clinical and polysomnographic course of childhood narcolepsy with cataplexy. Brain. 2013;136:3787–95.
39. Aran A, Lin L, Nevsimalova S, et al. Elevated anti-streptococcal antibodies in patients with recent narcolepsy onset. Sleep. 2009;32:979–83.
40. Natarajan N, Jain SV, Chaudhry H, et al. Narcolepsy-cataplexy: is streptococcal infection a trigger? J Clin Sleep Med. 2013;9:269–70.
41. Challamel MJ, Mazzola ME, Nevšímalová S, et al. Sleep. 1994;17 Suppl 8:S17–20.
42. Pisko J, Pastorek L, Buskova J, et al. Nightmares in narcolepsy – under-investigated symptom? Sleep Med. 2014;15:967–72.
43. Nevsimalova S, Prihodova I, Kemlink D, et al. REM behavior disorder (RBD) can be one of the first symptoms of childhood narcolepsy. Sleep Med. 2007;8:784–6.

44. Vernet C, Arnulf A. Narcolepsy with long sleep time: a specific entity? Sleep. 2009;32:1229–35.
45. Kotagal S, Krahn LE, Slocumb N. A putative link between childhood narcolepsy and obesity. Sleep Med. 2004;5:147–50.
46. Inocente CO, Lavault S, Lecendreux M, et al. Impact of obesity in children with narcolepsy. CNS Neurosci Ther. 2013;19:521–8.
47. Lammers GJ, Pijl H, Iestra J, et al. Spontaneous food choice in narcolepsy. Sleep. 1996;19:75–6.
48. Kok SW, Overeem S, Visscher TL, et al. Hypocretin deficiency in narcoleptic humans is associated with abdominal obesity. Obes Res. 2003;11:1147–54.
49. Plazzi G, Parmeggiani A, Mignot E, et al. Narcolepsy-cataplexy associated with precocious puberty. Neurology. 2006;66:1577–9.
50. Poli F, Pizza F, Mignot E, et al. High prevalence of precocious puberty and obesity in childhood narcolepsy with cataplexy. Sleep. 2013;36:175–81.
51. Inocente CO, Gustin MP, Lauvault S, Perret AG, Christol N, et al. Quality of life in children with narcolepsy. CNS Neurosci Ther. 2014;20:763–71.
52. Kubota H, Kanbayashi T, Tanabe Y, et al. Decreased cerebrospinal fluid hypocretin-1 levels near the onset of narcolepsy in 2 prepubertal children. Sleep. 2003;26:555–7.
53. Savvidou A, Knudsen S, Olsson-Engman M, et al. Hypocretin deficiency develops during onset of human narcolepsy with cataplexy. Sleep. 2013;36:147–8.
54. Mignot E, Hayduk R, Black J, et al. HLA DQB1*0602 is associated with cataplexy in 509 narcoleptic patients. Sleep. 1997;20:1012–20.
55. Kotagal S, Hartse KM, Walch JK. Characteristics of narcolepsy in pre-teenaged children. Pediatrics. 1990;85:205–9.
56. Han F, Lin L, Li J, et al. Presentation of primary hypersomnia in Chinese children. Sleep. 2011;5:627–32.
57. Jambhekar SK, Com G, Jones E, et al. Periodic limb movements during sleep in children with narcolepsy. J Clin Sleep Med. 2011;7:597–601.
58. Dauvilliers Y, Montplaisir Molinari N, et al. Age at onset of narcolepsy in two large populations of patients in France and Quebeck. Neurology. 2001;57:2029–33.
59. Dauvilliers Y, Gosselin A, Paquet J, et al. Effect of age on MSLT results in patients with narcolepsy-cataplexy. Neurology. 2004;62:46–50.
60. Aran A, Einen M, Lin L, et al. Clinical and therapeutic aspects of childhood-narcolepsy-cataplexy: a retrospective study of 51 children. Sleep. 2010;33:1457–64.
61. Nevsimalova S, Roth B, Zouhar A, Zemanova H. The occurrence of narcolepsy-cataplexy and periodic hypersomnia in early childhood. In: Koella WP, Obal F, Schulz H, Wisser P, editors. Sleep '86. Stuttgart: Gustav Fisher Verlag; 1988. p. 399–401.
62. Bouvier E, Arnulf I, Claustrat B, et al. Do children with idiopathic narcolepsy have a long sleep time? Sleep. 2009;32(Suppl):A97.
63. Mignot E. Genetic and familial aspects of narcolepsy. Neurology. 1998;50 Suppl 1:S16–22.
64. Martinez-Orozco FJ, Vicario JL, Villalibre-Valderrey I, et al. J Sleep Res. 2014;23:414–9.
65. Nevšímalová S, Mignot E, Šonka K, Arrigoni JL. Genetic aspects of narcolepsy-cataplexy in the Czech Republic. Sleep. 1997;20:1021–6.
66. Peyron C, Faraco J, Rogers W, et al. A mutation in a case of early onset narcolepsy and a generalized absence of hypocretin peptides in human marcoleptic brains. Nat Med. 2000;6:991–7.
67. Guilleminault C, Fromherz S. Narcolepsy. diagnosis and management. In: Kryger MH, Roth T, Dement WC, editors. Principles and practice of sleep medicine. 4th ed. Philadelphia: Elsevier Sounders; 2007. p. 780–90.
68. Greenhil LL, Pliszka S, Dulcan MK, et al. Practice parameter for the use of stimulant medication in the treatment of children, adolescents, and adults. J Am Acad Child Adolesc Psychiatry. 2002;41 Suppl 2:26S–49.
69. Lecendreux M, Bruni O, Franco P, et al. Clinical experience suggests that modafinil is an effective and safe treatment for paediatric narcolepsy. J Sleep Res. 2012;21:481–3.

70. Davies M, Wilton L, Shakir S. Safety profile of modafinil across a range of prescribing indications, including off-label use, in a primary care setting in England. Drug Saf. 2013;36:237–46.
71. Lecendreux M, Poli F, Oudertte D, et al. Tolerance and efficacy of sodium oxybate in childhood narcolepsy with cataplexy: a retrospective study. Sleep. 2012;35:709–11.
72. Mansukhani MP, Kotagal S. Sodium oxybate in the treatment of childhood narcolepsy-cataplexy: a retrospective study. Sleep Med. 2012;13:606–10.
73. Kotagal S. Hypersomnia in children. Sleep Med Clin. 2012;7:379–89.
74. American Academy of Sleep Medicine. International classification of sleep disorders. Diagnostic and coding manual. 2nd ed. Westchester: American Academy of Sleep Medicine; 2005.
75. Billiard M. From narcolepsy with cataplexy to idiopathic hypersomnia without long sleep time. Sleep Med. 2009;10:943–4.
76. Sonka K, Susta M, Billiard M. Narcolepsy with and without cataplexy, idiopathic hypersomnia with and without long sleep time: a cluster analysis. J Sleep Res. 2015;16:225–31.
77. Roth B, Nevsimalova S, Sagova V, et al. Neurological, psychological and polygraphic findings in sleep drunkenness. Schweiz Arch Neurol Neurochir Psychiatr. 1981;129:209–22.
78. Billiard M, Merle C, Carlander B, et al. Idiopathic hypersomnia. Psychiatr Clin Neurosci. 1998;52:125–9.
79. Kanbayashi T, Inoue Y, Chiba S, et al. CSF hypocretin-1 (orexin-A) concentration in narcolepsy with and without cataplexy and idiopathic hypersomnia. J Sleep Res. 2002;11:91–3.
80. Nevsimalova S, Blazejova K, Illnerova H, et al. A contribution to pathophysiology of idiopathic hypersomnia. In: Ambler Z, Nevsimalova S, Kadanka Z, Rossini PM, editors. Clinical neurophysiology at the beginning of the 21st century. Suppl Clin Neurophysiol. 2000;53:366–70.
81. Billiard M, Dauvilliers Y. Idiopathic hypersomnia. Sleep Med Rev. 2001;5:349–58.
82. Billiard M. Idiopathic hypersomnia. In: Thorpy MJ, Billiard M, editors. Sleepiness: causes, consequences and treatment. Cambridge: Cambridge University Press; 2011. p. 126–35.
83. Nevsimalova-Bruhova S, Roth B. Heredofamilial aspects of narcolepsy and hypersomnia. Schweiz Arch Neurol Neurochir Psychiat. 1972;110:45–54.
84. Janackova S, Motte J, Bakchine S, Sforza E. Idiopathic hypersomnia: a report of three adolescent-onset cases in a two-generation family. J Child Neurol. 2011;26:522–5.
85. Nevsimalova S. Idiopathic hypersomnia. In: Chokroverty S, Billiard M, editors. Sleep medicine. a comprehensive guide to its development, clinical milestones, and advances in treatment. New York: Springer; 2015. p. 223–8.
86. Lavault S, Dauvilliers Y, Drouot X, et al. Benefit and risk of modafinil in idiopathic hypersomnia vs. narcolepsy. Sleep Med. 2011;12:550–6.
87. Mayer G, Benes H, Young P, et al. Modafinil in the treatment of idiopathic hypersomnia without long sleep time – a randomized, double-blind, placebo-controlled study. J Sleep Res. 2015;24:74–81.
88. Remdurg S. Kleine-Levin syndrome: etiology, diagnosis, and treatment. Ann Indian Acad Neurol. 2010;13:241–6.
89. Arnulf I, Zeitzer JM, File J, et al. Kleine-Levin syndrome: a systematic review of 186 cases in the literature. Brain. 2005;2763–76.
90. Arnulf I, Lin L, Gadoth N, et al. Kleine-Levin syndrome: a systematic study of 108 patients. Ann Neurol. 2008;63:482–92.
91. Ramnath B, Kalaniti K. Kleine-Levin syndrome. Indian Pediatr. 2008;45:1007.
92. Nevšímalová S, Roth B, Zouhar A, Zemanová H. The occurrence of narcolepsy-cataplexy and periodic hypersomnia in infancy and early childhood. In: Koella WP, Obal F, Schultz H, Visser P, editors. Sleep 1986. Stuttgart: Gustav Fischer Verlag; 1988. p. 399–401.
93. Huang YS, Lin YH, Guilleminault C. Polysomnography in Kleine-Levin syndrome. Neurology. 2008;70:795–801.
94. Sethi S, Bhargava SC. Kleine-Levin syndrome and encephalitis. Indian J Pediatr. 2002;69:999–1000.

95. Das A, Radhakrishnan A. A case of PANDAS with Kleine-Levin type hypersomnia. Sleep Med. 2012;13:319–20.
96. Huang JC, Liao HT, Yeh GC, Hung KL. Distribution of HLA-DQB1 alleles in patients with Kleine-Levin syndrome. J Clin Neurosci. 2012;19:628–30.
97. Dauvilliers Y, Baumann CR, Carlander B, et al. CSF hypocretin-1 levels in narcolepsy, Kleine-Levin syndrome, and other hypersomnias and neurological conditions. J Neurol Neurosurg Psychiat. 2003;74:1167–73.
98. Kas A, Lavault S, Habert MO, Arnulf I. Feeling unreal: a functional imaging study in patients with Kleine-Levin syndrome. Brain. 2014;137:2077–87.
99. Huang YS, Guilleminault C, Kao PF, Liu FY. SPECT findings in Kleine-Levin syndrome. Sleep. 2005;28:955–60.
100. Billiard M, Jaussent I, Dauvilliers Y, Besset A, et al. Recurrent hypersomnias: a review of 339 cases. Sleep Med Rev. 2011;15:247–57.
101. Loganathan S, Manjunath S, Jhirwal OP, et al. Lithium prophylaxis in Kleine-Levin syndrome. J Neuropsychiatry Clin Neurosci. 2009;21:107–8.
102. Mukaddes NM, Kora ME, Bilge S. Carbamazepine for Kleine-Levin syndrome. J Am Acad Child Adolesc Psychiatry. 1999;38:791.
103. Itokawa K, Fukui M, Ninomiya M, et al. Gabapentin for Kleine-Levin syndrome. Inter Med. 2009;48:1183–5.
104. Ortega-Albas JJ, Diaz JR, Lopez-Bernabe R, et al. Treatment of Kleine-Levin syndrome with sodium oxybate. Sleep Med. 2011;12:730–1.
105. Osorio MB, Kurowski BG, Beebe D, et al. Association of daytime somnolence with executive functioning in the first 6 months after adolescent traumatic injury. PM R. 2013;5:554–662.
106. Milroy G, Dorris L, McMillan TM. Sleep disturbance following mild traumatic brain injury in childhood. J Pediatr Psychol. 2008;33:242–7.
107. Stores G, Stores R. Sleep disorders in children with traumatic brain injury: a case of serious neglect. Dev Med Child Neurol. 2013;55:797–805.
108. Owens JA, Fernando S, Mc Guinn M. Sleep disturbance and injury risk in young children. Behav Sleep Med. 2005;3:18–31.
109. Li Y, Jin H, Owens JA, Hu C. The association between sleep and injury among school-aged children in rural China: a case control study. Sleep Med. 2008;9:142–8.
110. Rafii F, Oskouie F, Shoghi M. The association between sleep and injury among school-aged children in Iran. Sleep Dis. 2013. http://dx.doi.org/10.1155/2013/891090.
111. Nevsimalova S, Malinova V. Cataplexy and sleep disorders in Niemann-Pick disease type C. Curr Neurol Neurosci Rep. 2015;15:522–9.
112. Rosen GM, Bendel AE, Neglia JP, et al. Sleep in children with neoplasms of the central nervous system: a case review of 14 children. Pediatrics. 2003;112:e46–54.
113. Gapstur R, Gross CR, Ness K. Factors associated with sleep-wake disturbances in child and adult survivors of pediatric brain tumors: a review. Oncol Nurs Forum. 2009;36:723–31.
114. Verberne LM, Maurice-Stam H, Grootenhuis MA, et al. Sleep disorders in children after treatment for a CNS tumour. J Sleep Res. 2012;21:461–9.
115. Poretti A, Grotzer MA, Ribi K, et al. Outcome of craniopharyngioma in children: long-term complications and quality of life. Dev Med Child Neurol. 2004;46:220–9.
116. Muller HL, Muller-Stover S, Gebhardt U, et al. Secondary narcolepsy may be a causative factor of increased daytime sleepiness in obese childhood craniopharyngioma patients. J Pediatr Endocrinol. 2006;19 Suppl 1:423–9.
117. Marcus CL, Trescher WH, Halbower AS, Lutz J. Secondary narcolepsy in children with brain tumors. Sleep. 2002;25:435–9.
118. Muller HK, Handwerker G, Gebhardt U, et al. Melatonin treatment in obese patients with childhood craniopharyngioma and increased daytime sleepiness. Cancer Causes Control. 2006;17:583–9.

119. Muller HK, Handwerker G, Wollny B, et al. Melatonin secretion and increased daytime sleepiness in childhood craniopharyngioma patients. J Clin Endocrinol Metab. 2002;87:3993–6.
120. Kothare SV, Kaleyias J. Sleep and epilepsy in children and adolescents. Sleep Med. 2010;11:674–85.
121. Izumi N, Mizuguchi H, Umehara, et al. Evaluation on efficacy and sedative profiles of H(1) antihistamines by large-scale surveillance using the visual analogue scale (VAS). Allergol Intern. 2008;57:257–63.

Chapter 14
Parasomnias in Children

Paola Proserpio and Lino Nobili

Abstract Parasomnias are undesirable physical events or experiences that occur during sleep. They are classified on the basis of the sleep stage during which each of the parasomnias tends to occur: NREM-related parasomnias also defined as disorders of arousal (confusional arousals, sleepwalking, sleep terrors, and sleep-related eating disorder), REM-related parasomnias (REM sleep behavior disorder, recurrent isolated sleep paralysis, and nightmare disorder), and other parasomnias (exploding head syndrome, sleep-related hallucinations, and sleep enuresis). Parasomnias include several clinical features, with different complexity of behaviors, usually associated with autonomic nervous system changes and skeletal muscle activity.

The current pathophysiological theories consider parasomnias as state dissociation, characterized by the coexistence of wake- and sleeplike activity within cortical and subcortical areas of the brain. Although parasomnias are not usually associated with a primary complaint of insomnia or excessive sleepiness, they are considered clinical disorders because of possible resulting injuries, adverse health, and psychosocial effects.

Most of the parasomnias can be diagnosed based on history alone. Only the REM sleep behavior disorder requires video-polysomnographic documentation as one of the essential diagnostic criteria. However, polysomnographic recordings can be useful also in other parasomnias especially when the differential diagnosis is difficult or in the case of suspected comorbidities with other sleep disorders. Patient education and behavioral management represent the main treatment approaches to the patient with parasomnias. A pharmacological treatment may be useful when episodes are frequent and persist despite resolution of possible inducing factors, are associated with a high risk of injury, or cause secondary consequences.

Keywords Confusional arousals • Sleepwalking • Sleep terrors • REM-related parasomnias • Sleep enuresis • State dissociation • Nocturnal frontal lobe epilepsy

P. Proserpio, MD • L. Nobili, MD, PhD (✉)
Department of Neuroscience, Centre of Sleep Medicine, Centre for Epilepsy Surgery, Niguarda Hospital, Milan, Italy
e-mail: paola.proserpio@tiscali.it; Lino.nobili@ospedaleniguarda.it

© Springer International Publishing Switzerland 2017
S. Nevšímalová, O. Bruni (eds.), *Sleep Disorders in Children*,
DOI 10.1007/978-3-319-28640-2_14

Introduction

The term "parasomnia" derives from the Greek "para" meaning "around" and the Latin "somnus" meaning "sleep" and was coined in 1932 by the French researcher Henri Roger who gave a scrupulous descriptions of sleep terror and somnambulistic episodes in his monograph entitled "Les Troubles du Sommeil-Hypersomnies, Insomnies, and Parasomnies."

In accordance with the third edition of International Classification of Sleep Disorder (ICSD3) [1], parasomnias are defined as "undesirable physical events or experiences that occur during entry into sleep, within sleep, or during arousal from sleep." There are several possible ways to classify the parasomnias. The most widely accepted classification is that suggested by the American Academy of Sleep Medicine [1], which is based on the sleep stage during which each of the parasomnias tends to occur (Table 14.1).

The current pathophysiological theories consider parasomnias as state dissociation, characterized by the coexistence of wake- and sleeplike activity within cortical and subcortical areas of the brain. The normally distinct three essential states of human consciousness – wake, NREM sleep, and REM sleep – are modulated by a complex neural system, with functionally distinct but integrated components, that allows an unambiguous separation between these states. However, recent studies showed that brain-sleep state may be spatially nonuniform and sleep and wakefulness may not be temporally distinct behavioral states but rather part of a continuum resulting from the complex interaction between diffuse neuromodulatory systems and intrinsic properties of the different thalamocortical modules [2]. This interaction may account for the occurrence of dissociated activity across different brain structures characterizing both physiological and pathological conditions [3].

Although these disorders occur predominantly or exclusively during sleep, they are not usually associated with a primary complaint of insomnia or excessive sleepiness. However, they are considered clinical disorders because of possible resulting injuries, adverse health, and psychosocial effects. The clinical consequences of the parasomnias can affect the patient, the bed partner, or both.

Parasomnias include several clinical features, with different complexities of behaviors, usually associated with autonomic nervous system changes and skeletal

Table 14.1 Classification of parasomnias

NREM-related parasomnias (disorders of arousal)	REM-related parasomnias	Other parasomnias
Confusional arousals	REM sleep behavior disorder	Exploding head syndrome
Sleepwalking	Recurrent isolated sleep paralysis	Sleep-related hallucinations
Sleep terrors	Nightmare disorder	Sleep enuresis
Sleep-related eating disorder		

Reproduced with permission from ICSD3

muscle activity. For this reason they are considered a different entity from the "sleep-related movement disorders" that include a wide range of predominantly simple motoric activities (myoclonic, repetitive, rocking, rhythmic, grinding, cramping, fragmentary, dystonic, or dyskinetic movements or tremors) which are not usually associated with dream mentation or experiential concomitants.

Most of the parasomnias can be diagnosed based on history alone. Considering the ten core categories of parasomnias listed in the ICSD3, only the REM sleep behavior disorder requires video-polysomnographic documentation as one of the essential diagnostic criteria. However, polysomnographic recordings can be useful also in other parasomnias especially when the differential diagnosis is difficult or in the case of suspected comorbidities with other sleep disorders.

NREM-Related Parasomnia

NREM-related parasomnia or "disorders of arousal" (DoA) are the subgroup of parasomnias arising from NREM sleep. Diagnostic criteria from the ICSD3 are shown in Table 14.2. This group is composed of confusional arousals, sleep terrors, sleepwalking, and sleep-related eating disorder (SRED). More than one type may coexist within the same patient. These parasomnias occur primarily in childhood and normally cease by adolescence, but the onset or persistence during adulthood is well recognized. Especially in children, they are considered benign phenomena. However sometimes DoA can be characterized by complex behavior with potentially violent or injurious features or can result in the complaint of excessive daytime sleepiness. Evaluation and treatment are therefore recommended for patients whose activities are potentially violent or are very disturbing to other family members. Finally, because other parasomnias, particularly the REM sleep behavior disorder and nocturnal seizures, can perfectly mimic disorders of arousal, extensive

Table 14.2 NREM-related parasomnias and diagnostic criteria

Criteria A–E must be met
A. Recurrent episodes of incomplete awakening from sleep
B. Inappropriate or absent responsiveness to efforts of others to intervene or redirect the person during the episode
C. Limited (e.g., a single visual scene) or no associated cognition or dream imagery
D. Partial or complete amnesia for the episode
E. The disturbance is not better explained by another sleep disorder, mental disorder, medical condition, medication, or substance use
Notes
1. The events usually occur during the first third of the major sleep episode
2. The individual may continue to appear confused and disoriented for several minutes or longer following the episode

Reproduced with permission from ICSD3

video-polysomnographic recordings can provide corroborative documentation in support of the clinical diagnosis.

Considering that SRED occurs almost exclusively during adulthood, this subtype of NREM parasomnia will be briefly described separately at the end of this chapter.

Epidemiology

NREM parasomnias are generally considered a common pediatric sleep disorder that tends to decrease with development. Same individual may experience more than one type of arousal parasomnias. However, epidemiological figures for these co-occurrences are yet to be determined.

Almost all children have confusional arousals on occasion; in particular, during the preschool age, they frequently experience minor episodes of partial awakening from sleep, which might not even come to parental attention. For this reason, epidemiological studies on confusional arousal are scanty. In children, Laberge et al. [4] found that about 17 % of children between 3 and 13 years are experiencing occasional or frequent episodes of confusional arousals. In another study, Ohayon et al. observed that confusional arousal affected 4.2 % of the general population, decreasing from 6.1 % in the 15–24 age group to 3.3 % in the 25–34 and stabilizing around 2 % after 35 years old [5].

The prevalence of sleepwalking in children ranges from 3 to 14.5 % [6, 7]; most episodes usually resolve after the age of 10 years. A strong familial occurrence has often been reported although the genetical basis of this phenomenon has yet to be clarified. Recently the first genetic locus for sleepwalking at chromosome 20q12-q13.12 has been described [8].

Sleep terrors have the greatest incidence in preschool children. Laberge et al. [4] reported an overall prevalence of sleep terrors of 17.3 % in children between 3 and 13 years. In another longitudinal study, the frequency of this sleep disorder was 39.8 % in age group 2.5–6 years, with a peak at ages 2.5, 3.5, and 4 years [7].

The prevalence of NREM parasomnias in adults is unknown, but mostly represents a continuation of episodes after adolescence, sometimes after having been symptom-free for several years. A recent population-based cross-sectional study in 1,000 randomly selected young adults (18 years and older) showed a lifetime prevalence of confusional arousals of 18.5 % and actual prevalence (in the previous 3 months) of 6.9 %. For sleepwalking these prevalences were 22.4 % and 1.7 %, and for sleep terrors they were 10.4 % and 2.7 %, respectively [9].

Pathophysiology

It is generally considered that disorders of arousal derive from a breakdown of boundaries between wakefulness and sleep regulatory systems. Apart from the phenomenon of state dissociation, other mechanisms seem to contribute to the appearance of these sleep disorders, such as activation of innate behaviors and loco-motor centers, arousal instability, internal and external triggering mechanisms, and genetic and psychopathological influences. Finally, due to the frequent association with perinatal risk factors and developmental comorbidities, a disorder of sleep maturation has been also hypothesized [10].

The Phenomenon of State Dissociation in Arousal Parasomnias

Intracerebral stereo-EEG (S-EEG) investigations conducted in epileptic patients during the presurgical evaluation have shown that physiological NREM sleep can be characterized by the coexistence of wake-like and sleeplike EEG patterns in different cortical areas [11]. These local cortical activations (lasting on average 5–10 s) can occur in the absence of any behavioral manifestation.

In 2009, Terzaghi et al. described an episode of a confusional arousal captured during a S-EEG exploration. During the event, local fast wake-like EEG activations in the motor and cingulated cortices contrasted with the persistence or increase of sleeplike delta activities in the frontal and parietal associative cortices [12]. In a more recent study [13], S-EEG recording during a confusional arousal showed the occurrence of a local activation in the motor, cingulate, insular, temporo-polar, and amygdalar cortices, while a simultaneous persistence of slow waves was observed in the frontal and parietal dorsolateral cortices as well as sleep spindles in the hippocampal cortex. Finally, a third episode of confusional arousal was recently recorded in another drug-resistant epileptic patient during a right temporo–parietal–occipital S-EEG exploration [14]. Interestingly, the nucleus ventralis intermedius (VIM) of the thalamus had also been sampled by one distal electrode contact. During the episode, the activity recorded from the VIM showed a slight decrease in delta power and a clear-cut emergence of beta activity, which normally characterizes wake thalamic EEG.

Interestingly, the electrophysiological patterns observed in these three cases are in accordance with data previously obtained with ictal SPECT in sleepwalking which showed decreased regional cerebral blood flow in the frontoparietal cortices associated with the activation of the cingulate cortex and the absence of a deactivation of the thalamus during sleepwalking [15].

From a speculative perspective, typical features of arousal parasomnias could be explained by the coexistence of an activation of the amygdalo–temporo–insular areas disengaged from the prefrontal control cortex (emotional activation, such as fear), with the persistence of the deactivation of the hippocampal and frontal associative cortices (amnesia for the event). Interestingly, functional studies have shown that sleep deprivation, a condition that can facilitate the occurrence and increase the complexity of somnambulistic events recorded during recovery sleep, can induce an activation of the amygdala, significantly strengthening its connectivity with autonomic activating centers of the brainstem and reducing the connectivity with the prefrontal cortex [6]. The fundamental cause of "pathological" state dissociation is still unknown, but probably influenced by genetic and maturational factors.

The presence of local dissociated states during physiological sleep could suggest a possible adaptive role of this phenomenon. Indeed, a lower arousal threshold during NREM sleep in humans may have been selected, because it increases the probability of survival, facilitating motor behaviors in the case of sudden awakenings. We could hypothesize that subjects with NREM parasomnias could show a pathological increased arousability of some local neuronal networks (such as motor and limbic cortex), in contrast with an increased sleep pressure in other cortical areas. Accordingly, a transcranial magnetic stimulation study found an increased excitability of the human motor cortex during wakefulness in a group of sleepwalkers [16].

There are no definitive data about the involvement of specific neurotransmitters in the pathophysiology of arousal disorders. Sleepwalking may be associated with abnormalities in the metabolism of serotonin considering its frequent association with migraine and Tourette syndrome and the observation that several factors, known to induce the occurrence of sleepwalking, such as fever, lithium, and antidepressants, activate the serotoninergic system. Based on the results of a transcranial magnetic stimulation study in sleepwalkers, an involvement of cholinergic and GABA pathways has been supposed [16]. Finally, a possible role of the hypocretin hypothalamic system, known to play a major role in vigilance state stabilization, cannot be excluded.

Neurophysiologic Features and Alteration of Sleep Continuity in NREM Parasomnias

A peculiar feature of subjects who experience NREM parasomnia is the presence of increased arousals and cyclic alternating pattern (CAP) rate during slow-wave sleep, even on nights without episodes (for detail see "diagnosis" section). The increased number of awakenings determines a chronic condition of intra-night slow-wave activity (SWA) deprivation that is reflected in an alteration of NREM sleep continuity and in a different dynamics of SWA throughout the night. Indeed, during the first sleep cycles, patients with NREM parasomnia show a decrease of SWA values with respect to control subjects and a lack of the typical exponential decaying trend of SWA during the consecutive sleep cycles. Moreover, it has been shown that a SWA rebound and a normalization of the SWA profile in sleepwalkers are not obtained even after sleep deprivation. Contrarily, sleep deprivation results in more awakenings and an increased frequency of clinical manifestations during recovery sleep [6]. These data suggest that abnormal arousal reactions persist in sleepwalkers even after sleep deprivation.

Activations of Innate Behaviors and Locomotor Centers

Animal and human data seem to suggest that part of the "emotional" and motor clinical features of parasomnias could result from a release of inhibition of "central pattern generators" (CPGs) [17]. CPGs are "functional neural organizations" which regulate innate behavioral automatisms and survival behaviors and located in the spinal cord, mesencephalon, pons, and bulb. The cortex itself can also operate as a CPG, and this could explain the occurrence of previously learned behaviors during arousal parasomnias.

Genetic Influences

Genetic factors have long been suggested to be involved in the occurrence of arousal parasomnias, although the pattern of inheritance of NREM parasomnias is still unknown. About 80 % of sleepwalkers have at least one family member affected by this parasomnia, and the prevalence of somnambulism is higher in children of parents with a history of sleepwalking [18]. A twin study found a concordance rate of sleepwalking 1.6 times greater in monozygotic vs. dizygotic twins for childhood sleepwalking and approximately 5.3 times greater for adult sleepwalking [19]. A small series indicates that somnambulism may be associated with excessive transmission of the HLA-DQB1*05 and *04 alleles [20]. Bisulli et al. found a high frequency of arousal disorders in patients with nocturnal frontal lobe epilepsy (NFLE), suggesting that both disorders can show an abnormal (possibly cholinergic) arousal system as a common pathophysiologic mechanism [21].

Precipitating Influences

There are different conditions that may induce the occurrence of a dysfunction of the limit between sleep and wakefulness, thus triggering the occurrence of arousal parasomnias. Different studies showed that arousal disorders are more likely to occur in genetically predisposed individuals in the presence of an increased pressure for slow-wave sleep and factors favoring arousals or fragmenting sleep [22]. Frequently these two main triggering factors, sleep fragmentation and sleep deprivation, work together in a vicious circle. In particular, factors that deepen sleep encompass different conditions, such as sleep deprivation, fever, and sedative and psychotropic medications (non-benzodiazepine hypnotics, antidepressants, neuroleptics, and sodium oxybate). On the other hand, sleep fragmentation can be caused by sleep disorder (sleep apnea, periodic leg movements), fever, stress, and external stimuli such as noise or touch. Finally, an increased incidence of NREM parasomnia in patients with either nocturnal or diurnal epilepsy has been reported; the increase of arousal instability induced by epileptic discharges may favor the occurrence of NREM parasomnias.

NREM Parasomnias and Psychopathology

Not all studies agree on the extent that psychological factors may contribute to arousal parasomnias. Some studies suggest that NREM parasomnias in childhood are mainly related to developmental and genetic predisposing factors, while their persistence or onset in adulthood can be triggered by psychological factors [23]. An epidemiological study demonstrated a high percentage of subjects with concurrent diagnoses of parasomnia and mood or anxiety disorders [24]. On the other hand, the observation that a successful treatment of a comorbid depressive disorder in adult patients with night terrors and sleepwalking had no effects on the course of parasomnias seems to suggest that the concurrent psychopathology does not play an essential role. Overall current data suggest a lack of a definitive association between a history of major psychological trauma, severe psychopathology, and sleepwalking/night terrors.

Clinical Features

Although representing distinct disorders, some researchers consider NREM parasomnias as a single continuum, ranging from confusional arousals with low motor and autonomic activation, on the one hand, to sleepwalking characterized by intense motor activity and mild autonomic activation, on the other hand. According to this theory, night terrors fall between these two, with intense autonomic discharge and mild motor activation [25]. Patients who experience one of these three phenomena are prone to demonstrate the others as well. In particular, episodes sometimes combine elements of all three, and a child might display a sequence of confusional arousals in early childhood and sleepwalking later, followed by sleep terrors in late childhood and adolescence. Alternatively, features of all three forms can occur at any one stage of development.

There are common features to these disorders (Tables 14.3 and 14.4). Although they may occur during any NREM sleep stage, these events generally occur out of deep NREM sleep (N3) and, thus, most often take place in the first third of the night when these sleep stages are most represented. Any factor that deepens sleep (sleep deprivation, stress, febrile illness, medications, alcohol) or is associated with arousals (external or internal stimuli, like the presence of sleep-disordered breathing,

Table 14.3 Clinical features of NREM parasomnia	General clinical features
	Common in childhood
	Decrease with increasing age
	Episodes in the first third of the night
	A state between sleep and waking during the event, disorientation, and confusion
	Presence of triggering factors
	Long episode duration (minutes)
	Minimal recall of the event
	Strong familial pattern

Table 14.4 A comparison of different clinical features of NREM parasomnia

	Confusional arousal	Sleepwalking	Sleep terror
Age of onset	2–10 years	4–12 years	18 months–10 years
Peak time of occurrence	First third of night	First third of night	First third of night
Ictal behavior	Whimpering, some articulation, sitting up in bed, inconsolable	Screaming, agitation, flushed face, sweating, inconsolable	Walking about the room or house, may be quiet or agitated, unresponsive to verbal commands
Motor activity	Low	Complex	Rarely complex
Autonomic activity	Low	Mild	Intense
Complications	Rare (aggressions)	Possible (violence)	Occasional (escape)
Typical duration	<1 min	1–20 min	5–20 min

natural termination of a sleep cycle, mental activity, or others) may increase the occurrence of NREM parasomnias. During the episode, patients are usually unresponsive to the environment, and they are typically completely or partially amnestic after the event, with little or no recall either immediately afterward or the next morning. Finally, the presence of a positive family history is another aspect helpful to identify NREM parasomnia.

Confusional Arousal

Confusional arousals are defined as episodes characterized by mental confusion or confused behavior that occurs while the patient is in bed, in the absence of terror or ambulation outside of the bed [1].

They occur mainly in infants and toddlers (probably most of whom have such episodes to some extent, at least in mild form) and almost invariably before the age of 5.

An episode may begin with mumbling, moaning, or whimpering, gradually increasing movements which then progress to agitated and confused behavior with marked perspiration, crying (perhaps intense, but not screaming), calling out, or thrashing about. Sometimes this causes the child to fall out of bed, although injuries are less likely than in the other arousal disorders. The child's eyes may be open or closed. Talking may also occur. The child may be partially aware of the environment and thus may be confused and combine reality with imagination, e.g., the child may sit up in the bed and put a toy in his mouth thinking that it is a dummy/pacifier. Typically, although appearing to be awake, the child does not respond when spoken to and may seem to "stare right through" his parents. Any forceful attempts to intervene may meet with severe resistance and even aggression.

Each episode usually lasts 5–15 min (sometimes much longer) before the child calms down spontaneously and returns to restful sleep. Enuresis may occur during or after an episode.

Sleepwalking

Sleepwalking is a series of complex behaviors that are usually initiated during arousals from slow-wave sleep and culminate in leaving the bed in an altered state of consciousness.

Actually, sleepwalking, also known as somnambulism, can consist of very complex motor activity, of which walking is just one element. Indeed, the symptoms and manifestations that characterize sleepwalking can show great variations both within and across predisposed patients. Movements can be repetitive and purposeless (e.g., sitting up in bed, pointing at a wall, fingering bedsheets) but also complex and meaningful (e.g., rearranging furniture, cooking or eating, getting dressed, etc.). Eyes are usually open and the sleepwalker's emotional expression can range from calm to extremely agitated. Given the heterogeneous nature of sleepwalking episodes, their duration can vary from a few seconds to dozens of minutes. Associated mental activity often includes misperception and relative unresponsiveness to external stimuli, confusion, perceived threat, and variable retrograde amnesia [6]. In a significant proportion of patients, short, unpleasant dreamlike mentations may occur during sleepwalking episodes [26].

Episodes of sleepwalking in children are rarely violent and their movements are often slow. If restrained, the child may attempt to avoid the other person but does not put up aggressive resistance. On the other hand, the most serious complication of sleepwalking in adulthood is represented by injuries and violent behavior; the number of legal cases of sleep-related violence involving sleepwalking is on the rise [22].

Sleep Terrors

Sleep terrors are characterized by episode of extreme fear or terror and agitation with prominent motor activities that arise abruptly from sleep. The episode begins suddenly with vocalization, which can be screaming or crying, sometimes associated with sitting up in bed, thrashing, agitation, confusion, a facial expression of fear, and sympathetic activation (tachycardia, flushing, mydriasis, and sweating). Patients are only partially responsive to the environment during episodes, and there is little or no recall of the event the morning after the event. Cases reported with violent behaviors appear related more to involuntary contact or provocation by another person, particularly if attempts are made to block or restrain the individual [27].

Sleep terrors usually last a few minutes but can range anywhere from 30 s to 30 min. They can occur more than once a night and up to several times per week.

Diagnosis

As in other sleep disorders, the first step in a clinical encounter with a patient with abnormal behaviors when asleep is taking a good history. An adequate general and hypnic anamnesis with the patient and bed partner is paramount, taken directly or aided by a questionnaire. There are no available standardized sleep questionnaires for parasomnias; however, other associated symptoms can be assessed by this modality. Sleep questionnaires can be helpful to the physician to collect more quickly extensive information regarding sleep–wake habits. For examples of screening questionnaires for pediatric sleep, see Owens et al. and Archbold et al. [28, 29]. Sleep diaries can highlight irregularities of sleep/wake schedules and help determine whether episodes are triggered by sleep deprivation. Finally, a videotape of a typical episode recorded by parents at home may be very helpful to the clinician.

A clear clinical history can be sufficient to diagnose the presence of NREM parasomnia in the majority of cases, but in others only video-polysomnographic (vPSG) recording can clarify the nature of the disorder. Indeed, although accordingly with the ICSD3, vPSG is not necessary for the diagnosis of arousal disorders, this diagnostic technique is recommended: (1) in cases in which the clinical history is not completely suggestive of NREM parasomnia; (2) in the presence of injurious or extremely disruptive behaviors; (3) when there may be associated sleep disorder (sleep apnea, periodic limb movement, etc.); or (4) when the parasomnia is associated with medical, psychiatric, or neurological symptoms or findings [30, 31].

There are no consistently robust features in terms of overall sleep architecture and normal cycling among sleep stages that can result highly suggestive of patients with NREM parasomnia. However, some unusual sleep-related features have been described as characterizing the sleep of patients suffering from arousal disorders. These include hypersynchronous delta waves, irregular buildup of slow-wave activity, and NREM sleep instability.

The hypersynchronous delta (HSD) activity is defined as continuous high-voltage (>150 microV) delta waves occurring during slow-wave sleep (Fig. 14.1) or immediately prior to an episode [32] and has been investigated for a long time as a possible diagnostic sign of a NREM parasomnia. However, careful studies analyzing HSD prior to arousal disorder episodes have yielded mixed to poor results [32, 33]. Indeed, an increased number of HSD have been reported, but HSD was absent in many sleepwalkers before episodes of complex behaviors [34]. Additionally, HSD is also present in patients without history of sleepwalking but with sleep apnea or periodic leg movements [33–35]. In summary, data indicate that this electroencephalographic pattern does not appear to be a sensitive or specific diagnostic sign for a NREM parasomnia in adults and even less in children [27].

The sleep of patients with arousal disorders is characterized by an inability to maintain consolidated periods of slow-wave sleep probably due to an abnormality in the neural mechanisms responsible for the regulation of this sleep stage [36]. The increased frequency of somnambulic episodes during post-deprivation recovery sleep confirms the view that sleepwalkers suffer from a dysfunction of the mechanisms responsible for sustaining stable slow-wave sleep [37].

The cyclic alternating pattern (CAP) is a phenomenon of changing patterns in sleep that often cycle and alternate every 20–30 s and expresses the organized complexity of arousal-related phasic events in NREM sleep, thus representing a measure of NREM instability [38, 39]. Recently this pattern has been studied in patients

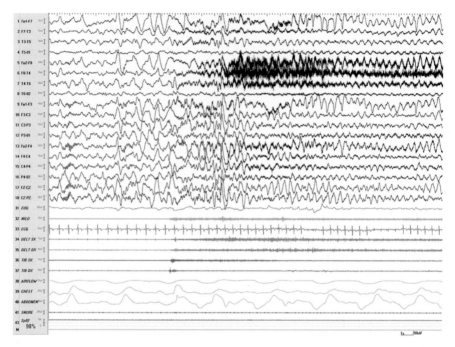

Fig. 14.1 Sleep EEG recording of an episode of confusional arousal in an 8-year-old child, occurring in N3 sleep stage. Notice the presence of a burst of delta waves immediately preceding the onset of the episode (corresponding to the increase of muscle tone) and the persistence of a hypersynchronous delta activity mainly expressed over the frontal regions. *EOG* electrooculogram, *MILO* chin, *ECG* electrocardiogram, *DELT SX* left deltoid muscle, *DELT DX* right deltoid muscle, *TIB SX* left anterior tibial muscle, *TIB DX* right anterior tibial muscle

with NREM parasomnia. The important finding was a higher CAP rate in patients with sleepwalking/sleep terrors in comparison with controls; the instability of NREM sleep in these patients was present also during non-sleepwalking nights [37, 40, 41]. Similarly, polysomnographic recordings have shown that, compared with controls, sleepwalkers experience a higher number of microarousals and arousals during slow-wave sleep [42].

In summary, these data indicate that NREM parasomnias are characterized by an increase in NREM sleep instability and arousal oscillations together with an inability to maintain stable and consolidated slow-wave sleep (for more details see Pathophysiology section).

Differential Diagnosis

NREM parasomnia needs to be distinguished from other parasomnias (in particular RBD and nightmare disorder), nocturnal panic attacks, and sleep-related seizures.

REM Behavior Disorder (RBD)

There is often considerable overlap of features between the disorders of arousal (in particular sleepwalking) and the RBD. However, this overlap can be observed much more frequently in adults than in children, where RBD is very rare. In general, the main features that allow distinguishing RBD from an arousal disorder are the dream enactment behavior, the usual occurrence during the second half of the night, and the absence of mental confusion upon awakening. Some patients may meet the diagnostic criteria for both NREM and REM parasomnias; these patients are diagnosed with "parasomnia overlap disorder."

Nightmares

Nightmares can sometimes resemble sleep terrors (for differential diagnostic features, see Table 14.5). Nightmares occur within REM sleep and are therefore more prominent in the second half of the night; children arousing from a nightmare usually become fully alert quickly, respond positively to comforting, and may offer a detailed description of dream content after awakening the following morning. Compared to sleep terrors, nightmares are characterized by lower levels of autonomic activation (e.g., palpitations or dyspnea), vocalization, and mobility, but are often associated with much more anxiety and subsequently difficulty returning to sleep [43, 44].

Table 14.5 Differential diagnosis between sleep terror and nightmares

	Sleep terror	Nightmares
Peak time of occurrence	First third of the night (from SWS)	Last third of the night (from REM sleep)
Sex	Males > females	In children males = females
Age	4–12 (peak at 5–7)	Any age (frequent at age 3–6)
Prevalence	3–4 % in children	10–20 % in children
Ictal behavior	Heartbreaking cry, screams	Scary awakening
Consciousness	Disoriented, confused	Fully alert after awakening
Vocalization	Common	Rare
Autonomic activity	Intense	Low/mild
Amnesia	Frequent	Absent
Dream recall	Absent	Present (scary vivid dream)
Familial history	Present	Absent
Complications	Potentially injurious and violent	Rarely injurious or violent
Predisposing factors	Sleep deprivation, febrile illness	Stress, traumatic events, personality disorders
Treatment	Safety, avoid predisposing factors, benzodiazepines	None, psycho-/behavioral therapy

Nocturnal Panic Attacks

Nocturnal panic attacks consist in waking from sleep in a state of panic, with intense fear or discomfort. They are frequent in patients with panic disorder, with 44–71 % reporting at least one such attack, and sometimes they can be hardly distinguishable from sleep terrors [45]. As sleep terrors, they can more frequently occur in the first third of the night, during late stage 2 or early stage 3 sleep. However, sleep panic attacks can be distinguished from arousal disorders because patients do not become physically agitated or aggressive during the attack; moreover, immediately after the episodes, they appear oriented, can vividly recall their attack, and usually have difficulty returning to sleep [45].

Nocturnal Frontal Lobe Epilepsy

Nocturnal frontal lobe epilepsy (NFLE) is a syndrome of heterogeneous etiology, encompassing genetic, lesional, and cryptogenetic forms [46–48]. NFLE is usually considered a benign clinical epileptic syndrome because seizures occur almost exclusively during sleep, and in the majority of patients, the pharmacological treatment is effective; however, severe and drug-resistant forms, occasionally associated with mental retardation, have been described [49].

During 1990s, the definition of autosomal dominant nocturnal frontal lobe epilepsy (ADNFLE) was introduced for the first time because of the observation of the occurrence of sleep-related motor seizures in different individuals of the same family [50].

The first genetic studies in ADNFLE families identified different mutations in the gene coding for neuronal nicotinic acetylcholine receptors (nAChRs). In the following years, ADNFLE was quickly recognized as a genetically heterogeneous disorder as most of the described families show mutations in different genes, not involved in the cholinergic system (for a review see Nobili et al. [48]).

The findings of a genetic alteration of the cholinergic system may give some insights into understanding the pathogenesis of this disorder. Indeed, the nAChR is known to exert a modulating effect in the regulation of NREM and REM stability and of arousal oscillations. On the other hand, a mutation of the nicotinic receptors has shown to facilitate the occurrence of an unbalanced excitation/inhibition circuitry within the GABAergic reticular thalamic neurons, thus generating seizures through the synchronizing effect of spontaneous oscillations in thalamocortical connections [51]. Thus, it seems that a genetic alteration observed in NFLE might facilitate both the epileptogenesis and the occurrence of arousal instability [52]. With these assumptions, the high prevalence of parasomnias in the personal and family history of individuals with NFLE [21] might rely on a common alteration of the arousal regulating system.

Considering the clinical aspects, in NFLE patients seizures usually begin before the age of 20 years, with a peak during childhood, although onset during adulthood has been also reported; seizure frequency is usually high. A distinctive characteristic of NFLE, common to the sporadic and the familial form, is that, in the space of a single night, NFLE patients may show a large number of different sleep-related motor attacks of increasing complexity and duration. These include:

1. Short-lasting (2–4 s) stereotyped movements involving the limbs, the axial musculature, and/or the head [53].
2. Paroxysmal arousals (PAs), characterized by abrupt episodes of arousals (5–10 s in duration) sometimes accompanied by stereotyped movements, vocalization, frightened expression, and fear [54].
3. Major attacks, lasting 20–30 s, characterized by asymmetric tonic or dystonic posturing or complex movements such as pelvic thrusting, pedaling, choreoathetoid, and ballistic movements of the limbs [47].
4. Epileptic nocturnal wandering, consisting of ictal deambulatory behaviors often associated with frightened expression and fear [55].

In recent years it has been shown that sleep-related complex motor attacks may also originate from the temporal lobe [56, 57], the insular–opercular region [58], and the posterior cerebral regions [59].

Considering the electrophysiological features, interictal and ictal scalp EEG abnormalities in NFLE patients are often scanty or absent, probably due to the inaccessibility of much of the frontal lobes to surface electrodes and to the presence of movement artifacts related to seizures [47, 49].

Taking into account the similarities and the possible coexistence of parasomnias in people with NFLE, the differential diagnosis between these disorders appears sometimes complicated, especially if it is only based on anamnestic investigations. A reliable semeiological description of motor events occurring during the night is often difficult to collect from a witness or sleep partner because observers may be lacking or, if present, not fully reliable or awake when attacks occur.

Main anamnestic differences between NFLE and NREM parasomnias are summarized in Table 14.6.

Different questionnaires and scales have been reported in the literature to help differentiate these disorders on the basis of clinical features. Indeed, in 2006 Derry et al. [60] developed the frontal lobe epilepsy and parasomnia (FLEP) scale in order to establish how reliably features from the history might distinguish NFLE from parasomnias. Although initially reported to have a sensitivity of 1 and specificity of 0.9, Manni et al. [61] challenged the usefulness of the scale after studying a tertiary sleep center population. They found that the FLEP scale risked misdiagnosing some patients, especially NFLE subjects presenting episodes of nocturnal wandering. More recently, Bisulli et al. [62] identified two major anamnestic patterns (i.e., dystonic posturing or hyperkinetic behavior) for NFLE diagnosis with a high specificity and unsatisfactory sensitivity. In addition, they found four minor features that may increase the specificity of these clinical items when associated with one of the two major patterns: unstructured vocalization, experience of an aura preceding the motor attack, duration less than 2 min, and a history of tonic–clonic seizures during sleep. This study confirms the weakness of the clinical history alone in differentiating NFLE from parasomnias and underlines the need of future efforts to develop a

Table 14.6 Differential diagnosis between NREM parasomnia and nocturnal frontal lobe epilepsy

	NREM parasomnia	NFLE
Age at onset	3–8 years	Any age (peak in childhood)
Familial history	Frequently present	Possible
Peak time of occurrence	Usually during the first third	Any time
Sleep-stage onset of episodes	NREM sleep (usually N3)	NREM sleep (usually N2)
Frequency during one night	Usually one episode/night	Several episodes/night
Frequency	Sporadic	Almost every night
Duration	1–10 min	Seconds to 3 min
Evolution	Tend to disappear	Stable, increased frequency, rare remission
Predisposing factors	Frequent (sleep deprivation, febrile illness)	Rare
Stereotypic motor pattern	No	Yes
Consciousness	Usually impaired	Usually preserved
Amnesia	Frequent	Unconstant

reliable algorithm to aid physicians in the diagnostic process of paroxysmal motor sleep disorders.

Many experts consider vPSG the "gold-standard" test for diagnosing paroxysmal sleep-related events, but it is expensive, with a limited availability, and does not always capture the event in a single-night recording. Moreover, interictal EEG fail to disclose epileptiform abnormalities in a substantial percentage of NFLE patients [49]. Conversely, interictal epileptiform abnormalities may occur in some parasomnias. Finally, even when the nocturnal episode has been recorded, the diagnosis can remain doubtful because ictal scalp EEG often fails to disclose epileptiform abnormalities or because the episode captured is a minor motor event for which the diagnosis is not reliable, even among experts.

To make video analysis of nocturnal paroxysmal events more reliable, a diagnostic algorithm focusing on the semeiological features of the arousal parasomnias and NFLE has recently been proposed [63]. In their work, Derry et al. noticed that the discrepancy between historical account and recorded events was more evident in NREM parasomnias than in NFLE. Moreover, the clinical features of the initial arousal behaviors (abrupt or slow movements) were indistinguishable between the two conditions, thus confirming that epileptic minor events and paroxysmal arousals cannot be easily differentiable from non-epileptic events on the basis of video-EEG analysis. In contrast, the clinical features of the evolution and the offset of the events could better differentiate NFLE from parasomnias. Finally, the presence of a coherent speech and a verbal interaction with the neighboring individuals during the episode, the possibility to modify the event by the actions of individuals present, and the absence of a clear and distinct offset of the attack seemed to be highly indicative of a NREM parasomnia.

Despite the limits of vPSG, the possibility of analyzing the video of the nocturnal attack remains an important diagnostic tool, making home video recording a useful adjunct [64].

Treatment

To date, no properly powered randomized controlled trials assessing medical and psychological treatment efficacy have been conducted in patients with NREM parasomnia. Indeed, current treatment recommendations are based only on small clinical trials as well as clinical and anecdotal evidence [65–67]. Patients should therefore be advised that prescribed drugs are considered "off-label."

Parasomnic attacks in healthy children and adolescents are often benign and normally require no treatment. Reassuring the patient and significant others about the generally benign nature of the episodes is sometimes sufficient. Especially in the case of sleepwalking, environmental safety issues should be discussed with the parents and represent a first-line approach. Physicians should always evaluate the possible presence of favoring and precipitating factors, including inadequate lifestyle, coexisting sleep disorders, and drugs. Pharmacotherapy should be considered only when the episodes are frequent or dangerous to the patient or others or when they cause undesirable secondary consequences, such as excessive daytime sleepiness, or cause distress to the patient or family.

Reassurance and Environmental Safety

In the majority of NREM parasomnic episodes during childhood, the most disturbing characteristics may sometimes be limited to what is experienced by an observing parent. In these cases, reassurance on the typically benign nature of episodes is often enough. Relatives should be also aware that most affected children outgrow the condition by late adolescence or sooner.

Moreover, parents should avoid any attempt at interrupting the episode because this practice may increase confusion and precipitate a dramatic or even violent reaction. Indeed, efforts to shorten parasomnic events may lead to aggressive behaviors because of the physical proximity and provocation [27, 68]. It is preferable to wait until the episode is over and then guide the child quietly back to bed [67].

Modifications of the environment may be necessary depending on the characteristics of the episodes to minimize the risk of injury. Safety recommendations should be addressed and tailored to each individual. Preventive measures can include locating the patient's bedroom on the ground floor, blocking access to stairs and kitchen, covering windows with heavy curtains, placing mattresses on the floor, using sleeping bags to reduce wandering, and eliminating any potentially dangerous objects [43, 67].

Bedroom door alarms may be used to signal the occurrence of a wandering episode; however it has been shown that a loud stimulus can worsen the behavior of the sleepwalker [69].

Predisposing and Triggering Factors

As mentioned above, all the conditions increasing the amount of slow-wave sleep increase the likelihood of occurrence a parasomnic episode [70]. Indeed, a careful history about sleep patterns and duration should be collected, including evaluation of the night-to-night stability of sleep achieved, periods of relative sleep deprivation, occurrence of recuperative sleep, and nap history [43]. Sleep hygiene should be recommended, including advising routine naps for children <4 years of age to ensure adequate sleep.

Moreover, considering that arousal induced by whatever external or internal stimuli (noise, light, pain, nocturia) could precipitate an episode, specific measures to identify and remove these triggers will lessen the arousals and consequently help in resolution of the parasomnias [67, 71]. In particular, when parasomnic episodes become frequent and intractable or are associated with daytime mood or behavioral disturbance, the possibility of comorbid sleep disordered, especially sleep apnea, but also periodic limb movements and gastroesophageal reflux, must be recognized and treated [67, 71].

Non-pharmacological Treatment: Psychological Interventions and Anticipatory Awakenings

A variety of non-pharmacological treatments has been recommended for long-term management of NREM parasomnias, including hypnosis, autogenic training, relaxation therapy, psychotherapy, and cognitive behavioral therapy. However, the evidence for these methods is based mainly on anecdotal data and case reports [67]. Hypnosis (including self-hypnosis) has been found to be effective in both children and adults presenting with chronic sleepwalking and sleep terrors [72, 73]. However, hypnosis in children can be often difficult, and individuals show varying degrees of susceptibility for this therapeutic approach.

Anticipatory awakening or scheduled awakening is another behavioral technique that can be recommended as an effective therapy when the episodes occur nightly and consistently at or about the same time each night. Since arousal parasomnia tends to be clustered into the first third of night sleep, in particular during slow-wave sleep, momentary awakening of the child by the parents, 15–20 min prior to the usual time of occurrence, may shift the child into a lighter state of sleep, thereby aborting the event. During the scheduled awakening, the parent should comfort the child. Anticipatory awakening seems to be effective in about 60 % of cases [66]. This technique can represent an important therapeutic option, particularly if the family is reluctant to administer a drug to the child and inclined toward non-pharmacologic management. The disadvantages are that it requires nightly vigil and intervention by the parents; also, sometimes the interruption itself may provoke a frank parasomnia [66].

Pharmacological Treatment

Clinicians should consider therapy only if the episodes cause undesirable secondary consequences, such as excessive daytime sleepiness, or cause distress to the patient or family. Pharmacologic interventions include benzodiazepines such as diazepam 5–10 mg or clonazepam 0.5–2 mg [74] and tricyclics such as imipramine or clomipramine [67]. The effectiveness of benzodiazepines may relate to sedative effects or to decreases in slow-wave sleep.

Other serotoninergic antidepressants, in particular paroxetine, have been reported to be particularly effective in the treatment of sleep terrors. On the other hand, paroxetine has been shown to favor episodes of sleepwalking thus suggesting possible distinct pathophysiological mechanisms between sleep terrors and sleepwalking [74].

An open pharmacological trial of L-5-hydroxytryptophan (2 mg/kg at bedtime) suggests its efficacy in the treatment of sleep terrors. L-5-Hydroxytryptophan is a precursor of serotonin that may modify central serotoninergic system dysfunction or enhance production of sleep-promoting factors [75]. Finally, some case studies have suggested that melatonin therapy, at 5 mg, half an hour before bedtime, may be helpful for patients with sleepwalking and sleep terrors [76].

Sleep-Related Eating Disorder (SRED)

SRED consists of "recurrent episodes of involuntary eating and drinking during arousals from sleep, associated with diminished levels of consciousness and subsequent recall, with problematic consequences" [1]. Episodes typically occur during partial arousals from sleep during the first third of the night, with impaired subsequent recall [77]. This disorder is potentially harmful; problematic features of the recurrent sleep-related eating include the following: consumption of abnormal combinations of food or toxic substances, sleep-related injurious behaviors performed while in pursuit of food [78, 79], adverse health consequences (weight gain, various metabolic problems), and daytime sleepiness.

The prevalence of SRED in the general population is unknown. Winkelman et al. reported that 16.7 % of individuals who were part of an inpatient eating disorder program, 8.7 % of those in an outpatient eating disorder program, 4.6 % of college students, 1.0 % of obese individuals in a weight loss program, and 3.4 % of those in an outpatient depression clinic reported behavior consistent with SRED [80]. SRED is found predominantly in women, and the average age of onset is approximately 22–27 years, with a mean of approximately 12–16 years before clinical presentation [80, 81].

A history of other parasomnias, especially sleepwalking, is frequently reported. Patients with SRED share several clinical commonalities with sleepwalkers plus previous or current eating behavior problems. It suggests that they have specialized a former sleepwalking behavior toward sleep-related eating because they are more vulnerable to eating behavior problems during the daytime [82].

Other sleep disorders can be associated with SRED, in particular restless legs syndrome (RLS), periodic limb movement of sleep (PLMS), and sleep apnea [80, 81]. Most of these sleep disorders can increase arousals during sleep and precipitate NREM parasomnia episodes in predisposed individuals. Several psychiatric conditions have been associated with SRED, including depression, bipolar disorder, anxiety, posttraumatic stress disorder, and history of repeated abuse. Finally, many drugs have been implicated in the initiation of SRED, including zolpidem, triazolam, amitriptyline, olanzapine, and risperidone [83].

Considering the management of SRED, a treatment of possibly associated sleep disorders is essential. Some drugs have been reported to be effective for the treatment of SRED such as topiramate and dopaminergic agents alone or in combination with benzodiazepines (mainly clonazepam) or opiates [83, 84].

REM-Related Parasomnia

REM Sleep Behavior Disorder (RBD)

Physiologic REM sleep is characterized by an activated brain state in combination with skeletal muscle paralysis. In RBD, normal atonia is lost, and patients present recurrent episodes of dream-enacted behaviors that can vary from small hand movements to violent activities, such as punching, kicking, or leaping out of bed. RBD is also associated with electromyography (EMG) abnormalities during REM sleep, including an excess of muscle tone and/or an excess of phasic EMG twitch activity during this sleep stage. A change in the pattern and frequency of dream recall is frequently described, and dreams can often have a negative emotional content. Accordingly with ICSD3, RBD requires polysomnography for making a diagnosis [1]. The key features of RBD on polysomnography are preserved chin electromyographic tone, or "REM sleep without atonia" (RSWA), and video evidence of motor dream enactment in the form of increased physical activity, including aggressive or violent behaviors.

RBD has been considered for a long time a parasomnia that occurs almost exclusively in elderly men. However, it is now recognized as a disorder of all ages and both sexes. In adults, there is clear association of RBD with synucleinopathic degenerative disorders such as Parkinson disease, dementia with Lewy bodies, and multiple system atrophy. In a minority of cases, RBD represents a side effect of treatment with drugs such as antidepressants (tricyclics, selective serotonin reuptake inhibitors (SSRIs), and selective noradrenaline reuptake inhibitors) and lipophilic beta-blockers. Different animal and human studies have suggested that lesions or dysfunction in REM sleep and motor control circuitry in the pontomedullary structures cause RBD phenomenology, and degeneration of these structures might

Table 14.7 Etiology of rapid eye movement sleep behavior disorder in childhood

Hypersomnias of central origin
Narcolepsy type 1
Narcolepsy type 2
Idiopathic hypersomnia
Neurodevelopmental–neurodegenerative disorders
Autism
Attention deficit disorder
Smith–Magenis syndrome
Moebius syndrome, juvenile
Parkinson disease
Tourette syndrome
Neurofibromatosis type 1
Structural brainstem abnormalities
Pontine glioma
Chiari malformation type 1
Drugs
Selective serotonin reuptake inhibitors
Tricyclic antidepressants

explain the presence of RBD years or decades before the onset of parkinsonism or dementia in people who develop neurodegenerative disorders [85].

Cases of RBD in childhood and adolescence are very infrequent, and the literature is composed only of single case reports or small case series [86–88]. Because of the rarity of these forms and the lack of long-term follow-up data, little is known about the natural history of early-onset RBD. RBD in children is virtually never idiopathic and is usually associated with narcolepsy or idiopathic hypersomnia, neurodevelopmental–neurodegenerative disorders, or structural brainstem abnormalities or represents a side effect of pharmacological agents, such as SSRI agents (Table 14.7).

RBD can occur in both children and adults with narcolepsy [89]. The prevalence of this parasomnia in narcolepsy, especially when associated with cataplexy, seems to be high, ranging from 36 to 60 % [90, 91]. RBD usually develops after hypersomnia and cataplexy onset; however, in a very few patients, especially during childhood, RBD can represent the first manifestation of the disease [92]. RBD in narcoleptic patients shows some distinct phenotypic features with respect to other RBD patients [90]. In particular, clinical severity is usually less aggressive and violent with a predominance of elementary jerks rather than complex behaviors and vocalizations; moreover there is no male predominance and an earlier onset. It has been hypothesized that hypocretin/dopaminergic system deficiency may lead to motor dyscontrol during REM sleep in narcolepsy, as hypocretin/dopaminergic neurons have wide projections to different nuclei that regulate REM sleep atonia (e.g., subcoeruleus nucleus) and the emotional content of dreams (e.g., central nucleus of the amygdala) [88].

In another group of patients, childhood RBD is associated with neurodevelopmental disabilities, such as autism. In autistic children, a decrease activation of GABA transmission has been described. GABA represents the main neurotransmitter of the ventral gigantocellular nucleus, and its decrease might predispose to a loss of the inhibition of spinal motor neurons during REM sleep [88].

Finally, RBD can be induced by specific drugs, such as selective serotonin reuptake inhibitors. During physiologic REM sleep, the serotoninergic neurons descending to motor neurons cease firing, leading to hypotonia. In this perspective, drugs that stimulate the serotonin system can induce RBD, possibly because they prevent normal sleep-related hypotonia [85].

RBD treatment is basically symptomatic. The main indications for RBD management encompass the preventive measures, a reevaluation of drugs that can precipitate or worsen RBD, and the use of drugs aimed at blunting the motor-behavior manifestations. Although no randomized double-blind trials exist, two agents have been shown to be beneficial: clonazepam (0.5–2 mg at bedtime) and melatonin (3–12 mg at bedtime). Clonazepam seems to have a suppressing effect on phasic locomotor activity and a positive influence on mental dream activity. The mechanism by which melatonin can restore the REM-related muscle atonia remains substantially unknown.

Considering childhood RBD, treatment is either not mentioned in some reports or given at unspecified dosages; however, in the short term, it seems to be modestly responsive to benzodiazepines or melatonin [88].

Recurrent Isolated Sleep Paralysis

Recurrent isolated sleep paralysis (RISP) is defined as "an inability to perform voluntary movements at sleep onset (hypnagogic or predormital form) or on waking from sleep (hypnopompic or postdormital form) in the absence of a diagnosis of narcolepsy" [1]. During the episodes consciousness is preserved and full recall is present. Hallucinations such as a feeling of the presence of others nearby, pressure on the chest, or hearing footsteps are common. A single episode usually lasts seconds to minutes and spontaneously resolves or can be halted by external auditory or tactile stimulation from a bed partner. The sensation of being paralyzed can cause intense anxiety. Although diaphragmatic function is not affected, difficulties in breathing may be reported.

RISP is considered to represent a condition of state dissociation, with a persistence of REM sleep into wakefulness.

Due to the differences in the definition used and in sampling methods, estimates of the prevalence vary widely, between 6 and 40 %. The lifetime prevalence of sleep paralysis, based on a large systematic review, is estimated to be 7.6 % of the general population, 28.3 % of students, and 31.9 % of psychiatric patients [93]. No consistent sex differences have emerged and the mean age of onset is 14–17 years.

Main predisposing factors for RISP are sleep deprivation and irregular sleep–wake schedules. The episodes seem to occur most frequently in the supine position. An association with anxiety/psychiatric disturbances has been described.

The management of RISP consists in reassurance about the benign nature of the episodes and in the avoidance of sleep deprivation and other triggering factors. Recurrent episodes may be treated with REM-suppressing agents such as low doses of tricyclic agents, clonidine, or clonazepam.

Nightmare Disorder

Nightmare disorder is characterized by "recurrent, highly dysphoric dreams, which are disturbing mental experiences that generally occur during REM sleep and that often result in awakening" [1]. Full alertness upon arousal and intact recall of the frightening dream are generally characteristic of the episodes. As REM sleep is more represented in the second half of the night, episodes tend to occur more frequently in the early hours of the morning. Nightmare content consists often in dream sequences that seem vivid and real. Emotions are characteristically negative and most frequently involve anxiety and fear but also anger, rage, embarrassment, and disgust. Monsters or other fantastical imageries often characterize the dreams of young children, whereas adolescent and adults may experience more realistic images derived from daytime stressors or traumatic events. Dream descriptions in preschool age children are usually short and simple, while older children may elaborate the dream content by adding fantastic features. There is rarely any physical movement during dreams because of the REM-induced atonia; somatic manifestations of anxiety such as tachycardia, sweating, and tachypnea may occur. The episodes are generally brief but there may be post-awakening anxiety and difficulty returning to sleep.

Occasional nightmares are very common in children, ranging from 60 to 75 % [94]. However, occasional nightmares do not constitute a nightmare disorder. In preadolescent children the prevalence of nightmare disorder was estimated to be 1.8–6 % [95]. Nightmare onset typically occurs between ages 3 and 6. The prevalence of nightmares decreases as children aged, although they are still common among adults. Close to a third of adults with recurrent nightmares have onset of the symptom during childhood. Nightmares are commonly seen in those who have been physically or sexually abused and in those suffering from posttraumatic stress disorder. A strong association with anxiety disorders has been also described.

Therapy with beta-blockers and dopaminergic agonists and withdrawal from REM-suppressing medications, such as selective serotonin reuptake inhibitors, tricyclic antidepressants, hypnotics, and alcohol, may precipitate or increase the severity of nightmares.

The diagnosis of nightmares is relatively simple, although it is important to ascertain with detail the main features of the event to rule out other sleep disorders, particularly sleep terrors (for details see the Differential Diagnosis section in NREM Parasomnia chapter).

Occasional nightmares do not require specific treatments but only behavioral suggestions such as reassurance of children about the unreal nature of dreams and avoidance of television viewing within 2–3 h of bedtime. Recurrent nightmares may benefit from psychological, pharmacological, or combined treatments, although studies in this field are scanty.

Rescripting techniques, in which parents/therapist and children discuss the dream and invent less frightening ending, can be helpful. Similarly, desensitization toward dream content can help the child to feel more in control of the nightmares, which may also serve to reduce anxiety. Encouraging children to write about or draw their dreams may also yield positive results.

Prazosin, risperidone, and trazodone are the most widely used drugs in treating nightmares.

Other Parasomnias

Exploding Head Syndrome (EHS)

Exploding head syndrome is characterized by a "sudden, loud imagined noise or sense of a violent explosion in the head occurring as the patient is falling asleep or waking during the night" [1, 96]. The abnormal sensation usually lasts a few seconds and is usually accompanied by a sense of fright. There have been reports of associated perceptions of a flash of light, a myoclonic jerk, or a brief stab of head pain. Patients range from having one episode in a lifetime to recurrent episodes per night. In this last case, an insomnia complaint may develop as a result of the recurring arousals.

In the majority of patients, predisposing factors are not recognized; however, some subjects report increased numbers of attacks when under personal stress or overtired. EHS can precede other neurological conditions, such as migraine attacks or sleep paralysis.

There are little systematic epidemiological data on this sleep disorder. It has been hypothesized to have a typical age of onset of over 50 years and to be more common in women and in those suffering from ISP. However, a recent study conducted in 211 undergraduate students using semi-structured diagnostic interviews assessing for both EHS and ISP showed that 18 % of the sample experienced lifetime exploding head syndrome and 16.6 % presented recurrent episodes without a female prevalence. An association with ISP was found in 36.89 % of subjects [97].

The neurophysiologic mechanisms underlying EHS are unknown. An asynchronous switch-off of different cortical regions (visual, acoustic, motor), leading to a prominent burst of neuronal activity, is the most popular pathogenetic hypothesis.

The cornerstone of management in EHS is reassurance and education, as this is a benign condition that remits over time in most patients. Some case reports describe the efficacy of tricyclic antidepressants (clomipramine) and calcium channel blockers (flunarizine) in patients with recurrent EHS.

Sleep-Related Hallucinations

Sleep-related hallucinations are "hallucinatory experiences that occur at sleep onset (hypnagogic) or on awakening from sleep (hypnopompic)" [1]. They are predominantly visual but may include auditory, tactile, or kinetic phenomena. Complex nocturnal visual hallucinations may represent a distinct form of sleep-related hallucinations. They typically occur following a sudden awakening, without recall of a preceding dream. They usually take the form of complex, vivid, relatively immobile images of people or animals, sometimes distorted in shape or size. These hallucinations may remain present for many minutes but usually disappear if ambient illumination is increased.

Hypnagogic and hypnopompic hallucinations can be associated with narcolepsy, but a high prevalence in the normal population is also described. Studies reported a prevalence of 25–37 % for hypnagogic hallucinations and of 7–13 % for hypnopompic hallucinations. Both hypnagogic and hypnopompic hallucinations are more common in younger persons and occur slightly more frequently in women than in men.

On the contrary, complex nocturnal visual hallucinations are often associated with a variety of underlying disorders typical of the elderly, such as visual loss (Charles Bonnet syndrome), Lewy body disorders, and pathology of the mesencephalon and diencephalon (peduncular hallucinosis).

Little objective information is available regarding the management of sleep-related hallucinations. Most often reassurance is sufficient. Tricyclic antidepressants have been suggested for hypnagogic and hypnopompic hallucinations.

Sleep Enuresis

Sleep enuresis (SE) is characterized by "recurrent involuntary voiding that occurs during sleep. In primary SE, recurrent involuntary voiding occurs at least twice a week during sleep after 5 years of age in a patient who has never been consistently dry during sleep for six consecutive months. SE is considered secondary in a child or adult who had previously been dry for six consecutive months and then began wetting at least twice a week. Both primary and secondary enuresis must be present for a period of at least three months" [1]. Primary and secondary SE is considered distinct phenomena with different etiologies and courses. SE is defined as *monosymptomatic* when the subject has no associated daytime symptoms of bladder dysfunction (such as wetting, increased voiding frequency, urgency, jiggling, squatting, and holding maneuvers). But, usually, when a meticulous history is obtained, the majority of children have at least some light daytime void symptoms, and their SE is classifiable as *non-monosymptomatic* [98].

SE is not specific to one stage of sleep and can occur during either NREM or REM sleep. Most enuretic episodes happen during the first half of the night.

From a developmental point of view, complete control of the bladder at night is usually achieved by the age of 5 years; thus bed-wetting in toddlers is physiologic.

The prevalence of NE is between 6 and 10 % at age 7, decreasing to 2 % at 15 years and 0.5–2 % in adults. Approximately 75–90 % of patients with SE have a primary form, while 10–25 % have secondary NE. SE is more frequent in boys than in girls under 11 years of age. After 11 years there is no difference between sexes. This sex-related difference can be due to a different time of sex-related brain or bladder development. The spontaneous annual remission during childhood is about 15 %, and this natural history should be kept in mind when counseling parents about the prognosis of the disorder.

There seems to be a strong genetic predisposition for primary SE. The reported prevalence is 77 % when both parents were enuretic as children and 44 % when one parent has a history of enuresis.

Sleep disorders that fragment sleep such as sleep apnea and periodic leg movements are frequently associated with SE, and treatment of these disorders may cure or reduce their incidence.

While primary SE is a typical childhood disorder, secondary SE can occur at any age.

Indeed, secondary SE is more commonly associated with organic factors such as the following: urinary tract infections, malformations of the genitourinary tract, extrinsic pressure on the bladder (such as chronic constipation or encopresis), medical conditions that result in an inability to concentrate urine (diabetes mellitus or insipidus, sickle cell disease), increased urine production secondary to excessive evening fluid intake (caffeine ingestion, diuretics, or other agents), neurologic diseases (spinal cord abnormalities with neurogenic bladder or seizures), and psychosocial stressors (parental divorce, neglect, physical or sexual abuse, and institutionalization).

Current pathophysiological model hypothesizes that SE results from three interrelated factors: nocturnal polyuria, decreased nocturnal bladder storage ability, and poor arousal to the stimulus of a full bladder. In particular, different studies hypothesized that children with primary SE should show a delay in achieving the normal increase in vasopressin release during sleep, thus developing nocturnal polyuria that exceeds the bladder capacity. If these children do not arouse to the sensation of a full bladder, primary SE can occur. In particular, children with enuresis are often described as "deep sleepers", and their arousal threshold seems to be more elevated in all sleep stages with respect to controls [98].

The management of NE starts from some simple strategies, such as lifting or wakening, rewarding dry nights, bladder training (including retention control training), and fluid restriction.

Alarm systems that alert and awaken the child if any moisture is detected are considered a first-line treatment, and its effect seems to be more gradual but sustained with respect to drugs [99].

The established drug therapy of polyuric bed-wetting is desmopressin, a synthetic analog of the antidiuretic hormone arginine (vasopressin) that decreases nocturnal urine production and increases urinary osmolality. Desmopressin is particularly helpful for short-term use, when a rapid response is needed and seems to have some positive effects in about 70 % of treated children [99]. Finally imipramine and oxybutynin may control enuresis by decreasing the parasympathetic tone of the bladder detrusor muscle.

References

1. American Academy of Sleep Medicine. International classification of sleep disorders. Darien: American Acad. of Sleep Medicine; 2014.
2. Nobili L, De Gennaro L, Proserpio P, Moroni F, Sarasso S, Pigorini A, et al. Local aspects of sleep: observations from intracerebral recordings in humans. Prog Brain Res. 2012;199:219–32.
3. Mahowald MW, Cramer Bornemann MA, Schenck CH. State dissociation, human behavior, and consciousness. Curr Top Med Chem. 2011;11(19):2392–402.
4. Laberge L, Tremblay RE, Vitaro F, Montplaisir J. Development of parasomnias from childhood to early adolescence. Pediatrics. 2000;106(1 Pt 1):67–74.
5. Ohayon MM, Priest RG, Zulley J, Smirne S. The place of confusional arousals in sleep and mental disorders: findings in a general population sample of 13,057 subjects. J Nerv Ment Dis. 2000;188(6):340–8.
6. Zadra A, Desautels A, Petit D, Montplaisir J. Somnambulism: clinical aspects and pathophysiological hypotheses. Lancet Neurol. 2013;12(3):285–94.
7. Petit D, Touchette E, Tremblay RE, Boivin M, Montplaisir J. Dyssomnias and parasomnias in early childhood. Pediatrics. 2007;119(5):e1016–25.
8. Licis AK, Desruisseau DM, Yamada KA, Duntley SP, Gurnett CA. Novel genetic findings in an extended family pedigree with sleepwalking. Neurology. 2011;76(1):49–52.
9. Bjorvatn B, Grønli J, Pallesen S. Prevalence of different parasomnias in the general population. Sleep Med. 2010;11(10):1031–4.
10. Nevsimalova S, Prihodova I, Kemlink D, Skibova J. Childhood parasomnia – a disorder of sleep maturation? Eur J Paediatr Neurol EJPN Off J Eur Paediatr Neurol Soc. 2013;17(6):615–9.
11. Nobili L, Ferrara M, Moroni F, De Gennaro L, Russo GL, Campus C, et al. Dissociated wake-like and sleep-like electro-cortical activity during sleep. Neuroimage. 2011;58(2):612–9.
12. Terzaghi M, Sartori I, Tassi L, Didato G, Rustioni V, LoRusso G, et al. Evidence of dissociated arousal states during NREM parasomnia from an intracerebral neurophysiological study. Sleep. 2009;32(3):409.
13. Terzaghi M, Sartori I, Tassi L, Rustioni V, Proserpio P, Lorusso G, et al. Dissociated local arousal states underlying essential clinical features of non-rapid eye movement arousal parasomnia: an intracerebral stereo-electroencephalographic study: *local sleep and NREM parasomnia.* J Sleep Res. 2012;21(5):502–6.
14. Sarasso S, Pigorini A, Proserpio P, Gibbs SA, Massimini M, Nobili L. Fluid boundaries between wake and sleep: experimental evidence from Stereo-EEG recordings. Arch Ital Biol. 2014;152(2–3):169–77.
15. Bassetti C, Vella S, Donati F, Wielepp P, Weder B. SPECT during sleepwalking. Lancet. 2000;356(9228):484–5.
16. Oliviero A, Marca G, Tonali PA, Pilato F, Saturno E, Dileone M, et al. Functional involvement of cerebral cortex in adult sleepwalking. J Neurol. 2007;254(8):1066–72.
17. Tassinari CA, Cantalupo G, Högl B, Cortelli P, Tassi L, Francione S, et al. Neuroethological approach to frontolimbic epileptic seizures and parasomnias: the same central pattern generators for the same behaviours. Rev Neurol (Paris). 2009;165(10):762–8.
18. Hublin C, Kaprio J, Partinen M, Heikkila K, Koskenvuo M. Prevalence and genetics of sleepwalking a population-based twin study. Neurology. 1997;48(1):177–81.

19. Hublin C, Kaprio J. Genetic aspects and genetic epidemiology of parasomnias. Sleep Med Rev. 2003;7(5):413–21.
20. Lecendreux M, Bassetti C, Dauvilliers Y, Mayer G, Neidhart E, Tafti M. HLA and genetic susceptibility to sleepwalking. Mol Psychiatry. 2003;8(1):114–7.
21. Bisulli F, Vignatelli L, Naldi I, Licchetta L, Provini F, Plazzi G, et al. Increased frequency of arousal parasomnias in families with nocturnal frontal lobe epilepsy: a common mechanism? Epilepsia. 2010;51(9):1852–60.
22. Siclari F, Khatami R, Urbaniok F, Nobili L, Mahowald MW, Schenck CH, et al. Violence in sleep. Brain. 2010;133(12):3494–509.
23. Szelenberger W, Niemcewicz S, Dąbrowska AJ. Sleepwalking and night terrors: psychopathological and psychophysiological correlates. Int Rev Psychiatry. 2005;17(4):263–70.
24. Ohayon MM, Guilleminault C, Priest RG. Night terrors, sleepwalking, and confusional arousals in the general population: their frequency and relationship to other sleep and mental disorders. J Clin Psychiatry. 1999;60(4):268–76; quiz 277.
25. Derry C. Nocturnal frontal lobe epilepsy vs parasomnias. Curr Treat Options Neurol. 2012;14(5):451–63.
26. Oudiette D, Leu S, Pottier M, Buzare M-A, Brion A, Arnulf I. Dreamlike mentations during sleepwalking and sleep terrors in adults. Sleep. 2009;32(12):1621.
27. Pressman MR. Factors that predispose, prime and precipitate NREM parasomnias in adults: clinical and forensic implications. Sleep Med Rev. 2007;11(1):5–30.
28. Owens JA, Spirito A, McGuinn M. The Children's Sleep Habits Questionnaire (CSHQ): psychometric properties of a survey instrument for school-aged children. Sleep. 2000;23(8):1043–51.
29. Archbold KH, Pituch KJ, Panahi P, Chervin RD. Symptoms of sleep disturbances among children at two general pediatric clinics. J Pediatr. 2002;140(1):97–102.
30. Aldrich MS, Jahnke B. Diagnostic value of video-EEG polysomnography. Neurology. 1991;41(7):1060–6.
31. Kushida CA, Littner MR, Morgenthaler T, Alessi CA, Bailey D, Coleman J, et al. Practice parameters for the indications for polysomnography and related procedures: an update for 2005. Sleep. 2005;28(4):499–521.
32. Pilon M, Zadra A, Joncas S, Montplaisir J. Hypersynchronous delta waves and somnambulism: brain topography and effect of sleep deprivation. Sleep. 2006;29(1):77–84.
33. Schenck CH, Pareja JA, Patterson AL, Mahowald MW. Analysis of polysomnographic events surrounding 252 slow-wave sleep arousals in thirty-eight adults with injurious sleepwalking and sleep terrors. J Clin Neurophysiol Off Publ Am Electroencephalogr Soc. 1998;15(2):159–66.
34. Pressman MR. Hypersynchronous delta sleep EEG activity and sudden arousals from slow-wave sleep in adults without a history of parasomnias: clinical and forensic implications. Sleep. 2004;27(4):706–10.
35. Guilleminault C, Kirisoglu C, da Rosa AC, Lopes C, Chan A. Sleepwalking, a disorder of NREM sleep instability. Sleep Med. 2006;7(2):163–70.
36. Gaudreau H, Joncas S, Zadra A, Montplaisir J. Dynamics of slow-wave activity during the NREM sleep of sleepwalkers and control subjects. Sleep. 2000;23(6):755–60.
37. Zadra A, Pilon M, Montplaisir J. Polysomnographic diagnosis of sleepwalking: effects of sleep deprivation. Ann Neurol. 2008;63(4):513–9.
38. Terzano MG, Parrino L. Origin and significance of the Cyclic Alternating Pattern (CAP). REVIEW ARTICLE. Sleep Med Rev. 2000;4(1):101–23.
39. Parrino L, Ferri R, Bruni O, Terzano MG. Cyclic alternating pattern (CAP): the marker of sleep instability. Sleep Med Rev. 2012;16(1):27–45.
40. Guilleminault C, Lee JH, Chan A, Lopes M-C, Huang Y, da Rosa A. Non-REM-sleep instability in recurrent sleepwalking in pre-pubertal children. Sleep Med. 2005;6(6):515–21.
41. Zucconi M, Oldani A, Ferini-Strambi L, Smirne S. Arousal fluctuations in non-rapid eye movement parasomnias: the role of cyclic alternating pattern as a measure of sleep instability. J Clin Neurophysiol Off Publ Am Electroencephalogr Soc. 1995;12(2):147–54.

42. Espa F, Ondze B, Deglise P, Billiard M, Besset A. Sleep architecture, slow wave activity, and sleep spindles in adult patients with sleepwalking and sleep terrors. Clin Neurophysiol Off J Int Fed Clin Neurophysiol. 2000;111(5):929–39.
43. Mason TBA, Pack AI. Sleep terrors in childhood. J Pediatr. 2005;147(3):388–92.
44. Fisher C, Kahn E, Edwards A, Davis DM. A psychophysiological study of nightmares and night terrors. The suppression of stage 4 night terrors with diazepam. Arch Gen Psychiatry. 1973;28(2):252–9.
45. Craske MG, Tsao JCI. Assessment and treatment of nocturnal panic attacks. Sleep Med Rev. 2005;9(3):173–84.
46. Oldani A, Zucconi M, Asselta R, Modugno M, Bonati MT, Dalpra L, et al. Autosomal dominant nocturnal frontal lobe epilepsy. A video-polysomnographic and genetic appraisal of 40 patients and delineation of the epileptic syndrome. Brain J Neurol. 1998;121(Pt 2): 205–23.
47. Provini F, Plazzi G, Tinuper P, Vandi S, Lugaresi E, Montagna P. Nocturnal frontal lobe epilepsy. A clinical and polygraphic overview of 100 consecutive cases. Brain. 1999;122(Pt 6):1017–31.
48. Nobili L, Proserpio P, Combi R, Provini F, Plazzi G, Bisulli F, et al. Nocturnal frontal lobe epilepsy. Curr Neurol Neurosci Rep. 2014;14(2):424.
49. Nobili L, Francione S, Mai R, Cardinale F, Castana L, Tassi L, et al. Surgical treatment of drug-resistant nocturnal frontal lobe epilepsy. Brain. 2007;130(Pt 2):561–73.
50. Scheffer IE, Bhatia KP, Lopes-Cendes I, Fish DR, Marsden CD, Andermann F, et al. Autosomal dominant frontal epilepsy misdiagnosed as sleep disorder. Lancet. 1994;343(8896):515–7.
51. Klaassen A, Glykys J, Maguire J, Labarca C, Mody I, Boulter J. Seizures and enhanced cortical GABAergic inhibition in two mouse models of human autosomal dominant nocturnal frontal lobe epilepsy. Proc Natl Acad Sci USA. 2006;103(50):19152–7.
52. Xu J, Cohen BN, Zhu Y, Dziewczapolski G, Panda S, Lester HA, et al. Altered activity-rest patterns in mice with a human autosomal-dominant nocturnal frontal lobe epilepsy mutation in the beta2 nicotinic receptor. Mol Psychiatry. 2011;16(10):1048–61.
53. Terzaghi M, Sartori I, Mai R, Tassi L, Francione S, Cardinale F, et al. Sleep-related minor motor events in nocturnal frontal lobe epilepsy. Epilepsia. 2007;48(2):335–41.
54. Nobili L, Francione S, Mai R, Tassi L, Cardinale F, Castana L, et al. Nocturnal frontal lobe epilepsy: intracerebral recordings of paroxysmal motor attacks with increasing complexity. Sleep. 2003;26(7):883–6.
55. Plazzi G, Tinuper P, Montagna P, Provini F, Lugaresi E. Epileptic nocturnal wanderings. Sleep. 1995;18(9):749–56.
56. Nobili L, Cossu M, Mai R, Tassi L, Cardinale F, Castana L, et al. Sleep-related hyperkinetic seizures of temporal lobe origin. Neurology. 2004;62(3):482–5.
57. Vaugier L, Aubert S, McGonigal A, Trebuchon A, Guye M, Gavaret M, et al. Neural networks underlying hyperkinetic seizures of "temporal lobe" origin. Epilepsy Res. 2009;86(2–3): 200–8.
58. Proserpio P, Cossu M, Francione S, Tassi L, Mai R, Didato G, et al. Insular-opercular seizures manifesting with sleep-related paroxysmal motor behaviors: a stereo-EEG study. Epilepsia. 2011;52(10):1781–91.
59. Proserpio P, Cossu M, Francione S, Gozzo F, Lo Russo G, Mai R, et al. Epileptic motor behaviors during sleep: anatomo-electro-clinical features. Sleep Med. 2011;12 Suppl 2:S33–8.
60. Derry CP, Davey M, Johns M, Kron K, Glencross D, Marini C, et al. Distinguishing sleep disorders from seizures: diagnosing bumps in the night. Arch Neurol. 2006;63(5):705–9.
61. Manni R, Terzaghi M, Repetto A. The FLEP scale in diagnosing nocturnal frontal lobe epilepsy, NREM and REM parasomnias: data from a tertiary sleep and epilepsy unit. Epilepsia. 2008;49(9):1581–5.
62. Bisulli F, Vignatelli L, Naldi I, Pittau F, Provini F, Plazzi G, et al. Diagnostic accuracy of a structured interview for nocturnal frontal lobe epilepsy (SINFLE): a proposal for developing diagnostic criteria. Sleep Med. 2012;13(1):81–7.

63. Derry CP, Harvey AS, Walker MC, Duncan JS, Berkovic SF. NREM arousal parasomnias and their distinction from nocturnal frontal lobe epilepsy: a video EEG analysis. Sleep. 2009;32(12):1637–44.
64. Nobili L. Can homemade video recording become more than a screening tool? Sleep. 2009;32(12):1544–5.
65. Harris M, Grunstein RR. Treatments for somnambulism in adults: assessing the evidence. Sleep Med Rev. 2009;13(4):295–7.
66. Kotagal S. Treatment of dyssomnias and parasomnias in childhood. Curr Treat Options Neurol. 2012;14(6):630–49.
67. Attarian H. Treatment options for parasomnias. Neurol Clin. 2010;28(4):1089–106.
68. Mahowald MW, Schenck CH. Insights from studying human sleep disorders. Nature. 2005;437(7063):1279–85.
69. Pilon M, Montplaisir J, Zadra A. Precipitating factors of somnambulism: impact of sleep deprivation and forced arousals. Neurology. 2008;70(24):2284–90.
70. Provini F, Tinuper P, Bisulli F, Lugaresi E. Arousal disorders. Sleep Med. 2011;12:S22–6.
71. Kotagal S. Parasomnias in childhood. Sleep Med Rev. 2009;13(2):157–68.
72. Hauri PJ, Silber MH, Boeve BF. The treatment of parasomnias with hypnosis: a 5-year follow-up study. J Clin Sleep Med JCSM Off Publ Am Acad Sleep Med. 2007;3(4):369–73.
73. Hurwitz TD, Mahowald MW, Schenck CH, Schluter JL, Bundlie SR. A retrospective outcome study and review of hypnosis as treatment of adults with sleepwalking and sleep terror. J Nerv Ment Dis. 1991;179(4):228–33.
74. Howell MJ. Parasomnias: an updated review. Neurotherapeutics. 2012;9(4):753–75.
75. Bruni O, Ferri R, Miano S, Verrillo E. L -5-Hydroxytryptophan treatment of sleep terrors in children. Eur J Pediatr. 2004;163(7):402–7.
76. Jan JE, Freeman RD, Wasdell MB, Bomben MM. A child with severe night terrors and sleepwalking responds to melatonin therapy. Dev Med Child Neurol. 2004;46(11):789.
77. Schenck CH, Mahowald MW. Review of nocturnal sleep-related eating disorders. Int J Eat Disord. 1994;15(4):343–56.
78. Howell MJ, Schenck CH, Crow SJ. A review of nighttime eating disorders. Sleep Med Rev. 2009;13(1):23–34.
79. Schenck CH, Hurwitz TD, Bundlie SR, Mahowald MW. Sleep-related eating disorders: polysomnographic correlates of a heterogeneous syndrome distinct from daytime eating disorders. Sleep. 1991;14(5):419–31.
80. Winkelman JW, Herzog DB, Fava M. The prevalence of sleep-related eating disorder in psychiatric and non-psychiatric populations. Psychol Med. 1999;29(6):1461–6.
81. Schenck CH, Hurwitz TD, O'Connor KA, Mahowald MW. Additional categories of sleep-related eating disorders and the current status of treatment. Sleep. 1993;16(5):457–66.
82. Brion A, Flamand M, Oudiette D, Voillery D, Golmard J-L, Arnulf I. Sleep-related eating disorder versus sleepwalking: a controlled study. Sleep Med. 2012;13(8):1094–101.
83. Auger RR. Sleep-related eating disorders. Psychiatry Edgmont. 2006;3(11):64.
84. Howell MJ, Schenck CH. Treatment of nocturnal eating disorders. Curr Treat Options Neurol. 2009;11(5):333–9.
85. Arnulf I. REM sleep behavior disorder: motor manifestations and pathophysiology. Mov Disord Off J Mov Disord Soc. 2012;27(6):677–89.
86. Kotagal S. Rapid eye movement sleep behavior disorder during childhood. Sleep Med Clin. 2015;10(2):163–7.
87. Stores G. Rapid eye movement sleep behaviour disorder in children and adolescents. Dev Med Child Neurol. 2008;50(10):728–32.
88. Lloyd R, Tippmann-Peikert M, Slocumb N, Kotagal S. Characteristics of REM sleep behavior disorder in childhood. J Clin Sleep Med. 2012;8(2):127–31.
89. Buskova J, Nevsimalova S, Kemlink D, Sonka K. REM sleep without atonia in narcolepsy. Neuro Endocrinol Lett. 2009;30(6):757–60.
90. Dauvilliers Y, Jennum P, Plazzi G. Rapid eye movement sleep behavior disorder and rapid eye movement sleep without atonia in narcolepsy. Sleep Med. 2013;14(8):775–81.

91. Mattarozzi K, Bellucci C, Campi C, Cipolli C, Ferri R, Franceschini C, et al. Clinical, behavioural and polysomnographic correlates of cataplexy in patients with narcolepsy/cataplexy. Sleep Med. 2008;9(4):425–33.
92. Schenck CH, Mahowald MW. Motor dyscontrol in narcolepsy: rapid-eye-movement (REM) sleep without atonia and REM sleep behavior disorder. Ann Neurol. 1992;32(1):3–10.
93. Sharpless BA, Barber JP. Lifetime prevalence rates of sleep paralysis: a systematic review. Sleep Med Rev. 2011;15(5):311–5.
94. Zadra A, Donderi DC. Nightmares and bad dreams: their prevalence and relationship to well-being. J Abnorm Psychol. 2000;109(2):273–81.
95. Steinsbekk S, Berg-Nielsen TS, Wichstrøm L. Sleep disorders in preschoolers: prevalence and comorbidity with psychiatric symptoms. J Dev Behav Pediatr JDBP. 2013;34(9):633–41.
96. Sharpless BA. Exploding head syndrome. Sleep Med Rev. 2014;18(6):489–93.
97. Sharpless BA. Exploding head syndrome is common in college students. J Sleep Res. 2015;24(4):447–9.
98. Harari MD. Nocturnal enuresis. J Paediatr Child Health. 2013;49(4):264–71.
99. Caldwell PHY, Deshpande AV, Gontard AV. Management of nocturnal enuresis. BMJ. 2013;347:f6259.

Chapter 15
Sleep and Epilepsy

Sejal V. Jain and Sanjeev V. Kothare

Abstract Sleep and epilepsy are common bedfellows. Sleep influences seizures and epilepsy in terms of frequency and occurrence of interictal spikes and occurrence, timing, and threshold of seizure. On the other hand, epilepsy can worsen sleep architecture and severity of sleep disorders. Thus a vicious cycle is set. Additionally, antiepileptic drugs also influence sleep. So sleep complaints/disorder also should be considered when selecting appropriate antiepileptic drugs. Moreover, sudden unexpected death in epilepsy (SUDEP) occurs in sleep and is most likely associated with cardiorespiratory changes in sleep, occurring ictally or postictally. Furthermore, poor sleep is associated with worsened quality of life, neurocognitive and behavioral functioning, and memory deficits on top of preexisting worsening due to epilepsy itself. Improving sleep and treatment of sleep disorders improve seizure frequency and overall well-being in patients with epilepsy. Hence, sleep evaluation and management are important in patient with epilepsy. In this chapter, we have discussed these interactions.

Keywords Sleep architecture • Obstructive sleep apnea • SUDEP • BECTS • Sleep disorders • ESES • NFLE • JME • Serotonin • Cyclic alternating pattern

Epilepsy affects 1 % of the population in the USA and causes significant impact on society [1]. In layman's terms, recurrent unprovoked seizures define epilepsy. A few years ago, the International League Against Epilepsy (ILAE) redefined epilepsy to be more inclusive and to advocate early treatment. Based on the new definition, (1) two or more unprovoked seizures, occurring more than 24 h apart, or (2) a single

S.V. Jain, MD (✉)
Division of Neurology, Banner University Medical Center,
1501 N Campbell Ave, Tucson, AZ 85724-5023, USA
e-mail: svjain2012@gmail.com; sejal1_in@yahoo.com

S.V. Kothare, MD
Department of Neurology, Comprehensive Epilepsy & Sleep Center, NYU Langone Medical Center, New York, NY, USA
e-mail: sanjeev.kothare@nyumc.org

© Springer International Publishing Switzerland 2017
S. Nevšímalová, O. Bruni (eds.), *Sleep Disorders in Children*,
DOI 10.1007/978-3-319-28640-2_15

unprovoked seizure (reflex seizure) with at least 60 % chances of recurrence or (3) diagnosis of an epileptic syndrome is diagnosed as epilepsy [2]. The diagnosis is based on clinical history and specific diagnostic tests that identify patterns for seizure occurrence. One such testing modality is electroencephalogram (EEG), which as the name suggests measures the electrical potentials of the pyramidal neurons. The abnormal activity which is linked to epilepsy is spike-wave discharges or interictal epileptiform discharges (IEDs), the presence of which may be helpful in diagnosing an event as a seizure. Based on the cerebral location, frequency of occurrence, morphology, and amplitude of abnormalities on EEG, certain epilepsy syndromes are identified. One example is benign epilepsy with centrotemporal spikes [BECTS or benign Rolandic epilepsy (BRE)], which is discussed later in the chapter. Additionally, rhythmic, evolving EEG patterns that disrupt the normal electrical background activity constitute most seizures electrographically. In the last two decades, there has been significant advancement in treatment of epilepsy as several new drugs and a few new devices have become available. Despite these, epilepsy largely remains incurable and in about a third of the patients, uncontrollable. Moreover, significant comorbidities have also been reported, one of which is coexisting sleep disorders and sleep problems.

Sleep and epilepsy are interrelated. This is well known since the ancient times. Aristotle wrote that sleep is similar to epilepsy and in the same way that sleep is to epilepsy. In 1885, Gower described that 21 % of children had nocturnal seizures. He also reported that nocturnal seizures occurred at specific times in sleep. Ferre described that seizures affected sleep [3–5]. The effects of sleep and epileptiform discharges were first described by Gibbs and Gibbs in 1947 [3–5]. In this chapter, we discuss these interactions.

Effect of Sleep on EEG, Seizures, and Epilepsy

Sleep activates interictal epileptiform discharges (IEDs). Studies in adults with focal epilepsy show that the spike frequency increases with increasing depth of NREM sleep besides the field of discharge, which also increases [6, 7]. On the other end, spike frequency and the field are reduced in REM sleep [8]. Due to both of these phenomena, REM-related IEDs can help to identify the seizure focus [9, 10]. Studies in children have shown that some children may have spikes only during sleep [11]. In children, the IEDs in focal epilepsies are more common during N1 and N2 stages of sleep [12].

Seizures are also known to occur during specific sleep stages. It is well documented that seizures are rare in REM sleep. A recent study reevaluated and confirmed that REM sleep was protective for seizure occurrence by reviewing 42 studies. The study showed that seizures in N1, N2, and N3 were 87, 68, and 51 times more common than in REM sleep, respectively. Even compared to wakefulness, both generalized and focal seizures were less common in REM sleep. Moreover, EEG of certain epilepsy syndromes such as BECTS and electrical status epilepticus during sleep (ESES) had marked improvement in REM sleep [13]. Additionally, sleep also influences epilepsy based on the location of seizure origin. In a study, 78 % of frontal lobe seizures were sleep related, while only 20 % of temporal lobe seizures were sleep related [14]. The temporal lobe seizures were more likely to generalize in sleep [15]. Furthermore, sleep can provide a differential diagnosis for psychogenic non-epileptic seizures (PNES) from epileptic seizures as PNES do not occur in sleep, so occurrence of events during sleep helps to diagnose seizures [16].

Just like sleep and other bodily functions, seizures also follow circadian rhythms. Studies show that tonic and tonic-clonic seizures occurred more frequently in sleep, while clonic, absence, atonic seizures and myoclonic seizures occurred in wakefulness. Epileptic spasms had two peaks at 6–9 am and 3–6 pm in wakefulness [17]. Seizures of temporal lobe origin occurred mainly between 1100 and 1700, while frontal seizures were seen mostly between 2300 and 0500 [18]. In another study, occipital seizures peaked at 1600–1900, parietal and frontal peaked at 0400–0700, and temporal seizures peaked bimodally at 0700 and 1600–1900 [19]. The proof that this is not just time based but actually based on circadian rhythm was provided by a study correlating dim light melatonin onset (DLMO) with seizure occurrence. In the study, temporal seizures occurred most frequently during the times 6 h before DLMO and frontal seizures mainly in 6–12 h after the DLMO [20]. Since these studies were performed in a hospital epilepsy monitoring unit setting, which may not represent a true sleep-wake cycle for subjects, a study evaluated circadian pattern of seizure occurrence on ambulatory EEG where patients are in the home environment. In this cohort, frontal lobe seizures occurred more frequently between 12 am and 12 pm, and temporal lobe seizures occurred more frequently between 12 pm and 12 am. Moreover, frontal lobe seizures clustered between 5:15 and 7:30 am, while temporal lobe seizures clustered between 6:45 and 11:56 pm [21]. Furthermore, sunlight may also affect seizure occurrence as complex partial seizures were less likely to occur on bright sunny days, than dull days in a study [22].

This information on circadian pattern of seizure occurrence is very helpful for treatment strategies. There is possibility of light therapy and changing the circadian pattern for treatment of epilepsy. Additionally, a study suggested that differential dosing with two-third dose in the evening for predominantly nocturnal seizures led to seizure freedom in 64.7 % of patients, while 88.2 % experienced more than 50 % reductions in seizures [23]. There was mild increase in nocturnal peak levels as compared to daytime levels with the differential dosing. This approach may also be helpful in reducing side effects of antiepileptic drugs (AEDs).

Sleep deprivation is one of the most commonly reported seizure precipitating factors in children with intractable epilepsy [24]. Additionally, patients with JME are very sensitive to seizure occurrence due to sleep deprivation. However, there is still some controversy whether sleep deprivation increases IEDs. In general, activation is seen even if no sleep is recorded on the EEG, and hence, most EEG laboratories have established protocols for sleep-deprived EEGs. Sleep deprivation is also known to induce seizures in certain epilepsies and in patients with no history of seizures [12, 25, 26].

There are several mechanisms hypothesized to explain the activated IEDs and seizures in sleep. During NREM sleep neuronal networks are hypersynchronized. This helps to propagate the IEDs which are also believed to be generated by the same thalamocortical circuit similar to the sleep-specific architecture such as spindle and slow waves. During REM sleep, this synchronization is absent which reduces the spread of IEDs.

The second theory relates to a cyclic alternating pattern (CAP), described in sleep EEG which is a marker of unstable sleep. This pattern is present in NREM sleep and at the transition from NREM to REM sleep. The pattern is defined by two phases, first is phase A, of transient events, and second is phase B, the background rhythm in between. Additionally, CAP phase A is further divided into (1) phase of synchrony (A1 subtype), which comprises of delta bursts, K-complex sequences, vertex sharp transients, and polyphasic bursts with <20 % of EEG desynchrony; (2) phase of a mixture of slow and fast rhythms (A2 subtype), which includes polyphasic bursts with 20–50 % of EEG desynchrony; and (3) phase of rapid low-voltage rhythms (A3 subtype), which includes K-alpha, EEG arousals, and polyphasic bursts with >50 % of EEG desynchrony. Each CAP cycle begins with phase A and ends with phase B and lasts 2–60 s in duration. At least two such cycles form CAP sequence. CAP sequences are intermixed with non-CAP, which is the absence of CAP for more than 60 s, and represent stable sleep. CAP sequences, particularly, phases A2 and A3, have 87 % of the arousals seen in NREM sleep. CAP rate is calculated as the percentage ratio of total CAP time to non-REM sleep time, which is a measure of arousal instability and has been used as a measure for restorative sleep in sleep disorders [27].

CAP cycles have also been evaluated in patients with epilepsy. In genetic generalized epilepsy, higher CAP rate is reported along with spikes occurring during phase A1. In lesional temporal lobe epilepsy, higher IEDs are seen during CAP cycle, specifically, during phase A1 as compared to non-CAP. Ninety-one percent of secondarily generalized focal lesional bursts are identified in CAP, while 96 % of all the generalized IEDs are found in CAP phase A [28]. Additionally, seizures also occurred during CAP cycle and in phase A than in phase B [29]. Moreover, in children with BECTS, CAP analysis showed reduced instability due to the presence of spikes which replaced the phase A1 and suggested that the centrotemporal spikes may disrupt the physiological synchronization mechanism [30]. In children with drug-resistant epilepsy, an increase of CAP rate in N2 was noted as compared to children with BECTS. Additionally, an increase in A1 index in N1 and N2 and significant reduction of A3 index in N1 were noted [31].

Based on these data, it is hypothesized that both CAP and IEDs are derived from similar if not the same anatomical pathways (thalamocortical). It is believed that CAP sequence triggers paroxysmal bursts like IEDs and IEDs promote the generation of phase A and, hence, increase instability. On the other hand, non-CAP part of sleep is unfavorable to IED generation due to reduced arousals [28].

Adenosine is also implicated in the complex relationships of sleep and epilepsy. Extracellular adenosine is antiepileptic, exerting its effects through pre- and postsynaptic adenosine receptors. The adenosine level depends upon the adenosine kinase (ADK) activity. Increased activity of ADK reduces adenosine and increases neuronal excitability. This endogenous adenosine mechanism is disrupted in chronic epilepsy. In studies, ADK activity was found to be overexpressed in mesial temporal sclerosis and temporal lobe epilepsy. Additionally, there was decreased expression of level of A_1 receptors [32]. Moreover, adenosine is essential in regulation of sleep homeostasis. In the event of disrupted system, poor sleep is noted [33]. So dysregulated adenosine system may also be a factor causing poor sleep in patients with chronic epilepsy.

Sleep-Related Epilepsy Syndromes

Certain epilepsy syndromes are related to sleep-wake cycle or occur depending on sleep state or arousal from sleep. These are termed sleep-related epilepsies and include the following.

West Syndrome [34]

It is characterized by epileptic spasm, hypsarrhythmia, and developmental delay. The onset occurs at 3–12 months of age. The spasms are flexor or extensor movements of the head, trunk, and limbs, which are brief and typically occur in clusters. The classic EEG pattern of hypsarrhythmia is characterized by very high amplitude multifocal spikes occurring over a chaotic background. This pattern is often seen in NREM sleep at the onset of the disorder and sometimes exclusively. Additionally, the associated epileptic spasms occur in clusters soon after awakening, which is pseudo-normalization of the EEG during that time. Treatment is recommended as early as possible after the diagnosis. Adrenocorticotrophic hormone and vigabatrin are approved treatment options.

Panayiotopoulos Syndrome [34]

It is an age-related benign focal epilepsy syndrome with usual onset between 3 and 6 years of age. Seizures are characterized by nausea, visual changes, and prominent autonomic symptoms with preserved consciousness. Majority of seizures occur in sleep (70%) or up on awakening (13%). These seizures can last from 30 min to several hours (autonomic status). EEG most commonly shows occipital discharges; however, temporal and parietal discharges are also seen. The ictal EEG shows theta waves intermixed with spikes or fast activity in anterior or posterior head region. The prognosis is good with resolution within 1–2 years of onset.

Benign Epilepsy with Centrotemporal Spikes (BECTS) [34]

BECTS or benign Rolandic epilepsy is the most common epilepsy in childhood. The onset occurs between 3 and 13 years of age and remission occurs by 16 years of age. The typical seizures are hemifacial sensory or motor and associated with speech slurring and drooling. Consciousness is typically preserved. They may progress to unilateral arm and leg and occasionally to generalization. About 70 % of seizures occur in sleep. EEG shows characteristic spikes and wave discharges in fronto-central and temporal head region occurring independently or synchronously with a horizontal dipole. The IEDs are amplified in NREM sleep. The seizure frequency and severity is disproportionate to the amount of IEDs. Cognitive behavioral and sleep problems have been associated with the syndrome. Treatment with focal antiepileptic drugs is effective and long-term prognosis is good.

Electrical Status Epilepticus During Sleep (ESES) and Related Disorders [34]

ESES is characterized by spike and wave discharges occurring almost continuously during slow-wave sleep. This pattern is associated with seizures and cognitive dysfunction. The term continuous spike-wave discharges during sleep (CSWS) was coined to dissociate clinical connotation from "status epileptics" in the ESES terminology. These terms are used interchangeable in literature many times. The syndromes are age-dependent epileptic encephalopathies with peak onset at 2–4 years of age. The seizure onset is prior to typical EEG pattern. Generalized tonic-clonic seizures as well as daytime atypical absences are seen. Tonic seizures are not seen. Cognitive deficits and behavioral problems are associated with the syndrome and may occur as an acute regression or insidious development after months of seizure onset. Daytime EEG may show focal or generalized spikes and sleep EEG shows spike-wave index of 85–100 % during NREM sleep. Additionally, recognition of normal sleep architecture is difficult. Treatment of spikes may improve cognitive function and should be started immediately and aggressively after the diagnosis. Treatment options are high-dose benzodiazepines, steroids, valproic acid, levetiracetam, immunoglobulins, etc. The prognosis is dependent upon etiology, duration, and treatment response.

Landau-Kleffner Syndrome It is a disorder characterized by acquired receptive aphasia due to auditory agnosia and epilepsy. The EEG shows almost continuous spike and wave discharges in unilateral or bilateral temporal region during NREM sleep. In addition to language, cognitive and behavioral problems can also be associated. Onset is between 2 and 8 years with regression. Treatment of EEG spikes improves language function. Treatments are similar to ESES treatments.

Atypical Benign Partial Epilepsy/Pseudo-Lennox Syndrome The syndrome is characterized by similar presentation as benign focal epilepsies but associated ESES EEG pattern and mental deficits. The prognosis and treatments are similar to ESES.

The presence of GRIN2A mutations in ESES, Landau-Kleffner syndrome, and BECTS suggests that these syndromes possibly occur as a continuum.

Juvenile Myoclonic Epilepsy [34]

JME affects 1–2% of general population worldwide. It is closely linked to sleep as most seizures occur upon awakening and sleep deprivation is a strong trigger for seizure occurrence. The age of onset is from 12 to 18 in 79% of patients. The characteristic seizures are myoclonic jerks that occur upon or soon after awakenings and may progress to generalized tonic-clonic seizures. The myoclonic seizures may be missed at the onset as they are thought to be clumsiness (dropping things) or tics/twitches. The diagnosis is typically made after a generalized tonic-clonic seizure (GTC), and upon obtaining further history, the myoclonic seizures become evident. About 20% of patients have absence seizure which may suggest a poor prognosis for seizure freedom if these occur at the onset of the epilepsy. The characteristic EEG pattern is polyspikes and waves and/or spike and wave discharges occurring at 2.5–3.5 Hz. Treatment with valproic acid and other broad-spectrum AEDs is recommended. Prognosis for seizure control on AEDs is good, with majority of the patients requiring lifelong treatment.

Nocturnal Frontal Lobe Epilepsy [34]

Nocturnal frontal lobe epilepsy represents an epilepsy syndrome which is misdiagnosed as parasomnia often. The onset is in adolescence or young adulthood. Three clinical seizure patterns were described which are (1) paroxysmal arousals, (2) nocturnal paroxysmal dystonia, and (3) episodic nocturnal wandering. The autosomal dominant type, called as autosomal dominant nocturnal frontal lobe epilepsy (ADNFLE), is associated with mutations in nicotinic acetylcholine receptor (CHRNA4) and in other genes (KCNT1 and DEPDC5). The clinical manifestations can vary between individuals in the family, but for the same individual, the seizures are stereotypic. Complex behaviors and sleep-related violent behaviors may also be present in addition to above-described pattern. The corresponding EEG findings include ictal epileptiform abnormalities predominantly over frontal areas in 31.6% of patients or rhythmic ictal slow-wave activity over larger anterior cortical areas in another 47.4%. A third of patients also have associated non-REM parasomnias [35].

Effect of Seizures and Epilepsy on Sleep

A seizure occurring in sleep causes significant reduction of REM sleep and sleep efficiency and increases N1. If the seizure occurs before the first REM cycle, the REM sleep and sleep efficiency are further reduced. Decrease in total sleep time due to reduced REM sleep and increased wake times have also been reported [36].

Epilepsy also affects sleep. In adults with epilepsy, increased N1 and decreased N3 and REM were seen [37]. Additionally, increase in sleep instability in terms of stage shifts and sleep fragmentation caused by increased arousals and wake times was seen [36]. Fragmented sleep was more common in temporal lobe epilepsy as compared to frontal lobe or generalized epilepsy [36, 38]. In children with refractory focal epilepsy, decreased time in bed, total sleep time, and increased N3 were seen [39]. In children with generalized epilepsy, increased N1% and REM sleep latency were seen [40]. In children with epileptic encephalopathies, fragmented sleep, increased REM latency, and reduced total sleep times were seen [41]. In children with refractory epilepsy with a brain lesion, reduction in total sleep time and sleep latency and an increase in REM latency and wake times have been described [31]. In children with tuberous sclerosis, increased arousals, wake time, increased N1, and reduced REM sleep were seen [42]. As discussed above, poor quality of sleep essentially creates a sleep-deprived state which then can precipitate seizures. Additionally, reduction in REM sleep and increased N1 sleep also perpetuates seizures, which further reduces REM sleep.

Effect of Antiepileptic Drugs (AEDs) on Sleep

Various studies in healthy adults and patients with epilepsy show that AEDs also affect sleep architecture. In healthy adults, clobazam reduced sleep latency. Clobazam also reduced arousals and wake time, similar to levetiracetam, phenobarbital, tiagabine, and pregabalin. Carbamazepine reduced sleep latency, arousal, and wake times. Gabapentin increased REM sleep, while carbamazepine, levetiracetam, and phenobarbital reduced it. Levetiracetam, carbamazepine, tiagabine, and pregabalin enhanced slow-wave sleep. Lacosamide did not affect sleep architecture in healthy adults [43]. The effects of antiepileptic drugs in patients with epilepsy are shown in Table 15.1. Even though there are reports of AEDs increasing sleepiness, in objective studies this was not identified for zonisamide, lamotrigine, topiramate, and vigabatrin. Valproic acid, phenobarbital, and high-dose levetiracetam objectively caused sleepiness in studies [44].

Non-medication treatments of epilepsy have also been shown to influence sleep. VNS improved daytime sleepiness and slow-wave sleep. Epilepsy surgery improved total sleep time (TST) and reduced arousals if the seizure frequency was also improved. Ketogenic diet also improved nocturnal sleep. As discussed above, improved seizure frequency may affect the sleep architecture by itself. Hence, when evaluating effects of AEDs on sleep architecture, it is important to note that many of

Table 15.1 Effect of antiepileptic drugs on sleep architecture

	TST	N1	N2	N3	REM	SL	WASO	Arousals	Sleepiness
Carbamazepine	–	–	–	↑	–	–	–	–	NA
ETH	–	↑	–	↓	↑	–	–	–	NA
Gabapentin	–	↓	–	↑	↑	–	–	↓	NA
Lamotrigine	–	–	↑/–	↓/–	↑/–	–	–	–	–
Levetiracetam	–	–	↑	↓	–	–	–	–	↑
Phenobarbital	–	–	↑	–	↓	↓	–	↓	↓
Phenytoin	–	↑	↓	↓/↑	↓	↓	–	–	NA
Pregabalin	–	↓	–	↑	–	–	–	–	NA
Topiramate	–	–	–	–	–	–	–	–	–
Valproic acid	↑	↑	–	–	↑	↓	↓	↓	↑
Vigabatrin	–	–	–	–	–	–	–	–	–
Zonisamide	–	–	–	–	–	–	–	–	–

TST total sleep time (also included is sleep efficiency in this column), *SL* sleep latency, *WASO* wakefulness after sleep onset; sleepiness was measured by mostly multiple sleep latency test (MSLT), but also maintenance of wakefulness test (MWT)

these studies did not analyze effects on sleep independent of improved seizure frequency [44].

Several AEDs have been implicated in either precipitating or worsening of sleep disorders. Vagus nerve stimulator use has been associated with sleep-related breathing disorders such as obstructive sleep apnea and central apneic patterns [45, 46]. AEDs such as benzodiazepine and phenobarbital have been suggested to worsen obstructive sleep apnea [47]. Depakote is also suggested to worsen OSA; however, this was not found in a study [48]. Felbamate and lamotrigine have been thought to worsen insomnia [47]. A recent study suggested that zonisamide by affecting carbonic anhydrase activity and causing weight loss may improve obstructive sleep apnea in obese adults with epilepsy [49].

Antiepileptic drugs significantly affect sleep architecture; hence the selection of AED for an individual patient should be customized, i.e., in a patient with insomnia, gabapentin may be useful. In a patient with higher risk of sleep apnea, proper sleep evaluation and treatment should be undertaken and continued before VNS is implanted and stimulation is increased to rapid cycling. Felbamate and possibly lamotrigine should be avoided or administered early in the evening in patients with insomnia. Valproic acid and phenobarbital should be avoided in children with excessive sleepiness in addition to sleep evaluation.

Sleep Disorders in Epilepsy and Impact of Treatment of Sleep Disorders on Epilepsy

Sleep disorders are common in epilepsy and many of the disorders have a higher prevalence than the general population.

Questionnaire-Based Studies for Sleep Problems

Studies using questionnaires have shown that children with epilepsy have higher sleep problems than siblings or healthy controls. Difficulty initiating and maintaining sleep and co-sleeping were more common in children with epilepsy as compared to siblings [50–54]. Even in children with new onset seizures, sleep problems were present in 45% and were associated with worse neuropsychological functioning [51]. Among epilepsy-related factors, nocturnal seizures and seizure frequency contributed toward higher sleep problems [50]. In younger children, sleep-related anxieties were more common, while in older children, poor sleep was associated with poor daytime behavior [55]. Additionally in a study, higher sleep problems were associated with worse quality of life [53].

Sleep Apnea

In adults with refractory epilepsy, obstructive sleep apnea was noted in a third of the patients [56]. Several other studies have suggested higher prevalence of OSA in epilepsy as compared to general population [22, 48]. In children with epilepsy, screened with clinical history and questionnaires for OSA, 80% had obstructive apnea [57]. In retrospective studies in patients referred to sleep lab, sleep-disordered breathing is reported in 40% of children [58]. In another study, uncontrolled epilepsy was a risk factor for obstructive sleep apnea as compared with primary snoring [48]. Obstructive index increased with increasing number of antiepileptic drugs [48]. Additionally, children with epilepsy had higher number of arousals, prolonged sleep latency, and higher O_2 desaturations as compared to controls with higher severity of OSA [58].

Central Sleep Apnea (CSA)

A retrospective study suggested that children with abnormal MRI of the brain are at higher risk of central sleep apnea [59]. No other data exist in children. In adults with epilepsy, OSA and mixed apnea were more prevalent than CSA. CSA was more common in males and in focal epilepsy [60]. Central apneas are also associated with seizures [31].

Restless Leg Syndrome (RLS)/Periodic Limb Movement Disorder (PLMD)

In retrospective studies in cohort of children referred to sleep lab, PLMs/PLMD was found in 5–10% [58, 61]. In studies in adults with epilepsy, 15% had PLMD and 17% had PLMs in sleep [62, 63]. In adult patients with epilepsy, RLS was identified in

18–35 % [62, 64]. No data exist on RLS in children with epilepsy. This may be due to difficulties in diagnosing children with RLS due to difficulty obtaining history from younger children, confusing the diagnosis with growing pains and studies focusing on referrals to sleep lab. As RLS and PLMD coexist in children, it is possible that some of the studies may have included the children with combination of the disorders.

Insomnia

Insomnia is under-recognized in children with epilepsy. In a study, 82 % of surveyed providers used melatonin or a hypnotic for sleep problems, prior to referral to a sleep specialist [61]. In children with epilepsy referred for sleep evaluation, insomnia was identified in 11 % [61]. In adult with epilepsy, 40–55 % subjects had insomnia [51, 65]. Sleep maintenance insomnia is more common (52 %) than sleep onset insomnia (34 %) [64]. Insomnia correlates with number of AEDs and higher scores on depression scales. Insomnia and poor sleep quality predict poorer quality of life [66].

Parasomnia

Parasomnias are common in children, especially in younger children. Hence, just by mere association, these are common in children with epilepsy also. This presents challenges for diagnosis in nocturnal epilepsy. Additionally, in patients with nocturnal frontal lobe epilepsy (NFLE), 30 % also have arousal parasomnia [67]. Hence, evaluation with careful history and video EEG monitoring may be needed for accurate diagnosis in these children. Some of the differentiating features include onset parasomnia seen in children younger than 10 years of age, whereas seizures of NFLE start at a later age, and parasomnia events are longer, have different behavior patterns, and occur during earlier part of the night, out of N3. On the other end, NFLE seizures are brief and highly stereotypic, may occur multiple times in the night, and are usually out of N1/N2 [68].

Sleepiness

Sleepiness is very common in children with epilepsy, present in 28–48 % of patients. However, referrals for sleep evaluations are limited for this complaint. The reason may be that most neurologists attribute sleepiness to antiepileptic drugs [61]. However, prospective studies in adults with epilepsy suggest that sleepiness is correlated with sleep apnea and RLS symptoms, habitual snoring, observed apneas, recurrence of seizures, neck circumference, and anxiety also [62, 69, 70]. Similarly, in children with epilepsy, 46.2 % of children with epilepsy had sleepiness which was associated with sleep disorders and not with the epilepsy syndrome, AEDs, and the presence or absence of seizure freedom [71].

Impact of Treatment of Sleep Disorders

OSA

There are several studies showing that treatment of OSA improves seizure frequency. A retrospective review in adult patients with OSA and epilepsy, treated with CPAP at least for 6 months, showed decreased seizure frequency. More than half of the CPAP-compliant subjects became seizure-free. In the non-compliant group, no significant differences were seen [72]. CPAP also improved IEDs in wakefulness and sleep except for REM sleep [73]. In a randomized study, 50 % responder rate was 28 % on CPAP as compared to 15 % of controls [74]. A recent study showed that the odds of more than 50 % reduction or seizure freedom in PAP-treated subjects were 9.9 and 3.91 times compared to untreated OSA and no OSA, respectively. PAP-treated subjects had 32.3 times the odds of having 50 % or more seizure reduction compared with the untreated OSA and 6.13 times compared with no OSA [75]. Additionally, treatment of underlying OSA with adenotonsillectomy resulted in improvement in seizure frequency [76].

Melatonin

A few randomized studies evaluated the effect of treatment of insomnia with melatonin in epilepsy. In a study, significant improvement was seen in sleep questionnaire total sleep score on melatonin [77]. In a study in children and young adults, no improvement was seen on actigraphy or sleep diary [78]. However, seizure frequency was significantly reduced. In another study, sleep latency was reduced on melatonin on sleep logs [79]. In a class I study, sleep latency and WASO were improved significantly. Additionally, there was some improvement in sleep efficiency (3.8 %) on polysomnography, total sleep time on actigraphy, and sleep duration and later wake times based on sleep diary on melatonin. Moreover, N3% was increased on melatonin. There was a trend toward improvement in epileptiform discharges [80].

Sudden Unexpected Death in Epilepsy (SUDEP), Sleep, and Cardiorespiratory Abnormalities

SUDEP is defined as a "sudden, unexpected, witnessed or unwitnessed, non-traumatic and non-drowning death in patients with epilepsy with or without evidence for a seizure and excluding documented status epilepticus in which postmortem examination does not reveal a toxicologic or anatomic cause for death"

[81]. The incidence depends on the age, the seizure frequency, and the type of epilepsy and could be as high as 6.0–9.3 per 1000 patient-years among patients with refractory surgery evaluated for or treated with epilepsy surgery or vagus nerve stimulation for epilepsy [82]. The incidence in children is estimated to be 1–2/10,000 patient-years, with a slight male preponderance [83]. Up to 70 % of these deaths occur in sleep, and hence, it is a concern for sleep providers as they may be evaluating patients at risk for it. A variety of risk factors and mechanisms have been suggested and there is no one accepted theory for causation. In children, the risk factors are believed to be major neurological impairment, refractory seizures, and generalized tonic-clonic seizures. In a study, half of the children with SUDEP had symptomatic epilepsy [83]. In children with epilepsy but without neurological handicap, risk of death was similar to general population [84]. Since most deaths occur after seizures, it is believed that it is related to events occurring during or after seizures. One of the mechanisms thought to be responsible for SUDEP is respiratory and cardiac changes during seizures. The respiratory abnormalities include central and obstructive apneas, hypoventilation, hypercapnia, and desaturation with acidosis, bradypnea, and tachypnea [85]. Respiratory abnormalities such as central apnea or hypopneas were noted in 53 % of the seizures, and oxygen desaturation below 90 % occurred in a third of the seizures. Additionally, there was substantial increase in CO_2 levels [86]. In studies in pediatric epilepsy, risk factors for ictal central apnea were younger age, temporal lobe seizures, left hemispheric seizures, symptomatic generalized seizures, longer seizures, desaturation, ictal bradycardia, and more antiepileptic drugs. Similarly, desaturation was more prevalent in longer-duration seizures, ictal apnea, ictal bradycardia, and more AEDs [87]. The cardiac abnormalities include postictal changes in heart rate variability caused by sympathetic activation, ictal bradycardia, asystole, repolarization, anomalies (prolonged or shortened QTc interval), and atrial fibrillation [85]. In pediatric epilepsy, ictal bradycardia was more prevalent in male patients, longer-duration seizures, desaturation, and more AEDs [87]. Additionally, children with Dravet syndrome have also been shown to be at higher risk due to decrease in heart rate variability presumably caused by sodium channel mutations [88, 89]. Moreover, postictal EEG suppression may be another mechanism which is more common in adults [85, 90]. Dysfunction in the serotonin system has been linked to epilepsy. Additionally, respiratory changes such as apnea or hypoventilation are common with generalized seizures. Serotonergic system also plays an important role in breathing control. Additionally, in animal model of epilepsy, SSRIs have been shown to reduce post-seizure respiratory arrest [86]. Hence, SSRIs may have a role in SUDEP prevention.

Behavior, Quality of Life, and Memory, Sleep, and Epilepsy

Poor memory, behavior, and quality of life along with psychiatric problems are common in patients with epilepsy. Sleep problems can worsen these [25]. Even in children with new onset seizures, sleep disturbances are associated with higher behavioral problems as well as poorer neuropsychological function [51].

Other studies have shown more behavioral problems and poorer psychological functioning in children with sleep problems than without sleep problems [25, 55]. Additionally, psychiatric problems and depression are also associated with epilepsy. In a recent study, suicidal ideation was also linked to poor sleep quality in patients with epilepsy [91]. Moreover, patients with epilepsy and sleep problems have poorer quality of life as compared to patients without sleep problems [92–94]. These have been seen in the domains of physical cognitive and social function [53]. Furthermore, sleep enhances memory consolidation. Slow-wave sleep enhances declarative memories, while REM sleep improves procedural and emotional memory. Hence, poor sleep can affect memory in children with epilepsy. In a recent study, children with idiopathic focal epilepsies had poorer sleep-related memory consolidation. This also correlated with IEDs in NREM sleep [95]. Hence, sleep problems worsen the other comorbidities of epilepsy, and adequate treatments should be performed for sleep problems and sleep disorders.

Conclusion

Sleep and epilepsy are interrelated and worsening of one worsens the other and sets up a vicious cycle. Epilepsy comorbidities of poor behavior, quality of life, and memory are further worsened by poor sleep. Moreover, sleep disorders are very common and treatment of them may improve seizure control. Hence, education on improving sleep quality and screening, evaluation, and treatment for sleep problems should be a part of routine care in patients with epilepsy.

References

1. Kwan P, Brodie MJ. Early identification of refractory epilepsy. N Engl J Med. 2000;342(5):314–9.
2. Fisher RS, Acevedo C, Arzimanoglou A, Bogacz A, Cross JH, Elger CE, et al. ILAE official report: a practical clinical definition of epilepsy. Epilepsia. 2014;55(4):475–82. doi:10.1111/epi.12550.
3. Bazil CW, Malow BA, Sammaritano MR. Sleep and epilepsy: the clinical spectrum. 1st ed. Amsterdam: Elsevier; 2002.
4. Lüders H, Dinner DS. Epilepsy and sleep: physiological and clinical relationships. San Diego: Academic; 2001.
5. Kotagal P. The relationship between sleep and epilepsy. Semin Pediatr Neurol. 2001; 8(4):241–50.
6. Malow BA, Lin X, Kushwaha R, Aldrich MS. Interictal spiking increases with sleep depth in temporal lobe epilepsy. Epilepsia. 1998;39(12):1309–16.
7. Sammaritano M, Gigli GL, Gotman J. Interictal spiking during wakefulness and sleep and the localization of foci in temporal lobe epilepsy. Neurology. 1991;41(2 (Pt 1)):290–7.
8. Foldvary-Schaefer N, Grigg-Damberger M. Sleep and epilepsy. Semin Neurol. 2009;29(4):419–28. doi:10.1055/s-0029-1237115.

9. Malow BA, Aldrich MS. Localizing value of rapid eye movement sleep in temporal lobe epilepsy. Sleep Med. 2000;1(1):57–60.
10. Rocamora R, Andrzejak RG, Jimenez-Conde J, Elger CE. Sleep modulation of epileptic activity in mesial and neocortical temporal lobe epilepsy: a study with depth and subdural electrodes. Epilepsy Behav. 2013;28(2):185–90. doi:10.1016/j.yebeh.2013.04.010.
11. Shinnar S, Kang H, Berg AT, Goldensohn ES, Hauser WA, Moshe SL. EEG abnormalities in children with a first unprovoked seizure. Epilepsia. 1994;35(3):471–6.
12. Kothare SV, Kaleyias J. Sleep and epilepsy in children and adolescents. Sleep Med. 2010;11(7):674–85. doi:10.1016/j.sleep.2010.01.012. S1389-9457(10)00214-5 [pii].
13. Ng M, Pavlova M. Why are seizures rare in rapid eye movement sleep? Review of the frequency of seizures in different sleep stages. Epilepsy Res Treat. 2013;2013:932790. doi:10.1155/2013/932790.
14. Crespel A, Coubes P, Baldy-Moulinier M. Sleep influence on seizures and epilepsy effects on sleep in partial frontal and temporal lobe epilepsies. Clin Neurophysiol. 2000;111 Suppl 2:S54–9. doi:S1388245700004028 [pii].
15. Herman ST, Walczak TS, Bazil CW. Distribution of partial seizures during the sleep – wake cycle: differences by seizure onset site. Neurology. 2001;56(11):1453–9.
16. Bazil CW, Walczak TS. Effects of sleep and sleep stage on epileptic and nonepileptic seizures. Epilepsia. 1997;38(1):56–62.
17. Zarowski M, Loddenkemper T, Vendrame M, Alexopoulos AV, Wyllie E, Kothare SV. Circadian distribution and sleep/wake patterns of generalized seizures in children. Epilepsia. 2011;52(6):1076–83. doi:10.1111/j.1528-1167.2011.03023.x.
18. Hofstra WA, Spetgens WP, Leijten FS, van Rijen PC, Gosselaar P, van der Palen J, et al. Diurnal rhythms in seizures detected by intracranial electrocorticographic monitoring: an observational study. Epilepsy Behav. 2009;14(4):617–21. doi:10.1016/j.yebeh.2009.01.020.
19. Durazzo TS, Spencer SS, Duckrow RB, Novotny EJ, Spencer DD, Zaveri HP. Temporal distributions of seizure occurrence from various epileptogenic regions. Neurology. 2008;70(15):1265–71. doi:10.1212/01.wnl.0000308938.84918.3f.
20. Hofstra WA, Gordijn MC, van der Palen J, van Regteren R, Grootemarsink BE, de Weerd AW. Timing of temporal and frontal seizures in relation to the circadian phase: a prospective pilot study. Epilepsy Res. 2011;94(3):158–62. doi:10.1016/j.eplepsyres.2011.01.015.
21. Pavlova MK, Woo Lee J, Yilmaz F, Dworetzky BA. Diurnal pattern of seizures outside the hospital: is there a time of circadian vulnerability? Neurology. 2012;78(19):1488–92. doi:10.1212/WNL.0b013e3182553c23.
22. Baxendale S. Seeing the light? Seizures and sunlight. Epilepsy Res. 2009;84(1):72–6. doi:10.1016/j.eplepsyres.2008.11.015.
23. Guilhoto LM, Loddenkemper T, Vendrame M, Bergin A, Bourgeois BF, Kothare SV. Higher evening antiepileptic drug dose for nocturnal and early-morning seizures. Epilepsy Behav. 2011;20(2):334–7. doi:10.1016/j.yebeh.2010.11.017.
24. Fang PC, Chen YJ, Lee IC. Seizure precipitants in children with intractable epilepsy. Brain Dev. 2008;30(8):527–32.
25. van Golde EG, Gutter T, de Weerd AW. Sleep disturbances in people with epilepsy; prevalence, impact and treatment. Sleep Med Rev. 2011. doi:10.1016/j.smrv.2011.01.002. doi:S1087-0792(11)00004-9 [pii].
26. Malow BA. Sleep deprivation and epilepsy. Epilepsy Curr. 2004;4(5):193–5. doi:10.1111/j.1535-7597.2004.04509.x.
27. Parrino L, Ferri R, Bruni O, Terzano MG. Cyclic alternating pattern (CAP): the marker of sleep instability. Sleep Med Rev. 2012;16(1):27–45. doi:10.1016/j.smrv.2011.02.003.
28. Parrino L, Smerieri A, Spaggiari MC, Terzano MG. Cyclic alternating pattern (CAP) and epilepsy during sleep: how a physiological rhythm modulates a pathological event. Clin Neurophysiol. 2000;111 Suppl 2:S39–46.
29. Manni R, Zambrelli E, Bellazzi R, Terzaghi M. The relationship between focal seizures and sleep: an analysis of the cyclic alternating pattern. Epilepsy Res. 2005;67(1-2):73–80. doi:10.1016/j.eplepsyres.2005.08.008.

30. Bruni O, Novelli L, Luchetti A, Zarowski M, Meloni M, Cecili M, et al. Reduced NREM sleep instability in benign childhood epilepsy with centro-temporal spikes. Clin Neurophysiol. 2010;121(5):665–71. doi:10.1016/j.clinph.2009.12.027.

31. Pereira AM, Bruni O, Ferri R, Palmini A, Nunes ML. The impact of epilepsy on sleep architecture during childhood. Epilepsia. 2012;53(9):1519–25. doi:10.1111/j.1528-1167.2012.03558.x.

32. Boison D. Adenosine dysfunction in epilepsy. Glia. 2012;60(8):1234–43. doi:10.1002/glia.22285.

33. Boison D, Aronica E. Comorbidities in neurology: is adenosine the common link? Neuropharmacology. 2015;97:18–34. doi:10.1016/j.neuropharm.2015.04.031.

34. Schmitt B. Sleep and epilepsy syndromes. Neuropediatrics. 2015;46(3):171–80. doi:10.1055/s-0035-1551574.

35. Jain SV, Kothare SV. Sleep and epilepsy. Semin Pediatr Neurol. 2015;22(2):86–92. doi:10.1016/j.spen.2015.03.005.

36. Touchon J, Baldy-Moulinier M, Billiard M, Besset A, Cadilhac J. Sleep organization and epilepsy. Epilepsy Res Suppl. 1991;2:73–81.

37. Marzec ML, Selwa LM, Malow BA. Analysis of the first night effect and sleep parameters in medically refractory epilepsy patients. Sleep Med. 2005;6(3):277–80. doi:10.1016/j.sleep.2005.01.002. doi:S1389-9457(05)00023-7 [pii].

38. Crespel A, Baldy-Moulinier M, Coubes P. The relationship between sleep and epilepsy in frontal and temporal lobe epilepsies: practical and physiopathologic considerations. Epilepsia. 1998;39(2):150–7.

39. Nunes ML, Ferri R, Arzimanoglou A, Curzi L, Appel CC, Costa da Costa J. Sleep organization in children with partial refractory epilepsy. J Child Neurol. 2003;18(11):763–6.

40. Maganti R, Sheth RD, Hermann BP, Weber S, Gidal BE, Fine J. Sleep architecture in children with idiopathic generalized epilepsy. Epilepsia. 2005;46(1):104–9. doi:10.1111/j.0013-9580.2005.06804.x. doi:EPI06804 [pii].

41. Carotenuto M, Parisi P, Esposito M, Cortese S, Elia M. Sleep alterations in children with refractory epileptic encephalopathies: a polysomnographic study. Epilepsy Behav. 2014;35:50–3. doi:10.1016/j.yebeh.2014.03.009.

42. Bruni O, Cortesi F, Giannotti F, Curatolo P. Sleep disorders in tuberous sclerosis: a polysomnographic study. Brain Dev. 1995;17(1):52–6.

43. Hudson JD, Guptill JT, Byrnes W, Yates SL, Williams P, D'Cruz O. Assessment of the effects of lacosamide on sleep parameters in healthy subjects. Seizure. 2015;25:155–9. doi:10.1016/j.seizure.2014.10.012.

44. Jain SV, Glauser TA. Effects of epilepsy treatments on sleep architecture and daytime sleepiness: an evidence-based review of objective sleep metrics. Epilepsia. 2014;55(1):26–37. doi:10.1111/epi.12478.

45. Parhizgar F, Nugent K, Raj R. Obstructive sleep apnea and respiratory complications associated with vagus nerve stimulators. J Clin Sleep Med. 2011;7(4):401–7. doi:10.5664/JCSM.1204.

46. Khurana DS, Reumann M, Hobdell EF, Neff S, Valencia I, Legido A, et al. Vagus nerve stimulation in children with refractory epilepsy: unusual complications and relationship to sleep-disordered breathing. Child's Nerv Syst ChNS Off J Int Soc Pediatr Neurosurg. 2007;23(11):1309–12. doi:10.1007/s00381-007-0404-8.

47. Bazil CW. Effects of antiepileptic drugs on sleep structure: are all drugs equal? CNS Drugs. 2003;17(10):719–28. doi:17103 [pii].

48. Jain SV, Horn PS, Simakajornboon N, Glauser TA. Obstructive sleep apnea and primary snoring in children with epilepsy. J Child Neurol. 2012. doi:10.1177/0883073812440326. doi:0883073812440326 [pii].

49. Eskandari D, Zou D, Karimi M, Stenlof K, Grote L, Hedner J. Zonisamide reduces obstructive sleep apnoea: a randomised placebo-controlled study. Eur Respir J. 2014;44(1):140–9. doi:10.1183/09031936.00158413.

50. Batista BH, Nunes ML. Evaluation of sleep habits in children with epilepsy. Epilepsy Behav. 2007;11(1):60–4. doi:10.1016/j.yebeh.2007.03.016. doi:S1525-5050(07)00100-X [pii].

51. Byars AW, Byars KC, Johnson CS, DeGrauw TJ, Fastenau PS, Perkins S, et al. The relationship between sleep problems and neuropsychological functioning in children with first recognized seizures. Epilepsy Behav. 2008;13(4):607–13.
52. Cortesi F, Giannotti F, Ottaviano S. Sleep problems and daytime behavior in childhood idiopathic epilepsy. Epilepsia. 1999;40(11):1557–65.
53. Wirrell E, Blackman M, Barlow K, Mah J, Hamiwka L. Sleep disturbances in children with epilepsy compared with their nearest-aged siblings. Dev Med Child Neurol. 2005;47(11):754–9. doi:10.1017/S0012162205001581.
54. Ong LC, Yang WW, Wong SW, alSiddiq F, Khu YS. . Sleep habits and disturbances in Malaysian children with epilepsy. J Paediatr Child Health. 2010;46(3):80–4. doi:10.1111/j.1440-1754.2009.01642.x.
55. Stores G, Wiggs L, Campling G. Sleep disorders and their relationship to psychological disturbance in children with epilepsy. Child Care Health Dev. 1998;24(1):5–19.
56. Malow BA, Levy K, Maturen K, Bowes R. Obstructive sleep apnea is common in medically refractory epilepsy patients. Neurology. 2000;55(7):1002–7.
57. Becker DA, Fennell EB, Carney PR. Daytime behavior and sleep disturbance in childhood epilepsy. Epilepsy Behav. 2004;5(5):708–15.
58. Kaleyias J, Cruz M, Goraya JS, Valencia I, Khurana DS, Legido A, et al. Spectrum of polysomnographic abnormalities in children with epilepsy. Pediatr Neurol. 2008;39(3):170–6. doi:10.1016/j.pediatrneurol.2008.06.002. doi:S0887-8994(08)00265-8 [pii].
59. Kritzinger FE, Al-Saleh S, Narang I. Descriptive analysis of central sleep apnea in childhood at a single center. Pediatr Pulmonol. 2011;46(10):1023–30. doi:10.1002/ppul.21469.
60. Vendrame M, Jackson S, Syed S, Kothare SV, Auerbach SH. Central sleep apnea and complex sleep apnea in patients with epilepsy. Sleep Breathing Schlaf Atmung. 2014;18(1):119–24. doi:10.1007/s11325-013-0858-8.
61. Jain SV, Simakajornboon N, Glauser TA. Provider practices impact adequate diagnosis of sleep disorders in children with epilepsy. J Child Neurol. 2012. doi:10.1177/0883073812449692. doi:0883073812449692 [pii].
62. Malow BA, Bowes RJ, Lin X. Predictors of sleepiness in epilepsy patients. Sleep. 1997;20(12):1105–10.
63. Malow BA, Fromes GA, Aldrich MS. Usefulness of polysomnography in epilepsy patients. Neurology. 1997;48(5):1389–94.
64. Khatami R, Zutter D, Siegel A, Mathis J, Donati F, Bassetti CL. Sleep-wake habits and disorders in a series of 100 adult epilepsy patients – a prospective study. Seizure. 2006;15(5):299–306. doi:10.1016/j.seizure.2006.02.018. doi:S1059-1311(06)00044-6 [pii].
65. Lopez MR, Cheng JY, Kanner AM, Carvalho DZ, Diamond JA, Wallace DM. Insomnia symptoms in South Florida military veterans with epilepsy. Epilepsy Behav. 2013;27(1):159–64. doi:10.1016/j.yebeh.2013.01.008.
66. Vendrame M, Yang B, Jackson S, Auerbach SH. Insomnia and epilepsy: a questionnaire-based study. J Clin Sleep Med. 2013;9(2):141–6. doi:10.5664/jcsm.2410.
67. Bisulli F, Vignatelli L, Naldi I, Licchetta L, Provini F, Plazzi G, et al. Increased frequency of arousal parasomnias in families with nocturnal frontal lobe epilepsy: a common mechanism? Epilepsia. 2010;51(9):1852–60. doi:10.1111/j.1528-1167.2010.02581.x.
68. Derry CP, Duncan JS, Berkovic SF. Paroxysmal motor disorders of sleep: the clinical spectrum and differentiation from epilepsy. Epilepsia. 2006;47(11):1775–91. doi:10.1111/j.1528-1167.2006.00631.x. doi:EPI631 [pii].
69. Manni R, Politini L, Sartori I, Ratti MT, Galimberti CA, Tartara A. Daytime sleepiness in epilepsy patients: evaluation by means of the Epworth sleepiness scale. J Neurol. 2000;247(9):716–7.
70. Giorelli AS, Neves GS, Venturi M, Pontes IM, Valois A, Gomes Mda M. Excessive daytime sleepiness in patients with epilepsy: a subjective evaluation. Epilepsy Behav. 2011;21(4):449–52. doi:10.1016/j.yebeh.2011.05.002.
71. Maganti R, Hausman N, Koehn M, Sandok E, Glurich I, Mukesh BN. Excessive daytime sleepiness and sleep complaints among children with epilepsy. Epilepsy Behav. 2006;8(1):272–7. doi:10.1016/j.yebeh.2005.11.002. doi:S1525-5050(05)00464-6 [pii].

72. Vendrame M, Auerbach S, Loddenkemper T, Kothare S, Montouris G. Effect of continuous positive airway pressure treatment on seizure control in patients with obstructive sleep apnea and epilepsy. Epilepsia. 2011;52(11):e168–71. doi:10.1111/j.1528-1167.2011.03214.x.
73. Pornsriniyom D, Shinlapawittayatorn K, Fong J, Andrews ND, Foldvary-Schaefer N. Continuous positive airway pressure therapy for obstructive sleep apnea reduces interictal epileptiform discharges in adults with epilepsy. Epilepsy Behav. 2014;37:171–4. doi:10.1016/j.yebeh.2014.06.025.
74. Malow BA, Foldvary-Schaefer N, Vaughn BV, Selwa LM, Chervin RD, Weatherwax KJ, et al. Treating obstructive sleep apnea in adults with epilepsy: a randomized pilot trial. Neurology. 2008;71(8):572–7.
75. Pornsriniyom D, Kim H, Bena J, Andrews ND, Moul D, Foldvary-Schaefer N. Effect of positive airway pressure therapy on seizure control in patients with epilepsy and obstructive sleep apnea. Epilepsy Behav. 2014;37:270–5. doi:10.1016/j.yebeh.2014.07.005.
76. Segal E, Vendrame M, Gregas M, Loddenkemper T, Kothare SV. Effect of treatment of obstructive sleep apnea on seizure outcomes in children with epilepsy. Pediatr Neurol. 2012;46(6):359–62. doi:10.1016/j.pediatrneurol.2012.03.005.
77. Gupta M, Aneja S, Kohli K. Add-on melatonin improves sleep behavior in children with epilepsy: randomized, double-blind, placebo-controlled trial. J Child Neurol. 2005;20(2):112–5.
78. Goldberg-Stern H, Oren H, Peled N, Garty BZ. Effect of melatonin on seizure frequency in intractable epilepsy: a pilot study. J Child Neurol. 2012;27(12):1524–8. doi:10.1177/0883073811435916.
79. Coppola G, Iervolino G, Mastrosimone M, La Torre G, Ruiu F, Pascotto A. Melatonin in wake-sleep disorders in children, adolescents and young adults with mental retardation with or without epilepsy: a double-blind, cross-over, placebo-controlled trial. Brain Dev. 2004;26(6):373–6.
80. Jain SV, Horn PS, Simakajornboon N, Beebe DW, Holland K, Byars AW, et al. Melatonin improves sleep in children with epilepsy: a randomized, double-blind, crossover study. Sleep Med. 2015;16(5):637–44. doi:10.1016/j.sleep.2015.01.005.
81. Nashef L. Sudden unexpected death in epilepsy: terminology and definitions. Epilepsia. 1997;38(11 Suppl):S6–8. doi:10.1111/j.1528-1157.1997.tb06130.x.
82. Devinsky O. Sudden, unexpected death in epilepsy. N Engl J Med. 2011;365(19):1801–11. doi:10.1056/NEJMra1010481.
83. Camfield P, Camfield C. Sudden unexpected death in people with epilepsy: a pediatric perspective. Semin Pediatr Neurol. 2005;12(1):10–4.
84. Berg AT, Nickels K, Wirrell EC, Geerts AT, Callenbach PM, Arts WF, et al. Mortality risks in new-onset childhood epilepsy. Pediatrics. 2013;132(1):124–31. doi:10.1542/peds.2012-3998.
85. Kothare SV, Singh K. Cardiorespiratory abnormalities during epileptic seizures. Sleep Med. 2014;15(12):1433–9. doi:10.1016/j.sleep.2014.08.005.
86. Richerson GB, Buchanan GF. The serotonin axis: shared mechanisms in seizures, depression, and SUDEP. Epilepsia. 2011;52 Suppl 1:28–38. doi:10.1111/j.1528-1167.2010.02908.x.
87. Singh K, Katz ES, Zarowski M, Loddenkemper T, Llewellyn N, Manganaro S, et al. Cardiopulmonary complications during pediatric seizures: a prelude to understanding SUDEP. Epilepsia. 2013;54(6):1083–91. doi:10.1111/epi.12153.
88. Skluzacek JV, Watts KP, Parsy O, Wical B, Camfield P. Dravet syndrome and parent associations: the IDEA League experience with comorbid conditions, mortality, management, adaptation, and grief. Epilepsia. 2011;52 Suppl 2:95–101. doi:10.1111/j.1528-1167.2011.03012.x.
89. Delogu AB, Spinelli A, Battaglia D, Dravet C, De Nisco A, Saracino A, et al. Electrical and autonomic cardiac function in patients with Dravet syndrome. Epilepsia. 2011;52 Suppl 2:55–8. doi:10.1111/j.1528-1167.2011.03003.x.
90. Pavlova M, Singh K, Abdennadher M, Katz ES, Dworetzky BA, White DP, et al. Comparison of cardiorespiratory and EEG abnormalities with seizures in adults and children. Epilepsy Behav. 2013;29(3):537–41. doi:10.1016/j.yebeh.2013.09.026.
91. Wigg CM, Filgueiras A, Gomes Mda M. The relationship between sleep quality, depression, and anxiety in patients with epilepsy and suicidal ideation. Arq Neuropsiquiatr. 2014;72(5):344–8.

92. de Weerd A, de Haas S, Otte A, Trenite DK, van Erp G, Cohen A, et al. Subjective sleep disturbance in patients with partial epilepsy: a questionnaire-based study on prevalence and impact on quality of life. Epilepsia. 2004;45(11):1397–404.
93. Xu X, Brandenburg NA, McDermott AM, Bazil CW. Sleep disturbances reported by refractory partial-onset epilepsy patients receiving polytherapy. Epilepsia. 2006;47(7):1176–83.
94. Piperidou C, Karlovasitou A, Triantafyllou N, Terzoudi A, Constantinidis T, Vadikolias K, et al. Influence of sleep disturbance on quality of life of patients with epilepsy. Seizure. 2008;17(7):588–94. doi:10.1016/j.seizure.2008.02.005. doi:S1059-1311(08)00057-5 [pii].
95. Galer S, Urbain C, De Tiege X, Emeriau M, Leproult R, Deliens G, et al. Impaired sleep-related consolidation of declarative memories in idiopathic focal epilepsies of childhood. Epilepsy Behav. 2014;43C:16–23. doi:10.1016/j.yebeh.2014.11.032.

Chapter 16
Sleep in Neurological and Neurodevelopmental Disorders

Soňa Nevšímalová and Oliviero Bruni

Abstract Sleep problems are highly prevalent in children suffering from diverse neurological diseases. There is a close relationship between the degree of brain abnormality and impaired ability to generate physiological sleep-wake cycles and normal sleep architecture. This chapter summarizes clinical features and management of sleep pathologies in different neurological diseases. Cerebral palsy and neurodevelopmental disorders such as mental retardation, motor coordination disorder, developmental dysphasia, and learning disabilities are reviewed, as well as attention deficit/hyperactivity disorder and autism spectrum disorders. Attention is focused on sleep complaints in chromosomal abnormalities and various genetic programming malformations of the nervous system. Sleep disturbances can be a leading symptom (increasing with the severity of the disease) in many neurometabolic and/or neurodegenerative diseases. Children suffering from neuromuscular diseases are at increased risk of sleep-related breathing disorders, and their management has a substantial role in the patients' life longevity.

Keywords Sleep disorders • Cerebral palsy • Neurodevelopmental disabilities • Mental retardation • Autistic spectrum disorders • Chromosomal abnormalities • Neurometabolic and neuromuscular diseases

Introduction

Sleep quality in children is extremely important for brain development and synaptic plasticity during further life. There is considerable evidence that different sleep stages have a role to play in learning and memory and in the development of

S. Nevšímalová, MD, DSc (✉)
Department of Neurology, Charles University and General Teaching Hospital,
Katerinska 30, Prague, Czech Republic
e-mail: sona.nevsimalova@lf1.cuni.cz

O. Bruni, MD
Department of Developmental and Social Psychology, S. Andrea Hospital, Sapienza University, Via dei Marsi 78, Rome, Italy
e-mail: oliviero.bruni@uniroma1.it

© Springer International Publishing Switzerland 2017
S. Nevšímalová, O. Bruni (eds.), *Sleep Disorders in Children*,
DOI 10.1007/978-3-319-28640-2_16

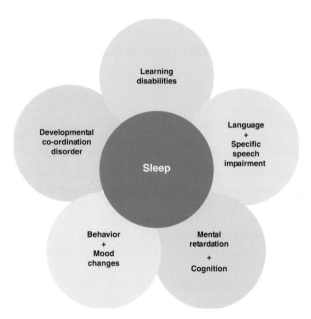

Fig. 16.1 Sleep and its disorganization are connected with all intellectual functions including cognition, learning disabilities, language, and developmental dysphasia, with developmental coordination disorder as well as behavior and mood changes

neuronal plasticity. However, the consequences of sleep disorders in structural and functional damaged brain structures are connected not only with intellectual capacity, but they influence mood changes, such as irritability, aggression, and depression, leading frequently to hyperactivity and conduct problems. Relationships between sleep and these functions are closely interconnected (Fig. 16.1).

Sleep disturbances in children with brain damage are highly prevalent and have different etiologies and medical, neurologic, and psychiatric comorbidities. Furthermore, unlike age-related sleep disturbances in typically developing children, sleep disorders in patients with neurodevelopmental disorders tend to be chronic, lasting into adolescence or adulthood.

The clinical picture of sleep disorders in these children could be directly linked to the brain damage, to a specific genetic syndrome, to hormonal and neurotransmitter dysfunction, or to altered perception of the "zeitgebers" (light-dark cycle, dietary schedule, maternal inputs, etc.) [1]. Sleep problems have a major impact not only on the child, but they affect the whole family's health and well-being.

Cerebral Palsy

Cerebral palsy (CP) affects approximately 1 in 500 live-born infants (more frequently in the developing countries), and the main risk is prematurity. The condition is nonprogressive and arises most commonly as the result of perinatal asphyxia and hypoxic-ischemic encephalopathy or intraventricular hemorrhage. The location of injury predicts the type of motor symptoms; the clinical picture is usually divided in four groups: diplegia, hemiplegia, quadriplegia, and dyskinesia [2, 3].

Children with CP are at increased risk of sleep disturbances for their motor involvement, as well as for a high association with different comorbidities. Severe developmental delay and mental retardation accompany CP in 31 %, seizure in 21 %, and blindness in 11 % patients [4]. Patients with more severe CP have a greater likelihood of sleep dysfunction. Spasticity, contractures, limitation of movement, and associated pain due to a high degree of functional motor impairment contribute to abnormal positioning during sleep. Severe CP can be associated with scoliosis and restricted lung volume and at risk for sleep-related hypoventilation. Abnormalities of the structure and tone of the upper airways may contribute to obstructive sleep apnea. The prevalence of sleep-disordered breathing is under-recognized and undertreated. Respiratory disorders, severe motor disability, seizures, and intellectual status may be associated with unexpected death during sleep in affected children [5].

Comorbid epilepsy strongly correlates with sleep disorders: nocturnal seizures disrupt sleep continuity, while certain antiepileptic drugs alter the sleep structure and, at the same time, influence daytime alertness. Blindness or severe visual impairment can affect the timing and maintenance of sleep through their effect on melatonin secretion and the lack of light perception. Intellectual disability and behavioral problems predispose to inconsistent bedtime routine and poor sleep hygiene [6, 7]. Romeo et al. [2] found in a detailed study of 165 children with CP that almost half of them (42 %) suffer at least from one sleep disorder. The most frequent complaints were sleep initiation and maintenance disorders (22 %), followed by sleep-wake transition disorder such as hypnic jerks, rhythmic movement disorder, hyperkinesias and bruxism (15 %), sleep breathing disorders (14 %), disorders of excessive somnolence 13 %, and disorders of arousal including sleepwalking, sleep terrors, and nightmares (10 %). There was no significant difference in the questionnaire data (Sleep Disturbance Scale for Children, SDSC) among the four classical types of CP. However, a group of dyskinetic CP children that is connected with structural or functional lesion of basal ganglia presented a more significant score for sleep-wake transition disorder (represented mainly by sleep-related movement disorders) than other children with hemiplegia, quadriplegia, or diplegia. The authors found also a significant correlation with sleep disorders and active epilepsy, mental retardation, and severity of motor CP involvement [2].

Anatomical factors such as upper airway hypotonia, adenotonsillar hypertrophy, glossoptosis, and midface anatomy or mandibular alterations, together with abnormal central control of respiration, can aggravate obstructive sleep disorder. Scoliosis and restricted lung volumes may increase the risk of sleep-related hypoventilation. A questionnaire-based survey of 233 children with CP found habitual snoring in 63 % and sleep apnea in 19.7 % [8]. In another study Wiggs et al. [9] found that 14.5 % of the 173 children with CP had a pathologic score for sleep-related breathing disorders on the Sleep Disturbance Scale for Children.

A few studies on sleep organization in children with CP showed abnormal sleep EEG pattern, absence or alteration of phasic sleep EEG events, difficult differentiation of stages NREM and REM, extremely low incidence of sleep spindles or presence of "extreme spindles," or an abnormally high percentage of wake after sleep onset [10].

No sleep interventions specifically designed to improve sleep of children with CP are reported in the literature, and only melatonin remains a commonly prescribed drug for disturbed sleep in children with CP. Treatment of OSA with adenotonsillectomy or CPAP may improve sleep and quality of life in children with CP [11].

To sum up, sleep disorders are common in children with CP, and different factors, such as motor or cognitive impairment, behavioral problems, or epilepsy, are important risk factors for the development of sleep disorders. Parenting children with CP is associated with an increased risk of psychological stress developing in the primary caregivers, usually the mothers. Children's sleep disturbances are, therefore, frequently connected with poor maternal sleep quality and depression [12]. The optimal management in children with CP is based not only on the determination and therapy of the physical features of the disease itself; the diagnosis and treatment of comorbid sleep disorders are very important too. A combination of pharmacological treatment (including melatonin), behavioral intervention, and respiratory support should be involved in the complex care.

Neurodevelopmental Disorders

Mental Retardation

Sleep problems are reported to occur in 13–86% of individuals with intellectual disabilities depending on the study design, participant characteristics, and definition of sleep problems [14]. The most prevalent problems include setting difficulties, long sleep latencies, night waking, and shortened sleep duration with early morning waking. There is a trend for sleep problems and daytime sleepiness to occur more frequently with more severe levels of mental retardation. Besides altered macrostructure, changes were found also in the sleep microstructure, particularly in cyclic alternating pattern (CAP) [14].

Recent studies on the relationship between CAP and cognitive and memory performances support the idea that EEG slow components (A1) play a role in sleep-related cognitive processes and could obviously be altered in mental retardation [15]. In two groups of children with mental retardation, i.e., fragile X (fraX) and Down syndrome, CAP analysis showed a decrease of CAP rate in slow-wave sleep (SWS) and a decreased A1 index (EEG slow oscillations) and an increase of A2 and A3 percentages (i.e., arousals) in both groups, compared to normal controls. Similar results were found in children with autistic spectrum disorder and mental retardation. Therefore, it seems that the decrease in the CAP rate and in A1 mainly in SWS represents a sleep microstructural pattern typical of intellectual disability [16].

However, there is a controversy about whether sleep problems in mentally retarded children are related more to their general medical problems and brain lesions rather than to the mental retardation itself. Some recent studies [17] strongly support the hypothesis that general medical conditions are mainly coresponsible for the sleep patterns in mentally retarded children.

Mental retardation has a wide spectrum of clinical diagnoses. Tietze et al. [18] found, in a cohort of 214 children with severe mental retardation and sleep disturbances, that 25 % of them were children with cerebral palsy, 13 % with genetic syndromes, and 11 % with metabolic disorders. However, the diagnosis was either not established or was caused by a global developmental delay almost in one-third of the whole patients' cohort.

The relationship between sleep and optimal cognitive and physical function is bidirectional. Sleep problems in developmentally disabled children are associated with a number of associated clinical outcomes: poor communication and academic skills, poor self-help skills, incontinence, daytime behavioral problems, and epilepsy [3]. Blankenburg et al. [19] recommended a specific questionnaire (SNAKE) for the diagnosis of sleep disturbances in children with severe psychomotor impairment. The questionnaire evaluates symptoms and consequences of sleep disturbances, as well as conditions that are known to have a direct or indirect impact on sleep in affected children. It takes into account the patient's impaired or limited perception, intellectual ability, limited behavioral repertoire, motor impairment due to underlying disease, and the environmental impact of the disease that makes it less conducive to sleep (e.g., nursing care, artificial ventilation, etc.). The questionnaire is based on the ICSD-2 classification for sleep problems, and it should be completed by parents or nursing personnel over a 4-week period of child's sleep.

Sleep problems are often complex and usually difficult to treat in individuals with mental retardation. The management of sleep disorders in mentally retarded children should include an early intervention program [20] and a pharmaceutical approach with different drugs, with melatonin as the most widely used medicine. Melatonin is increasingly prescribed to many children with mental retardation using a wide range of doses and demonstrating efficacy in improving sleep quality by reducing sleep-onset latency or by slightly increasing total sleep time. These effects appear to be stronger in children with visual impairment, mental retardation, attention deficit, and autism [21].

A meta-analysis of nine randomized and placebo-controlled trials including a total of 183 individuals with neurodevelopmental disorders showed that melatonin decreases sleep latency by a mean of 34 min, increases total sleep time by a mean of 50 min, and less significantly decreases the number of awakenings per night [22]. A recent placebo-controlled study in 146 children (aged 3–15 years) with intellectual disability showed similar results [23].

In spite of the heterogeneity of the studies, regarding patient groups, melatonin preparations, dosage, and timing of administration, the results of different studies [13, 21] indicate that melatonin is effective and safe in the treatment of sleep problems in intellectually disabled individuals.

Developmental Coordination Disorder

Children with developmental coordination disorder experience significant difficulty in the performance of every body's movement skills (particularly clumsiness) in the absence of obvious neurological, sensory, or intellectual impairment. The condition has a reported prevalence of at least 2% in population studies [24]. The biological background is currently unknown; however, it is frequently found in children with a history of perinatal risk factors (e.g., low birth weight), and genetic factors probably play an important role, too. Affected children show more sleep disturbances than the healthy ones. Particular problems include bedtime resistance, parasomnias, and daytime sleepiness [25]. Scabar et al. [26] found in six out of eight children with severe type of this disorder rolandic spikes during sleep and propose a close link between developmental coordination disorder, so-called benign rolandic epilepsy, and specific language impairment.

Specific Language Impairment (Developmental Dysphasia)

Specific language impairment includes both developmental expressive and receptive language disorder and affects 3–5% children's population. The resulting language difficulties interfere with social communication and with successful performance of daily activities including school results. Neurological findings are usually normal; however, a mild hypotonia can be seen. The disorder is very frequently associated with developmental coordination and learning disabilities; neuroimaging abnormalities and EEG changes have been observed, too [27].

Dlouha and Nevsimalova [28] examined a group of 100 children with specific language impairment (69 boys, 31 girls, mean age 6.3 ± 1.2 years). Most of them had signs of mild coordination disorder, borderline or mild decrease intellectual capacity was found in nine children, and learning disabilities (dyslexia, dysgraphia) had developed in 21 out of 33 school children. Epileptic discharges were found in 48 cases in waking EEG, and polysomnography verified epileptiform discharges in 20 out of 26 children (77%) (Fig. 16.2). In one case, even continual spike-wave discharges during sleep (electrical status epilepticus during sleep, ESES) were found. Severe epileptiform discharges during sleep were seen as a neurophysiological continuity leading to neurocognitive impairment and particularly language disorder in a wide spectrum of diseases including benign rolandic epilepsy and Landau-Kleffner syndrome [29].

---➤

Fig. 16.2 A 7-year-old girl with developmental dysphasia. (**a**) Generalized epileptic discharges during wakefulness before nocturnal polysomnographic recording starts. (**b**) Stage 1, NREM sleep with sharp wave discharges predominating above the left centro-temporo-parietal regions

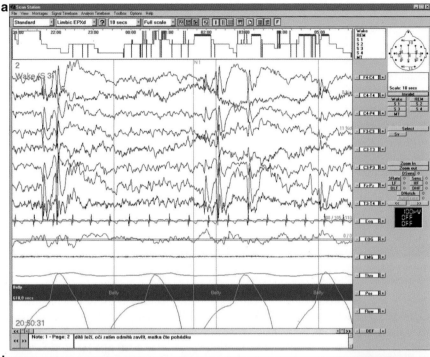

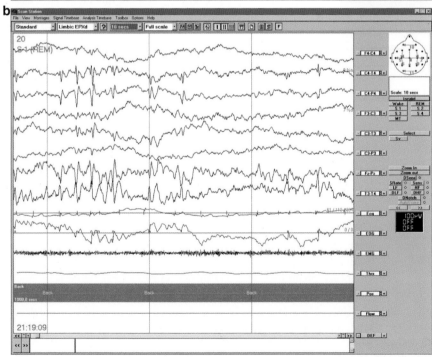

Learning Disabilities

Learning disabilities (dyslexia, dysgraphia, dysorthographia, dyscalculia) affect up to 5–7 % school children, and they are frequently associated with other developmental disorders. The most frequent learning disability is developmental dyslexia. It is characterized by a difficulty in accurate and/or fluent world recognition and by poor spelling and decoding abilities. Although sleep plays a key role in the processes of learning and memory, almost no studies are available on sleep in children with this disorder. Bruni et al. [30] found a clear increase in spindle activity and sigma power (11–15 Hz frequency) while examining nocturnal sleep in 19 children with developmental dyslexia. A relationship was found between increased sleep spindle activity and the severity of dyslectic impairment, supporting an important role of NREM sleep and spindles in sleep-related neurocognitive processing.

Furthermore, CAP analysis revealed an increase in total CAP rate and EEG slow oscillation (A1) index in stage N3. A correlation analysis between CAP parameters and cognitive-behavioral measures showed a significant positive correlation between the A1 index in N3 with Verbal IQ, full-scale IQ, and Memory and Learning Transfer reading test, while CAP rate in N3 was positively correlated with verbal IQ [30]. In order to explain this finding, the authors hypothesize that to overcome reading difficulties, dyslexic subjects overactivate thalamocortical and hippocampal circuitry to transfer information between cortical posterior and anterior areas. The overactivation of the ancillary frontal areas may account for the CAP rate modifications and mainly for the increase of CAP rate and the A1 index in N3 that seem to be correlated with IQ and reading abilities [30].

Attention Deficit/Hyperactivity Disorder (ADHD)

ADHD is a highly prevalent childhood-onset neuropsychiatric condition, with an estimated worldwide prevalence of approximately 5 % in school-age children. The syndrome is defined by a persistent and age-inappropriate pattern of inattention, hyperactivity-impulsivity, or both. ADHD is frequently comorbid with other neuro-developmental disorders including coordination disorder, specific language impairment, and learning difficulties [31].

As many as 70 % of children with ADHD have been reported having mild to severe sleep problems including sleep-onset insomnia (the most often reported problem), bedtime resistance, night awakenings, difficulties in morning awakenings, sleep disorder breathing, and daytime sleepiness [32]. Objective studies showed that children with ADHD had significant differences vs. control children for sleep-onset latency, apnea-hypopnea index, sleep efficiency, and higher levels of daytime sleepiness on the Multiple Sleep Latency Test (MSLT) supporting the hypothesis of disorders of vigilance in ADHD [33, 34]. Both subjective and objective sleep/alertness alteration presented in ADHD children [35, 36] are suggested to

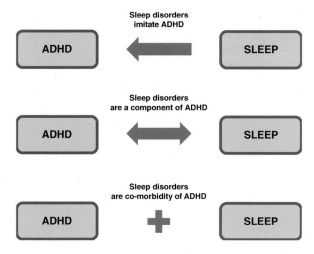

Fig. 16.3 A comprehensive view on a relationship between sleep disturbances and attention deficit/hyperactivity disorder (ADHD) (Adapted from Owens et al. [37]). Sleep disturbances may imitate ADHD, may be a component of ADHD, and/or may be a comorbidity of ADHD

be a result of changes in the micro- rather than macro-sleep architecture [33]. Generally speaking, the relationship between sleep disturbances and ADHD is very complicated [37]. Sleep disturbances may mimic ADHD, may be the consequence, or may contribute to ADHD – like phenotypes, as Fig. 16.3 illustrates. Several comorbid sleep disorders – particularly periodic limb movements (PLMs) and restless leg syndrome (RLS) – take part in the clinical picture of ADHD.

The next chapter (17) brings a more comprehensive view of sleep disorders in ADHD and its comorbidities.

Autistic Spectrum Disorders

Autistic spectrum disorders (ASD) are a set of neurodevelopmental disorders characterized by varying degrees of impairment in communication skills, social interaction, and restricted, repetitive, and stereotyped patterns of behavior. The prevalence varies between 0.2 and 0.7 % in the whole population [38, 39].

Parental surveys show a 50–80 % prevalence of sleep problems in children with ASD mainly represented by insomnia [40]. Sleep disturbance in these children seems to be correlated with aggressive behavior, developmental regression, internalizing problems [41], and anxiety and sensory over-responsibility [42]. Sleep disorders were reported either in ASD children with severe mental retardation or in high-functioning subjects [40].

Children with a history of developmental regression have a more disturbed sleep pattern than children without regression [43] and demonstrate a higher degree of sleep disruption either at a macrostructural or microstructural level [38, 44]. Circadian abnormalities in ASD children might be a result of genetic abnormalities related to melatonin synthesis and its role in modulating synaptic transmission. In ASD, there is an overall reduction in nocturnal melatonin secretion or a delay in its secretion at night. Low levels of melatonin and/or its urinary metabolic derivatives correlate with sleep problems and autistic behaviors [45]. This is probably the cause of the difficulties in falling asleep and of the irregular sleep-wake rhythms [46]. Recently, a bifurcation of the sleep-wake cycle with increased sensitivity to external noise and short sleep duration causing irregular sleep-onset and wake-up times has been suggested [43].

Several studies have demonstrated effectiveness of behavioral interventions for sleep-onset and maintenance problems [39]. Consistent sleeping environment and routine should be maintained to help the child relax down to sleep. The management of sleep disturbance in ASD children depends on the type of sleep disorder, but behavioral therapy associated to melatonin supplementation is the most used since ASD children have endogenous melatonin deficiency [47].

A more detailed description of sleep studies in ASD is described in the next chapter (17).

Chromosomal Abnormalities and Microdeletion Syndrome

Sleep problems are highly prevalent in children suffering from diverse genetic syndromes featured by autosomal, gonosomal, and/or microdeletion changes. The main sleep characteristics involve nocturnal sleep complaints (mainly night awakenings and sleep apnea); however, also tiredness or even excessive daytime sleepiness has been reported [48].

Down Syndrome

Down syndrome is one of the most common autosomal abnormalities occurring in 0.9 per 1000 live births, its probability being directly proportional to increasing maternal age. Typically phenotypic features are accompanied by delayed psycho-motor development with generalized hypotonia and impaired cognitive performance. The most frequent cause rests in trisomy chromosome 21, translocation of the long arm of an extra chromosome 21 to chromosome 14 or 22, and/or mosaicism of trisomy 21.

The leading sleep complaints are sleep-related breathing disorder and insomnia. The prevalence of obstructive sleep apnea (OSA) is higher than 50%, the obstruction being caused by an anatomically narrow upper airway due to midfacial and mandibular hypoplasia, relative macroglossia, glossoptosis, and frequent adenotonsillar hypertrophy. Other factors predisposing to OSA include obesity and generalized hypotonia with upper airway muscle malfunction. However, changes were found also in the sleep architecture. The patients have a reduced quantity of REM sleep and decreased REM sleep density. Sleep fragmentation and arousals independent of respiratory events and PLMs and even RLS have also been reported. Daytime sleepiness is therefore a consequence of poor nocturnal sleep quality. From the therapeutic point of view, management of OSA as well as behavioral methods is usually recommended to decrease sleep problems [49, 50].

Recently, the practice parameters from the American Academy of Pediatrics recommended to discuss with parents, at least once during the first 6 months of life, symptoms of obstructive sleep apnea, uncommon sleep positions, frequent night awakening, daytime sleepiness, and behavior problems [51].

Fragile X Chromosome

Fragile X chromosome is the most common cause of sex chromosomal abnormalities with a rate of occurrence 1:4000 live births in males. It is the most frequent cause of inherited mental retardation in boys due to X-linked trinucleotide repeat disorders (Xq27.3). The characteristic face features (elongated face, large ears, and protruding jaw) are accompanied by macroorchidism. Cognitive and language features comprise a deficit consistent with the level of mental retardation; behavioral changes include increased social avoidance, anxiety, and hyperactivity [52].

Very few studies evaluated the presence of sleep disorders in patients with fragile X. Kronk et al. [53] reported a prevalence of 32–50% of significant sleep problems with the more frequent complaints represented by sleep-onset difficulties and frequent awakenings during the night.

Data obtained from the Fragile X Clinical and Research Consortium Database (FXCRC) showed that 27% of parents reported sleep problems in affected children, and also OSA has been reported to be a frequent complaint [54]. A variable sleep duration and sleep fragmentation are sporadically observed [49]. Some sleep studies showed a correlation between REM sleep deficit and the level of mental retardation [52].

In an interesting study, Gould et al. [55] found increased levels of melatonin across the circadian cycle in young fragile X individuals, possibly explaining the difficulties in maintaining consistent sleep and increased number of night wake episodes. Clonidine has been reported to have a beneficial effect on hyperactivity and abnormal sleep patterns [56]; behavioral therapy was also used with a benefit [57].

Prader-Willi Syndrome

Prader-Willi syndrome (PWS) is a genetic disorder affecting in 1:10,000–25,000 live births. The genetic defect is linked to a deletion in the paternally inherited chromosome 15q11–q13 in 70–75% of individuals, to a maternal uniparental disomy in

20–25 % of cases, and to abnormal methylation of the imprinting center on chromosome 15 in 1–2 %.

PWS is characterized by obesity, small status, hyperphagia, hypogonadism, mental retardation, and behavioral disorder. The most frequent sleep complaints include breathing disorders, particularly OSA, and daytime sleepiness. The risk factors for OSA are obesity and mass loading of the chest wall, facial dysmorphism, and hypotonia. Abnormality of central respiratory control also predisposes to central apneas.

OSA seems to be a feature that appears during development; in fact, infants with PWS, when compared with older children, were more likely to experience central sleep apnea than obstructive events [58]. With age obesity increasing and OSA emerging, a recent review analyzing 14 studies in children with PWS reported an OSA prevalence of 79.91 %: 53.07 % had mild, 22.35 % moderate, and 24.58 % severe OSA. Adenotonsillectomy was found to be effective in reducing OSA for some children, but residual OSA was present in the majority of cases after surgery [59].

Although OSA may have a role in decreased vigilance during the day, excessive daytime sleepiness (EDS) is primary caused by hypothalamic dysfunction. Decreased level of hypocretin-1 in the cerebrospinal fluid [60] can support a potential involvement of hypothalamic dysfunction.

Different polysomnographic studies have been carried out to evaluate sleep in PWS subjects showing a decrease of sleep and REM latency and the presence of sleep-onset REM periods (SOREMPs), corroborating the hypothesis of a primary disorder of vigilance [61].

Reviewing the relevant literature, Camfferman et al. [62] found EDS in 74 out of 110 cases and cataplexy-like symptoms in 13 out of 63 patients. However, no convincing correlation was found between OSA severity and EDS.

Growth hormone (GH) therapy in children with PWS may determine hypertrophy of tonsils or adenoids, increase OSA, and may be responsible for sudden death in PWS subjects [63]. A recent paper, however, showed a decrease in the respiratory disturbance index and the central apnea index. The authors [63] concluded that long-term GH treatment in patients with PWS is generally safe and recommended annual polysomnography and adenotonsillar evaluation.

CPAP (or BiPAP) is commonly prescribed for sleep-disordered breathing, while most patients benefit from modafinil to counteract excessive daytime sleepiness [62].

Angelman Syndrome

Angelman syndrome (AS) is a neurodevelopmental genetic disorder caused by the absence or loss of function of the maternally inherited allele at the 15q11-q13 domain; it occurs in 1:12,000–20,000 individuals and accounts for 6 % of all children with severe cognitive disability and epilepsy [64]. AS is called "happy puppet syndrome" because of the patients' characteristic jerky movements, happy disposition, and frequent laughter. Microcephaly, severe mental retardation, and epileptic seizures accompany the clinical picture [65].

A variety of sleep abnormalities are reported including prolonged sleep latency, frequent nocturnal awakenings, involuntary movements, bruxism, snoring, and a higher rate of parasomnias (enuresis, sleep terrors, sleepwalking) [66]. Nocturnal sleep time is reduced and some children have abnormal sleep-wake cycles with short periods of diurnal and nocturnal sleep [49].

Polysomnographic studies showed a reduction in sleep efficiency and in REM sleep, while the percentage of SWS was found to be significantly higher, due to the presence of the 1–3 Hz bursts that represent the typical EEG pattern of the syndrome. No respiratory abnormalities were found; however, a tendency to an increase in the periodic limb movement index (PLMI) was observed [67].

In children with AS, treatment with sleep hygiene, behavioral therapy, associated with melatonin was documented to be effective. Melatonin before bedtime promotes less fragmented sleep and helps to regulate sleep-wake cycles [68]. A recent research in children with AS reported that the nighttime serum melatonin levels were significantly low in AS patients and with delayed melatonin peak showing the delayed sleep phase syndrome (DSPS) [69].

Williams Syndrome

Williams syndrome (WS) is a disorder marked by an unusual elfin-like facies, hyperacusis, infantile hypercalcemia, and significant physical and mental retardation. The condition is caused by a heterozygous deletion in chromosome 7q11.23 and its incidence is estimated at 1:10,000.

There are only few studies dealing with sleep problems in these patients. While in children the attention has been focused on night sleep complaints and predominantly on PLMs [70], Goldman et al. [71] used actigraphy to examine overnight sleep pattern in 23 adolescents and young adults and completed their sleep data with a structured questionnaire: although free to spend 9 h in bed, nearly all the subjects were tired and almost 80 % were sleepy during the day.

Smith-Magenis Syndrome

Smith-Magenis syndrome (SMS) is characterized by mental retardation with distinctive behavioral characteristics, dysmorphic features, and an abnormal circadian pattern of melatonin ascribed to an interstitial deletion of chromosome 17 (17p11.2). The prevalence is estimated at 1:25,000 live births [72].

Sleep disturbances are seen in 65–100 % cases, and all affected children display a phase shift in their circadian rhythm of melatonin secretion. Prominent sleep problems include early sleep onset, repeated and prolonged awakening during the night, and early sleep offset. Most patients exhibit morning tiredness, temper tantrums when tired, and naps during the day (Fig. 16.4).

Actigraphic studies indicated a sleep disturbance that begins as early as 6 months of age, with fragmented sleep and reduced 24-h sleep compared with healthy control subjects [73]. This finding was corroborated by polysomnographic studies which revealed reduced sleep time in virtually all SMS patients [74].

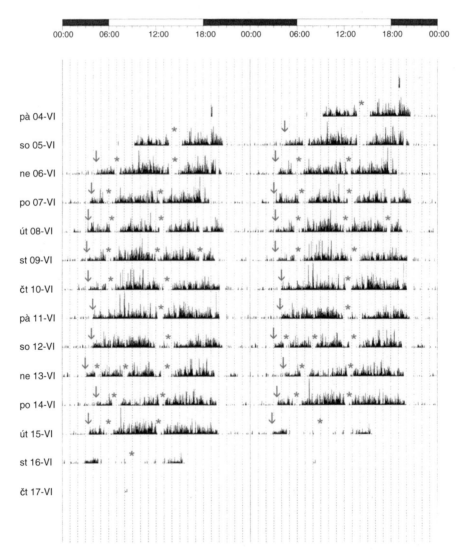

Fig. 16.4 A 7-year-old boy with Smith-Magenis syndrome: the actigraphic recording shows early awakenings from nocturnal sleep (marked by *arrowheads*) and many excessive daytime sleep attacks (marked by *asterisks*)

The disorder of circadian rhythm in SMS is related to disturbed regulation of downstream circadian clock genes and explains sleep disturbance and abnormal daytime behavior with hyperactivity. The mechanism of the quantitatively normal, but rhythmically abnormal, melatonin secretion is, as yet, unknown [75]. A series of studies have found that 96% of SMS children had inverted endogenous melatonin secretion, peaking in the day rather than at night [76, 77]. The best recommended treatment is a combination of evening melatonin administration and morning β1-adrenergic antagonist (acebutolol) to reduce the daytime production of this hormone [78].

Rett Syndrome

Rett syndrome (RS) is a severe neurological disorder with an incidence of 1:10,000 girls. It is one of the most frequent causes of mental retardation in female patients. It is generally caused by mutation in the MECP2 (methyl-CpG binding protein 2) gene (Xq28). Almost 300 mutations have been recorded [79]. The disorder is characterized by progressive intellectual and neurological impairments beginning after apparently normal psychomotor development. Early signs of RS typically manifest at the age of 6–18 months. Characteristic features comprise microcephaly, stereotyped hand movements (hand-wringing or washing), severely impaired language functioning, autistic behavior, regress of motor and intellectual functions, epilepsy, and attacks of breathing disturbance during wakefulness.

Several studies show that sleep patterns are changed from infancy. The affected girls sleep longer during the day and, on the other hand, wake and laugh in the middle of night. Their sleep onset is very irregular and total daytime sleep remains prolonged instead of showing the normal age-related physiological decline. The immature sleep pattern seems to be a consequence of arrested brain development. Frequent daily napping has been reported almost in 80% of affected patients and found to increase with the age [80].

Polysomnographic studies revealed lower sleep efficiency, long sleep-onset latency, and short total sleep time, but also increased wakefulness after sleep onset (WASO), decreased REM sleep, fewer spindles, and K complexes similar to other forms of mental retardation [81, 82]. Alterations in sleep architecture including tonus changes in NREM as well as REM sleep were found [83, 84]. Patients with RS commonly show irregular breathing during wakefulness consisting of episodes of hyperventilation interspersed with breath-holding spells, sometimes associated with severe oxygen desaturation.

Respiratory disturbances during the night are very frequent [85–87]. Hagebeuk et al. [86] found in a group of 12 RS girls combined central and obstructive apneas in five patients, in another three prevailed central apnea, and in further two obstructive one. Only two cases showed normal respiratory functions.

A recent study showed, in a sample of more than 300 cases followed over 12 years, that the prevalence of any sleep disturbance was very high (more than 80%) and decreased with age (less common in individuals aged more than 18 years) [88].

Night laughing represented the most frequent problem occurring in 60–88 % of younger girls followed by night screaming.

Behavioral insomnia and nighttime behaviors in RS are usually treated with a combination of behavioral treatments and oral melatonin (2.5–7.5 mg) that reduced mean sleep latency [89, 90].

Management of breathing sleep disorder is necessary almost in all RS cases, sometimes including 1–2 h per day of continuous positive airway pressure (CPAP) while awake.

Coffin-Lowry Syndrome

Coffin-Lowry syndrome is a rare disorder characterized by moderate to severe mental retardation, facial dysmorphism, tapering digits, and skeletal deformity. The gene is located on Xp22.2 [91]. The characteristic features are stimulus-induced drop episodes, accompanied by sudden loss of muscle tone, and induced by unexpected tactile or auditory stimuli. No epileptiform activity was proven in any reported case. Drop attacks are not induced by emotion (as in true cataplectic attacks), and recovery is immediate. The attacks last only a few seconds and always lead to fall. The pathophysiology of these cataplexy-like drop attacks remains unclear [92]. Sleepiness has not been described in any case. Treatment with conventional antiepileptic medication proved ineffective. Sporadically clomipramine and/ or tiagabine – a potent GABA-uptake inhibitor – was used with a benefit [92, 93].

Norrie Disease

Norrie disease is a rare X-linked microdeletion syndrome (Xp11.3–p11.4) characterized by infantile blindness, pseudotumorous retinal dysgenesis, and ocular atrophy. It is associated commonly with mental retardation, sensorineural deafness, dysmorphic features, and occasionally with atonic seizures. Sleep studies are extremely rare. Vossler et al. [94] described three boys with this syndrome and found them to have cataplexy and abnormal REM sleep with no other signs of narcolepsy. The authors verified the congenital absence of monoamine oxidase (MAO) in these patients and suppose its indirect responsibility for cataplexy and REM sleep disturbance.

Some other congenital syndromes such as *Möbius, Pierre-Robin, Treacher-Collins, Goldenhar, and/or centrofacial dysgenesia* also belong to neuroembryological and/or genetic programming malformations of the nervous system. Their difficulties are primarily connected with upper airway obstruction and subsequent sleep disorder breathing difficulties. Noninvasive breathing support (BiPAP) followed by individually chosen surgical treatment manages usually a necessary benefit.

Neurometabolic Diseases

Metabolic and/or degenerative diseases affecting the central nervous system usually result from a single mutant gene coding for an enzymatic protein mostly involved in the catabolic pathway. The defective gene in metabolic diseases is normally expressed in one or more organs (not necessarily in the nervous system), where chemical analyses of tissues often have a diagnostic value. Most of them belong to the group of lysosomal or so-called storage diseases [95].

Storage lysosomal diseases are characterized by an accumulation of undergraded macromolecules within lysosomes. The most common representatives are the glycogen storage diseases – glycogenosis (Pompe disease), mucopolysaccharidosis and mucolipidosis, glycoproteinosis together with sphingolipidosis, and neuronal ceroid lipofuscinosis. Almost all are autosomal recessive inherited diseases; the combined prevalence of all lysosomal storage diseases is 1:6600–1:7700 live births [95].

Pompe Disease

Pompe disease results from acid α-glucosidase deficiency; its incidence is estimated at 1:40,000 individuals. The infantile form is usually fatal before the age of 2 years, and the juvenile form progresses more slowly, but all patients develop involvement of respiratory muscles – predominantly of the diaphragm. Enzyme replacement therapy is the only causal treatment improving significantly the prognosis and diminishing breathing difficulties. Obstructive sleep apnea and hypoventilation are common without causal treatment in both patients' groups, and noninvasive ventilation support is indicated [96, 97].

Mucopolysaccharidosis

Mucopolysaccharidoses are heterogeneous syndromes consisting of mental and physical retardation, typical facies features with the large head, multiple skeletal deformities, hepatosplenomegaly, and clouding of the cornea in Hunter and Hurler syndrome. The syndrome comprises seven major entities, which are distinguishable by their clinical picture, genetic transmission, enzyme defect, and urinary mucopolysaccharide pattern.

OSA is the most common sleep disorder in all types. Upper airway obstruction has multiple causative factors, and progressive respiratory disease may severely affect morbidity and mortality [98]. Children are more severely affected than adult patients [99]. Retropalatal and retroglossal spaces were found to be significantly smaller in children than in adults. Adenoid hypertrophy was found to have a significant role to play in all examined children.

The most frequent and probably specific sleep disturbances have been found in the commonest mucopolysaccharidosis, Sanfilippo syndrome. These patients have extremely irregular sleep pattern, with several sleep episodes of variable duration and irregular round-the-clock distribution [100]. Guerrero et al. [101] examined urine melatonin excretion in 12 patients with Sanfilippo syndrome and found a significantly lower melatonin excretion at night and significantly higher concentration in the morning with keeping a slightly higher level also during the day compared to the controls. Analysis of the circadian rhythm alteration may explain the cause of sleep disorders found in these patients, and melatonin can be recommended as a benefit treatment.

Niemann-Pick Disease

Niemann-Pick disease is a heterogeneous syndrome comprising different forms (A–D). However, its type C (NP-C) with sphingomyelinase activity deficit is one of the most frequent recessively inherited lysosomal storage sphingolipidoses. The prevalence is 1:150,000, and about 95 % of NP-C patients have mutation in NPC1 gene (18q11). Three main clinical forms are distinguished: infantile with early onset and rapid progression, late infantile/juvenile with slower progression, and variant with a late onset. The most common late infantile/juvenile form is characterized by vertical supranuclear ophthalmoplegia, cerebellar ataxia, dystonia, dysarthria, dysphagia, and intellectual deterioration. Cataplexy is a frequent symptom, and spleen enlargement or hepatosplenomegalia is expressed in all patients.

Several sleep studies [102–105] were done in NPC1 patients. Night sleep is interrupted with frequent arousals, disorganized, shortened, and of low efficiency. The MSLT shows shortened mean sleep latency (independent of the presence or absence of cataplexy). A decreased value of CSF hypocretin was found to be independent of the presence of cataplexy. Vankova et al. [102] found in five NP-C patients altered sleep patterns including sudden increase in muscle tone during delta sleep, electroencephalographic sigma activity connected with rapid eye movements and muscle atonia, presence of alpha-delta sleep, and atypical K complexes as well as spindle activity. All patients exhibited fragmentary myoclonus (Fig. 16.5).

According to Vanier [106] only about 10 % of NPC1 cases have clinically evident cataplectic attacks. However, cataplexy as a leading sleep disorder symptom was recently described by many authors [104, 107, 108]. Nevsimalova and Malinova [109] found cataplexy in four out of nine patients with late infantile and in one out of three patients with infantile NP-C form, while cataplexy was absent in juvenile or adult cases. Cataplectic attacks were found more frequently in children than in adults also by further authors [110]. Therefore, Challamel et al. [111] recommend to rule out NPC1 disease in all children with frequent cataplectic attacks.

Miglustat® represents a new possibility of NP-C treatment; its benefit was exceptionally observed also on cataplectic attacks [112].

Neuronal Ceroid Lipofuscinosis

Neuronal ceroid lipofuscinosis (NCL) is characterized by the accumulation of auto-fluorescent storage material within lysosomes, leading to neuronal death. The major clinical subtypes are infantile, late infantile, early juvenile, juvenile, and the adult forms, all transmitted in an autosomal recessive manner [95].

   Late infantile neuronal ceroid lipofuscinosis is one of the most common variants. It is caused by a genomic defect in chromosome 11p15.5, the Finish variant of late infantile NCL, which is also known as the early juvenile form of 13q22. Clinical features include progressive visual failure, intellectual deterioration, cerebellar

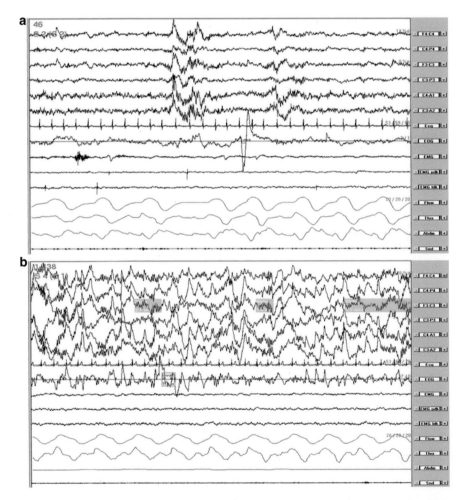

Fig. 16.5 A 14-year-old girl with Niemann-Pick disease type C. (**a**) REM sleep with rapid eye movements, muscle twitches, and sigma activity. (**b**) NREM sleep, stage 3 with diffuse penetration of alpha rhythm. (**c**) Alpha-delta sleep. (**d**) NREM sleep, stage 2 with fragmental myoclonus

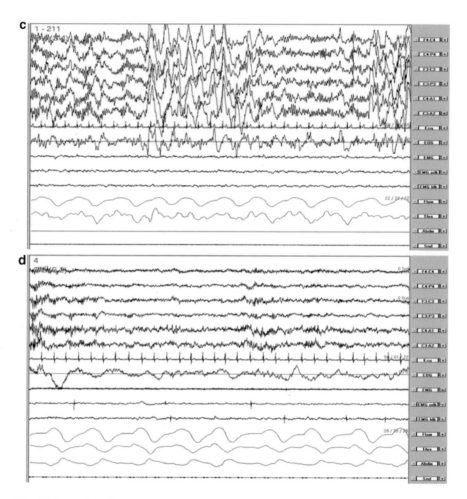

Fig. 16.5 (continued)

symptoms with ataxia, epilepsy, and frequent myoclonic jerks. Clinical decline leads to coma vigile and premature death. Sleep studies [113] show in the initial phase an excess of night sleep and frequent daytime naps. Later on, the longest sleep period was frequently shifted into daytime hours. Fragmented diurnal rest activity patterns with no distinct rhythm are seen during disease progression. The internal circadian timing system may be damaged also due to visual deterioration.

Juvenile neuronal ceroid lipofuscinosis is mapped to chromosome 16p12.1. Its clinical features include progressive loss of vision, usually leading to blindness between 8 and 13 years of age, intellectual deterioration, extrapyramidal and cerebellar symptoms, and epilepsy. Common sleep disturbances are reported in more than half of the patients. The most typical are daytime sleepiness [114], settling problems, nocturnal awakenings, and nightmares. Polysomnography showed significantly reduced total sleep time, sleep efficiency, percentage of REM sleep, and NREM stage 2. Treatment with melatonin before bedtime may help to slightly improve the circadian rhythm [114].

Neuromuscular Diseases

Neuromuscular diseases include a wide spectrum of motor unit diseases starting with the affection of motor neuron in the brainstem and spinal cord and spinal muscular atrophies (SMA), continuing through myasthenic syndromes, congenital myopathies, muscle dystrophies, and myotonic syndromes, and ending with Charcot-Marie-Tooth (CMT) disease, called also as hereditary motor and sensory polyneuropathy (HMSN).

Patients suffering from neuromuscular diseases are at an increased risk of sleep-disordered breathing (SDB) disorders such as OSA and hypoventilation, as well as central sleep apnea. SDB increases particularly due to diaphragmatic weakness and can precede abnormalities during wakefulness by months to years. Hypoventilation becomes more severe as the disease progresses, but SDB can be seen in some cases still in early stages of neuromuscular diseases (Fig. 16.6). Sleep-related hypoxemia is predominantly seen in REM sleep, because of the loss of accessory muscle contribution to breathing in coping with diaphragmatic weakness. REM-related desaturations are also frequently associated with recurring apnea and hypopnea. These apneas are most commonly central origin, but obstructive apnea can develop if upper airway muscle contraction is impaired [115]. Later on, SDB appears also during NREM sleep. A decrease in blood oxygen saturation can reach a value between 60 and 80 %, a quantity connected with compensatory increased breathing effort and nocturnal awakening reactions. Noninvasive nocturnal breathing support is the adequate treatment for SDB in all the types of neuromuscular diseases [116].

Nocturnal sleep-related ventilatory alterations lead to sleep inertia in the morning with headaches, daytime somnolence, fatigue, and inappropriate napping. Children are also at higher risk for developing complications as pulmonary hypertension, cor pulmonale, and neurocognitive dysfunction that impair their quality of life and may lead to significant morbidity and increased mortality [115, 117].

Spinal Muscular Atrophy (SMA)

Spinal muscular atrophy is transmitted by an autosomal recessive gene and manifested by widespread muscular denervation and atrophy. The incidence is 1:10,000–25,000. Three main clinical variants exist in children: infantile (SMA 1) with the most rapid course, intermediate (SMA 2) which makes approximately one-half of all cases, and juvenile (SMA 3) with much slower progression. All forms are caused by mutations in a survival motor neuron gene 1 (SMN1) located at chromosome 5q11.2–q13.3 [118].

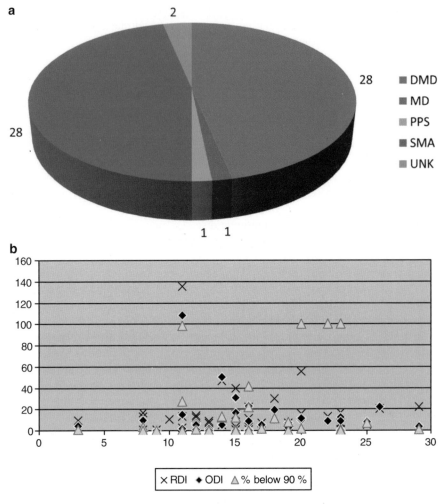

Fig. 16.6 Neuromuscular diseases followed-up in our Prague Sleep Center (Kemlink D. et al., unpublished data). (**a**) A survey of a cohort of 60 children, adolescents, and young adults with neuromuscular diseases: *DMD* Duchenne muscle dystrophy, *MD* myotonic dystrophy, *PPS* post-poliomyelitic syndrome, *SMA* spinal muscular atrophy type 2 and 3. (**b**) An age-related polysom-nographic (PSG) respiratory findings in 34 patients from the abovementioned cohort. *RDI* respiratory disturbance index, *ODI* oxygen desaturation index, *% below 90 %* the percentage of the total recorded time spent below 90 % of oxygen saturation level. The graph shows no age-related dependence on the severity of the patients' respiratory parameters

There are very few studies of sleep patterns in patients with SMA and especially in subjects with SMA1. In a polysomnographic study of 32 neuromuscular patients, four with a form of SMA, sleep architecture revealed an increase in stage 1 sleep coupled with a decrease or absence of REM sleep [119]. Another study on seven SMA children (six with SMA type 1.5–1.8, one with SMA type 2) showed impaired sleep architecture, in whom nocturnal noninvasive ventilation (NIV) resulted in a significant improvement of sleep architecture with higher sleep efficiency, increased deep sleep, longer REM sleep, and significantly fewer EEG arousals [120].

A recent study on SMA1 patients indicates the presence of an abnormal sleep microstructure in SMA1 patients, characterized by a reduction of A2 and A3 CAP subtypes (corresponding to arousals). The authors hypothesize that SMA1 patients have reduced arousability during NREM sleep, which could be interpreted as additional evidence of central nervous system involvement in this disease and might represent an additional risk factor for the premature death of these patients, which is frequently attributed to the rapid progress of weakening of muscles and respiratory failure [121].

SDB is a classical feature particularly in SMA 1 and 2. The intercostal muscles in these cases are more affected than the diaphragm, resulting in paradoxical breathing (inspiratory efforts cause the rib cage to move inward as the abdomen moves outward). Thoracoabdominal asynchrony is present during the inspiratory and expiratory phases in both REM and NREM sleep [122].

In the past 20 years, NIV has been used as a standard method for increasing the duration and quality of life of the affected children. Nocturnal sleep architecture is consolidated and daytime functioning improves. Both the growth and development of lung parenchyma are positively influenced, and chest wall deformity either slows down growing or starts reversing its progression [115, 123].

Congenital Myasthenic Syndromes

The congenital myasthenic syndromes represent a group of heterogeneous disorders that can be classified into presynaptic, synaptic, or postsynaptic according to the site of the transmission defect. The manifestations can be severe from birth with weak cry, congenital hypotonia with generalized weakness, and feeble suck or can combine in various degrees ptosis, ophthalmoparesis, easy fatigability, and proximal pattern of muscle weakness.

The presence of sleep hypoventilation syndrome has been reported [115], and therefore, polysomnographic evaluation and NIV positive pressure ventilation can be indicated.

Congenital Muscular Dystrophies

Congenital muscular dystrophies are genetically and clinically heterogeneous group of autosomal recessive disorders, presenting with muscle weakness and hypotonia at birth or within the first few months of life. The diagnosis is possible at the molecular level; the course of disease is usually slowly progressive.

Patients are at risk of SDB including central apneas/hypopneas, awakenings, as well as of poor quality of sleep and epileptic seizures. Pinard et al. [124] examined sleep structure in a group of 20 children and adolescents and found frequent awakenings with decreased total sleep time and decreased REM duration in all the cases. Increased apnea-hypopnea index was noticed in 13 out of 20 children, and in a half of the patients (10 out of 20) nocturnal paroxysmal activity was found. Association of nocturnal paroxysmal activity with apnea-hypopnea syndrome was noticed in eight of these ten children. Systematic screening of SDB and sleep quality should be, though, a part of routine management.

Duchenne Muscular Dystrophy

Duchenne muscular dystrophy (DMD) is the most frequent progressive muscular dystrophy in childhood. It belongs to a group of dystrophinopathies, resulting from mutation in the dystrophin gene, located on the short arm of the X chromosome (Xp21) and transmitted in a sex-linked recessive manner. The incidence of DMD of approximately 1:3000 up to 1:6000 male births [118] makes it the most widespread neuromuscular disease. The clinical picture includes classic myopathic features (difficulty in climbing stairs, rising from the floor, progressive muscle wasting with increased lordosis, and diminished tendon reflexes). In contrast to general atrophy, there is striking pseudohypertrophy of the calves. At about the age of 10–12 years, the children start being wheelchair bound and developing cardiomyopathy. After the introduction of the palliative steroid therapy, the median age for the loss of ambulation has increased by approximately two years. However, the prognosis depends also on respiratory care. Over the past 20 years, improvement in ventilatory support and multidisciplinary care has improved the survival rate of DMD patients till their 30s [125].

Signs of early respiratory insufficiency are usually first detectable in sleep; hence, polysomnographic examination is indispensable there. Annual monitoring is recommended if vital capacity declines to <65 %; the patients should undergo twice yearly a visit to a pulmonary and cardiology pediatric specialists and somnologist after confinement to a wheelchair, after their vital capacity falls below 80 % and/or after the age of 10 years [115]. Increased risk for SDB includes hypopnea, central and obstructive apnea, and hypoxemia. Suresh et al. [126] presume a bi-phase presentation SDB, with OSA found in the first decade and hypoventilation more commonly seen at the beginning of the second decade. However, the patients' sleep can also be influenced by medication and/or physical factors. Disorders of initiating and maintaining sleep were significantly more frequent in children treated by steroids. The need to start a career where immobility forms to obstacle seems to be a major burden on the quality of sleep, and sleep disturbances are strongly associated with immobility [125]. Gradually increasing number of nocturnal awakenings leads to daytime sleepiness and morning headaches and can contribute to cognitive impairment. Although SDB treatment with NIV support is very important, the treatment should take into account its complexity as the aim to improve quality of life and reduce the high morbidity and early mortality associated with DMD.

Myotonic Dystrophy

Myotonic dystrophy, particularly type 1, is the most frequent adult-onset muscular dystrophy characterized, besides clear neurological symptoms, by fatigue and daytime sleepiness [127]. The inheritance is autosomal dominant with amplification of a trinucleotide repeat localized at the chromosome 19q13.2. The clinical severity depends on the number of repeats. The congenital form is usually related to a maternal transmission and shows the greatest number of repeats. Facial diplegia and dysmorphic craniomandibular structures aggravate respiratory difficulty. Mixed central and obstructive apneas have been reported in children with congenital myotonic dystrophy [115].

Besides the presence of frequent central apnea, not only in REM sleep but occurring throughout all the sleep stages, and less frequent obstructive events [128], there is impairment of neural respiratory control indicated by abnormal response to hypoxia and hypercapnia, which is due to the CNS involvement. The excessive daytime sleepiness, often described in children with the initial stage of the myopathy, is probably independent of the apnea-hypopnea index, oxygen desaturations, or sleep fragmentation, occurring because of the direct effect of CNS lesions as indicated by the cognitive and neuropsychological deficits [129].

Charcot-Marie-Tooth Disease (CMT)

CMT represents a widely heterogeneous group of diseases as regards the genetic background, mode of transmission, and clinical and neurophysiological manifestation. As the most common form, CMT1 is characterized by progressive peroneal muscular atrophy and transmitted as a rule by an autosomal dominant trait of inheritance. Their prevalence is 3.8 per 10,000 in population, with most cases located at the chromosome 17p11.2 [95]. The clinical picture varies from very mild up to the quite severe wheelchair-bound handicapped phenotype.

Restrictive pulmonary impairment has been described in association with phrenic nerve dysfunction, diaphragm dysfunction, or thoracic cage abnormalities. Sleep disturbances may be associated with paresthesia, muscle cramps, or RLS. Fatigue, and reduced sleep quality, has been described in adult patients; the references about children are scarce. Sleep apnea was found to be common in CMT patients, and the apnea-hypopnea index correlated with disease severity. Since causative treatment for CMT is not available, sleep-related symptoms should be recognized and treated in order to improve quality of life [130]. Bi-level positive airway pressure (BiPAP) is more appreciate treatment than positive airway pressure (CPAP). The prominence of peripheral neuropathy as a cause of the RLS in CMT may justify treatment with neuropathic medication (e.g., gabapentin) better than dopaminergic agents [131].

Conclusions

Sleep disturbances in children with neurodevelopmental disabilities are highly prevalent and tend to be chronic. A specific sleep phenotype could be characteristic of a particular disorder and can represent a clinical clue for the diagnosis.

The clinical evaluation of children with neurodevelopmental disabilities should always comprise a detailed investigation of sleep problems, disturbances, and complaints reported by parents. Also the contributing factors to sleep disorders should be analyzed (either psychiatric or medical) in order to choose the best treatment for sleep disorders that are often overlooked and considered as a minor issue in relation to the general condition of the child. A comprehensive awareness of sleep disorders in these patients becomes essential for the appropriate recognition and effective treatment.

References

1. Angriman M, Caravale B, Novelli L, et al. Sleep in children with neurodevelopmental disabilities. Neuropediatrics. 2015;46:199–210.
2. Romeo DM, Brogna C, Quintiliani M, et al. Sleep disorders in children with cerebral palsy: neurodevelopmental and behavioral correlate. Sleep Med. 2014;15:213–2018.
3. Lipton J. Sleep and circadian dysfunction in children with mental retardation or cerebral palsy. In: Kothare SV, Kotagal S, editors. Sleep in childhood neurological disorders. New York: Demos Medical; 2011. p. 235–44.
4. Fitzgerald DA, Follett J, Van Asperen PP. Assessing and managing lung disease and sleep disordered breathing in children with cerebral palsy. Paediatr Respir Rev. 2009;10:18–24.
5. Karatas AF, Miller EG, Miller F, et al. Cerebral palsy patients discovered dead during sleep: experience from a comprehensive tertiary pediatric center. J Pediatr Rehabil Med. 2013;6:225–31.
6. Atmawidjaja RW, Wong SW, Yang WW, Ong LC. Sleep disturbance in Malaysian children with cerebral palsy. Dev Med Child Neurol. 2014;56:681–5.
7. Newman CJ, O'Regan M, Hensey O. Sleep disorders in children with cerebral palsy. Dev Med Child Neurol. 2006;48:564–8.
8. Shintani T, Asakura K, Ishi K, et al. Obstructive sleep apnea in children with cerebral palsy. Nihon Jibiinkoka Gakkai kaiho. 1998;101:266–71.
9. Wiggs L, Stores G. Severe sleep disturbance and daytime challenging behaviour in children with severe learning disabilities. J Intellect Disabil Res JIDR. 1996;40:518–28.
10. Shibagaki M, Kiyono S, Takeuchi T. Nocturnal sleep in mentally retarded infants with cerebral palsy. Electroenceph Clinical Neurophysiol. 1985;61:465–71.
11. Hsiao KH, Nixon GM. The effect of treatment of obstructive sleep apnea on quality of life in children with cerebral palsy. Res Dev Disabil. 2008;29:133–40.
12. Wayte S, McCaughey E, Holley S, et al. Sleep problems in children with cerebral palsy and their relationship with maternal sleep and depression. Acta Pediatr. 2012;101:618–23.
13. Braam W, Smits MG, Ridded R, et al. Exogenous melatonin for sleep problems in individuals with intellectual disability: a meta-analysis. Dev Med Child Neurol. 2009;51:340–9.
14. Miano S, Bruni O, Arico D, et al. Polysomnographic assessment of sleep disturbances in children with developmental disabilities and seizures. Neurol Sci. 2010;31:575–83.
15. Parrino L, Ferri R, Bruni O, Terzano MG. Cyclic alternating pattern (CAP): the marker of sleep instability. Sleep Med Rev. 2012;16:27–45.

16. Bruni O, Novelli L, Miano S, et al. Cyclic alternating pattern: a window on pediatric sleep. Sleep Med. 2010;11:628–36.
17. Ghanizadeh A, Faghih M. The impact of general medical condition on sleep in children with mental retardation. Sleep Breath. 2011;15:57–62.
18. Tietze AL, Zernikow B, Michel E, Blankenburg M. Sleep disturbances in children, adolescents and young adults with severe psychomotor impairment: impact on parental quality of life and sleep. Dev Med Child Neurol. 2014;56:1187–93.
19. Blankenburg M, Tietze AL, Hechler T, et al. Snake: the developmental and validation of a questionnaire on sleep disturbances in children with severe psychomotor impairment. Sleep Med. 2013;14:339–51.
20. Bonuck K, Grant R. Sleep problems and early developmental delay: implications for early intervention programs. Intellect Dev Disabl. 2012;50:41–52.
21. Bruni O, Alonso-Alconada D, Besag F, et al. Current role of melatonin in pediatric neurology: clinical recommendations. Eur J Paediatr Neurol. 2015;19:122–33.
22. Braam W, van Geijlswijk, Keijzer H, et al. Loss of response to melatonin treatment is associated with slow melatonin metabolism. J Intellect Disabil Res. 2010;54:547–55.
23. Gringras P, Gamble C, Jones AP, et al. Melatonin for sleep problems in children with neurodevelopmental disorders: randomised double masked placebo controlled trial. BMJ. 2012;345:e6664.
24. Lingham R, Hunt L, Golding J, et al. Prevalence of developmental coordination disorder in the DSM-IV at 7 years of age: a UK population based study. Pediatrics. 2009;123: e693–700.
25. Barnett AL, Wiggs L. Sleep behaviour in children with developmental co-ordination disorder. Child Care Health Dev. 2011;3:403–11.
26. Scabar A, Devescovi R, Blason L, et al. Comorbidity of DCD and SLI: significance of epileptiform activity during sleep. J Compil. 2006;32:733–9.
27. Echenne B, Cheminal R, River F, et al. Epileptic electroencephalographic abnormalities and development dysphasias: a study of 32 patients. Brain Dev. 1992;14:216–25.
28. Dlouhá O, Nevšímalová S. EEG changes and epilepsy in developmental dysphasia. Clinical Neurophysiology at the Beginning of the 21st Century. Suppl Clin Neurophysiol. 2000; 53:271–4.
29. Sanchez Fernandez I, Loddenkemper T, Peters JM, Kothare SV. Electrical status epilepticus in sleep: clinical presentation and pathophysiology. Pediatr Neurol. 2012;47:390–410.
30. Bruni O, Ferri R, Novelli L, et al. Sleep spindle activity is correlated with reading abilities in developmental dyslexia. Sleep. 2009;32:1333–40.
31. Cortese S. The neurobiology and genetics of Attention-Deficit/Hyperactivity Disorder (ADHD): what every clinician should know. Eur J Paediatr Neurol. 2012;16:422–33.
32. Cortese S, Faraone SV, Konofal E, Lecendreux M. Sleep in children with attention-deficit/hyperactivity disorder: metaanalysis of subjective and objective studies. J Am Acad Child Adolesc Psychiatry. 2009;48:894–908.
33. Miano S, Donfrancesco R, Bruni O, et al. NREM sleep instability is reduced in children with attention-deficit/hyperactivity disorder. Sleep. 2006;29:797–803.
34. Prihodova I, Paclt I, Kemlink D, et al. Sleep disorders and daytime sleepiness in children with attention-deficit/hyperactivity disorder: a two night polysomnographic study with a multiple sleep latency test. Sleep Med. 2010;11:922–8.
35. Calhoun SL, Fernandez-Medoza J, Vgontzas AN, et al. Learning, attention/hyperactivity, and conduct problems as sequelae of excessive daytime sleepiness in a general population of young children. Sleep. 2012;35:627–32.
36. Cortese S. Sleep and ADHD: what we know and what we do not know. Sleep Med. 2015;16:5–6.
37. Owens JA. The ADHD and sleep conundrum redux: moving forward. Sleep Med Rev. 2006;10:377–9.
38. Miano S, Ferri R. Epidemiology and management of insomnia in children with autistic spectrum disorders. Pediatr Drugs. 2010;12:75–84.

39. Vriend JL, Corkum PV, Moon EC, Smith IM. Behavioral interventions for sleep problems in children with autism spectrum disorders: current findings and future directions. J Paediatr Psychol. 2011;36:1017–29.
40. Richdale AL, Schreck KA. Sleep problems in autism spectrum disorders: prevalence, nature, and possible biopsychosocial aetiologies. Sleep Med Rev. 2009;13:403–11.
41. Kotagal S, Broomall E. Sleep in children with autism spectrum disorder. Pediatr Neurol. 2012;47:242–51.
42. Mazurek MO, Petroski GF. Sleep problems in children with autism spectrum disorder: examining and contributions of sensory over-responsibility and anxiety. Sleep Med. 2015;16: 270–9.
43. Cortesi F, Giannotti F, Ivanenko A, Johnson K. Sleep in children with autistic spectrum disorder. Sleep Med. 2010;11:659–64.
44. Giannotti F, Cortesi F, Cerquiglini A, et al. Sleep in children with autism with and without autistic regression. J Sleep Res. 2011;20:338–47.
45. Rossignol DA, Frye RE. Melatonin in autism spectrum disorders: a systematic review and meta-analysis. Dev Med Child Neurol. 2011;53:783–92.
46. Miano S, Bruni O, Elia M, et al. Sleep in children with autistic spectrum disorder: a questionnaire and polysomnographic study. Sleep Med. 2007;9:64–70.
47. Andersen IM, Kaczmarska J, McGrew SG, Malow BA. Melatonin for insomnia in children with autism spectrum disorders. J Child Neurol. 2008;23:482–5.
48. Nevsimalova S. Genetic disorders and sleepiness. In: Thorpy MJ, Billiard M, editors. Sleepiness: causes, consequences and treatment. New York: Cambridge University Press; 2011. p. 335–50.
49. Rack MJ. Sleep disorders associated with mental retardation. In: Culebras A, editor. Sleep disorders and neurologic diseases. 2nd ed. New York: Informa Healthcare; 2007. p. 27–37.
50. Stores G, Stores R. Sleep disorders and their clinical significance in children with Down syndrome. Dev Med Child Neurol. 2013;55:126–30.
51. Bull MJ, Committee on G. Health supervision for children with Down syndrome. Pediatrics. 2011;128:393–406.
52. Harvey MT, Kennedy CH. Polysomnographic phenotypes in developmental disabilities. Int J Dev Neurosci. 2002;20:443–8.
53. Kronk R, Bishop EE, Raspa M, et al. Prevalence, nature, and correlates of sleep problems among children with fragile X syndrome based on a large scale parent survey. Sleep. 2010;33:679–87.
54. Kidd SA, Lachiewicz A, Barbouth D, et al. Fragile X syndrome: a review of associated medical problems. Pediatrics. 2014;134:995–1005.
55. Gould EL, Loesch DZ, Martin MJ, et al. Melatonin profiles and sleep characteristics in boys with fragile X syndrome: a preliminary study. Am J Med Genet. 2000;95:307–15.
56. Hagerman R. Fragile X: treatment of hyperactivity. Pediatrics. 1997;99:753.
57. Weiskop S, Richdale A, Matthews J. Behavioural treatment to reduce sleep problems in children with autism or fragile X syndrome. Dev Med Child Neurol. 2005;47:94–104.
58. Cohen M, Hamilton J, Narang I. Clinically important age-related differences in sleep related disordered breathing in infants and children with Prader-Willi Syndrome. PLoS One. 2014;9:e101012.
59. Sedky K, Bennett DS, Pumariega A. Prader Willi syndrome and obstructive sleep apnea: co-occurrence in the pediatric population. J Clin Sleep Med: JCSM. 2014;10:403–9.
60. Nevsimalova S, Vankova J, Stepanova I, et al. Hypocretin deficiency in Prader-Willi syndrome. Eur J Neurol. 2005;12:70–2.
61. Bruni O, Verrillo E, Novelli L, Ferri R. Prader-Willi syndrome: sorting out the relationships between obesity, hypersomnia, and sleep apnea. Curr Opin Pulm Med. 2010;16:568–73.
62. Camfferman D, McEvoy RD, O'Donoghue F, Lushington K. Prader Willi syndrome and excessive daytime sleepiness. Sleep Med Rev. 2008;12:65–75.
63. Berini J, Spica Russotto V, Castelnuovo P, et al. Growth hormone therapy and respiratory disorders: long-term follow-up in PWS children. J Clin Endocrinol Metab. 2013;98:E1516–23.

64. Bird LM. Angelman syndrome: review of clinical and molecular aspects. Appl Clin Genet. 2014;7:93–104.
65. Menkes JH, Falk E. Chromosomal anomalies and contiguous-gene syndromes. In: Menkes JH, Sarnat HB, Maria BL, editors. Child neurology. 7th ed. Philadelphia: Lippincott Williams and Wilkins; 2006. p. 227–57.
66. Bruni O, Ferri R, D'Agostino G, et al. Sleep disturbances in Angelman syndrome: a questionnaire study. Brain Dev. 2004;26:233–40.
67. Miano S, Bruni O, Elia M, et al. Sleep breathing and periodic leg movement pattern in Angelman Syndrome: a polysomnographic study. Clin Neurophysiol. 2005;116:2685–92.
68. Zhdanova IV, Wurtman RJ, Wagstaff J. Effect of a low dose of melatonin on sleep in children with Angelman syndrome. J Pediatr Endocrinol Metab. 1999;12:57–67.
69. Takaesu Y, Komada Y, Inoue Y. Melatonin profile and its relation to circadian rhythm sleep disorders in Angelman syndrome patients. Sleep Med. 2012;13:1164–70.
70. Arens R, Wright B, Elliot J, et al. Periodic limb movement in sleep in children with Williams syndrome. J Pediatr. 1998;133:670–4.
71. Goldman SE, Malow BA, Newman KD, et al. Sleep patterns and daytime sleepiness in adolescents and young adults with Williams syndrome. J Intellect Disabil Res. 2009;53:182–8.
72. Shelley BP, Robertson MM. The neuropsychiatry and multisystem features of the Smith-Magenis syndrome: a review. J Neuropsychiatry Clin Neurosci. 2005;17:91–7.
73. Gropman AL, Duncan WC, Smith AC. Neurologic and developmental features of the Smith-Magenis syndrome (del 17p11.2). Pediatr Neurol. 2006;34:337–50.
74. Potocki L, Glaze D, Tan DX, et al. Circadian rhythm abnormalities of melatonin in Smith-Magenis syndrome. J Med Genet. 2000;37:428–33.
75. Novakova M, Nevsimalova S, Prihodova I, et al. Alteration of the circadian clock in children with Smith-Magenis syndrome. J Clin Endocrinol Metab. 2012;97:E312–8.
76. De Leersnyder H. Inverted rhythm of melatonin secretion in Smith-Magenis syndrome: from symptoms to treatment. Trends Endocrinol Metab. 2006;17:291–8.
77. De Leersnyder H. Smith-Magenis syndrome. Handb Clin Neurol. 2013;111:295–6.
78. De Leersnyder H, Verloes A. Le syndrome de Smith-Magenis. Devenir. 2008/3;20:197–209.
79. Menkes JH. Heredodegenerative diseases. In: Menkes JH, Sarnat HB, Maria BL, editors. Child neurology. 7th ed. Philadelphia: Lippincott Williams and Wilkins; 2006. p. 163–226.
80. Young D, Nagarajn L, de Klerk N, et al. Sleep problems in Rett syndrome. Brain Dev. 2007;29:609–16.
81. Glaze DG, Frost Jr JD, Zoghbi HY, Percy AK. Rett's syndrome: characterization of respiratory patterns and sleep. Ann Neurol. 1987;21:377–82.
82. Marcus CL, Carroll JL, McColley SA, et al. Polysomnographic characteristics of patients with Rett syndrome. J Pediatr. 1994;125:218–24.
83. Nomura Y. Early behavior characteristics and sleep disturbance in Rett syndrome. Brain Dev. 2005;27 Suppl 1:S35–42.
84. Carotenuto M, Esposito M, D'Aniello A, et al. Polysomnographic findings in Rett syndrome: a case-control study. Sleep Breath. 2013;17:93–8.
85. D'Orsi G, Demaio V, Scarpelli F, et al. Central sleep apnoea in Rett syndrome. Neurol Sci. 2009;30:389–91.
86. Hagebeuk EEO, Bijlmer RP, Koelman JH, Poll-The BT. Respiratory disturbance in Rett syndrome: don't forget to evaluate upper airway obstruction. J Child Neurol. 2012;27:888–92.
87. Hagebeuk EEO, Van den Bossche RAS, De Weerd AW. Respiratory and sleep disorders in female children with atypical Rett syndrome caused by mutations in the CDKL5 gene. Dev Med Child Neurol. 2013;55:480–4.
88. Wong K, Leonard H, Jacoby P, et al. The trajectories of sleep disturbances in Rett syndrome. J Sleep Res. 2015;24:223–33.
89. Nomura Y. Neurophysiology of Rett syndrome. Brain Dev. 2001;23 Suppl 1:S50–7.
90. McArthur AJ, Budden SS. Sleep dysfunction in Rett syndrome: a trial of exogenous melatonin treatment. Dev Med Child Neurol. 1998;40(3):186–92.

91. Trivier E, De Cesare D, Jacquot S, et al. Mutation in the kinase Rsk-2 associated with Coffin-Lowry syndrome. Nature. 1996;384:567–70.

92. Nelson GB, Hahn JS. Stimulus-induced drop episodes in Coffin-Lowry syndrome. Pediatrics. 2003;111:e197–202.

93. Caraballo R, Tesi Rocha A, Medina C, Fejerman N. Drop episodes in Coffin-Lowry syndrome: an unusual type of startle response. Epileptic Disord. 2000;2:173–6.

94. Vossler DG, Wyler AR, Wilkus RJ, et al. Cataplexy and monoamine oxidase deficiency in Norrie disease. Neurology. 1996;46:1258–61.

95. Menkes JH, Wilcox WR. Inherited metabolic diseases of the nervous system. In: Menkes JH, Sarnat HB, Maria BL, editors. Child neurology. 7th ed. Philadelphia: Lippincott Williams and Wilkins; 2006. p. 29–141.

96. Kansagra S, Austin S, DeArmey S, et al. Polysomnographic findings in infantile Pompe disease. Am J Med Genet Part A. 2013;161A:3196–200.

97. Mellies U, Stehling F, Dohna-Schwake C, et al. Respiratory failure in Pompe disease: treatment with noninvasive ventilation. Neurology. 2005;64:1465–7.

98. Leighton SEJ, Papsin B, Vellodi A, et al. Disordered breathing during sleep in patients with mucopolysacharidoses. Int J Pediatr Otorhinolaryngol. 2001;58:127–38.

99. Santamaria F, Andreucci MV, Parenti G, et al. Upper airway obstructive disease in mucopolysacharidoses: polysomnography, computed tomography and nasal endoscopy findings. J Inherit Metab Dis. 2007;30:743–9.

100. Fraser J, Wraith JE, Delatycki MB. Sleep disturbance in mucopolysaccharidoses type III (Sanfilippo syndrome): a survey of managing clinicians. Clin Genet. 2002;62:418–21.

101. Guerrero JM, Pozo D, Diaz-Rodrigues JL, et al. Impairment of the melatonin rhythm in children with Sanfilippo syndrome. J Pineal Res. 2006;40:192–3.

102. Vankova J, Stepanova I, Jech R, et al. Sleep disturbances and hypocretin deficiency in Niemann. Pick disease type C. Sleep. 2003;26:427–30.

103. Kanabayashi T, Abe M, Fujimoto S, et al. Hypocretin deficiency in Niemann-Pick type C with cataplexy. Neuropediatrics. 2003;34:52–3.

104. Nishino S, Kanbayashi T. Symptomatic narcolepsy, cataplexy and hypersomnia, and their implications in the hypothalamic hypocretin/orexin system. Sleep. 2005;9:269–310.

105. Oyama K, Takahashi T, Shoji Y, et al. Niemann-Pick disease type C: cataplexy and hypocretin in cerebrospinal fluid. Tokohu J Exp Med. 2006;209:263–7.

106. Vanier MT. Biochemical studies in Niemann-Pick disease. I. Major sphingolipids of liver and spleen. Biochim Biophys Acta. 1883;750:178–84.

107. Smit LS, Lammers GJ, Castman-Berrevoets CE. Cataplexy leading to the diagnosis of Niemann-Pick disease type C. Pediatr Neurol. 2006;35:82–4.

108. Pedroso JL, Fusao EF, Ladeia-Frota C, et al. Teaching video neuroimages: gelastic cataplexy as the first neurologic manifestation of Niemann-Pick disease type C. In: MSV Elkind, editor. Resident and Fellow Section, American Academy of Neurology. 2012; p. e189.

109. Nevsimalova S, Malinova V. Cataplexy and sleep disorders in Niemann-Pick disease type C. Curr Neurol Neurosci Rep. 2015;15:522–9.

110. Patterson MC, Vecchio D, Prady H, et al. Miglustat for treatment of Niemann-Pick C disease: a randomized controlled study. Lancet Neurol. 2007;6:765–72.

111. Challamel MJ, Mazzola ME, Nevšímalová S, et al. Sleep. 1994;17 Suppl 8:S17–20.

112. Zarowski M, Steinborn B, et al. Treatment of cataplexy in Niemann-Pick disease type C. Eur J Paediatr Neurol. 2011;15:84–7.

113. Kirevski E, Partinen M, Santavuori P. Sleep and its disturbance in a variant form of late infantile neuronal ceroid lipofuscinosis (CLN5). J Child Neurol. 2001;16:707–13.

114. Kirevski E, Partinen M, Salmi T, et al. Sleep alteration in juvenile neuronal ceroid-lipofuscinosis. Pediatr Neurol. 2000;22:347–54.

115. Alves RSC, Resende MBD, Skomro R, et al. Sleep and neuromuscular disorders in children. Sleep Med Rev. 2009;13:133–48.

116. Culebras A. Sleep disorders and neuromuscular disorders. In: Culebras A, editor. Sleep disorders and neurologic diseases. 2nd ed. New York: Informa Healthcare; 2007. p. 387–403.

117. Arens R, Muzumdar H. Sleep, sleep disorders breathing, and nocturnal hypoventilation in children with neuromuscular disorders. Paediatr Respir Rev. 2010;11:24–30.
118. Sarnat HB, Menkes JH. Diseases of the motor unit. In: Menkes JH, Sarnat HB, Maria BL, editors. Child neurology. 7th ed. Philadelphia: Lippincott Williams and Wilkins; 2006. p. 969–1024.
119. Pradella M. Sleep polygraphic parameters in neuromuscular diseases. Arq Neuropsiquiatr. 1994;5:476–83.
120. Mellies U, Dohna-Schwake C, Stehling F, Voit T. Sleep disordered breathing in spinal muscular atrophy neuromuscular disorders. Neuromuscul Disord. 2004;14:797–803.
121. Verrillo E, Bruni O, Pavone M, et al. Sleep architecture in infants with spinal muscular atrophy type 1. Sleep Med. 2014;15:1246–50.
122. Chiarini Testa MB, Pavone M, Berini E, et al. Sleep-disordered breathing in spinal muscular atrophy types 1 and 2. Am J Phys Med Rehabil. 2005;84:666–70.
123. Petrone A, Pavone M, Ciarini Testa MB, et al. Noninvasive ventilation in children with spinal muscular atrophy types 1 and 2. Am J Phys Med Rehabil. 2007;86:216–21.
124. Pinard JM, Azabou E, Essid N, et al. Sleep-disordered breathing in children with congenital muscular dystrophies. Eur J Paed Neurol. 2012;16:619–24.
125. Bloetzer C, Jeannet PY, Lynch B, Newman CJ. Sleep disorders in boys with Duchenne muscular dystrophy. Acta Paediatr. 2012;101:1265–9.
126. Suresh S, Wales P, Dakin C, et al. Sleep-related breathing disorder in Duchenne muscular dystrophy: disease spectrum in paediatric population. J Paediatr Child Health. 2005;41:500–3.
127. Hermans MCE, Merkies ISJ, Laberge L, et al. Fatigue and daytime sleepiness scale in myotonic dystrophy type 1. Muscle Nerve. 2013;47:89–95.
128. Cirignotta F, Mondim S, Zucconi M, et al. Sleep related breathing impairment in myotonic dystrophy. J Neurol. 1988;235:80–5.
129. Ono S, Kurisaki H, Sakuma A, Nagao K. Myotonic dystrophy with alveolar hypoventilation and hypersomnia: a clinicopathological study. J Neurol Sci. 1995;128:225–31.
130. Boentert M, Dziewas R, Heidbreder A, et al. Fatigue, reduced sleep quality and restless legs syndrome in Charcot-Marie-Tooth disease: a web-based survey. J Neurol. 2010;257:646–52.
131. Aboussouan LS, Lewis RA, Shy ME. Disorders of pulmonary functions, sleep and the upper airway in Charcot-Marie-Tooth disease. Lung. 2007;185:1–7.

Chapter 17
Sleep in Children with Psychiatric and Behavioral Problems

Rosalia Silvestri and Irene Aricò

Abstract Sleep is commonly affected in psychiatric and behavioral pediatric disorders, contributing to children's disability and parental burden. Difficulties initiating and maintaining sleep, often non-restorative in quality, frequent parasomnias, such as disorders of arousals, enuresis, and nightmares; sleep-related movement disorders such as bruxism, restless legs syndrome (RLS), and periodic limb movement during sleep (PLMS); snoring; and sleep apnea may all interfere with sleep consolidation and daytime performance both at school and daycare. Alterations of slow-wave sleep (SWS), both in terms of macro- and microstructural aspects, are common to almost all disorders, whereas rapid eye movement (REM) sleep is more impacted by mood and autism spectrum disorders (ASDs), often correlating with relational and emotional profiles rather than with cognitive problems. In said disorders, subjective complaints always override objective findings from all-night actigraphic or polysomnographic (PSG) recordings. In particular, sleep latency (SL) and total sleep time (TST) are severely affected only in the acute manic and psychotic phases and in early ASDs, whereas infranight awakenings and slow-wave sleep (SWS) fragmentation appear to be the hallmarks of these disorders, reflecting an impaired maturational process affecting mostly the frontal lobes and their connectivity.

Keywords Sleep • Anxiety • Depression • Bipolar disorder • ASD • ADHD

R. Silvestri (✉)
Department of Clinical and Experimental Medicine, Sleep Medicine Center,
AOU G. Martino, Via Consolare Valeria,
Messina 98125, Italy
e-mail: rsilvestri@unime.it; rosalia.silvestri@unime.it

I. Aricò
Department of Clinical and Experimental Medicine, AOU G. Martino,
Via Consolare Valeria, Messina 98125, Italy
e-mail: Irene.arico77@gmail.com

© Springer International Publishing Switzerland 2017
S. Nevšímalová, O. Bruni (eds.), *Sleep Disorders in Children*,
DOI 10.1007/978-3-319-28640-2_17

Introduction

There appears to be a complex bidirectional relationship between psychiatric disorders and sleep problems in children and adolescents. Numerous studies have been carried out addressing the influence of poor sleep on the development and burden of psychiatric morbidity. Both old [1] and more recent epidemiologic studies [2] indicate significant nighttime problems such as bedtime resistance, fear of the dark, need for co-sleeping, restless sleep, snoring, and several parasomnias including nightmares and sleep terrors, enuresis, and excessive movements during sleep (see Table 17.1).

Some complaints appear to be more common within specific psychiatric diagnosis, whereas others seem to be largely distributed across all psychiatric disorders. Often, the severity of sleep inadequacy carries a negative prognosis for the resolution of the psychiatric condition, heralding in most cases recurrent symptomatic episodes.

Objective evaluation of sleep via traditional or ambulatory PSG and/or actigraphic recordings has been limited to few cases [3].

The same scarcity of sleep data can be observed in many studies considering specific therapeutic interventions addressing sleep, whether cognitively behavioral or pharmaceutical in nature.

Little is known about safety of hypnotics in the pediatric population; many commonly used drugs among adults may even exert paradoxical effects in children. Furthermore, psychotropic drugs addressing the primary psychiatric condition may negatively affect sleep continuity and be responsible for unpleasant oneiric potentiation [4, 5] or induce comorbid sleep disorders such as RLS or periodic limb

Table 17.1 Sleep in children with psychiatric disorders

Disorders	Subjective children data	Objective data
Anxiety disorders	Parental reports of bedtime fears and rituals, need for co-sleeping and transitional objects. Nighttime waking, nightmares, DOA	Reduced SL and SWS Increased WASO Less consistently Reduced REM-L and TST
Mood disorders		
MDD	Insomnia, worries, hypersomnia	Increased SL and REM density, WASO Reduced REM-L and SWS
Bipolar	Decreased need for sleep/hyperactivity (mania phase)	Increased N1 Reduced SWS Longer TST and reduced SL between episodes
Schizophrenia	Insomnia, EDS	Decreased SE; TST and SWS, REM-L and REM density

movement disorder (PLMD). Indeed, the latter has been reportedly enhanced by most selective serotonin reuptake inhibitors (SSRIs) and dual serotonin and nor-adrenalin reuptake inhibitors (SNRIs) [6].

Anxiety Disorders and Sleep

Up to 20 % of the pediatric population [7] suffers from a diagnosable anxiety disorders according to the most recent DSM-5 classification [8], not considering previously included diagnoses such as post-traumatic stress disorder (PTSD) and obsessive-compulsive disorders (OCDs).

The incidence of children encountering significant stressful anxiety without otherwise meeting conditions for being properly classified among current diagnostic criteria for anxiety disorders is thought to be quite elevated.

A relatively recent report [9] estimates a prevalence of transient sleep problems in 85 % against 50 % of chronically impaired sleep, in children with anxiety disorders.

Typical habits of anxious children vary with age and cultural diversities, ranging from bedtime fears and rituals to requests for transitional objects, crying, and co-sleeping.

Nocturnal awakenings are the most consistent marker of all anxiety disorders [2].

Family habits and parental conflicts or psychopathology significantly interfere with anxiety symptoms, favoring the development of sleep disorders. In particular, lack of structure and inconsistent parenting styles may negatively influence the development of correct maturational skills such as self-soothing at bedtime, thus depriving the child of early opportunities to achieve this imperative ability [10]. Nighttime fears and recurrent nightmares may be emblematic of traumatic abusive experiences, albeit generally present in most anxiety disorders.

In addition, sleep-related symptoms in anxiety disorders vary across the life span, being expressed as bedtime fears and refusal in younger children or as disruptive nightmares with prominent sleep fragmentation in adolescents [2].

The severity of sleep problems correlates with functional impairment within anxiety disorders, with early sleep disruption holding a predictive negative value for the development of anxiety disorders but not for depression in later years [10, 11]. Longitudinal community-based studies give rise to the concern that anxious children may often underreport their sleep problems in comparison to depressed kids [12], thus rendering parental reports and objective findings crucial to diagnosis [13].

Separation anxiety disorder (SAD) is by far the most common anxiety disorder in very young children, accounting for most of the referrals in the field. Ninety-seven percent of these children experience sleep problems, most commonly initial insomnia and bed refusal without the presence of a significant attachment figure. These children also experience more awakenings and frequent enuretic episodes besides typical disorders of arousal such as sleepwalking and night terrors [14].

Generalized anxiety disorder (GAD) is, instead, characterized by more generic worries about school and home in this age group, with a lifetime prevalence estimated of approximately 5 % [8]. Sleep problems are overly common, being reported by 90 % of the pediatric population with GAD. To simplify, they could be summarized as generating a "hyperarousal" state leading to difficulties in both initiating and maintaining sleep, nightmares, as well as difficulties waking up in the morning and daytime somnolence [9, 15]. A few objective studies offer conflicting results about sleep structure in anxiety disorders. Forbes et al. [13] found a prolonged SL, more awakenings, and reduced slow-wave sleep (SWS) when comparing healthy and depressed subjects. Alfano et al. [16] also indicated a reduced REM latency in the control group. In fact, a recent meta-analysis [17] reported very similar objective findings in polygraphically recorded anxious and depressed children.

Children with PTSD have been exposed to and reexperience a traumatic event. They manifest increased stimuli reaction, avoidance of trauma-related stimuli, hyperarousal, and, sometimes, dissociative behavior. Approximately 14 % of children exposed to traumatic events develop PTSD. Trauma may be related to physical or sexual abuse or to disastrous experiential events such as hurricanes, earthquakes, and terrorist attacks. All PTSD subjects are five times more likely to show sleep disruption after 3 years from the event [18]. A few actigraphic studies confirmed sleep fragmentation and poor quality sleep [19] and significantly increased SL with enhanced nocturnal activity [20].

OCD has a lifetime prevalence of 1–2 %, 0.8 % within the pediatric population [8]. Bedtime routines may be extenuatingly long and interfere with sleep onset especially, but also with sleep continuity by promoting a high rate of waking after sleep onset (WASO). Also TST is inversely related to the severity of compulsions [21]. The one and only, very dated, PSG study in OCD adolescents revealed decreased sleep efficiency (SE) with increased SL [22]. The importance of a genetic component has been demonstrated by exposing high-risk (one parent with a diagnosis of social anxiety) versus normal-risk children to different emotional facial stimuli. Frontal, temporal, and limbic areas were selectively overactivated during exposure in high-risk versus typical-risk children. These are the same areas that are thought to be potentially responsible for nightmares and hyperarousal during sleep [23].

Pediatric Depression and Sleep

Major depressive disorder (MDD) presents with pervasive sadness, loss of interest, and pleasure leading to significant impairments in social and academic life [8]. Additional symptoms in children include irritability, behavioral dysregulation, and failure to gain weight. MDD prevalence increases with age from 1 % in early years up to 8 % in adolescence, often with a recurrent course [2]. Two-ninth of the descriptive features of MDD in the DSM-5 are related to sleep alterations such as insomnia or, conversely, hypersomnia. The latter is rare in pediatric depression; however, when co-occurring with insomnia, it carries a negative and dire prognosis [24]. Insomnia is usually associated with psychomotor agitation and restlessness, rumination, and worries, whereas hypersomnia correlates with psychomotor delay, hopelessness, and decreased vital energy. All of these symptoms strictly reflect mood oscillations which are influenced in a bidirectional way. In fact, in a prospective cohort study run on a community-based sample, insomnia at baseline increased by two- to threefolds the risk for MDD; conversely, MDD increased the occurrence of subsequent insomnia by the same measure. Early persistent sleep problems hold a negative prognostic value, predicting the development of anxiety and mood disorders later in adult life [25].

In examining special subgroups with suicidal ideation, 87 % of the sample was reported to suffer from persistent sleep problems [26]. Dated objective PSG measures carried out in pediatric populations revealed reduced REM and increased SL, increased REM density, and reduced and fragmented SWS [27, 28]. A more recent meta-analysis, however, found a significant difference of increased sleep latency in over 31 % of depressed children compared to normal controls. In addition, intra- and interhemispheric temporal coherence was decreased in the same percentage of patients [17]. Actigraphy, on the other hand, was only able to detect a blunted diurnal activity with delay of reaction phase in depressed children [29].

Maturational and gender-related factors are also powerful modulators of sleep features. Females, in fact, do not differ from healthy controls, whereas males exhibit the shortest REM latencies, fewer SWS, and highest arousals and transitional phases [30]. Greater REM density and longer SL were significantly associated with hospitalization and suicidality [31]. Adolescent female patients show the most drastic PSG changes compared to males. Trazodone and fluoxetine have both been employed for the treatment of adolescents with MDD, alone or in combination [32]. Hypnotic agents should be used judiciously and for short periods in this age group, so as to avoid excessive daytime sedation and worsening of comorbid disorders [33].

Sleep and Bipolar Disorders

Pediatric patients experience different bipolar symptoms from adults. Especially in prepubescent children, rapid or even continuous cycling is common with both manic and depressive overlapping. The hallmark of bipolar disorder is mania co-occurring with a decreased need for sleep along with other key symptoms including grandiosity, hypersexuality, and racing thoughts and ideas. Few studies report sleep features in early-onset bipolar disorder, and they all reflect a core symptom: decreased need for sleep paralleling the most severe mood episodes [34].

Only two studies collected PSG data. Rao et al. [35] found increased transitional phases and reduced SWS, but no significant differences as far as REM sleep. On the other hand, another study that assessed children via the Child Behavior Checklist revealed increased WASO and lower REM sleep compared to the control group [36].

Two actigraphic studies [37, 38] showed opposite results: decreased SE and duration with prolonged SL versus longer TST and less activity in between episodes coupled with a subjective report of unrefreshing fragmented sleep. Shorter SL and longer TST were also observed in unaffected children with a familial risk for bipolar disorders [38].

Pediatric Schizophrenia and Sleep

Fortunately, the incidence of early schizophrenia in children under the age of 15 is very low, being less than 1 in 10,000 children. The DSM-5 [8] does not include sleep disturbances among the diagnostic features. However, insomnia is the most common side effect in young schizophrenics. Co-occurrence of insomnia and excessive daytime sleepiness (EDS) predicted psychotic episodes in adolescents and potential risk of psychosis based on specific structured rating instruments [39]. Sleep dysfunction in a subsequent study on "ultrahigh-risk" (UHR) adolescents was found to correlate more with negative rather than positive symptoms [40]. No PSG studies are available so far in children with schizophrenia. In adults, SWS reduction and disrupted architecture are thought to be trait markers of the disease, correlating with severity of psychotic symptoms and lasting over remission [41]. Reduced SE and TST along with increased SL and decreased REM density and latency comprise other important and confirmed features [42].

Several non-pharmacological approaches are available for the treatment of sleep problems in pediatric psychiatric disorders. They include cognitive behavioral therapy (CBT) often combined with medications [43], sleep hygiene, and behavioral intervention to address maladaptive sleep habits. For very young children, correct seeking-and-reward consequence systems to promote adaptive behaviors work best [44]. Avoiding presleep frightening TV contents and creating self-soothing rituals may quell bedtime anxiety. Sleep consolidation, instead, is promoted by delaying bedtime, as suggested by bed restriction therapy (BRT), in order to favor sleep pressure in keeping with the sleep homeostasis predicate [45, 46]. More specific techniques may be employed to avoid negative presleep worries and rumination by planning a session of positive relaxing thoughts through imagery distraction [47].

Autism Spectrum Disorder and Sleep

Autism spectrum disorders (ASDs) refer to a gamut of developmental disorders impacting communication and social skills, characterized by the expression of restricted repetitive stereotyped behaviors. This category includes autistic and Asperger disorders in addition to pervasive developmental disorder (PDD) not otherwise specified. A substantial increment in ASD diagnosis has been observed over the last decades, with an estimated prevalence rate of almost 70/10,000, likely due

Table 17.2 Sleep in children with ASDs and ADHD

	Subjective complaints	Sleep structure	CAP
ASDs	Bedtime refusal and difficulties setting limits, restlessness, labored breathing, nighttime waking	Decreased TST and SWS Increased SL and REM-L Increased PLMs index REMWA	Decreased CAP rate in SWS Decreased A1 Increased A2, A3
ADHD	Restlessness, insomnia, bed tantrums, sleepwalking and terrors, enuresis, bruxism	Normal or increased SWS Increased WASO Increased PLMs index with or without arousal OSA Decreased SL on MSLT	Decreased CAP rate in SWS Decreased A1 Increased A2, A3

CAP cyclic alternating pattern, *DOA* disorders of arousal, *EDS* excessive daytime sleepiness, *MSLT* multiple sleep latency test, *PLMs* periodic limb movements, *REM-L* REM latency, *REMWA* REM without atonia, *SE* sleep efficiency, *SL* sleep latency, *SWS* slow-wave sleep, *TST* total sleep time, *WASO* wake after sleep onset

to increased awareness, genetic and environmental factors, and the extension of ASD diagnosis to less severe and uncommon forms of the disorder. Sleep problems are often experienced by ASD subjects (see Table 17.2). Children comprise up to 80 % of the whole ASD population. ASD seems to represent an independent risk factor for the occurrence of sleep disorders, besides that conferred by intellectual deficit alone [48]. Insomnia is the most common complaint from parents of ASD children. Initial as well as maintenance and early morning insomnia may coexist in varying associations. Mostly behavioral insomnia of childhood, either limit setting or sleep association type, seems to recur in these children where behavioral problems perpetuate innate neurobiological deficits linked to serotonin and glutamate domains [33]. Circadian rhythmicity is also dysfunctional due to an abnormal melatonin regulation, thus contributing to a delayed phase shift with melatonin rising in the morning rather than at nighttime. Several objective abnormalities have been detected in these children's PSGs regarding microstructural aspects of both REM and NREM sleep [49]. They also exhibit reduced TST and REM latency, with a lower cyclic alternating pattern (CAP) rate in SWS due to selectively reduced percentage of A1 subtypes. This parallels what is seen in other mental retardation (MR) disorders where IQ and cognitive abilities negatively relate to the A1 percentage. A previous study from the same group [50] compared ASD sleep with that of normal children and children with MR and fragile X syndrome, showing reduced REM latency and increased transitional (ST1) phases in ASD compared to normal controls, whereas sleep findings almost overlapped with those observed in fragile X subjects. Interestingly, mental abilities correlated with tonic variables such as TST and WASO, whereas communicational skills and activity levels were significantly related to REM variables. In other words, cognition separates from verbal/

communication skills, the former being mainly affected by alterations of SWS and the latter by REM sleep alteration. Within the ASD gamut, children with high-functioning Asperger disorder exhibit significantly higher A1 subtype percentage, akin to normal controls, compared to autistic children [51], showing a positive correlation of A1 percentage with verbal IQ and performance IQ as far as their duration is concerned. ASD does not seem to be an independent risk factor for obstructive sleep apnea (OSA), unless local risk factors such as adenotonsillar hypertrophy or craniofacial malformations are at stake. For this reason, PSG is warranted whenever an organic primary sleep disorder is suspected. This also includes the possible occurrence of PLMS, which several authors report as highly prevalent (nearly 50 %) in ASD children compared to controls. ASD children have been also reported to exhibit low serum ferritin levels [52] compared to normal subjects, and, as known, this is an independent risk factor for sleep-related movement disorders including PLMS and RLS.

Gastrointestinal problems linked to a deficient serotonin metabolism are highly prevalent in ASD [53] and may impact both sleep and iron absorption. ASD children also exhibit several parasomnias including arousal disorders, enuresis, and nightmares. REM without atonia, akin to what is seen in older adults with REM behavior disorder (RBD), has been reported in a case series [54]. Bedtime clonazepam, as in typical RBD, improved both daytime and nighttime behavior in these children.

Treating insomnia in ASD children may be a challenge [55]. Complete versus gradual extinctions are the most used behavioral techniques. Behavioral interventions such as chronotherapy [56], massage, and dental appliances [57] for the management of OSA often require additional pharmacotherapy. One to 3 mg of melatonin represents the safest and most efficient treatment for the majority of ASD-related sleep problems. Extended release melatonin may be selectively indicated for sleep maintenance insomnia [58].

Attention-Deficit/Hyperactivity Disorder (ADHD)

ADHD has an increasing prevalence, recently estimated around 12 %, especially in the Western world. According to the DSM-5 [8], ADHD refers to an impairment in three major areas: attention, hyperactivity, and impulsivity. Three major clinical/phenomenological subtypes are generally recognized: predominantly hyperactive-impulsive type (H), predominantly inattentive (I), and a combined type (C). Both gender and age play a major role in the phenotypic expression of this disorder, with an estimated 1:10 male prevalence, associated with more disruptive symptoms in this gender and a tendency to subside, but not completely disappear, by adult age.

Sleep disturbance is an important hallmark of ADHD with over 80 % of affected children reporting inadequate or altered sleep [59]. Most data deal with subjective children or parental reports and/or with actigraphic data, whereas only few data of PSG recordings are available. Several meta-analytic reviews [60–62] were published over the last decade, dealing with the many confounding factors affecting most of the relevant studies including gender, age, comorbid disorders, medication and diversity of methods, and data collection.

Subjective Reports

Subjective reports of sleep complaints in ADHD include initial insomnia with delayed sleep onset, which has been interpreted in some cases as delayed sleep phase. Endogen circadian alterations [63] along with forced ultradian cycling [64] have been quoted as possible responsible mechanisms.

More often, though, an increased sleep duration along with multiple nocturnal awakenings and parasomnias has been described [65]. In addition, increased EDS compared to normal controls has been reported [65, 66]. This might be related to sleep-disordered breathing (SDB) with snoring and mild apneas or to narcoleptic-like traits [67, 68]. Despite the fact that ADHD symptoms, in particular attention deficits, are common in narcolepsy, no conclusive evidence has been reached of narcoleptic traits in ADHD children [69].

Restlessness and increased number of movements during sleep in ADHD types H and C are almost unanimously reported [62, 70–72]. Multiple studies report an increased prevalence of PLMS in ADHD [67, 73]. RLS has instead been reported in up to 44 % of ADHD children [74] with a tendency to decrease with age. In fact, only a 20 % prevalence was reported in young adults [75]. Common underlying genetic and pathophysiological alterations in both ADHD and RLS may be related to iron deficiency [76, 77] and dopaminergic transmission [78].

Among sleep-related movement disorders (SRMDs), bruxism [71] and rhythmic movement disorders [79] also seem to occur with discrete frequency, the latter mostly in the inattentive (I) ADHD subgroup, with a tendency to persist beyond the usual age range in relation to its common occurrence [80].

According to some authors [71, 81, 82], there is an increased prevalence of parasomnias in ADHD children, whereas others report no differences in their prevalence compared to pediatric controls [70].

One possible explanation of these conflicting results, especially in relation to disorders of arousals (DOA), could be linked to the possible co-occurrence of SDB as a major precipitant of night terrors, sleepwalking, and confusional arousals. DOA have been reported in up to 50 % of an ADHD cohort via clinical interview [71] with confusional arousals being most common. According to both Gau et al. [81] and Silvestri et al. [71], cognitive deficits rather than behavioral symptoms are more indicative of children with DOA as opposed to children with increased nocturnal hyperactivity.

An increased prevalence of sleep talking [70, 83] and enuresis [83, 84] has been described in earlier reports. As far as REM parasomnias are concerned, frequent nightmares [65, 83] and one case of dream enactment in the context of overlap parasomnia disorder [71] were described. Parents of ADHD children often report snoring and apneas as occurring during the night [83, 85]. Respiratory events seem to be more common in Hispanic rather than Caucasian kids and appear to correlate with reported EDS and learning problems [86].

Objective Reports

Objective actigraphic studies [87, 88] and, even more so, video-PSG recordings in ADHD children are sparse compared to subjective reports, mainly due to the oppositional attitude of most of these subjects. Correspondence between subjective complaints and objective assessment is often inconsistent, especially when the latter is performed via actigraphic means. Video-PSG, instead, enables the recording of behavioral events and the assessment of both macro- and microstructural aspects of sleep. Certain alterations in the sleep structure of ADHD subjects are agreed upon by most researchers, as highlighted by a critical review [89]. These include a decreased REM percentage with increased REM latency in the (I) subgroup [71, 82]. Conversely, reduced REM latency was found by Cortese et al. [60] and by Kirov et al. [64, 90]. Age group and methodological issues, irrespective of whether or not an adaptation night was considered, differently affect TST. According to Sadeh et al. [62], TST is shorter with increased stage 1 in younger, severely affected children, especially in the H or C subgroups, in comparison to older (>9 years) subjects.

Microstructural aspects of sleep generally show an increase in sleep oscillations during the night, contributing to the formation of a "hypoarousal" phenotype linked to a decrease in SE [91]; however, while event-related arousals and phase shifts are common in H or C subgroups with OSA and PLMS [71, 83], an overall decrease of CAP rate in SWS with fewer A1 subtypes akin to the CAP features of narcolepsy is observed in ADHD children with normal apnea-hypopnea index (AHI) or PLMS index [82]. This represents a seminal observation for the possible interpretation of ADHD as a primary disorder of vigilance [92]. A recent study [93], however, did not confirm an alteration of CAP rate and/or CAP phases and subtypes, calling attention to the extreme variability within phenotypic expression.

Video-PSG confirms a generally higher AHI in ADHD versus normal children [60, 94]. However, severe OSA is rare in ADHD, whereas most authors agree on the association of only mild apneas to ADHD [69, 71, 95].

Factors such as race and craniofacial predisposition may play a pivotal role in sleep disorders in ADHD subjects. It appears that mild forms of OSA may contribute only to mild ADHD mimics, whereas severe OSA would generate EDS more than hyperactivity symptoms, impulse control disorders, and emotional liability. Adenotonsillectomy (AT) as opposed to pharmacological treatment led to a favorable outcome in these children [69, 96].

PLMS with an index >5 have been objectively recorded in up to 64 % of ADHD children [97] with positive probands holding a positive familial history for RLS. The latter's reported prevalence ranges from 44 % [74] to none [98] and has been shown to correlate with hyperactive and oppositional scores [71] and low ferritin. Iron supplementation [99], L-dopa [100], and, most recently, levetiracetam [101] have proved useful in the management of RLS symptoms in ADHD.

Therapeutic Management of Sleep Disorders in ADHD

Different clinical ADHD subtypes may benefit from carefully addressed pharmaceutical therapy. The hypoarousal/inattentive phenotype appears to mostly benefit from stimulants, adrenergic alpha1 agonists, modafinil, and bupropion, whereas SSRIs and venlafaxine may help comorbid depression. Atypical antipsychotic drugs such as risperidone [102] and atomoxetine, besides iron, vitamin D [103], and melatonin [104], have proven to be useful in severe cases of H or C ADHD subgroups with comorbid SRMDs. AT remains the treatment of choice for OSA in ADHD. Interestingly, most studies of stimulant therapeutic regimens report no effects on the magnitude of parental complaints [105], nor on objective sleep measures.

Conclusions

Most psychiatric and behavioral developmental disorders share a profound bidirectional relation with sleep. The latter is often significant, for it contributes strongly to patients' and parental burden. Specific management of sleep disorders often improves both symptoms and prognosis in the affected children. Special attention should therefore be allotted to sleep-related complaints. Consultation with experts in sleep medicine and objective instrumental sleep evaluations should be promoted when encountering difficult refractory cases.

References

1. Simonds JF, Parraga H. Sleep behaviors and disorders in children and adolescents evaluated at psychiatric clinics. J Dev Behav Pediatr. 1984;5(1):6–10.
2. Ivanenko A, Crabtree VM, O'Brien LM, et al. Sleep complaints and psychiatric symptoms in children evaluated at a pediatric mental health clinic. J Clin Sleep Med. 2006;2:42–8.
3. Ramtekkar U, Ivanenko A. Sleep in children with psychiatric disorders. Semin Pediatr Neurol. 2015;22(2):148–55.
4. Pace-Schott EF, Gersh T, Silvestri R, Stickgold R, Salzman C, Hobson JA. SSRI treatment suppresses dream recall frequency but increases subjective dream intensity in normal subjects. J Sleep Res J Sleep Res. 2001;10(2):129–42.
5. Silvestri R, Pace-Schott EF, Gersh T, Stickgold R, Salzman C, Hobson JA. Effects of fluvoxamine and paroxetine on sleep structure in normal subjects. J Clin Psychiatry J Clin Psychiatry. 2001;62(8):642–52.
6. Rottach KG, Schaner BM, Kirch MH, Zivotofsky AZ, Teufel LM, Gallwitz T, et al. Restless legs syndrome as side effect of second generation antidepressants. J Psychiatr Res. 2008;43(1):70–5.

7. Beesdo K, Knappe S, Pine DS. Anxiety and anxiety disorders in children and adolescents: developmental issues and implications for DSM-V. Psychiatr Clin N Am. 2009;32(3):483–524.
8. American Psychiatric Association. Diagnostic and statistical manual of mental disorders: DSM-5. Arlington: American Psychiatric Association; 2013.
9. Alfano CA, Ginsburg GS, Kingery JN. Sleep-related problems among children and adolescents with anxiety disorders. J Am Acad Child Adolesc Psychiatry. 2007;46(2):224–32.
10. Gregory AM, Caspi A, Eley TC, Moffitt TE, O'Connor TG, Poulton R. Prospective longitudinal associations between persistent sleep problems in childhood and anxiety and depression disorders in adulthood. J Abnorm Child Psychol J Abnorm Child Psychol. 2005;33(2):157–63.
11. Gregory AM, O'Connor TG. Sleep problems in childhood: a longitudinal study of developmental change and association with behavioral problems. J Am Acad Child Adolesc Psychiatry. 2002;41(8):964–71.
12. Alfano CA, Pina AA, Zerr AA, Villalta IK. Pre-sleep arousal and sleep problems of anxiety-disordered youth. Child Psychiatry Hum Dev Child Psychiatry Hum Dev. 2010;41(2):156–67.
13. Forbes EE, Bertocci MA, Gregory AM, Ryan ND, Axelson DA, Birmaher B, et al. Objective sleep in pediatric anxiety disorders and major depressive disorder. J Am Acad Child Adolesc Psychiatry. 2008;47(2):148–55.
14. Verduin TL, Kendall PC. Differential occurrence of comorbidity within childhood anxiety disorders. J Clin Child Adolesc Psychol. 2003;32(2):290–5.
15. Ivanenko A, Kushnir J, Alfano CA. Sleep in psychiatric disorders. Principles and practice of pediatric sleep medicine. 2nd ed: Elsevier Saunders, London. 2012. p. 369–77.
16. Alfano CA, Reynolds K, Scott N, Dahl RE, Mellman TA. Polysomnographic sleep patterns of non-depressed, non-medicated children with generalized anxiety disorder. J Affect Disord. 2013;147(1–3):379–84.
17. Augustinavicius JL, Zanjani A, Zakzanis KK, Shapiro CM. Polysomnographic features of early-onset depression: a meta-analysis. J Affect Disord. 2014;158:11–8.
18. Chemtob CM, Nomura Y, Abramovitz RA. Impact of conjoined exposure to the world trade center attacks and to other traumatic events on the behavioral problems of preschool children. Arch Pediatr Adolesc Med Arch Pediatr Adolesc Med. 2008;162(2):126.
19. Kovachy B, O'hara R, Hawkins N, Gershon A, Primeau MM, Madej J, et al. Sleep disturbance in pediatric PTSD: current findings and future directions. J Clin Sleep Med JCSM. 2013;9(5):501–10.
20. Glod CA, Teicher MH, Hartman CR, Harakal T. Increased nocturnal activity and impaired sleep maintenance in abused children. J Am Acad Child Adolesc Psychiatry. 1997;36(9):1236–43.
21. Alfano CA, Kim KL. Objective sleep patterns and severity of symptoms in pediatric obsessive compulsive disorder: a pilot investigation. J Anxiety Disord. 2011;25(6):835–9.
22. Rapoport J, Elkins R, Langer DH, et al. Childhood obsessive-compulsive disorder. Am J Psychiatr. 1981;138:1545–54.
23. Christensen R, Ameringen MV, Hall G. Increased activity of frontal and limbic regions to emotional stimuli in children at-risk for anxiety disorders. Psychiatry Res Neuroimaging. 2015;233(1):9–17.
24. Liu X, Buysse DJ, Gentzler AL, et al. Insomnia and hypersomnia associated with depressive phenomenology and comorbidity in childhood depression. Sleep. 2007;30:83–90.
25. Gregory AM, Rijsdijk FV, Lau JYF, et al. The direction of longitudinal associations between sleep problems and depression symptoms: a study of twins aged 8 and 10 years. Sleep. 2009;32:189–99.
26. Franić T, Kralj Ž, Marčinko D, Knez R, Kardum G. Suicidal ideations and sleep-related problems in early adolescence. Early Inter Psychiatry. 2013;8(2):155–62.
27. Goetz RR, Puig-Antich J, Ryan N, et al. Electroencephalographic sleep of adolescents with major depression and normal controls. Arch Gen Psychiatry. 1987;44(1):61–8.

28. Mendlewicz J, Kerkhofs M. Sleep electroencephalography in depressive illness. A collaborative study by the World Health Organization. Br J Psychiatry. 1991;159(4):505–9.
29. Armitage R, Hoffmann R, Emslie G, Rintelman J, Moore J, Lewis K. Rest-activity cycles in childhood and adolescent depression. J Am Acad Child Adolesc Psychiatry. 2004;43(6):761–9.
30. Robert JT, Hoffmann RF, Emslie GJ, Hughes C, Rintelmann J, Moore J, et al. Sex and age differences in sleep macroarchitecture in childhood and adolescent depression. Sleep. 2006; 29(3):351–8.
31. Goetz RR, Puig-Antich J, Dahl RE, Ryan ND, Asnis GM, Rabinovich H, et al. EEG sleep of young adults with major depression: a controlled study. J Affect Disord. 1991; 22(1–2):91–100.
32. Kallepalli BR, Bhatara VS, Fogas BS, Tervo RC, Misra LK. Trazodone is only slightly faster than fluoxetine in relieving insomnia in adolescents with depressive disorders. J Child Adolesc Psychopharmacol. 1997;7(2):97–107.
33. Ivanenko A, Johnson K. Sleep disturbances in children with psychiatric disorders. Semin Pediatr Neurol. 2008;15(2):70–8.
34. Lofthouse N, Fristad M, Splaingard M, Kelleher K. Parent and child reports of sleep problems associated with early-onset bipolar spectrum disorders. J Fam Psychol. 2007;21(1):114–23.
35. Rao U, Dahl RE, Ryan ND, Birmaher B, Williamson DE, Rao R, et al. Heterogeneity in EEG sleep findings in adolescent depression: unipolar versus bipolar clinical course. J Affect Disord. 2002;70(3):273–80.
36. Mehl RC, O'Brien LM, Dreisbach JK, Mervis CB, Gozal D. Correlates of sleep and pediatric bipolar disorder. Sleep. 2006;29(2):193–7.
37. Faedda GL, Teicher MH. Objective measures of activity and attention in the differential diagnosis of childhood psychiatric disorders. Essent Psychopharmacol. 2005;6:239–49.
38. Jones SH, Hare DJ, Evershed K. Actigraphic assessment of circadian activity and sleep patterns in bipolar disorder. Bipolar Disord. 2005;7(2):176–86.
39. Lee YJ, Cho S-J, Cho IH, Jang JH, Kim SJ. The relationship between psychotic-like experiences and sleep disturbances in adolescents. Sleep Med. 2012;13(8):1021–7.
40. Lunsford-Avery JR, Orr JM, Gupta T, Pelletier-Baldelli A, Dean DJ, Watts AKS, et al. Sleep dysfunction and thalamic abnormalities in adolescents at ultra high-risk for psychosis. Schizophr Res. 2013;151(1–3):148–53.
41. Sarkar S, Katshu MZUH, Nizamie SH, Praharaj SK. Slow wave sleep deficits as a trait marker in patients with schizophrenia. Schizophr Res. 2010;124(1–3):127–33.
42. Monti JM, Monti D. Sleep in schizophrenia patients and the effects of antipsychotic drugs. Sleep Med Rev. 2004;8(2):133–48.
43. Kennard B, Silva S, Vitiello B, Curry J, Kratochvil C, Simons A, et al. Remission and residual symptoms after short-term treatment in the Treatment of Adolescents With Depression Study (TADS). J Am Acad Child Adolesc Psychiatry. 2006;45(12):1404–11.
44. Owens JA, Palermo TM, Rosen CL. Overview of current management of sleep disturbances in children: II—behavioral interventions. Curr Ther Res. 2002;63:B38–52.
45. Mindell JA, Meltzer LJ. Behavioral sleep disorders in children and adolescents. Ann Acad Med Singapore. 2008;37(8):722–8.
46. Alfano CA, Zakem AH, Costa NM, Taylor LK, Weems CF. Sleep problems and their relation to cognitive factors, anxiety, and depressive symptoms in children and adolescents. Depress Anxiety. 2009;26:503–12.
47. Harvey AG, Payne S. The management of unwanted pre-sleep thoughts in insomnia: distraction with imagery versus general distraction. Behav Res Ther. 2002;40(3):267–77.
48. Couturier JL, Speechley KN, Steele M, Norman R, Stringer B, Nicolson R. Parental perception of sleep problems in children of normal intelligence with pervasive developmental disorders: prevalence, severity, and pattern. J Am Acad Child Adolesc Psychiatry. 2005;44(8):815–22.

49. Miano S, Bruni O, Elia M, Trovato A, Smerieri A, Verrillo E, et al. Sleep in children with autistic spectrum disorder: a questionnaire and polysomnographic study. Sleep Med. 2007;9(1):64–70.
50. Elia M, Ferri R, Musumeci SA, Gracco SD, Bottitta M, Scuderi C, et al. Sleep in subjects with autistic disorder: a neurophysiological and psychological study. Brain and Development. 2000;22(2):88–92.
51. Bruni O, Ferri R, Vittori E, Novelli L, Vignati M, Porfirio MC, et al. Sleep architecture and NREM alterations in children and adolescents with Asperger syndrome. Sleep. 2007;30(11):1577–85.
52. Youssef J, Singh K, Huntington N, Becker R, Kothare SV. Relationship of serum ferritin levels to sleep fragmentation and periodic limb movements of sleep on polysomnography in autism spectrum disorders. Pediatr Neurol. 2013;49(4):274–8.
53. Klukowski M, Wasilewska J, Lebensztejn D. Sleep and gastrointestinal disturbances in autism spectrum disorder in children. Dev Period Med. 2015;19(2):157–61.
54. Thirumalai SS, Shubin RA, Robinson R. Rapid eye movement sleep behavior disorder in children with autism. J Child Neurol. 2002;17(3):173–8.
55. Miano S, Ferri R. Epidemiology and management of insomnia in children with autistic spectrum disorders. Pediatr Drugs. 2010;12(2):75–84.
56. Piazza CC, Hagopian LP, Hughes CR, Fisher WW. Using chronotherapy to treat severe sleep problems: a case study. Am J Ment Retard Am J Mental Retard. 1998;102(4):358–66.
57. Fetner M, Cascio CJ, Essick G. Nonverbal patient with autism spectrum disorder and obstructive sleep apnea: use of desensitization to acclimate to a dental appliance. Pediatr Dent. 2014;36(7):499–501.
58. Jan JE, Hamilton D, Seward N, Fast DK, Freeman RD, Laudon M. Clinical trials of controlled-release melatonin in children with sleep-wake cycle disorders. J Pineal Res J Pineal Res. 2000;29(1):34–9.
59. Silvestri R, Aricò I. Sleep disorders diagnosis and management in children with attention deficit/hyperactivity disorder (ADHD). In: Idzikowski C, editor, Sleep disorders: INTECH Open Access Publisher, Rijeka, Croatia. ISBN 978-953-51-0293-9. 2014.
60. Cortese S, Konofal E, Yateman N, Mouren MC, Lecendreux M. Sleep and alertness in children with attention-deficit/hyperactivity disorder: a systematic review of the literature. Sleep. 2006;29(4):504–11.
61. Owens JA. The ADHD and sleep conundrum: a review. J Dev Behav Pediatr. 2005;26(4):312–22.
62. Sadeh A, Pergamin L, Bar-Haim Y. Sleep children with attention-deficit hyperactivity disorder: a meta-analysis of polysomnographic studies. Sleep Med Rev. 2006;10(6):381–98.
63. Van der Heijden KB, Smits MG, Gunning WB. Sleep-related disorders in ADHD: a review. Clin Pediatr (Phila). 2005;44(3):201–10.
64. Kirov R, Kinkelbur J, Heipke S, Kostanecka-Endress T, Westhoff M, Cohrs S, Ruther E, Hajak G, Banaschewski T, Rothenberger A. Is there a specific polysomnographic sleep pattern in children with attention deficit/hyperactivity disorder? J Sleep Res. 2004;13(1):87–93.
65. Owens JA, Maxim R, Nobile C, McGuinn M, Msall M. Parental and self-report of sleep in children with attention-deficit/hyperactivity disorder. Arch Pediatr Adolesc Med. 2000;154(6):549–55.
66. Marcotte AC, Thacher PV, Butters M, Bortz J, Acebo C, Carskadon MA. Parental report of sleep problems in children with attentional and learning disorders. J Dev Behav Pediatr. 1998;19(3):178–86.
67. Golan N, Shahar E, Ravid S, Pillar G. Sleep disorders and daytime sleepiness in children with attention-deficit/hyperactive disorder. Sleep. 2004;27(2):261–6.
68. Lecendreux M, Konofal E, Bouvard M, Falissard B, Mouren-Siméoni MC. Sleep and alertness in children with ADHD. J Child Psychol Psychiatry. 2000;41(6):803–12.
69. Walters AS, Silvestri R, Zucconi M, Chandrashekariah R, Konofal E. Review of the possible relationship and hypothetical links between attention deficit hyperactivity disorder (ADHD)

and the simple sleep related movement disorders, parasomnias, hypersomnias, and circadian rhythm disorders. J Clin Sleep Med. 2008;4(6):591–600.

70. Corkum P, Moldofsky H, Hogg-Johnson S, Humphries T, Tannock R. Sleep problems in children with attention- deficit/hyperactivity disorder: impact of subtype, comorbidity, and stimulant medication. J Am Acad Child Adolesc Psychiatry. 1999;38(10):1285–93.

71. Silvestri R, Gagliano A, Aricò I, Calarese T, Cedro C, Bruni O, Condurso R, Germanò E, Gervasi G, Siracusano R, Vita G, Bramanti P. Sleep disorders in children with Attention-Deficit/Hyperactivity Disorder (ADHD) recorded overnight by video-polysomnography. Sleep Med. 2009;10(10):1132–8.

72. Wagner J, Schlarb AA. Subtypes of ADHD and their association with sleep disturbances in children. Somnologie. 2012;16(2):118–24.

73. Gaultney JF, Terrell DF, Gingras JL. Parent-reported periodic limb movement, sleep disordered breathing, bedtime resistance behaviors, and ADHD. Behav Sleep Med. 2005;3(1):32–43.

74. Cortese S, Konofal E, Lecendreux M, Arnulf I, Mouren MC, Darra F, Dalla Bernardina B. Restless legs syndrome and attention-deficit/hyperactivity disorder: a review of the literature. Sleep. 2005;28(8):1007–13.

75. Zak R, Fisher B, Couvadelli BV, Moss NM, Walters AS. Preliminary study of the prevalence of restless legs syndrome in adults with attention deficit hyperactivity disorder. Percept Mot Skills. 2009;108(3):759–63.

76. Konofal E, Lecendreux M, Arnulf I, Mouren MC. Iron deficiency in children with attention-deficit/hyperactivity disorder. Arch Pediatr Adolesc Med. 2004;158(12):1113–5.

77. Picchietti D. Is iron deficiency an underlying cause of pediatric restless legs syndrome and of attention-deficit/hyperactivity disorder? Sleep Med. 2007;8(7–8):693–4.

78. Walters AS, Mandelbaum DE, Lewin DS, Kugler S, England SJ, Miller M. Dopaminergic therapy in children with restless legs/periodic limb movements in sleep and ADHD. Dopaminergic Therapy Study Group. Pediatr Neurol. 2000;22(3):182–6.

79. Dyken ME, Lin-Dyken DC, Yamada T. Diagnosing rhythmic movement disorder with video-polysomnography. Pediatr Neurol. 1997;16(1):37–41.

80. Stepanova I, Nevsimalova S, Hanusova J. Rhythmic movement disorder in sleep persisting into childhood and adulthood. Sleep. 2005;28(7):851–7.

81. Gau SS, Kessler RC, Tseng WL, Wu YY, Chiu YN, Yeh CB, Hwu HG. Association between sleep problems and symptoms of attention-deficit/hyperactivity disorder in young adults. Sleep. 2007;30(2):195–201.

82. Miano S, Donfrancesco R, Bruni O, Ferri R, Galiffa S, Pagani J, Montemitro E, Kheirandish L, Gozal D, Pia VM. NREM sleep instability is reduced in children with attention-deficit/hyperactivity disorder. Sleep. 2006;29(6):797–803.

83. O'Brien LM, Ivanenko A, Crabtree VM, Holbrook CR, Bruner JL, Klaus CJ, Gozal D. Sleep disturbances in children with attention deficit hyperactivity disorder. Pediatr Res. 2003;54(2):237–43.

84. Kaplan BJ, McNicol J, Conte RA, Moghadam HK. Sleep disturbance in preschool-aged hyperactive and non hyperactive children. Pediatrics. 1997;80(6):839–44.

85. Chervin RD, Dillon JE, Bassetti C, Ganoczy DA, Pituch KJ. Symptoms of sleep disorders, inattention, and hyperactivity in children. Sleep. 1997;20(12):1185–92.

86. Goodwin JL, Babar SI, Kaemingk KL, Rosen GM, Morgan WJ, Sherrill DL, Quan SF. Symptoms related to sleep- disordered breathing in white and Hispanic children: the Tucson Children's assessment of sleep apnea study. Chest. 2003;124(1):196–203.

87. Dagan Y, Zeevi-Luria S, Sever Y, Hallis D, Yovel I, Sadeh A, Dolev E. Sleep quality in children with attention deficit hyperactivity disorder: an actigraphic study. Psychiatry Clin Neurosci. 1997;51(6):383–6.

88. Wiggs L, Montgomery P, Stores G. Actigraphic and parent reports of sleep patterns and sleep disorders in children with subtypes of attention-deficit hyperactivity disorder. Sleep. 2005;28(11):1437–45.

89. Bullock GL, Schall U. Dyssomnia in children diagnosed with attention deficit hyperactivity disorder: a critical review. Aust N Z J Psychiatry. 2005;39(5):373–7.

90. Kirov R, Kinkelbur J, Banaschewski T, Rothenberger A. Sleep patterns in children with attention-deficit/hyperactivity disorder, tic disorder, and comorbidity. J Child Psychol Psychiatry J Child Psychol Psychiatry. 2007;48(6):561–70.

91. Gruber R, Grizenko N, Schwartz G, Bellingham J, Guzman R, Joober R. Performance on the continuous performance test in children with ADHD is associated with sleep efficiency. Sleep. 2007;30(8):1003–9.

92. Weinberg WA, Brumback RA. Primary disorder of vigilance: a novel explanation of inattentiveness, daydreaming, boredom, restlessness, and sleepiness. J Pediatr. 1990;116(5):720–5.

93. Prihodova I, Paclt I, Kemlink D, Skibova J, Ptacek R, Nevsimalova S. Sleep disorders and daytime sleepiness in children with attention-deficit/hyperactivity disorder: a two-night polysomnographic study with a multiple sleep latency test. Sleep Med. 2010;11(9):922–8.

94. Huang YS, Chen NH, Li HY, Wu YY, Chao CC, Guilleminault C. Sleep disorders in Taiwanese children with attention deficit/hyperactivity disorder. J Sleep Res. 2004;13(3):269–77.

95. Sangal RB, Owens J, Sangal J. Patients with attention-deficit/hyperactivity disorder without observed apneic episodes in sleep or daytime sleepiness have normal sleep on Polysomnography. Sleep. 2005;28:1143–8.

96. Huang YS, Guilleminault C, Li HY, Yang CM, Wu YY, Chen NH. Attention deficit/hyperactivity disorder with obstructive sleep apnea: a treatment outcome study. Sleep Med. 2007;8(1):18–30.

97. Picchietti DL, Underwood DJ, Farris WA, Walters AS, Shah MM, Dahl RE, Trubnick LJ, Bertocci MA, Wagner M, Hening WA. Further studies on periodic limb movement disorder and restless legs syndrome in children with attention-deficit hyperactivity disorder. Mov Disord. 1999;14(6):1000–7.

98. Gamaldo CE, Benbrook AR, Allen RP, Scott JA, Henning WA, Earley CJ. Childhood and adult factors associated with restless legs syndrome (RLS) diagnosis. Sleep Med. 2007;8:716–22.

99. Cortese S, Konofal E, Bernardina BD, Mouren MC, Lecendreux M. Sleep disturbances and serum ferritin levels in children with attention-deficit/hyperactivity disorder. Eur Child Adolesc Psychiatry. 2009;18(7):393–9. Sleep Med. 2013 Apr;14(4):359-66.

100. Ferri R, Bruni O, Novelli L, Picchietti MA, Picchietti DL. Time structure of leg movement activity during sleep in attention-deficit/hyperactivity disorder and effects of levodopa. Sleep Med. 2013;14(4):359–66.

101. Gagliano A, Aricò I, Calarese T, Condurso R, Germanò E, Cedro C, et al. Restless Leg Syndrome in ADHD children: levetiracetam as a reasonable therapeutic option. Brain and Development. 2011;33(6):480–6.

102. Reyes M, Croonenberghs J, Augustyns I, Eerdekens M. Long-term use of risperidone in children with disruptive behavior disorders and subaverage intelligence: efficacy, safety, and tolerability. J Child Adolesc Psychopharmacol. 2006;16(3):260–72.

103. Goksugur SB, Tufan AE, Semiz M, Gunes C, Bekdas M, Tosun M, Demircioglu F. Vitamin D status in children with attention-deficit-hyperactivity disorder. Pediatr Int. 2014;56(4):515–9.

104. Herman JH. Attention deficit/hyperactivity disorder and sleep in children. Sleep Med Clin. 2015;10(2):143–9.

105. Cohen-Zion M, Ancoli-Israel S. Sleep in children with attention-deficit hyperactivity disorder (ADHD): a review of naturalistic and stimulant intervention studies. Sleep Med Rev. 2004;8(5):379–402.

Chapter 18
Childhood Sleep and Medical Disorders

Teresa Paiva

Abstract Sleep is an important regulator of growth, metabolism, tissue repair, cell division, endocrine segregation, and immunologic functions. Therefore, many medical disorders are affected by sleep dysfunctions and impact upon sleep quality.

During the first two decades, sleep duration, sleep timing, and sleep characteristics are of utmost importance to an adequate children development being crucial for physical, mental, emotional, and behavioral equilibrium.

A number of medical conditions may give rise to sleep disturbances: asthma and allergies, hematologic diseases, metabolic disorders and obesity, gastrointestinal disorders, including colic and gastroesophageal reflux, chronic pain syndromes, cystic fibrosis, and other orphan genetic diseases.

Keywords Sleep • Children • Adolescents • Medical disorders • Allergic rhinitis • Asthma • Gastroesophageal reflux • Sickle cell anemia • Thalassemia • Headaches • Fibromyalgia • Chronic pain

Sleep is an important regulator of growth, metabolism, tissue repair, cell division, endocrine segregation, and immunologic functions. Therefore, many medical disorders are affected by sleep dysfunctions and impact upon sleep quality.

During the first two decades, sleep duration, sleep timing, and sleep characteristics are of utmost importance to an adequate children development being crucial for physical, mental, emotional, and behavioral equilibrium.

A number of medical conditions may give rise to sleep disturbances: asthma and allergies, hematologic diseases, metabolic disorders and obesity, gastrointestinal disorders, including colic and gastroesophageal reflux, chronic pain syndromes, cystic fibrosis, and other orphan genetic diseases.

T. Paiva, MD, PhD
CENC, Sleep Medicine Center, Lisbon, Portugal
e-mail: teresapaiva0@gmail.com

© Springer International Publishing Switzerland 2017
S. Nevšímalová, O. Bruni (eds.), *Sleep Disorders in Children*,
DOI 10.1007/978-3-319-28640-2_18

Asthma and Allergies

Allergic disorders affect children sleep. The causes of such impact vary: (1) the allergic symptoms awake the child inducing fragmented sleep or even insomnia, both in the child and the caregivers; (2) allergic disorders are associated with sleep disorders which disturb sleep; and (3) allergic disorders may be associated with behavioral changes which impact sleep due to poor sleep hygiene and decreased parental control.

The prevalence of asthma varies worldwide; in children it ranges from 3.5 % in China [1] to 8.3 % in the USA [2], while the prevalence of atopic eczema ranges from 7 % to 21 % in various countries [3].

Both the subjective and objective quality of sleep, verified by polysomnography, are decreased in nonobese asthmatic children without sleep apnea, mainly due to the reduction in slow-wave sleep [4]; furthermore, the sleep impact of asthma is increased whenever there is association with other sleep disorders, namely, sleep-disordered breathing (SDB) [1, 5, 6] and bruxism [7].

The association between asthma and SDB was verified in large epidemiologic studies and systematic reviews [1, 5]. SDB is among the factors associated with longer hospitalization in asthmatic children [8]; furthermore, SDB and sleep fragmentation may persist even in well-controlled children [9], while the poor control of asthma is associated with higher level of sleep problems [10].

Adenotonsillar hypertrophy is among the predisposing factors of SDB in asthmatic children [11], while persistent wheezing during daytime is a predictive factor of asthma in children with sleep disturbances [12].

Pruritus induced by atopic dermatitis, especially in severe cases, induces itching. Scratching is not interrupted during sleep; it occurs by bouts mostly during NREM stages N1 and N2 and also during REM [13]; whenever scratching induces severe skin lesions, parents' sleep may be severely affected due to the attempts to prevent skin damage in their children. Furthermore, sleep quality is severely impacted and severe cognitive deficits do exist; these deficits, mostly in verbal comprehension, perceptual reasoning, and working memory, are predicted by the eczema status [14].

Mouth breathing, both during daytime and during sleep, is significantly associated with atopic dermatitis in small children [15]; consequently in these cases, the presence of SDB must be properly evaluated.

Furthermore, allergic disorders may impact upon the children's school environment: the presence of persistent or late-onset rashes is significantly associated with being bullied, while the presence of persistent wheezing is associated with being "left out" [16].

Metabolic Disorders

Diabetes, hypothyroidism and other hormonal disorders, and obesity have clear-cut relationship with sleep.

The increased risk of type II diabetes and insulin resistance in children associated with sleep curtailment has been demonstrated [17].

Congenital Hypothyroidism

Congenital hypothyroidism strongly affects sleep; in infants from 1.5 to 18 months of age, and mostly in girls, daytime polysomnography showed a high prevalence of both central sleep apnea (43 %) and hypopnea (83 %), which decreased with age; furthermore, light stages of sleep were predominant with reduction of slow-wave sleep and no major changes in REM sleep [18].

Growth Hormone Deficiency

Growth hormone is mainly secreted during slow-wave sleep; therefore, children with chronic sleep reduction may have changes in the somatotropic system and the likelihood of low stature exists. In a study comparing polysomnography features of children with growth hormone deficiency and normal children, the reduction of the total sleep time and sleep efficiency, together with an increased rate of type A cyclic alternating pattern, was demonstrated [19].

Obesity

Obesity is becoming progressively more common among children and adolescent.

In obesity, the involvement of several complex metabolic and inflammatory mechanisms increases orexinogenic behaviors and dysfunctional satiety, which, acting as retroactive and maintaining feedback loops, induce dyslipidemia and insulin resistance which ultimately may lead to the metabolic syndrome [20].

Sleep plays an important role in these obesogenic mechanisms due to the imbalance between leptin, ghrelin, and orexin induced by sleep deprivation and via the erroneous dietary preferences in food and beverages, associated with reduced sleep duration [21] and late sleep timings [22]. Altogether these mechanisms increase the obesity risk [23].

The triangle of sleep curtailment, increased screen time, and sedentary behaviors leading to unhealthy dietary choices and consequently increased BMI is nowadays proved in many studies.

In fact, in a multicentric and multinational study involving several continents and ethnicities, the risk factors associated with excessive weight and obesity in these age groups are nocturnal sleep duration, low physical activity, TV time, health disorders, and unhealthy diet patterns [24].

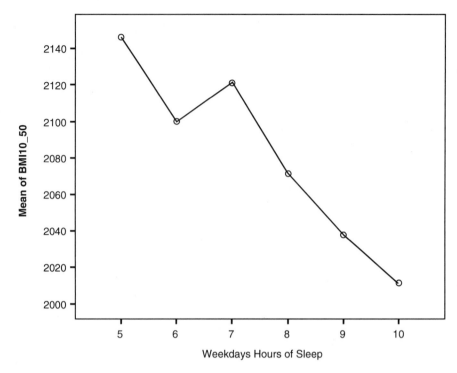

Fig. 18.1 Data from the Portuguese national survey – Health Behaviour in School-Aged Children (HBSC) [60], including 3476 students with a mean age of 14 years. The mean BMI is plotted against sleep duration in week days. Noticed the marked reduction in BMI for sleep durations equal or longer than 8 h

The sleep characteristics associated with increased body mass index (BMI) and obesity are short sleep duration [25–34], sleep variability, and erroneous sleep timings [22, 35] (see Fig. 18.1).

Furthermore, other sleep variables and sleep behaviors correlate with increased obesity risk. In preschoolers parental presence when falling asleep and short sleep duration are associated with increased BMI [36]; in schoolchildren shorter sleep duration, high-screen or TV viewing time, and low socioeconomic status were associated with increased BMI [26].

Cardiometabolic risk in adolescents has however gender differences, since the differences in cardiometabolic markers are statistically significant for girls: increased cholesterol and high-density lipoprotein (HDL) occur predominantly in the subgroups who go to bed late and rose early and in those which are sleepy and tired at least once a week [37].

The opposite pathway is also at stake: obesity is a risk factor for sleep disorders in children and adolescents, namely, for obstructive sleep apnea syndrome (OSAS). The relation with OSAS is bidirectional, since OSAS associated with short sleep duration is a risk factor for obesity [38].

Gastrointestinal Disorders

Gastroesophageal reflux (GER) is the passive transfer of gastric contents into the esophagus due to transient or chronic relaxation of the lower esophageal sphincter [39]. It may be present since birth, occurring in 51 % of the infants, but it is problematic in 14 % of them [40].

The recumbent sleep position increases the reflux and sleep complaints are common, with the child crying when lying down or having frequent awakenings, especially after a meal; frequent vomiting, spitting, and regurgitation are usually alerting symptoms, together with wet burps and wet hiccups and inconsolable crying after eating. Suffocation is a rare but possible complication, and swallowing fits, during which the agitated child turns around in bed, sweating, spitting, with associated swallowing movements, can justify the differential diagnosis with epileptiform seizures.

The association with OSAS is frequent; gastroesophageal reflux disease (GERD) is among the comorbidities of OSAS occurring in 30 % of the cases [41]; it is a predictor of complications of adenotonsillectomy [42] and is usually associated with residual OSAS after an adequate treatment [43]. GERD may also be associated with asthma and with obesity in children.

Hematologic Disorders

Sickle Cell Anemia

Sickle cell disease (SCD) is an inherited blood disorder associated with hemoglobin S; the red cells have a characteristic donut shape (the drepanocytes) and lack plasticity, and as a consequence they can block the blood vessels, provoking acute pain syndromes, bacterial infections, and tissue necrosis [44, 45].

The impact upon sleep is serious, since several factors contribute to it, namely, the pain episodes, anemia, and sleep-disordered breathing. Children have significantly higher rates of parent reported SDB and night wakings [46, 47], together with objective demonstration of polysomnographic features of OSAS [47].

Elevated periodic limb movements of sleep (PLMS) are common in children with SCD and are associated with sleep disruption and symptoms of restless legs syndrome (RLS) [48].

Thalassemia

Thalassemia is an inherited, mostly autosomal recessive, blood disorder associated with abnormal formation of hemoglobin, which results in abnormal transportation of oxygen and destruction of red cells. It predominates in Mediterranean countries (European, West Asia, and North Africa), South Asian countries, and Maldives.

Besides anemia it may be associated with other complications, namely, slower growth rates, bone deformities, and cardiovascular disorders. There are alpha, beta, delta, and combined variants of thalassemia.

Symptoms may develop with different severity levels, but they are present since early life. Children and adolescents with beta-thalassemia have increased number of arousals during sleep which is partially due to the presence of periodic limb movements of sleep; a similar picture occurs in sufferers from congenital dyserythropoietic anemia type 1 [49]. Furthermore, children with thalassemia have an estimated prevalence of OSAS of 8.3 %; sleep apnea occurs predominantly in children with high serum ferritin levels; furthermore, snoring and adenotonsillar lymphoid hyperplasia should be considered as alert factors for the presence of OSAS [50].

Chronic Pain Syndromes

Chronic pain in children and adolescents may be a consequence of another disorder, as it is the case for juvenile idiopathic arthritis (JIA) and sickle cell disease (SCD) or the major symptom of a specific disorder [51], as it is the case in chronic idiopathic headaches or fibromyalgia.

The relation between sleep and pain in pediatric populations has been described by Lewis and Dahl 1999 [52]; the relations are bidirectional: pain interrupts sleep, and the interrupted sleep induces a dysfunctional cascade affecting emotional, immunologic, anti-inflammatory, and somatic balance, which by themselves increase pain. The model of Valrie et al. includes also disease stage, sex, race/ethnicity/culture, and socio-contextual factors [51].

The prevalence of chronic pain in pediatric community populations is very high, varying between 25 and 40 % [53].

Poor sleep is a common comorbidity; sleep can be affected by the presence of nocturnal pain, by the existence of other symptoms of the underlying disorder, by the required medication, or by the eventual hospitalizations; sleep disturbances can include bedtime resistance, increased awakenings, poor sleep hygiene, and the presence of SDB and/or parasomnias [51].

The behavioral, emotional, and cognitive dysfunctions of poor sleep and the consequences upon school achievement and family equilibrium are well known and tend to increase the severity of the chronic pain condition.

More detailed descriptions will be given for headaches, chronic muscle skeletal pain, and fibromyalgia.

Headaches

In children and adults the relationships between headaches and sleep are mutual.

The links, headache sleep links, are related to common neurophysiological, neuroanatomical, and genetic substrates [54].

The prevalence of headache increases from childhood to adolescence; it is similar in both genders before puberty, but afterward it is higher in females.

During adolescence frequent and chronic headaches are a common issue, affecting 22–32% of the teens [55–59]. Sleep deprivation [60], sleep habits, and sleep disorders [61–64] are among the important comorbidities of chronic headaches.

Furthermore, headaches are commonly associated with children sleep disorders [54], namely, obstructive sleep apnea [65], parasomnias [54, 65], periodic limb movements, restless legs [64], bruxism [66], and narcolepsy and hypersomnia [64].

Chronic Muscle Skeletal Pain Complaints

The prevalence of neck and shoulder pain is higher in girls; the risk factors are family history, school furniture, long sitting time, extended computer use, insufficient rest time, short sleep duration, transportation type, schoolbag weight, and smoking [67].

The prevalence of pain in the back, neck, and shoulders is high in adolescents and increases with sleep deprivation [60, 68, 69] and with irregular sleep schedules across weekdays and weekends [60].

The relations between chronic pain and insomnia are mutual, with insomnia being a risk for pain chronicity, while pain, poor sleep hygiene, and higher depressive symptoms are the main risks for insomnia persistence [70].

Fatigue and Fibromyalgia

Fatigue is rather frequent among children and adolescents [60] and occurs often associated with sleep disturbances [71, 72]. The risk factors for fatigue with poor clinical outcome are sleep problems, somatic complaints, blurred vision, pain in the arms or legs, back pain, constipation, and memory deficits, while the indicators of a good outcome are male gender and a physically active lifestyle [73].

The diagnosis of fibromyalgia in young ages is currently difficult due to the unspecific or vague complaints, but the prevalence of juvenile fibromyalgia syndrome (JFS) is relatively high, affecting 2–15% of the children, being higher in girls and increasing after the puberty.

The symptoms include sleep difficulties in initiating and maintaining sleep, nonrestorative sleep, generalized musculoskeletal pain, and daytime fatigue [74]; furthermore, there is a negative impact upon quality of life, increased rates of depression, and higher likelihood of missing school. Polysomnographic data of these patients demonstrates longer total sleep time, decreased slow-wave sleep, prolonged REM latency, and increased sleep fragmentation; actigraphy demonstrates a reduced activity during daytime [75].

The genetic components of fibromyalgia are currently described [76]; this together with the increased risk due to stressful events during childhood explains its relevance in young ages.

References

1. Li L, Xu Z, Jin X, Yan C, Jiang F, Tong S, Shen X, Li S. Sleep-disordered breathing and asthma: evidence from a large multicentric epidemiological study in China. Respir Res. 2015;16:56.
2. CDC report 2015. www.cdc.gov/asthma/asthmadata.htm.
3. Hanifin JM, Reed ML, Eczema Prevalence and Impact Working Group. A population-based survey of eczema prevalence in the United States. Dermatitis. 2007;18(2):82–91.
4. Teng YK, Chiang LC, Lue KH, Chang SW, Wang L, Lee SP, Ting H, Lee SD. Poor sleep quality measured by polysomnography in non-obese asthmatic children with or without moderate to severe obstructive sleep apnea. Sleep Med. 2014;15(9):1062–7.
5. Brockmann PE, Bertrand P, Castro-Rodriguez JA. Influence of asthma on sleep disordered breathing in children: a systematic review. Sleep Med Rev. 2014;18(5):393–7.
6. Goldstein NA, Aronin C, Kantrowitz B, Hershcopf R, Fishkin S, Lee H, Weaver DE, Yip C, Liaw C, Saadia TA, Abramowitz J, Weedon J. The prevalence of sleep-disordered breathing in children with asthma and its behavioral effects. Pediatr Pulmonol. 2015;50(11):1128–36.
7. Amato JN, Tuon RA, Castelo PM, Gavião MB, Barbosa TS. Assessment of sleep bruxism, orthodontic treatment need, orofacial dysfunctions and salivary biomarkers in asthmatic children. Arch Oral Biol. 2015;60(5):698–705.
8. Shanley LA, Lin H, Flores G. Factors associated with length of stay for pediatric asthma hospitalizations. J Asthma. 2015;52(5):471–7.
9. Yoon HK, Kang SG, Lee HJ, Yoo Y, Choung JT, Seo WH, Kim L. Apnea-related sleep fragmentation and poor vigilance in children with well-controlled asthma. J Sleep Res. 2014;23:189–95.
10. Koinis-Mitchell D, Kopel SJ, Boergers J, McQuaid EL, Esteban CA, Seifer R, Fritz GK, Beltran AJ, Klein RB, LeBourgeois M. Good sleep health in urban children with asthma: a risk and resilience approach. J Pediatr Psychol. 2015;40(9):888–903.
11. Evcimik MF, Dogru M, Cirik AA, Nepesov MI. Adenoid hypertrophy in children with allergic disease and influential factors. Int J Pediatr Otorhinolaryngol. 2015;79(5):694–7.
12. van der Mark LB, van Wonderen KE, Mohrs J, van Aalderen WM, ter Riet G, Bindels PJ. Predicting asthma in preschool children at high risk presenting in primary care: development of a clinical asthma prediction score. Prim Care Respir J. 2014;23(1):52–9.
13. Gupta MA, Gupta AK. Sleep-wake disorders and dermatology. Clin Dermatol. 2013;31(1):118–26.
14. Camfferman D, Kennedy JD, Gold M, Simpson C, Lushington K. Sleep and neurocognitive functioning in children with eczema. Int J Psychophysiol. 2013;89(2):265–72.
15. Yamaguchi H, Tada S, Nakanishi Y, Kawaminami S, Shin T, Tabata R, Yuasa S, Shimizu N, Kohno M, Tsuchiya A, Tani K. Association between mouth breathing and atopic dermatitis in Japanese children 2–6 years old: a population-based cross-sectional study. PLoS One. 2015;10(4):e0125916.
16. Teyhan A, Galobardes B, Henderson J. Child allergic symptoms and mental well-being: the role of maternal anxiety and depression. J Pediatr. 2014;165(3):592–9.e5.
17. Javaheri S, Storfer-Isser A, Rosen CL, Redline S. Association of short and long sleep durations with insulin sensitivity in adolescents. J Pediatr. 2011;158:617–23.
18. Terán-Pérez G, Arana-Lechuga Y, González-Robles RO, Mandujano M, Santana-Miranda R, Esqueda-Leon E, Calzada R, Ruiz ML, Altamirano N, Sánchez C, Velázquez-Moctezuma

J. Polysomnographic features in infants with early diagnosis of congenital hypothyroidism. Brain Dev. 2010;32(4):332–7.

19. Verrillo E, Bizzarri C, Cappa M, Bruni O, Pavone M, Ferri R, Cutrera R. Sleep characteristics in children with growth hormone deficiency. Neuroendocrinology. 2011;94(1):66–74.

20. Hakim F, Kheirandish-Gozal L, Gozal D. Obesity and altered sleep: a pathway to metabolic derangements in children? Semin Pediatr Neurol. 2015;22(2):77–85.

21. Hjorth MF, Quist JS, Andersen R, Michaelsen KF, Tetens I, Astrup A, Chaput JP, Sjödin A. Change in sleep duration and proposed dietary risk factors for obesity in Danish school children. Pediatr Obes. 2014;9(6):e156–9.

22. Thivel D, Isacco L, Aucouturier J, Pereira B, Lazaar N, Ratel S, Doré E, Duché P. Bedtime and sleep timing but not sleep duration are associated with eating habits in primary school children. J Dev Behav Pediatr. 2015;36(3):158–65.

23. Miller AL, Lumeng JC, LeBourgeois MK. Sleep patterns and obesity in childhood. Curr Opin Endocrinol Diabetes Obes. 2015;22(1):41–7.

24. Katzmarzyk PT, Barreira TV, Broyles ST, Champagne CM, Chaput JP, Fogelholm M, Hu G, Johnson WD, Kuriyan R, Kurpad A, Lambert EV, Maher C, Maia J, Matsudo V, Olds T, Onywera V, Sarmiento OL, Standage M, Tremblay MS, Tudor-Locke C, Zhao P, Church TS, ISCOLE Research Group. Relationship between lifestyle behaviors and obesity in children ages 9–11: results from a 12-country study. Obesity (Silver Spring). 2015;23(8):1696–702.

25. Kuriyan R, Bhat S, Thomas T, Vaz M, Kurpad AV. Television viewing and sleep are associated with overweight among urban and semi-urban South Indian children. Nutr J. 2007;6:25.

26. Padez C, Mourao I, Moreira P, Rosado V. Long sleep duration and childhood overweight/ obesity and body fat. Am J Hum Biol. 2009;21(3):371–6.

27. Moore M, Kirchner HL, Drotar D, Johnson N, Rosen C, Redline S. Correlates of adolescent sleep time and variability in sleep time: the role of individual and health related characteristics. Sleep Med. 2011;12(3):239–45.

28. Mitchell JA, Pate RR, España-Romero V, O'Neill JR, Dowda M, Nader PR. Moderate-to-vigorous physical activity is associated with decreases in body mass index from ages 9 to 15 years. Obesity (Silver Spring). 2013;21(3):E280–93.

29. Araújo J, Severo M, Ramos E. Sleep duration and adiposity during adolescence. Pediatrics. 2012;130(5):e1146–54.

30. Martinez SM, Tschann JM, Greenspan LC, Deardorff J, Penilla C, Flores E, Pasch LA, Gregorich SE, Butte NF. Is it time for bed? Short sleep duration increases risk of obesity in Mexican American children. Sleep Med. 2014;15(12):1484–9.

31. Taveras EM, Gillman MW, Peña MM, Redline S, Rifas-Shiman SL. Chronic sleep curtailment and adiposity. Pediatrics. 2014;133(6):1013–22.

32. Fatima Y, Doi SA, Mamun AA. Longitudinal impact of sleep on overweight and obesity in children and adolescents: a systematic review and bias-adjusted meta-analysis. Obes Rev. 2015;16(2):137–49.

33. Sijtsma A, Koller M, Sauer PJ, Corpeleijn E. Television, sleep, outdoor play and BMI in young children: the GECKO Drenthe cohort. Eur J Pediatr. 2015;174(5):631–9.

34. Chen G, Ratcliffe J, Olds T, Magarey A, Jones M, Leslie E. BMI, health behaviors, and quality of life in children and adolescents: a school-based study. Pediatrics. 2014;133(4):e868–74.

35. Scharf RJ, DeBoer MD. Sleep timing and longitudinal weight gain in 4- and 5-year-old children. Pediatr Obes. 2015;10(2):141–8.

36. Plancoulaine S, Lioret S, Regnault N, Heude B, Charles MA, Eden Mother-Child Cohort Study Group. Gender-specific factors associated with shorter sleep duration at age 3 years. J Sleep Res. 2015;24(6):610–20.

37. Berentzen NE, Smit HA, Bekkers MB, Brunekreef B, Koppelman GH, De Jongste JC, Kerkhof M, Van Rossem L, Wijga AH. Time in bed, sleep quality and associations with cardiometabolic markers in children: the Prevention and Incidence of Asthma and Mite Allergy birth cohort study. J Sleep Res. 2014;23(1):3–12.

38. Bonuck K, Chervin RD, Howe LD. Sleep-disordered breathing, sleep duration, and childhood overweight: a longitudinal cohort study. J Pediatr. 2015;166(3):632–9.

39. Kumar Y, Sarvananthan R. GORD in children. BMJ Clin Evid. 2008;2008:0310.
40. Nelson SP, Chen EH, Syniar GM, Christoffel KK. Prevalence of symptoms of gastroesophageal reflux during infancy. A pediatric practice-based survey. Pediatric Practice Research Group. Arch Pediatr Adolesc Med. 1997;151(6):569–72.
41. Ramgopal S, Kothare SV, Rana M, Singh K, Khatwa U. Obstructive sleep apnea in infancy: a 7-year experience at a pediatric sleep center. Pediatr Pulmonol. 2014;49(6):554–60.
42. McCormick ME, Sheyn A, Haupert M, Folbe AJ. Gastroesophageal reflux as a predictor of complications after adenotonsillectomy in young children. Int J Pediatr Otorhinolaryngol. 2013;77(9):1575–8.
43. Wasilewska J, Kaczmarski M, Debkowska K. Obstructive hypopnea and gastroesophageal reflux as factors associated with residual obstructive sleep apnea syndrome. Int J Pediatr Otorhinolaryngol. 2011;75(5):657–63.
44. http://www.who.int/mediacentre/factsheets/fs308/en/.
45. http://www.nhlbi.nih.gov/health/health-topics/topics/sca.
46. Daniel LC, Grant M, Kothare SV, Dampier C, Barakat LP. Sleep patterns in pediatric sickle cell disease. Pediatr Blood Cancer. 2010;55(3):501–7.
47. Goldstein NA, Keller R, Rey K, Rao S, Weedon J, Dastgir G, Mironov A, Miller ST. Sleep-disordered breathing and transcranial Dopplers in sickle cell disease. Arch Otolaryngol Head Neck Surg. 2011;137(12):1263–8.
48. Rogers VE, Marcus CL, Jawad AF, Smith-Whitley K, Ohene-Frempong K, Bowdre C, Allen J, Arens R, Mason TB. Periodic limb movements and disrupted sleep in children with sickle cell disease. Sleep. 2011;34(7):899–908. Erratum in: Sleep. 2012 Jun;35(6):725.
49. Tarasiuk A, Abdul-Hai A, Moser A, Freidman B, Tal A, Kapelushnik J. Sleep disruption and objective sleepiness in children with beta-thalassemia and congenital dyserythropoietic anemia. Arch Pediatr Adolesc Med. 2003;157(5):463–8. Erratum in: Arch Pediatr Adolesc Med. 2004 Feb;158(2):110.
50. Sritippayawan S, Norasetthekul S, Nuchprayoon I, Deerojanawong J, Desudchit T, Prapphal N. Obstructive sleep apnea among children with severe beta-thalassemia. Southeast Asian J Trop Med Public Health. 2012;43(1):152–9.
51. Valrie CR, Bromberg MH, Palermo T, Schanberg LE. A systematic review of sleep in pediatric pain populations. J Dev Behav Pediatr. 2013;34(2):120–8.
52. Lewin DS, Dahl RE. Importance of sleep in the management of pediatric pain. J Dev Behav Pediatr. 1999;20(4):244–52.
53. Stanford EA, Chambers CT, Biesanz JC, Chen E. The frequency, trajectories and predictors of adolescent recurrent pain: a population-based approach. Pain. 2008;138(1):11–21.
54. Dosi C, Figura M, Ferri R, Bruni O. Sleep and headache. Semin Pediatr Neurol. 2015;22(2):105–12.
55. Braz M, Barros Filho AA, Barros MB. Adolescent health: a population-based study in Campinas, São Paulo State, Brazil. Cad Saude Publica. 2013;29(9):1877–88. Portuguese.
56. Zwart JA, Dyb G, Holmen TL, Stovner LJ, Sand T. The prevalence of migraine and tension-type headaches among adolescents in Norway. The Nord-Trøndelag Health Study (Head-HUNT-Youth), a large population-based epidemiological study. Cephalalgia. 2004;24(5):373–9.
57. Perquin CW, Hazebroek-Kampschreur AA, Hunfeld JA, Bohnen AM, van Suijlekom-Smit LW, Passchier J, van der Wouden JC. Pain in children and adolescents: a common experience. Pain. 2000;87(1):51–8.
58. Dooley JM, Gordon KE, Wood EP. Self-reported headache frequency in Canadian adolescents: validation and follow-up. Headache. 2005;45(2):127–31.
59. Bellini B, Arruda M, Cescut A, Saulle C, Persico A, Carotenuto M, Gatta M, Nacinovich R, Piazza FP, Termine C, Tozzi E, Lucchese F, Guidetti V. Headache and comorbidity in children and adolescents. J Headache Pain. 2013;14:79.
60. Paiva T, Gaspar T, Matos MG. Sleep deprivation in adolescents: correlations with health complaints and health-related quality of life. Sleep Med. 2015;16(4):521–7.
61. Sillanpää M, Aro H. Headache in teenagers: comorbidity and prognosis. Funct Neurol. 2000;15 Suppl 3:116–21.

62. Bruni O, Novelli L, Guidetti V, Ferri R. Sleep and headaches during adolescence. Adolesc Med State Art Rev. 2010;21(3):446–56.
63. Paiva T. Sleep and headache. Handb Clin Neurol. 2011;99:1073–86.
64. Esposito M, Parisi P, Miano S, Carotenuto M. Migraine and periodic limb movement disorders in sleep in children: a preliminary case-control study. J Headache Pain. 2013;14:57.
65. Chang SJ, Chae KY. Obstructive sleep apnea syndrome in children: epidemiology, pathophysiology, diagnosis and sequelae. Korean J Pediatr. 2010;53(10):863–71.
66. Masuko AH, Villa TR, Pradella-Hallinan M, Moszczynski AJ, Carvalho Dde D, Tufik S, do Prado GF, Coelho FM. Prevalence of bruxism in children with episodic migraine – a case-control study with polysomnography. BMC Res Notes. 2014;7:298.
67. Shan Z, Deng G, Li J, Li Y, Zhang Y, Zhao Q. How schooling and lifestyle factors effect neck and shoulder pain?: a cross-sectional survey of adolescents in China. Spine (Phila Pa 1976). 2013;222C:34–41.
68. Haraldstad K, Sørum R, Eide H, Natvig GK, Helseth S. Pain in children and adolescents: prevalence, impact on daily life, and parents' perception, a school survey. Scand J Caring Sci. 2011;25(1):27–36.
69. Siu YF, Chan S, Wong KM, Wong WS. The comorbidity of chronic pain and sleep disturbances in a community adolescent sample: prevalence and association with sociodemographic and psychosocial factors. Pain Med. 2012;13(10):1292–303.
70. Palermo TM, Fonareva I, Janosy NR. Sleep quality and efficiency in adolescents with chronic pain: relationship with activity limitations and health-related quality of life. Behav Sleep Med. 2008;6(4):234–50.
71. Tham SW, Holley AL, Zhou C, Clarke GN, Palermo TM. Longitudinal course and risk factors for fatigue in adolescents: the mediating role of sleep disturbances. J Pediatr Psychol. 2013;38(10):1070–80.
72. Holmberg LI, Hellberg D. Behavioral and other characteristics of relevance for health in adolescents with self-perceived sleeping problems. Int J Adolesc Med Health. 2008;20(3):353–65.
73. Bakker RJ, Sinnema G, Kuis W, van de Putte EM. Exercise in social context contributes to a favourable outcome in fatigued children and adolescents. Arch Dis Child. 2009;94(12):999–1000.
74. Palermo TM, Kiska R. Subjective sleep disturbances in adolescents with chronic pain: relationship to daily functioning and quality of life. J Pain. 2005;6(3):201–7.
75. Davies S, Crawley E. Chronic fatigue syndrome in children aged 11 years old and younger. Arch Dis Child. 2008;93(5):419–21.
76. Ablin JN, Buskila D. Predicting fibromyalgia, a narrative review: are we better than fools and children? Eur J Pain. 2014;18(8):1060–6.

Index

© Springer International Publishing Switzerland 2017
S. Nevšímalová, O. Bruni (eds.), *Sleep Disorders in Children*,
DOI 10.1007/978-3-319-28640-2

Printed by Printforce, the Netherlands